VETERINARY ETHICS

ANIMAL WELFARE,
CLIENT RELATIONS,
COMPETITION AND COLLEGIALITY

VETERINARY ETHICS
ANIMAL WELFARE,
CLIENT RELATIONS,
COMPETITION AND COLLEGIALITY

SECOND EDITION

Jerrold Tannenbaum, M.A., J.D.

Clinical Associate Professor
Department of Environmental Studies
Tufts University School of Veterinary Medicine
North Grafton, Massachusetts

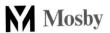 Mosby

St. Louis Baltimore Boston Carlsbad Chicago Naples New York Philadelphia Portland
London Madrid Mexico City Singapore Sydney Tokyo Toronto Wiesbaden

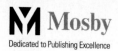
Mosby
Dedicated to Publishing Excellence

Publisher: Don Ladig
Executive Editor: Linda L. Duncan
Senior Developmental Editor: Penny Rudolph
Project Manager: Deborah Vogel
Production Editor: Mamata Reddy
Electronic Production Coordinator: Terri Schwaegel
Design Manager: Susan Lane
Cover Designer: Pati Pye

SECOND EDITION

Printed in the United States of America
Composition by Mosby Electronic Production, St. Louis
Printing/binding by R.R. Donnelley & Sons Company

Mosby–Year Book, Inc.
11830 Westline Industrial Drive
St. Louis, Missouri 63146

Library of Congress Cataloging in Publication Data

Tannenbaum, Jerrold.
    Veterinary ethics : animal welfare, client relations, competition
and collegiality / Jerrold Tannenbaum. — 2nd ed.
      p. cm.
    Includes index.
    ISBN 0-8151-8840-4
    1. Veterinary medicine—Moral and ethical aspects.   2. Veterinarians—Professional ethics.
3. Animal Welfare.
I. Title.
SF756.39.T36   1995
174′.9636—dc20
                                 95-10433
                                 CIP

95 96 97 98 99 / 9 8 7 6 5 4 3 2 1

For Nadine

Foreword

In my Foreword to what is now the first edition of *Veterinary Ethics*, I accurately predicted that it would prove so popular—and so useful—that subsequent editions would be necessary. I also wrote that the ethical dimension of veterinary medicine would "hit the reader squarely between the brain and the heart." A reader apparently unused to the metaphor wrote me and asked if that meant the neck!

This intellectually tough-minded but compassionate and readable book is the best single guide a veterinary medical student, practitioner, researcher, or faculty member can have to the world of ethics as applied to animals and human interaction with them.

Professor Tannenbaum is unusually well informed about the practice and theory of veterinary medicine. His analyses are clear, crisp, and fully documented. And he earns the reader's trust by his careful phrasing and unfailing good intention. New in this edition, the inclusion of provocative cases—a sort of problem-based learning—makes excruciatingly real some of the most difficult ethical dilemmas that veterinarians, ranchers, farmers, and companion animal owners face.

People who choose to become veterinarians tend to be modest, caring overachievers whose daily lives take place on what is often uncertain ethical footing. *Veterinary Ethics* will inform those lives, and the lives of those who care about animals, in a very special way.

Franklin M. Loew, Dean
Tufts University School of Veterinary Medicine
North Grafton, Massachusetts

~~~~~~~~~~~~~~~~~~~~~~~~~

Preface

∼ WHY VETERINARY ETHICS?

When the first edition of this book appeared in 1989, it was the first comprehensive treatment of veterinary ethics ever published. It remains the only comprehensive treatment of the subject. This fact has both necessitated and shaped the present edition.

Some people are surprised to learn that a book in veterinary ethics even exists. They are not surprised because they think that veterinarians are unethical. Nor does their amazement stem from the belief that people do not care about animals. Quite the contrary. It is obvious that when many people say they love their animals, they mean it literally. They will do almost anything to keep their treasured pets safe, healthy, and happy. When an animal becomes ill or is injured, personal or family life stops right then and there. No effort, and often no expense, is spared to obtain help. In such times of human as well as animal need, we can count on the gentle doctor to be there—in the animal hospital, surrounded by grateful clients and patients, doing his or her best, day in and day out.

When some people hear the words "veterinary ethics" they immediately think of James Herriot and are puzzled about why a *veterinarian* would have to worry about ethics. The fact that the profession is so often associated with this great man is a compliment of the highest order. Like Herriot, veterinarians are viewed as a paradigm of everything people value in professional behavior: hard work, dignity, modesty, ingenuity, compassion, clarity of purpose, and dedication to helping. The complex and nasty problems of life seem a world away from what veterinarians do. To suppose otherwise is almost to doubt whether there exists on our troubled planet any bastion, however small, of goodness and decency. Why would *veterinarians* need an ethics book? Veterinarians are the very embodiment of ethics!

Veterinarians are understandably flattered by such idealized portraits of their profession, but they also know better. They have long faced ethical conflicts that would make even the most conscientious physician cringe with horror. Built into the very essence of their professional role is a conflict: they serve both animals and people. This dual function can put veterinarians in an impossible position when what is good for the patient is not good for the client, or when helping the client means harming the patient. Physicians are understandably concerned about euthanasia. Veterinarians have always had to deal with it. Physicians are troubled about how economic considerations will affect medical choices. Veterinarians have always had to face this problem. And today the veterinary profession is confronted by forces, from within and without, that challenge traditional views about animals and animal doctors. Some of these challenges may threaten the ability of the profession to function competently or independently.

That a book on veterinary ethics *should* exist is apparent from what follows in this text. Here, I want to advise the reader what this book is intended to do and how it can be used.

∼ WHO SHOULD READ THIS BOOK

Everyone who ever has any contact with a veterinarian, or whose life is affected in some way by an animal that comes in contact with a veterinarian, should be interested in veterinary ethics. Therefore everyone should be interested in veterinary ethics. Everyone either owns an animal or is affected in some way by veterinary treatment of animals. Pet owners are certainly affected by what veterinarians do. But so are people who eat or wear animal products, who enjoy animal entertainments such as horse racing, who have benefited from medical research that has been conducted using animals, or who care about the environment, a major part of which consists of animals.

Many different kinds of people should therefore find a great deal of interest in this book. Pet owners, pet lovers, and pet breeders will learn much about a profession too many of them take for granted. Physicians and biomedical ethicists might consider the discussions of euthanasia and other aspects of veterinary practice that can both illuminate and be illuminated by issues relating to human medical care. Physicians and biomedical researchers who are concerned about ethical problems posed by animal research (some of which have a distinctive veterinary perspective) should also discover useful information. Farmers and animal husbandry scientists should be interested in the discussions of the concept of animal welfare and of ethical issues relating to farm and food animals. Environmentalists and environmental ethicists may receive assistance in responding to the increasing number of veterinarians who want to do their part to preserve the environment.

Although this book should be read by people outside of veterinary medicine, it is addressed directly to veterinarians and veterinary students. There are many other volumes dealing with ethical questions faced by other professions. Veterinarians are entitled to at least one book devoted to their distinctive ethical issues.

Considerations of space have necessitated certain limitations in the text. The book focuses on ethical questions facing private practitioners. I do not provide as extensive argumentation regarding many issues that are considered as would be possible in a longer work. This should not be a problem for the reader because the primary purpose of the text is to provide a comprehensive introduction to the subject that will stimulate readers to engage in their own further thought. The text does not discuss laws and official professional standards governing veterinary practice outside the United States. However, veterinarians in other lands will find the bulk of the discussion helpful. I encourage them to consider how the laws and professional codes of their countries and veterinary associations relate to the issues, most of which do, after all, transcend national borders.

∼ WHAT THIS BOOK AIMS TO DO

It is not the primary purpose of this book to answer ethical questions or to suggest what is right or wrong. Some readers may be puzzled by this statement because the book contains many of my own conclusions and recommendations. Indeed, I warn at various points that the very future of veterinary medicine as a profession will depend on its making certain ethical choices rather than others.

It is impossible to engage in ethical deliberation without expressing one's own value judgments and without drawing ethical conclusions. This is so because the fundamental purpose of ethical deliberation is the search for defensible values and conclusions. It is impossible to illustrate how this can be done without doing it. Whether one seems to be doing it right often turns on whether one's conclusions are satisfying.

Moreover, it would be pointless to spend a good deal of time worrying about ethical questions in veterinary medicine unless it matters how these questions are answered. One cannot consider many of these issues without thinking that answers are as important as questions and that certain answers are better (sometimes much better) than others.

I want each reader to regard this book as a personal companion, instigator, and interrogator. I mean this seriously. I will summarize salient arguments on different sides of various subjects, propose solutions or further questions, and challenge you to react and to state your own conclusions. My purpose is to ask about *everything*. The more obvious something might seem, the more vigorously I sometimes will ask about it. People who do not ask questions rarely find the right answers. It is almost always useful to ask why one believes what one does, indeed to challenge one's beliefs. For then one can come to a better and stronger appreciation of one's views, even if they are the correct views.

Some readers will undoubtedly disagree with certain of my conclusions about substantive issues. Whether we agree or disagree about such matters is not my major concern. My hope is that as a result of reading this book you will reach a deeper appreciation of the meaning and implications of your views. If you concur with positions taken here, I ask you to find better ways of arguing for these positions. If you differ with my conclusions, I challenge you, as you sit in the privacy of your reading chair or in the arena of a veterinary school classroom discussion, to show why I am wrong. The aim of this challenge is not to prove that my conclusions are correct, but to encourage *you* to make your own best arguments for your conclusions. Only if the best arguments are raised on all sides of an issue can the truth prevail.

∾ HOW TO USE THE BOOK

Because this is the only current text in veterinary ethics, it is designed for use in a variety of contexts. The book can be approached as a convenient reference guide for people who need information about ethical issues. Suppose, for example, that you are troubled by a competitor's Yellow Pages advertisement, want to know what if anything can be done about "superstore" veterinary clinics, believe that you have been unfairly criticized by a colleague, have been challenged by a client to explain the role of veterinarians in animal research, would like some information about the relevance of bovine growth hormone and genetic engineering to animal welfare, are thinking about inserting a "noncompete" clause into an associate veterinarian's employment contract, are distressed by a client who refuses to authorize euthanasia for a terminally ill animal that is suffering desperately, or would like to refresh your memory about the Veterinarian's Oath. The index will lead you to discussions of these and many other ethical matters that arise often in veterinary practice. These discussions, in turn, will refer you to sections of the book that provide background information about a selected topic and related subjects.

The text can be used by people who seek more extensive treatment of a general topic or set of ethical issues. For example, someone who wants to focus on the distinction between animal welfare and animal rights, the issue of competition among veterinarians, or the role of the American Veterinary Medical Association in articulating ethical rules for practitioners will find large portions of the book that concentrate on these and other general subjects. For those who want to approach the book with a more general ethical issue in mind, I would recommend reading Chapters 1 through 4 and 7 through 10 as early as possible. These chapters provide an overall road map of the book and of veterinary ethics. Chapter 10 is the central chapter of the book. It offers a way of approaching problems in veterinary ethics that I have found extremely effective in helping people to formulate sensible answers to difficult questions.

The book is also designed for use in veterinary school ethics courses. Instructors will find cases for class discussions in the body of the text and the Appendix. However, cases are not enough. A student's response to a case is only as good as the information and background that goes into the response. It is worse than a waste of time to present students with a case and to ask them what they think, if what they think has not yet been informed by consideration of underlying medical, conceptual, or ethical issues. To prepare students for truly educational class discussions of cases, the chapters are organized around topics that are readily assigned for home study.

Finally, the book can be read straight through as a comprehensive approach to veterinary ethics. After one of my talks, a veterinarian accosted me with a complaint about the first edition. He found the book extremely interesting, but wished it read more like a novel. It would, he said, be nice if he could come home after a busy day at the practice, sit in his easy chair with a cold drink, and "read some ethics." He could not do this because he sometimes had to go slowly when topics in philosophy or law were related in unexpected ways to questions he was facing all the time. He also kept putting the book down so that he could start an argument with someone about what he had just read. I guess, he said, this material is serious, like cardiology. We both laughed because he made the point superbly.

Any subject that raises so many difficult questions cannot make for light reading. I hope the book does not make the subject seem more difficult than it is. It would be irresponsible to make it seem easier or more pleasant than it is.

∽ THE CONVERSATION

Academic textbooks have a characteristic tone of aloofness and formality. Discussions are terse and matter-of-fact. Authors refer to themselves in the third person, if they refer to themselves at all. Each reader is expected to come away from the experience (if it can be called such) with exactly the same information as every other reader. All this is justified on the theory that textbooks convey truth. Truth, we all know, has nothing to do with the personal backgrounds or experiences of those who describe or receive it.

There surely is ethical truth. If people did not believe that certain ways of behaving were morally better than other ways they would not bother arguing about right and wrong. But at the same time, ethics is intensely personal. Each of us must decide for ourselves what we think is right and wrong. The questions we find pressing and the answers we find satisfying often have a great deal to do with what we have experienced and what we feel most deeply. This is not to say that ethical positions are merely expressions of personal preferences and that anyone's preferences are as good as anyone else's. Nevertheless, we all must struggle to find what is right both burdened and buoyed by how each of us has come to see the world in our own particular way.

This book attempts to establish a common framework that people with varying experiences and views can use to converse with each other about veterinary ethics. The central plea of the book is that each veterinarian and veterinary student *must* participate in this conversation. Your point of view is important and worthy of being heard. You must not think for a moment that you are caught up in "inevitable" developments that you, individually, have no power to affect. Important choices need to be made. Some of these choices will be made for you by others if you fail to make them yourself. *You* must participate in the conversation.

And now let us discuss!

Jerrold Tannenbaum

~~~~~~~~~~~~~~~~~~~~~~~~~~~~~~~~~~~~~~~

Acknowledgments

*T*his task could not have been undertaken without the assistance of many who shared with me their perspectives and concerns. To these veterinarians, scientists, representatives of state veterinary boards, and officers of veterinary medical associations, I offer my heartfelt appreciation. You cannot all be named here. I hope that you are pleased with the results.

Several people can and must be mentioned. Dean Franklin Loew has given me the opportunity to learn from as intelligent and spirited a group of veterinary students and faculty as exists anywhere. Without his encouragement and support, this book would never have been possible. To my students at Tufts University School of Veterinary Medicine—who challenged me to write the book and who have helped me to improve it—I give boundless thanks. Dr. Robert Shomer has been an inexhaustible fount of probing questions and experienced ideals. Dr. Lawrence Lamb and Jacqueline Lamb provided important insights and invaluable assistance with the manuscript.

Permission to reproduce portions of the following works by the author is gratefully acknowledged: "Ethics and Human-Companion Animal Interaction: A Plea for a Veterinary Ethics of the Human-Companion Animal Bond." *Veterinary Clinics of North America: Small Animal Practice*, Vol. 15, No. 2, pp. 431-447. Copyright © by and reprinted with permission from W.B. Saunders Company; "The Human/Companion Animal Bond: Cliché or Challenge?" *Trends*, Vol. 1, No. 5, pp. 45-50, 1985. Reprinted with permission of the American Animal Hospital Association; Tannenbaum J, Rowan AN: "Rethinking the Morality of Animal Research." *The Hastings Center Report*, Vol. 15, No. 5, pp. 32-43, 1985. Reproduced by permission. ©The Hastings Center; "Animal Rights: Some Guideposts for the Veterinarian." Originally published in the *Journal of the American Veterinary Medical Association* (June 1, 1986), reprinted in Chapter 12 with minor changes, with permission of the publisher; "Ethics and Animal Welfare: The Inextricable Connection." Originally published in the *Journal of the American Veterinary Medical Association* (April 15, 1991), reprinted in Chapter 13 with minor changes, with permission of the publisher; "Ethics and the Veterinary Technician." *Proceedings of the 17th Annual Seminar for Veterinary Technicians*, pp. 206-217. Copyright ©1988 by the Western Veterinary Conference. Reproduced with Permission.

Permission is also acknowledged to quote from James Herriot, *All Creatures Great and Small*. Bantam Books, St. Martin's Press, Inc., New York, 1973, p. 308. Copyright ©1972 by James Herriot. Reprinted by permission of Saint Martin's Press, Harold Ober Associates, David Higham Associates Ltd., and James Herriot.

Finally, I want to thank my wife Nadine and our departed friend Phillip. He motivated her to become a veterinarian. He enticed me away from careers in academic philosophy and law and onto the faculty of a veterinary school. Some hard-nosed types might find these statements hopelessly anthropomorphic, but such people clearly have not experienced life with a Yorkshire Terrier. How blessed a profession to be able to care for such as these!

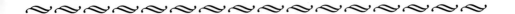

Table of Contents

PART ONE

The Nature
and Importance
of Veterinary Ethics

CHAPTER 1

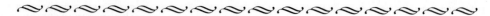

A Time for Veterinary Ethics

*V*eterinary ethics is important for every present and future veterinarian—and everyone whose animals come in contact with a veterinarian. There are three reasons this is so.

Virtually everything veterinarians do in their professional lives reflects moral choices. Each veterinarian should therefore want to make these choices knowledgeably and correctly.

Second, what makes veterinary medicine a true profession, as distinguished from a trade or occupation, is its endorsement of fundamental ethical values and its desire to make goodness of purpose as much a part of its mission as technical competence.

Finally, the profession of veterinary medicine faces numerous challenges that require ethical responses. These challenges are not abstract or academic. They affect all practitioners. Their resolution will determine how veterinarians provide for patients, clients, and themselves in the coming decades.

∾ THE NEED TO MAKE MORAL CHOICES
Ethical Decisions in Practice Situations

Some veterinarians believe that because theirs is a scientific discipline, they do not have to make value judgments. Ethics, some think, might be important to professors or animal rights agitators—but is not part of the day-to-day business of treating patients, dealing with clients, and earning a living. The following case demonstrates why this view is incorrect.

> *Case 1-1 A client appears in your hospital for the second time in 4 weeks with her 2-year-old dog. At the first visit, you diagnosed a moderate case of flea allergy dermatitis, dispensed an appropriate medication and flea powder, and advised the client to vacuum and powder her premises thoroughly for several weeks to prevent recurrence of the problem. As the client and the dog enter your examination room, it is apparent that the dog's condition has deteriorated. You believe the medication has not been applied as directed, and you doubt that the client has attempted to remove the fleas and their eggs from her home.*
>
> *She now tells you for the first time that the animal has been impossible to housebreak. She wants it put to sleep.*
>
> *What should you do?*

In this example moral choices are unavoidable. If you would immediately agree to euthanize the dog because the client has requested it, you probably would be expressing your adherence to several ethical positions, including the following:

- A companion animal has no inherent right to live.
- An animal's owner may have it killed if keeping it has become an inconvenience.
- The owner of a pet with a curable malady or behavioral problem need not take steps to remedy these problems but may just opt for euthanasia.
- It is proper for a veterinarian to euthanize a companion merely because its owner requests that it be killed.

Likewise, if you would try to persuade the client to address the dog's medical and behavioral problems, you would be expressing your belief in a number of other ethical principles, including, perhaps, the view that an animal like the one in the case ought not simply to be killed but deserves, at the very least, a second chance.

Many situations in veterinary practice present a large number of possible ethical choices. The following are just some of the choices that could be made in Case 1-1. One might:

- Euthanize the animal at the client's request.
- Ask the client whether she has followed your directions and inquire further about the housebreaking problem, hoping this will lead her to conclude on her own that the animal need not be put to sleep.
- Ask the client whether she has followed your directions and about the housebreaking problem and actively challenge her decision to euthanize the dog, but agree to euthanasia if she still wants it.
- Aggressively challenge the client about her failure to treat the dermatitis and insist that she make some serious attempts to do so before you agree to euthanize the animal.
- Ask her whether she will board the dog temporarily at your hospital and have you treat the skin condition and assess the housebreaking problem.
- Decline to euthanize the animal and ask for permission to place it with an animal shelter for adoption.
- Decline to euthanize the dog, and ask the client to permit you to place it out for adoption.
- Tell the client politely that, although you can understand her desire to euthanize the animal, it is against your personal principles to euthanize pets with curable conditions, and refer her to another practitioner or agency that will put the dog to sleep.
- Tell her that you think killing a curable animal is morally wrong and criticize her for her lack of concern about the life of her dog.

Some of these alternatives may well be morally wrong. That is not the point. The point is that, *whatever* your response to this case, you will be choosing only one or some of the possible alternatives. Whether you actually consider all the alternatives, your decision will reflect your views about what it is morally proper to do.

The Difficulty of Ethics

If ethically correct decisions in veterinary practice were always obvious, that there are usually many possible alternatives would not be troubling, and would not argue for a serious discipline of veterinary ethics. In almost all situations we face, there are many possible choices. However, most of these alternatives are so clearly unacceptable that we need not consider them seriously. If an acquaintance approaches me on the street and says hello, a proper response is to return the greeting. The fact that I might throw my briefcase in his face, or cry out to a police officer, "Thief! Stop him!" or do any of a thousand other awful things does not mean serious ethical deliberation regarding a proper response is justified.

Veterinary ethics is important and inescapable, because it is often far from obvious how veterinarians should act.

Several of the possible choices in Case 1-1 have some plausibility. It appears to be the client's fault that the dog's dermatitis has not improved, and the housetraining problem (if it exists at all) may be attributable to her as well. If these things are so, and if the dog's "problems" can readily be cured, one can argue that it would be unfair to the animal to deprive it of the opportunity to receive care and love from a more suitable owner. This argument may be stronger the longer the dog has been in the client's possession. There is some plausibility in suggesting that a companion animal that has been cared for and has been a functioning member of a human-companion animal bond for some time deserves extra consideration before it is killed at the whim of a now-dissatisfied owner.

However, even these suggestions raise further questions. Should the client be responsible for treating the dog if this would be a significant financial expense? If so, how great an expense can she be expected to bear under these circumstances? Is it wrong not to try to persuade the client, who might, with some education, make a good pet owner, to keep the animal? Should a veterinarian with a practice to run take the time and money to attempt to adopt out curable animals? Even if the dog should not yet be euthanized, why should the veterinarian be concerned with attempting to save it? The client could take the animal elsewhere, and by making a nuisance of herself, the practitioner may only risk losing her and other clients as well.

Veterinary Ethics and Conflicting Interests

The difficulty of veterinary ethics does not result just from an accumulation of problematic situations, such as that presented in Case 1-1. Ethical difficulties are an inescapable and inherent feature of veterinary practice itself.

I like to torment my veterinary students at the beginning of their required ethics course at Tufts University with a simple question: "Does a veterinarian serve the patient or the client?"

Typically, the class divides into two opposing factions. One group insists that veterinarians work for the patient. The other faction argues with equal zeal on behalf of the client. The debate continues for some time, often with considerable vehemence. Eventually, as exhaustion sets in and neither side has won the hoped-for approval of the instructor, the combatants realize that they have fallen into a trap.

Some students (and a few veterinarians) believe animals are so important that veterinarians must proclaim their undivided allegiance to *patients*. Clients, this group concedes, can be helped too, but satisfying a client is appropriate only if this results from helping the patient. Other students (and a few veterinarians) appear to think that one extreme claim requires an equally extreme response. This group maintains that animal owners are *the* focus of a veterinarian's efforts. Patients, they concede, may be helped too but only when doing so suits the needs of clients.

As every veterinarian who has practiced with a modicum of success knows, veterinarians typically serve *both* patients and clients. Obviously, a patient is important. But so is the client, who pays the bill and whose emotional or economic interests are often as much the focus of a veterinarian's craft as the needs of the patient.

The fact that veterinarians are the servants of two masters can make ethical issues in veterinary practice extremely difficult. The interests of patients sometimes conflict with those of clients. A doctor caught in the middle wants to do the best for both, but is sometimes unable to do so. For example, a pet's interest in being spared interminable suffering may conflict with the client's desire to keep it alive as long as possible. A patient's interest in being helped can conflict with a client's inability to pay for that help. As in Case 1-1, a patient's interest in a continuing and healthy life can conflict with a client's disinterest in the animal, or worse—hostility to it.

Such conflicts are common in veterinary practice. Thinking that these conflicts can be eliminated—by swearing allegiance to either patients or clients—is unrealistic and pointless. Veterinarians will always serve both patients and clients. Because the interests of people and their animals sometimes conflict, veterinarians will never be able to avoid ethical problems caused by such conflicts.

Some people believe that the devotion of veterinarians to people as well as animals is merely an accident of history that can be overcome with hard work and sufficient dedication to animals. This is a foolish view. The concern of veterinary medicine for both humans and animals reflects deep, unchangeable facts about humans and animals. Any society that has survived and prospered believes it is appropriate for people to use animals for a wide range of purposes. Any society that can lay claim to fundamental decency also believes some animals have interests of their own, and that these interests sometimes place ethical limitations on what people may do to animals.

Society *requires* a profession that attends to animal medical issues—sometimes in the service of people, sometimes in the service of animals, and sometimes in the service of both. If veterinarians could somehow decide to promote only animal interests, then another profession of animal doctors would quickly spring into existence. This new profession, like veterinary medicine, would serve the interests of both people and animals. This new profession, like veterinary medicine, would need to confront ethical issues resulting from conflicts of interests between people and their animals. This new profession would be indistinguishable from contemporary veterinary medicine.

The Range of Ethical Choices

Although Case 1-1 raises the sensitive issue of euthanasia, its lesson—that ethical choices are part of virtually anything one does—applies to almost all situations veterinarians face. As long as there are alternative approaches to a medical or practice management question, one can usually ask whether any one of these possible approaches is morally acceptable. Almost always, the approach chosen reflects a veterinarian's views about what is ethically correct, as the following case illustrates.

Case 1-2 Consider the next client and patient about to enter your examining room. This client had to make an appointment to see you. Was the number of days she waited appropriate to her needs and that of her animal? Do you have enough doctors on staff, and do they work an appropriate schedule so that she and other clients can obtain an appointment in a reasonable time? When the client arrived at your facility, how was she treated? Did she wait in surroundings that made her and her animal comfortable? Were adequate steps taken to protect her and her animal from diseases or untoward behavior of other clients' animals? Was she treated cour-

teously by your receptionist, and were her questions and concerns answered seriously and sympathetically? Was the time she waited to see you reasonable, given not only her needs but that of other patients and clients being attended to at the time?

When she enters with her animal into the examining room, how will she be treated? Will you listen to her carefully and respectfully? Will you examine her animal thoroughly and diligently? If there are various possible choices about how to proceed with the animal's care, will these be presented clearly, completely, compassionately, and respectfully? To what extent will you attempt to influence her decision? Will she be given enough time to think about the possible options? To what extent, if any, will you consider your own economic interests and that of your practice in making your recommendations? How will you respond if the client requests something that is not in your patient's best interests or refuses to authorize something that is? If she complains about another veterinarian who treated her animal, what will you say? If you see something another doctor has done to her animal that is puzzling or problematic, what will you say to her? What might you say to the other doctor?

Will you charge her a fair fee for your services?

When she leaves your hospital, will she be leaving a facility that offers services and products that are proper for a veterinarian to offer? Does the facility treat its inpatients humanely? Do these animals receive sufficient supervision and attention? Are treatments and surgeries performed meticulously and professionally with appropriate supplies and materials?

Will this client be leaving a facility that provides working hours and conditions for doctor and nonveterinarian employees that are decent and fair, and therefore conducive to the interests not just of those who work in the practice but of clients and their animals? Are these employees paid fairly? Does the facility present itself, professionally (for example, in its exterior physical appearance, client newsletters, and Yellow Pages listing) and with respect for the interests of patients, clients, and the public?

To be sure, this is not a "case" at all. It is a list (and an incomplete one at that) of various ways in which veterinarians deal with patients, clients, colleagues, coworkers, and the public. As this book demonstrates, all the questions raised in this "case" are to some extent ethical in nature. As will be seen, some of these questions, and a great many more that arise in everyday veterinary practice, are extremely difficult.

Making Choices Correctly and Confidently

Because veterinarians make many ethical choices, it is important for them to know what ethical choices they are making and why they are making these choices. It is important to know such things because one wants to act well. If one is making ethical choices, they should be the *right* choices. But it is impossible to know that one's choices are correct without knowing what they are, the reasons for them, and whether the reasons for them are good reasons. Knowing that one's choices are appropriate also promotes confidence about the worth and value of one's professional life. This, in turn, enables well-informed and confident responses to people who question one's choices.

The study of professional ethics is important, because it can assist in understanding and evaluating one's ethical choices.

⮜ ETHICS AND THE NATURE OF A PROFESSION

Attention to ethics is also important because veterinary medicine is a *profession*. There are many occupations and trades. However, very few ways of earning a living are recognized by society and the legal system as learned professions. The most important feature of the professions (which include, in addition to veterinary medicine, medicine, dentistry, nursing, and law) is that they are permitted to play a predominant role in the education and regulation of their members. This role, which is usually exercised through a national organization of members of each profession, includes accreditation and supervision of the profession's schools, providing continuing education for practitioners, support for and publication of research, and active cooperation with government agencies, including state licensing boards.

The professions develop and articulate two kinds of standards for their members: requirements for professional competence and principles of professional ethics. The task of articulating ethical standards is absolutely essential to their characterization as professions. All the learned professions have written codes of ethics, which state each profession's most fundamental moral values, and which are interpreted and enforced by internal quasijudicial bodies. Each of the ethics codes of the professions has a long history. These codes are presented to members of the professions and the public not only as a set of rules regarding how members ought to act, but also as a statement of how each profession defines its mission. In sum, a profession articulates certain ethical values and positions, the adoption of which becomes part of what it *means* to be a veterinarian, physician, dentist, nurse, or lawyer.

The study of professional ethics is crucial for all veterinarians because from the time they enter veterinary school, they absorb, accept, and eventually live by most if not all of the profession's ethical values. Sometimes by deliberate choice, but more often through a subtle process of osmosis from teachers and colleagues, these values become part of how they view themselves as veterinarians. Studying professional ethics can help practitioners and students understand which components of their behavior are derived from the profession's values. Studying professional ethics can assist veterinarians in defending these values when they ought to be defended, and in changing them when they ought to be changed.

～ CONTEMPORARY ETHICAL CHALLENGES TO VETERINARY MEDICINE

Finally, attention to ethics is important because veterinary medicine faces serious challenges that require answers to ethical questions. Some of these challenges come from within the profession. Others come from without, sometimes from people who reject the profession's oldest and most firmly held values. Many of these challenges arise, as we shall see, from changing attitudes toward animals and from the fact that veterinarians serve both human and animal masters.

This book is devoted to discussing these challenges and the ethical questions they raise. The following is a brief overview of several of them.

Elevation of the Status of Companion Animals

Today many veterinary patients enjoy a status that would have been unthinkable for any animals just a few generations ago. Pets—mainly cats, dogs, and birds, but increasingly horses and some exotic species as well—are valued companions and friends. Many are considered members of their owners' families.

This elevation of the status of pets in contemporary society has fueled the economic and scientific progress of veterinary medicine. People who are devoted to animals will seek good medical care for them and will spend money for such care. The demand for effective animal medical care enables veterinarians to offer it and necessitates research to develop it.

Unfortunately, the elevated status of many of these patients also raises serious ethical challenges for the profession. The more animals are valued, the more difficult it becomes for owners to request that they be euthanized when these animals can no longer be helped. It becomes more trying for clients who wish to assist their animals but cannot afford the fees a veterinarian must ask to provide such assistance. Veterinarians are caught in the middle of such problems, wanting to help both patient and client but sometimes being unable to do so.

As more animals are accorded a higher status, veterinarians must also consider what to do about animals that are not so highly valued. How, for example, should a profession committed to making the lives of animals longer and more enjoyable react when clients request euthanasia for healthy animals? How should a profession dedicated to animal health respond to those who perpetuate breed standards or request veterinary procedures that are not in patients' interests? What should veterinarians do about the tens of millions of unwanted cats and dogs killed each year in shelters and pounds?

Importance of the Human Side of the Human-Animal Bond

If there is an omnipresent veterinary "buzz word" of the last quarter of this century, it is "the human-companion animal bond." As we shall see, this "bond" raises important questions about whether animals that are supposedly part of the bond are being treated fairly. As we shall also see, a true bond is a two-sided relationship, and in the human-companion animal bond the human side is as important as the animal. This fact raises difficult ethical issues for veterinarians. Veterinarians are trained in animal medicine not human psychology. How should they deal with clients who are unable to approach an animal's situation knowledgeably or rationally? How does one respond to a client who is emotionally overwrought or grief-stricken? In general, how should one exercise one's enormous power to influence clients' decisions? Does the importance of the client in the veterinarian-patient-client relationship require the profession to rethink traditional notions that veterinarians are solely, or mainly, animal doctors and to expand training in client relations for practitioners and students? Can veterinarians promote the emotional attachment between people and companion animals and at the same time insist—when something goes wrong and they are sued—that animals are just pieces of ordinary property and clients therefore should not be compensated for emotional distress caused by veterinary malpractice?

The Advent of High-tech Veterinary Procedures

Ethical problems veterinarians face in attempting to serve both patients and clients are intensified by high-tech, advanced procedures. Stories about total hip replacements, cancer chemotherapy, root canals, hearing aids, intensive care units, and heart pacemakers for animals may sell newspapers and magazines, and they may give the profession valuable publicity. However, the increasing tide of technologically advanced medical treatments for animals raises traditional moral dilemmas to new levels. Many high-tech procedures are expensive. Some subject animals that would previously be put out of their misery to significant distress or, if "successful," to a diminished or poor quality of life. How should veterinarians deal with clients who insist on spending thousands of dollars for questionable ends, refuse to spend money when doing so would help their animal, or, when unable to afford the latest high-tech veterinary treatment, question the morality and rationality of providing such care to *animals*?

The Role of Food, Farm, and Sport Animal Practice

The elevation of the status of companion animals raises serious ethical issues for a profession many of whose patients are eaten, worn, or ridden or raced in competition—in short, viewed not as companions but economic resources. How should veterinarians reconcile the advanced, sometimes heroic, measures taken to save the lives of some animals with efforts to keep others alive until they can be profitably killed? How should a profession increasingly imbued with regard for individual companion animals react to the trend in food and farm animal practice to move away from a concern for the health of individual animals and toward the productivity of herds? How should food, farm, and sport animal practitioners respond to the growing demand in the profession and society for the promotion of animal welfare? What should be the veterinarian's role in areas, such as meat production or horse and dog racing, where no one may speak for the animal's interests unless the veterinarian does? Will equine doctors find some of their values and practices challenged, not just as more people appreciate the value of companion animals, but as more people keep horses *as* companion animals?

As Dean Franklin Loew observes in a seminal discussion, veterinary medicine has been transformed from a profession with agricultural roots, to one that is mainly urban and suburban.[1] This has happened because most clients are now in the cities and suburbs. However, the nature of the metamorphosis is more than demographic. Different values now predominate. The overwhelming majority of city and suburban animals are companion animals. Their relationships with their owners tend to be lengthy, intense, and decidedly nonexploitive (on both sides). What should be the role of agricultural veterinary medicine in an urban society? How will farm and food animal doctors respond if the public and most veterinarians come to view *all* animals through the growing urban and suburban prism?

The Emergence of Animal Welfare Science

One of the most potentially far-reaching developments to affect veterinary medicine is the recent emergence of animal welfare science. Veterinarians, physiologists, animal behaviorists, and ethologists have embarked on the creation of a new and distinct area of study. The scientific aim of this field is to discover basic facts about the biological and psychological needs of animals and to better understand what animals experience. The practical goal of animal welfare science is to improve the lives of animals consistent with their legitimate use by people.

Animal welfare science raises serious ethical issues, in part because, as we shall see, the very concept of welfare is an ethical one. This concept requires judgment about what animals ought (or ought not) to be allowed or compelled to experience. Taking animal welfare seriously also raises challenges to some traditional ways of using animals. Have veterinarians and producers paid sufficient attention to the welfare of food and farm animals? Are some uses of these animals inconsistent with even a minimally acceptable level of welfare? What should be the role of veterinarians in promoting the welfare of laboratory and research animals? Are veterinarians in various kinds of practice doing enough to alleviate pain and distress experienced by animals as a result of medical or surgical procedures? If protecting animal welfare sometimes makes promoting human happiness more difficult or expensive, to what extent (if at all) is it appropriate to compromise animal welfare?

Animal Activism and Challenges to Traditionally Accepted Uses of Animals

A set of major and potentially devastating challenges to veterinary medicine comes from so-called animal "rightists," "liberationists," and animal use "abolitionists." These people oppose the utilization of animals for food, on farms, for entertainment, and in research. Many believe it is wrong to breed or have companion animals. Although some claim to be friends of veterinary medicine, the ideal world envisioned by many animal activists would not contain a veterinary profession, because the vast majority of veterinarians participate in what they believe to be illegitimate uses of animals.

The profession must understand and fight the dangers of extreme positions. At the same time, veterinarians should avoid rejecting issues and positions just because these may sometimes be endorsed by opponents of the profession. Meeting the challenges of animal extremism will require veterinarians to be aware of philosophical concepts and scientific principles that reach far beyond the boundaries of day-to-day veterinary practice.

Competing Models of Practice

The most important fact of professional life for most veterinarians is that they must earn a living. Despite the high regard many people have for animals, this is not always an easy task. Veterinarians are not as well paid as members of other professions with comparable education, skill, and importance. It is not always easy to convince people to spend scarce discretionary income on medical care for animals.

Traditionally, veterinarians have been viewed as healers of their patients and friends of their clients. However, in response to the demands of the contemporary marketplace, there has arisen a new model of veterinary practice. This model views veterinary medicine as essentially a business, which includes the retailing of services and products that are not inherently veterinary in nature. Practitioners, according to this model, should sell whatever clients can be persuaded to buy and should compete aggressively against their colleagues just as other kinds of businesses compete against each other. Some advocates of this model welcome the ownership of veterinary practices by nonveterinarians, venture capitalists, and general business corporations.

There may be no more important choice for the profession than whether to endorse this new entrepreneurial model of practice or to build upon more traditional views of professional life.

Promotion and Collegiality

Intimately connected with the need to attract and keep clients are issues relating to promotion and competition. The law, as we shall see, severely restricts the ability of organized veterinary medicine and the state licensing boards to compel veterinarians to present themselves to the public in a dignified and professional manner. What kinds of activities designed to attract clients are ethically permissible? Can the veterinary profession prevent its image from being tainted by sleazy or deceptive promotion?

Does the legal freedom to compete require veterinarians to aggressively seek clients, including satisfied clients of other veterinarians? What may a veterinarian say about another doctor to obtain or keep clients? Is it appropriate for a practitioner to criticize the performance of a colleague to a client? Are there ethical limitations on what veterinary specialists may do to promote themselves and on how they may deal with general practitioners?

In short, are veterinarians colleagues or competitors?

Issues in Employer-Employee Relations

Most veterinarians work for or hire other veterinarians. Employer-employee relations are an essential part of veterinary ethics. Veterinary employers and employees spend much more time interacting with each other than they do with any individual patient or client. Many employed veterinarians are concerned about their working conditions, salaries, prospects for advancement, and ability to compete with former employers. Employers have an interest in motivating associate veterinarians to generate revenue and to respect practice policies regarding services and fees. Nonveterinarian practice staff raise issues of their own, complicating the ethical issues related to employer and employee veterinarians.

Employer-employee relations present important ethical challenges to the profession because such relations affect not only those who work in veterinary practices, but also patients and clients.

Changing Professional Demographics

The profession is changing at least as quickly as its patients and clients. Veterinarians, like animal owners, come increasingly from the cities and suburbs. At many veterinary colleges, students with backgrounds in liberal arts and the sciences now outnumber those with degrees in agriculture. However, the most striking change in the profession is the growing proportion of female members. In 1985 women comprised 50.8% of the total student body of veterinary schools in the United States.[2] Just 7 years later, their proportion in both U.S. and Canadian schools had risen to 64%,[3] and by 1994 women constituted more than three-fourths of the entering classes at several veterinary colleges. Some social scientists and observers of the profession believe that female veterinary students and practitioners are more concerned about the interests of patients and are more interested in animal welfare than their male counterparts. If this is so, there may be significant changes in the profession's emphasis as the proportion of female veterinarians increases. There may also be issues relating to how the profession can maintain appropriate earnings for all its members in a society that still tends to pay women less than men for equal work.

Widening Horizons

Finally, veterinary medicine at the close of the twentieth century is exploring new areas. Veterinarians are playing an expanding role in assisting developing nations to improve their economies and food supplies. As people and animals interact more closely, veterinarians assume ever greater importance in the field of public health. Increased attention to the environment, so much of which is comprised of animals, has led many in the profession to ask what contributions veterinarians can make to improve the lives of all that inhabit the planet.

These widening horizons of veterinary medicine are not without ethical challenges and dangers. How will the profession's traditional concern for animal health square with the predominant aim of many environmentalists to make the planet a better place for *people*? What role will the profession's traditional concern for the health and welfare of individual animals play in ecological programs in which the primary interest is to preserve groups or species of animals? Is it ethically appropriate for veterinarians to provide medical care for wild animals at all if this risks interfering with evolution and leaving species or individual treated animals less able to fend for themselves in their natural environments?

∾ ANIMAL WELFARE, CLIENT RELATIONS, COMPETITION AND COLLEGIALITY

The more vibrant, interesting, and important a profession, the more difficult it is to briefly characterize the ethical problems it faces. As all who enter it know—and as *everyone* who comes in contact with it *ought* to know—veterinary medicine is an extraordinarily vibrant, interesting, and important profession. It is therefore impossible to capture quickly the range, complexity, and difficulty of its ethical challenges. Nevertheless, three general themes emerge. These themes do not exhaust all of professional veterinary ethics, but they comprise a large part of it. These themes therefore provide the structural foundation around which this book is organized.

Veterinarians are animal doctors, whatever else they do, and however strongly they advocate and promote the interests of people. What distinguishes them from members of other healing professions and practitioners of other sciences is their expertise regarding the medical problems of animals. Whenever a veterinarian is acting as a veterinarian, an animal is involved. In addition, because veterinarians are committed by their professional Oath and fundamental ethical values to *care about* animals, animal welfare is a core concern of veterinary ethics. In recent years, this subject has gained increased importance as society and the profession endorse ever more strongly the moral imperative to treat animals decently.

Most veterinarians are doctors of patients that are owned by clients. A veterinarian in private practice does very little that will not affect and will not be affected by a client. However strongly they advocate the interests of patients, practitioners must also take into account the interests and needs of their clients. Relations with clients constitute another central focus of veterinary ethics.

Veterinarians are also members of a profession. They cooperate with each other in promoting public concern for animal health. They learn from each other about principles of medicine and management. They make and accept referrals in cooperative efforts to provide animals and clients the best services the profession can offer. For many years, I have had the good fortune to be able to talk with hundreds of veterinarians about ethical issues presented in everyday practice. I have learned that veterinarians are concerned about whether the traditional values of collegiality and cooperation will survive. Many resent aggressive competition, critical comments, and undignified commercialistic behavior by some practitioners. A central focus of this book is the issue of how veterinarians should behave toward their fellow veterinarians—because this sub-ject is important to so many veterinarians, and because how veterinarians relate to each other can affect greatly how they treat patients and clients.

This is truly a time for veterinary ethics.

REFERENCES

[1]Loew FM: Animals and the urban prism, *J Am Vet Med Assoc* 202:1658-1661, 1993.
[2]Enrollment declines in DVM-degree programs, *J Am Vet Med Assoc* 192:1028, 1988.
[3]Veterinary medical degree enrollment, 1992-1993, *J Am Vet Med Assoc* 202:1954, 1993.

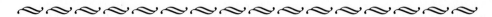

CHAPTER 2

The Four Branches of Veterinary Ethics

∿ VETERINARY ETHICS AND ANIMAL ETHICS

Ethics deals with what is morally good and bad, right and wrong, just and unjust. As a kind or branch of ethics, veterinary ethics shares these concerns. However, the term "veterinary ethics" does not have a single accepted usage and indeed, seems capable of two different interpretations.

By "veterinary ethics" one might mean ethics as it relates to animals, just as veterinary medicine is medicine relating to animals. In this sense, any moral issue concerning animals—whether it involves veterinarians—would be an issue of veterinary ethics. In this sense, whether people have a moral obligation to protect endangered wildlife or whether it is morally acceptable to wear animal fur are questions of veterinary ethics, because these are questions concerning what it is morally right to do with or to animals.

On the other hand, by "veterinary ethics," one might mean ethics as it relates directly to veterinarians and others (for example, veterinary students and technicians) directly involved in providing veterinary care. This is how veterinarians understand the term. Thus the official code of ethics of the profession, the American Veterinary Medical Association *Principles of Veterinary Medical Ethics*[1] is a document about ethical issues in veterinary practice.

In this book, "veterinary ethics" will be understood in the second, or professional, sense. The term "animal ethics" will be used to refer to the broader range of ethical issues involving animals, including ethical issues relating to veterinarians.

The focus of this text is *veterinary* ethics thus understood. However, there are important issues in veterinary ethics that cannot be tackled without venturing into the larger and sometimes extremely difficult realm of animal ethics. For example, if, as some people assert, animals and human beings have equal moral value (a claim in animal ethics), it would be wrong for people to eat or experiment on animals, and veterinarians who engage in food or laboratory animal practice would therefore be acting immorally (a claim in veterinary ethics). Likewise, how strong a role one thinks veterinarians should play in advocating the interests of animals will depend in part on how one ranks animals and people in the moral spectrum. The less value one accords to an animal patient, for example, the less one might oppose a client's wish to kill a healthy but no longer wanted pet.

Because some questions in veterinary ethics involve underlying issues in animal ethics, it is impossible for any book in veterinary ethics to provide complete and definitive answers to all questions in professional veterinary ethics. As we shall see, a fundamental question of animal ethics that touches many issues in veterinary ethics is precisely the issue of how much value animals have relative to people. Philosopher Robert Nozick observes that there has not been enough persuasive thinking, even by academic philosophers, about this question.[2] This does not mean that veterinarians (or society in general) should be racked by wholesale doubt about whether animals are being treated properly. Nozick notes that many of society's long-standing intuitions and attitudes concerning animals (for example, that they are not equal in value to human beings) are surely correct. What is needed, however, is more sophisticated philosophical and empirical underpinning of these attitudes. The implication for veterinary ethics is that while one will sometimes know that certain positions are correct, one may lack all the principles of animal ethics required to support these positions. There may also be times when one will be unable to answer a question in veterinary ethics because an underlying issue in animal ethics remains unsettled. We must expect that discussions and conclusions in veterinary ethics will be revised and refined as we develop greater sophistication in animal ethics.

"Ethics" and "Morality"

It is useful to clarify early on another matter of terminology. Some people attempt to distinguish between *ethics* and *morality*. They often base this distinction on the fact that the word "ethics" can be traced back to the ancient Greek term *ethikos*, which emphasized the character of the individual, while the word "morality" is derived from the Latin term *mores*, which referred to rules that groups of people (and ultimately, society at large) applied to its members. Following such a distinction, "veterinary ethics" might have something to do with the character of individual veterinarians. "Moral" aspects of veterinary medicine would pertain, perhaps, to values the profession has developed for its members or relations among veterinarians.

In this book, the terms "ethics" and "morality" are used synonymously. However these words may have been employed in the past, today, differentiation between the "ethical" and "moral" seems forced and unnatural. Indeed, among those who think that there is a difference, there is often disagreement about what this difference is supposed to be.[3,4] In fact, the overwhelming majority of speakers of the language, as well as most philosophers,[3] use the terms "ethical" and "moral" interchangeably. For example, the *Principles of Veterinary Medical Ethics* not only seeks to identify good individual character traits but also sets forth, on behalf of the entire society of veterinarians, rules concerning how doctors should behave toward each other and members of the public. When the code speaks about personal traits that each individual veterinarian should nurture, it refers to them as traits of "*moral* character."[5]

There seems little point in attempting to resurrect or invent artificial distinctions between ethics and morality or between veterinary ethics and veterinary morality. What is important is that the field of veterinary ethics considers issues of both individual character and group behavior.

～ THE FOUR BRANCHES OF VETERINARY ETHICS

Even when one conceives of veterinary ethics as ethics relating to veterinary medicine, there are four different things one might have in mind.

Descriptive Veterinary Ethics

By the "ethics" of a profession like veterinary medicine, one might mean the actual values or standards of the profession, that is, what members of the profession in fact think is right and wrong regarding professional behavior and attitudes. In this sense, understanding the "ethics" of a profession is a matter of describing its actual values and does not involve making value judgments about what is moral or immoral in that profession's behavior. (One can study the "ethics," in this sense, of a profession one believes to be utterly evil.) I shall call the study of the actual ethical views of veterinarians and veterinary students regarding professional behavior and attitudes *descriptive veterinary ethics*.

Official Veterinary Ethics

In speaking of the ethics of veterinarians or other professionals, one might also mean the official ethical standards formally adopted by organizations composed of these professionals and which these organizations attempt to impose upon their members. In this sense, also, one can understand (or appeal to) part of a profession's "ethics" without believing that the standards involved are morally correct. For example, some attorneys believe that they should sometimes be able to speak directly to the person suing their client, instead of dealing only with the opposing attorney; yet they would never do so because "legal ethics," the official bar association ethical rules, forbid it. I shall call the process of the articulation and application of ethical standards for veterinarians by the organized profession *official veterinary ethics*.

Administrative Veterinary Ethics

Another important source of moral standards for veterinarians are administrative government bodies that regulate veterinary practice and various activities in which veterinarians engage. What distinguishes the moral standards of such bodies from those of professional organizations is that only the former carry the force of law. If practitioners violate the ethical rules of the AVMA, the most severe penalty they can face is expulsion from this organization. However, violation of administrative standards can result in criminal or civil penalties—or if the administrative body is one's state board of registration, revocation or suspension of one's license to practice. I shall call the application of ethical standards to veterinarians by administrative government bodies *administrative veterinary ethics*.

Normative Veterinary Ethics

Finally, in speaking of veterinary ethics, one can mean the attempt to discover correct moral standards for veterinarians and others involved in providing veterinary care. In the philosophical literature, the term "normative ethics" is used to refer to the search for correct principles of good and bad, right and wrong, justice and injustice. I shall therefore call the activity of looking for correct norms for veterinary professional behavior and attitudes *normative veterinary ethics*.

～ THE IMPORTANCE OF ALL FOUR BRANCHES OF VETERINARY ETHICS

Clearly, the standards of descriptive, official, administrative, and normative ethics can differ. Practitioners' actual values can deviate from official or administratively imposed standards. Any of these can, in turn, differ from what is actually right.

Some students (and some ethics teachers as well) tend to equate professional ethics with normative professional ethics. They believe that the official standards of the profession are "just" what happens to be accepted by most members of the profession at the time, and they are eager to get to what is *really* right and wrong. Each year, several students in my course in veterinary ethics at Tufts University initially protest that it is a waste of time to study the AVMA *Principles of Veterinary Medical Ethics*. They suppose that once one determines what is actually right in veterinary practice, one need only make the official, administrative, and actual standards coincide with these correct moral principles.

Certainly, normative veterinary ethics is the most important of the four branches of veterinary ethics. Most veterinarians are interested in ethics because they want to determine how they really should behave and not just how their fellow professionals, official rules, or governmental bodies say they should. However, it would be a terrible mistake to underestimate the importance of the other branches of veterinary ethics.

For reasons that are explained in subsequent chapters, there will always be differences between official and administrative rules on the one hand and the principles of normative ethics on the other. This means that even the most moral of practitioners must study official and administrative standards to understand what they say. One reason practitioners should want to understand what they say is that they can get themselves into various kinds of trouble if they violate these standards. To be sure, it might not always be morally right to follow official or administrative standards. But it is a foolhardy practitioner indeed who does not know that in choosing to follow the dictates of one's conscience, one might be exposing oneself to the censure of colleagues, or worse.

It is also important to study official and administrative veterinary ethics, because there will always be such standards, and one cannot improve them without knowing what they are and how they have or have not worked.

Official veterinary ethics is especially useful in approaching normative veterinary ethics. The official rules indicate what ethical questions the profession has found most pressing, and they propose specific answers to many of these questions. Descriptive veterinary ethics also, can reveal the concerns of the profession and can help authors of official and administrative rules understand what standards might be necessary and whether proposed rules are likely to be accepted or resisted.

❧ THE TASKS AHEAD

This book concentrates primarily on normative veterinary ethics and secondarily on official veterinary ethics. The latter is worth considering in some detail because it is of such great practical importance to the profession, and currently, it is the most fully developed branch of veterinary ethics.

Much less can be said, at least at present, about administrative and descriptive veterinary ethics. As explained in Chapter 7, the most important source of administrative veterinary ethical standards are the state veterinary licensing boards. However, these boards vary in the extent to which they enforce ethical standards. Moreover, because few boards share their deliberations about individual cases with the public, it is extremely difficult to obtain an overall picture of the activity of the licensing boards in the ethical arena. Likewise, no treatment of veterinary ethics can yet give descriptive ethics the treatment it deserves. There has been relatively little empirical work describing the actual moral values of veterinarians. However, as activity in the other branches of veterinary ethics increases, interest in understanding how practitioners actually think about and deal with ethical issues should grow as well.

REFERENCES

[1]American Veterinary Medical Association: *Principles of Veterinary Medical Ethics*, 1993 Revision, *1994 AVMA Directory*, Schaumburg, IL, The Association, pp 42-46. The *Principles*, the latest revision of which are always included in the current annual *AVMA Directory*, are also available from the AVMA in booklet form.

[2]Nozick R: About mammals and people, *New York Times Book Review*, November 27, 1983, New York Times, p 11.

[3]Beauchamp TL, Childress JF: *Principles of Biomedical Ethics*, ed 3, New York, 1989, Oxford University Press, p 23 (stating that "*ethics* often refers to reflective and theoretical perspectives, whereas *morality* often refers to actual conduct and practice," but also conceding that the authors "often use the terms *moral* and *ethical* interchangeably").

[4]Williams B: *Ethics and the Limits of Philosophy*, Cambridge, MA, 1985, Harvard University Press, pp 6 and 177 (stating that morality is a narrower subsystem within ethics that emphasizes the notion of obligation, and that evokes the characteristic reaction of "blame between persons").

[5]American Veterinary Medical Association: *Principles of Veterinary Medical Ethics*, 1993 Revision, "Guidelines for Professional Behavior," paragraph 9, *1994 AVMA Directory*, Schaumburg, IL, The Association, p 42, emphasis supplied.

CHAPTER 3

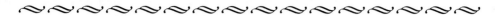

Veterinary Ethics and Religion

*V*eterinary ethics is made difficult by more than just animal ethics. This chapter considers how religious beliefs can affect views about how veterinarians ought to act. Chapter 4 examines the complicating effects of the law.

∾ RELIGIOUS AND METAPHYSICAL VIEWS ABOUT ANIMALS

There can be little doubt that some people, and some veterinarians, hold views about animals that are based at least in part on religious beliefs. As prominent veterinarian and author Dr. Robert M. Miller observes, many people believe "man has a right to utilize animals for his own welfare [because] the Bible says [so]."[1] Canadian laboratory animal specialist Dr. Harry Rowsell contends that "the Bible not only establishes man's dominion over animals, but urges us not to waste our resources, among which animals must be listed."[2] Laboratory animal specialist Dr. John Mulder argues that the Bible declares:

> All animals…subject to the uses and bounds established by human beings. However, sufficient instructions are provided suggesting compassionate as well as proper and humane use and care of animals. Although the Biblical position does not recognize animal rights it strongly advocates respect for animal life.[3]

People sometimes also make similar metaphysical claims (statements not directly or indirectly verifiable by experience or observation) about animals, claims that appear to be based on religious belief. One veterinarian, for example, states that animals have the right "to live their intended lives, which for some is to serve man."[4] A former AVMA President maintains that "animals are here for man to use but not abuse…Animals are here on earth to better the life of human beings which are more important in the overall than animal life."[5]

∾ THE RELIGIOUS PROBLEM

The fact that claims about ethical obligations concerning animals are sometimes based on religious belief can cause difficulties for normative veterinary ethics.

Different people can appeal to religion and reach diametrically opposing views about animals. For example, one Jewish theologian denies that God granted any rights to animals and concludes that His prohibition against cruelty to animals is based on a "concern for the moral welfare of the human agent rather than concern for the physical welfare of the animals, that is, the underlying concern is the need to purge inclinations of cruelty and to develop compassion in human beings."[6] Another Jewish scholar insists that God did give animals their own "status and rights," and that He demands "man obligate himself toward them, to consider their welfare and treat them with kindness and benevolence."[7] Among Christian thinkers, too, there is wide diversity of views about God's decrees regarding animals. These range from Cardinal Newman's statement that "(w)e have no duties toward the brute creation; there is no relation of justice between them and us…they can claim nothing at our hands; into our hands they are absolutely delivered,"[8] to the view of Anglican animal rights advocate Andrew Linzey that certain animals have moral rights because when they suffer they "share in the effects of the crucifixion of Christ and his victory over evil and negative forces."[9]

Different conclusions are sometimes reached about the very same religious texts. Two passages from Genesis play a central role in both Judaism and Christianity and are among the most frequently cited parts of the Bible relating to animals. The first chronicles the creation of animals on the fifth day:

> And God said: 'Let the earth bring forth the living creature after its kind, cattle, and creeping thing, and beast of the earth after its kind.' And it was so. And God made the beast of the earth after its kind, and the cattle after their kind, and everything that creepeth upon the ground after its kind; and God saw that it was good. And God said: 'Let us make man in our image, after our likeness; and let them have dominion over the fish of the sea, and over the fowl of the air, and over the cattle, and over all the earth, and over every creepeth thing that creepeth upon the earth.' And God created man in his own image, in the image of God created He him; male and female created He them. And God blessed them; and God said unto them: 'Be fruitful, and multiply, and replenish the earth, and subdue it; and have dominion over the fish of the sea, and over the fowl of the air, and over every living thing that creepeth upon the earth.'[10]

A second passage, in which God announced His covenant with the people and animals that would survive the flood, appears to reiterate the theme of the subservience of animals to people:

> And God blessed Noah and his sons, and said unto them: 'Be fruitful and multiply, and replenish the earth. And the fear of you and the dread of you shall be upon every beast of the earth, and upon every fowl of the air, and upon all wherewith the ground teemeth, and upon all the fishes of the sea: into your hand are they delivered. Every moving thing that liveth shall be for food for you; as the green herb have I given you all. Only flesh with the life thereof, which is the blood thereof, shall ye not eat…'
>
> And God spoke unto Noah, and to his sons with him, saying 'As for me, behold, I establish My covenant with you, and with your seed after you; and with every living creature that is with you, the fowl, the cattle, and every beast of the earth with you; of all that go out of the ark, even every beast of the earth…'[11]

Whatever else the Bible and other Jewish and Christian texts say about animals, at first glance, these passages appear to support Dr. Mulder's interpretation that animals are "subject to the uses and bounds established by human beings." There may be ample support elsewhere for Dr. Mulder's view that the Bible directs compassion toward animals. However, such a command does not emerge unequivocally from these passages, especially from God's statement to Noah that "fear of you and the dread of you shall be upon every beast of the earth." These words do not appear to call for great compassion or even high regard for animals.

However, some people see quite different messages in even these Biblical passages. William Paton, the British scientist and supporter of animal research, believes that the inclusion of the animals in God's covenant was intended to establish human "trustee-ship" over them, presumably on God's behalf.[12] An opponent of animal research draws support from the participation of animals in the covenant. Despite God's decla-ration that *animals* should fear *people* and shall be eaten by people, this writer finds in Genesis the principle that man should "do all in his power to reverence animal life."[13] Another religious advocate of animal rights also stresses God's agreement with both Noah and the animals, which in his view led the Hebrew sages to conclude that "the wall of partition between man and beast was rather thin, and the legal rights and priv-ileges of the latter must neither be neglected nor overlooked."[14] Even God's words to Noah regarding the eating of meat (which seem to be not a permission but a com-mandment) have been variously interpreted. Orthodox Judaism rejects the view that all animals "that liveth shall be for food for you," and follows instead specific directives to Moses prohibiting the eating of certain species.[15] One Christian scholar asserts that God allowed Noah and his descendants to eat meat as a concession to man's inherent sinfulness.[16] Another insists that "the diet assigned to men *and* beast by God the Creator is vegetarian."[17]

My aim in this discussion is not to attack the basing of ethical views relating to ani-mals on religious texts, nor is it to criticize any particular interpretation of even the texts quoted above. What these (and many other) differing interpretations of certain religious writings show is that any given reading of a text is likely to turn not only on the words of that text, but also on the interpreter's general theological views—some of which may come from other texts, and some from underlying religious beliefs with which the interpreter approaches texts. Indeed, there have been, within individual reli-gions themselves, sharp differences about the value of religious writings in general and the importance of certain texts in particular.

Clearly, no discussion of veterinary ethics can propose definitive interpretations of religious writings or choose among fundamental theological positions that can under-lie interpretations of these writings. Unfortunately, however, religious differences and different interpretations of religious teachings often produce differences in views about how people should treat animals. Someone who believes that God made animals to serve people may have no problem killing a pet no longer of interest to its owner. Someone who does not share this religious belief or who believes that God gave ani-mals a right to live, may reach a very different conclusion. Most veterinarians do not object to the sterilization of animals to prevent breeding, but to Orthodox Jews (including Orthodox Jewish veterinarians) this practice violates religious law. Hindus who believe eating meat to be a heinous sin will find much of food animal veterinary practice morally abhorrent.

It is extremely difficult to know what to do when people disagree on religious grounds about moral obligations concerning animals. If they are of the same religion, it may be possible for them to reach agreement about the meaning of a certain text or doctrine, but this might not always be possible. If they are of different religions, they may face the prospect of convincing each other that one of their religions is correct, and if some of them have no religious beliefs the task may be even more difficult. Even if they reach agreement about a correct course of action regarding animals, the reasons they give for their conclusions, if based on conflicting religious doctrines, might be incompatible.

❧ IS A COMPLETELY NONRELIGIOUS APPROACH POSSIBLE?

Many philosophers deal with these problems by setting them aside. They take the position that, whether there is a God or whatever God may or may not decree about moral matters, normative ethical issues can always be considered without the need to resort to religious arguments.

Different reasons have been given for the possibility of a purely secular normative ethics.

According to one approach, it cannot be the case that something is good because God wills it. Rather, God wills something *because* it is good. If things were otherwise, there would be no excellence in God's actions, for anything God willed would automatically be good. Therefore it is claimed, what is right and wrong is independent of and can be understood without reference to, God's will.[18]

In *The Case For Animal Rights*, Tom Regan provides the following argument for dispensing with appeals to a moral authority (like God) who might be the source of all right and wrong. Those of us who are not such authorities, Regan states:

> ...can have no reason for thinking that there is one unless the judgments of this supposed authority can be checked for their truth or reasonableness, and it is not possible to check for this unless what is true or reasonable can be known independently of reliance on what the supposed authority says. If, however, there must be some independent way of knowing what moral judgments are true or reasonable, the introduction of a moral authority will not succeed in providing a method for answering moral questions.[19]

These and other arguments for dispensing with religion in normative ethics cannot work against all religious attitudes about ethics. Many people believe that God's reasons are ultimately unknowable to people, who must receive them by faith.[20] Thus for many believers, it would not follow from God's choosing something because it is good that we mortals can fully understand why what is good is good. Likewise, insisting that one must have independent, nonreligious reasons for knowing whether God is right will strike many believers as inappropriate, again because they hold that people cannot fully appreciate God's ways. To refute the claim that only God knows why His ethical commandments are correct, one must engage in religious argument.

Those who maintain that ethical deliberation need never include consideration of religious claims have a special problem regarding religious beliefs about animals. Some of these beliefs go beyond mere claims about what is right and wrong in the treatment of animals. Some religious views concerning animals are claims about what animals in fact *are*. One such belief is that animals were made by God to serve human needs and desires. Another is that animals, unlike human beings, do not have immortal souls. If there is a secular, or purely empirical or scientific way of proving or disproving such claims, it is hard to imagine what it would be.

❧ ATTEMPTING A SECULAR NORMATIVE VETERINARY ETHICS

It is impossible then to engage in normative veterinary ethics and guarantee that we will never have to confront religious arguments or beliefs. This does not mean one must accept any or all religious justifications for ethical positions. But it does mean that differences in ethical views may sometimes reflect fundamental, and sometimes irreconcilable, differences in religious belief.

On the other hand, it is certainly beyond the scope of this book (or a veterinary school course in professional ethics) to engage in theological argument or to assess the validity of religious beliefs about the nature of animals and our moral obligations regarding them.

However, all might not be lost. There are several reasons nonreligious normative veterinary ethics seems possible.

First, many believers do think that what is good is independent of God's will and that moral issues can therefore be resolved without appeal to religion. The eminent rabbinical scholar J. David Bleich, for example, contends that although a Jew committed to following religious law will not look to secular ethics for guidance, secular ethics is possible:

> The Sages clearly recognized that the ethical moment of [Jewish law] consists of commandments which, 'Had they not been written, it would have been proper that they be written.' Thus [one Rabbi] states that in the absence of a revealed Torah 'we would have learned modesty from the cat, aversion to robbery from the ant, marital faithfulness from the dove, and conjugal deportment from the rooster.' Basic moral values are universal and not contingent on sectarian claims.[21]

Speaking of animal ethics Protestant theologian John B. Cobb, Jr. states that:

> Ethical questions can be discussed apart from questions relating to beliefs about God. In a time when all talk of God is problematic, this is fortunate. Broadening the scope of ethics to include serious consideration of the welfare and rights of other animals can and should be urged on its own merits.[22]

Second, people of differing religious beliefs (including those with no religious beliefs) quite often approach ethical argument with the same basic moral principles, even though these principles may have different religious (or nonreligious) sources. When this happens, religious differences can drop out—not because they are unimportant to the disputants, but because they are unnecessary to the process of discussion. Thus as Rabbi Bleich notes, the basic virtues, such as honesty, compassion, loyalty, and modesty are accepted at least in theory by almost everyone of whatever religious belief and view about the need to ground ethics in religion. Because most people start with these and other moral building blocks, and because it is these building blocks (and not specific religious commandments) on which arguments often turn, ethical discussion is usually possible.

Indeed, it may be easier for people of differing religious convictions to engage in normative *veterinary* ethics than in other kinds of ethical disputes, such as, for example, issues concerning abortion and euthanasia of terminally ill people. Most religions have a great deal to say about these fundamental issues of human life and death. But no religion provides voluminous specific guidance to those who provide medical care to animals. Thus regarding veterinary ethics, we seem forced to rely on basic moral principles that all good people may be able to accept, whatever their religious or theological persuasion.

In fact, people who have differing religious beliefs that relate directly to animals often do approach ethical issues concerning animals with the same basic general moral principles. Most people believe that although animals have less value than human beings, and can therefore often be used for legitimate human purposes, they should not be caused unnecessary pain. People who share this view can talk to each other and argue about what it requires. Yet, this same principle finds direct support in Jewish,[23] Christian,[24] and Hindu[25] doctrine. The principle can be endorsed by someone who believes that God made the animals for man's purposes as well as by someone who does not.

Many people with deeply held religious beliefs do think that normative veterinary ethics can proceed without appeal to religious doctrine. Thus Dr. Rowsell, whose Biblical interpretation is quoted previously, also offers nonreligious support for his views about the appropriate treatment of research animals. Dr. Mulder also asserts that the Biblical perspective on humane care and animal rights is "really quite rational" and "does not differ from most other current opinions."[26]

Nevertheless, anyone engaged in normative veterinary ethics must understand that differences in ethical positions may sometimes come down to fundamental differences in religious conviction. If this happens, our ability to pursue purely secular moral argument will end.

Ultimately, the best way to demonstrate that one can engage in normative veterinary ethics without appealing to religion is to do so in a way that is satisfying and helpful.

REFERENCES

[1]Miller RM: Animal welfare-yes! Humane laws-sure! Animal rights-no! *Calif Vet* 37:21, 1983.
[2]Roswell HC, McWilliam AA: The animal in research: Domination or stewardship? *Anim Reg Stud* 2:238, 1979/1980.
[3]Mulder JB: Letter. Who is right about animal rights? *Lab Anim Sci* 29:436, 1979.
[4]Marshall RT: Animal welfare, animal rights, expectations, *Calif Vet* 37:18, 1983.
[5]Rigdon CR: Interview, *Intervet* 21:14, 1985.
[6]Bleich JD: Judaism and animal experimentation. In Regan T, editor: *Animal Sacrifices*, Philadelphia, 1986, Temple University Press, p 67.
[7]Cohen NJ: *Tsa'ar Ba'ale Hayim: The Prevention of Cruelty to Animals, Its Bases, Development and Legislation in Hebrew Literature*, Jerusalem, 1976, Feldheim, p 105.
[8]Newman JH: *Sermons Preached on Various Occasions*, ed 2, quoted in Passmore J: The treatment of animals, *J Hist Ideas* 36:203, 1979.
[9]Linzey A: *Animal Rights*, London, 1976, SCM Press, p 76.
[10]Genesis 1:24-1:28: *The Holy Scriptures*, Philadelphia, 1955, The Jewish Publication Society of America, p 12.
[11]Genesis 9:1-9:10: *The Holy Scriptures*, Philadelphia, 1955, The Jewish Publication Society of America, p 12.
[12]Paton W: *Man and Mouse: Animals in Medical Research*, ed 2, 1993, Oxford, Oxford University Press, pp 253-255.
[13]Linzey A: The place of animals in creation: A Christian view. In Regan T, editor: *Animal Sacrifices*, Philadelphia, 1986, Temple University Press, p 129, quoting Phillips A: Respect for life in the Old Testament, *King's Theol Rev* Autumn 1983, p 32.
[14]Cohen NJ: *Tsa'ar Ba'ale Hayim: The Prevention of Cruelty to Animals, Its Bases, Development and Legislation in Hebrew Literature*, Jerusalem, 1976, Feldheim Publishers, p 1.
[15]Leviticus 11:1-47: *The Holy Scriptures*, Philadelphia, 1955, The Jewish Publication Society of America, pp 144-146.
[16]Baker JA: Biblical attitudes to nature. In Montefiore H editor: *Man and Nature*, London, 1975, Collins, p 96.
[17]Barth K: *Church Dogmatics*, vol 3, Part 2, Edinburgh, 1960, T and T Clark, pp 208-212, emphasis supplied; quoted in Linzey A: The place of animals in creation: A Christian view. In Regan T editor: *Animal Sacrifices*, Philadelphia, 1986, Temple University Press, p 126.
[18]For example, Plato: *Euthyphro*. In Hamilton E, Cairns H, editors: *Plato: The Collected Dialogues*, Princeton, 1961, Princeton University Press, pp 169-185.
[19]Regan T: *The Case for Animal Rights*, Berkely, 1983, University of California Press, p 126.
[20]Baillie J: *Our Knowledge of God*, New York, 1959, Scribners.
[21]Bleich JD: The *a priori* component of bioethics. In Rossner F, Bleich JD, editors: *Jewish Bioethics*, Brooklyn, 1985, Hebrew, p xix.
[22]Cobb JB: Beyond anthropocentrism in ethics and religion. In Morris RK, Fox MW, editors: *On the Fifth Day*, Washington, DC, 1978, Acropolis Books, p 148.
[23]Bleich JD: Judaism and animal experimentation. In Regan T, editor: *Animal Sacrifices*, Philadelphia, 1986, Temple University Press, pp 89-90.

24*See*, for example, Gaffney J: The relevance of animal experimentation to Roman Catholic ethical methodology. In Regan T, editor: *Animal Sacrifices*, Philadelphia, 1986, Temple University Press, pp 161-169. Even Cardinal Newman, who denied that people have direct duties to animals, believed that "we are bound not to treat them ill, for cruelty is an offense against that holy Law which our maker has written in our hearts, and is displeasing to him." Newman JH: *Sermons Preached on Various Occasions*, ed 2, quoted in Passmore J: The treatment of animals, *J Hist Ideas* 36:203, 1979.

25According to one Hindu scholar, human life "is a privilege because it is superior to the lives of animals and plants." One school of Hinduism therefore permits the medical uses of animals in science, "if and only if (1) the benefits humans receive far outweigh the pain animals endure, and (2) the use of animals is necessary (that is, the benefits are not otherwise obtainable)." Lal BK: Hindu perspectives on the use of animals in science. In Regan T, editor: *Animal Sacrifices*, Philadelphia, 1986, Temple University Press, pp 208-209.

26Mulder JB: Letter: Who is right about animal rights? *Lab Anim Sci* 29(4):436, 1979. Dr. Mulder's conclusion that the Bible does not recognize any animal rights may not follow from his statements about the text. Mulder asserts that although the Bible gives man "full authority over the animal kingdom," animals must be given "compassionate care and proper treatment," and "righteous people are admonished to show concern for the lives of their animals." As discussed in Chapter 12, such views are not necessarily incompatible with the ascription of moral rights to animals, although they need not reflect a belief in animal rights.

CHAPTER 4

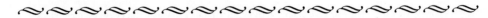

Veterinary Ethics and the Law

∾ THE DIFFERENCE BETWEEN ETHICAL AND LEGAL STANDARDS

One thing that makes ethics of great practical importance to veterinarians is the relationship between veterinary ethics and the law. A person may be able to choose (without penalty in this life at least) to ignore the dictates of any particular religion. However, we often have no such choice regarding the requirements of law. Indeed, what characterizes standards as rules of *law* is that the government can use its substantial power to force people to comply with these standards and can subject them to punishment or deprivation if they do not.

In considering how the law can affect ethical deliberation, there is an important fact one must always keep in mind: that something is required by law does not necessarily make it morally right or desirable. Laws are made by people, and they can be as morally bad as the people who make them. Therefore it is conceivable that there be situations in which the law would require veterinarians to do something, but their moral conscience will tell them something else.

Consider the following case:

Case 4-1 You practice in one of the states in which people are not permitted to own, and veterinarians are not permitted to provide routine (that is, nonemergency) veterinary care for ferrets. In your state, owning or treating a ferret is a misdemeanor, a criminal offense punishable by several months in jail or a fine. Your state's laws also prohibit ownership and treatment of skunks and raccoons.

Mrs. Jones appears in your examining room with her 6-month-old intact male pet ferret, Freddie. She purchased the animal from a pet shop in a neighboring state that permits private ownership of ferrets. She is very happy with the ferret, to which, she informs you, her 1-year-old son has already become quite attached. She asks you to give Freddie a general physical examination, to neuter him and remove his scent glands, and to make sure he gets "all the necessary vaccinations."

What should you do?

In formulating your response to this situation, you might want to consider the following facts:

- *Your state's veterinary practice act allows the veterinary licensing board to revoke or suspend the license of, or to subject to other kinds of discipline, any veterinarian who violates any of the state's laws relating to the practice of veterinary medicine.*
- *Your veterinary malpractice insurance policy contains an exclusionary clause which permits the insurance company to withhold coverage for any claim "arising out of or related to the intentional performance of a criminal act of the insured." Providing Freddie the treatment requested by Mrs. Jones is considered by the laws of your state an intentional performance of a criminal act.*

- *Although there is now an approved ferret rabies vaccine, many veterinarians are opposed to the keeping of ferrets as pets, on the grounds that they have bitten family members of owners, especially small children. Other veterinarians consider these claims overblown and believe that, when kept responsibly, ferrets are no more dangerous than dogs or cats.[1]*
- *Mrs. Jones is a good client and has over the years brought her pets to you regularly.*
  How relevant would be the following considerations to your response to the case?
- *Whether your state veterinary licensing board ignores the fact that veterinarians are treating ferrets, or has announced its intention to enforce legal restrictions on the routine treatment of these animals?*
- *Whether there are other veterinarians in your area who routinely treat ferrets and who would gladly accept Freddie as a patient and Mrs. Jones as a client?*
  Would your response to this case be different if Freddie were a raccoon? If so, why?

I have found that many practitioners and students believe this case presents a conflict between ethics and the law. Ethics, some will say, tells me to accept the ferret as a patient: I can help it and the client by doing so; I believe ferrets can make good pets if kept properly by responsible owners; and if I do not accept this patient another doctor will. I might even lose this client all together, for no good reason. At the same time, some doctors and students will say, the law forbids me to do something my conscience tells me is right.

At this point, among those who believe that ethics points toward accepting Freddie as a patient, there tend to be two different approaches. From the perceived conflict between law and ethics, some doctors and students would still decline the case. These people say that they respect the law and that the law must be obeyed. They also state that they want to make sure they follow the law's guidance in each situation they face in practice. Other doctors and students concede that they would want to take into account any potential danger to themselves that disobeying a legal prohibition, such as the one against treating ferrets, may present. However, they do not see any special or independent reason why the law should be followed: if the law is a good law it should be followed, but if it is a bad law, it should not be followed merely because it is law.

~ SHOULD ONE FOLLOW OR IGNORE THE LAW?

Both these reactions to the case—and to the relationship between ethics and the law—are simplistic. The law does not provide guidance for all situations in veterinary practice. Moreover, even when the law does dictate a particular approach and when this course of action seems morally questionable, one cannot dismiss this approach as "just the law." That the law sets forth a requirement or prohibition is itself of ethical significance.

Why One Cannot Always Follow the Law

If the dictates of the law could always be followed, people, when faced with an ethical problem, would only have to determine what the law says, and their questions would be answered. Unfortunately, this approach will not work.

The law is often ethically neutral

First, there are many situations in which the law is consistent with a number of different approaches. For example, it is perfectly legal for a veterinarian to euthanize a healthy animal no longer wanted by its owner, but it is also just as lawful to refuse to do this on ethical grounds. The law does not attempt to decide whether one should refuse on ethical grounds or what ethical grounds might or might not justify such a refusal.

Legal requirements can differ from correct normative standards.

A second reason is that sometimes the dictates of normative veterinary ethics might be morally preferable to legal standards. For example, assuming one has not held oneself out to the public as willing to accept certain kinds of cases and does not turn away a client because of racial or some other kind of legally prohibited discrimination, a veterinarian has no legal obligation to accept a patient (see Chapter 20). One can refuse to begin treating any animal simply because one does not feel like it. It seems clear, however, that it is sometimes morally wrong for a veterinarian to turn away an animal in need of care just because one feels like it. Official ethics also condemns such an attitude, at least regarding emergencies; the *Principles of Veterinary Medical Ethics* hold that "every practitioner has a moral and ethical responsibility to provide service when because of accidents or other emergencies involving animals it is necessary to save life or relieve suffering."[2]

Why One Cannot Ignore the Law

Although following the law will not always provide satisfactory guidance for approaching moral questions, it would also be wrong for veterinarians to ignore the law.

It can be morally wrong to disobey a bad law.

First, a strong argument can often be made that it is morally correct to obey a law which, in its intended application, may be a morally bad law. Violation of a particular bad law can sometimes lead to more general disregard for the law, which can, in turn, result in great harm.

POTENTIAL VIOLATION OF GOOD AS WELL AS BAD LAWS RELATING TO VETERINARY PRACTICE. In all states it is illegal for private citizens to possess and veterinarians to treat certain designated species of wildlife without permission from state government. Thus most states (including those that allow ferrets) prohibit the ownership and routine veterinary treatment of raccoons. At the time of this writing, private ownership of ferrets is prohibited in Massachusetts. Yet, many veterinarians in the state treat these animals. They argue that it makes no sense to prohibit ferrets in Massachusetts, when they are permitted just across the border in Connecticut.

Supposing only for the purpose of argument that a legal prohibition against treating ferrets is, taken by itself, unjustified, one must still consider the potential wider effects of disobeying such a law. Someone who feels justified in keeping or treating one kind of prohibited species may feel justified in judging for herself which species are appropriate to keep or treat. This may in turn result in some very bad decisions by veterinarians and clients to possess species which the law is indisputably correct in prohibiting. Thus there are already in Massachusetts (and doubtlessly in other states) veterinarians who treat not only ferrets but also skunks and raccoons and who already evidence a general disregard for the authority of the state to restrict possession of wild animals. If a general practice of keeping skunks and raccoons contributes to a rabies epidemic or results in injuries to people who do not know how dangerous these animals can be, those veterinarians who consider themselves above the law may have to share part of the blame.

WHERE WILL ILLEGALITY STOP? A number of philosophers have argued that the disobeying of even bad laws leads to a tendency to think that one is above the law, which in turn leads to wholesale violation of the law.[3] After one disobeys a particular law, one may disobey another, and yet another, until one adopts the general attitude that one always has the right to decide how to act irrespective of legal requirements. And just as an individual can begin to think and act above the law, so can larger numbers of people come to disobey the law as the attitude of deciding for themselves what laws to obey becomes commonplace. If veterinarians think they are free to decide for themselves what kinds of wild species they treat—the law be damned—will some feel comfortable about deciding for themselves whether to obey the requirements of their veterinary practice act and state licensing board? After all, if one knows better than the government what kinds of animals one can treat, mightn't one also know better than the government what kinds of surgery equipment to use in one's practice, how long to retain patient records, how to store controlled substances, and whether it is proper to dispense drugs labeled for veterinary use to one's friends or family? Thinking that one can disobey the law if one likes can become a habit. If this habit leads to the disobeying of good as well as bad laws, it can have very harmful consequences indeed.

It can be imprudent to ignore or disobey the law.

A second reason veterinarians engaged in ethical deliberation cannot ignore what the law might say about a particular issue is that it can be exceedingly imprudent to disobey the law. Disobeying the criminal law can result in a criminal prosecution, imprisonment, or fine. Disobeying the civil law can result in a malpractice or other kind of lawsuit. Disobeying either the criminal or civil law can lead to suspension or revocation of one's license to practice veterinary medicine by one's state board of registration. In short, ignoring the law can ruin one's professional and personal life. One may, of course, still decide that it is better to disobey the law. However, in light of the potential consequences of violating the law, one at least ought to know whether a certain course of action would be unlawful.

～ HOW TO WEIGH THE LAW IN ETHICAL DECISIONS

With these principles in mind, we are better equipped to respond to Case 4-1. A few general rules need to be added to structure one's thinking about the relevance of the law. The reader should also find useful the decision procedure for approaching ethical issues presented in Chapter 10.

There are, it must be emphasized, many ways in which the law can affect veterinary practice, and there are many different ethical issues involving veterinarians about which the law voices an opinion. Thus it is extremely difficult to state in general terms how much weight one should give legal standards in normative ethical deliberations. I have found it useful to ask the following questions in thinking through a problem in normative veterinary ethics that raises legal issues.

1. Is there a law that speaks to the ethical issue under consideration?

Although much of what we do in life is affected in some way by the law, quite often the law does not attempt to guide or restrict one's choices in ethical decisionmaking. For example, I have noted that the law permits a veterinarian to euthanize, or not to euthanize, a healthy animal (to attempt to change the client's mind or to take the animal and try to adopt it out, and so on). Where the law does not attempt to guide one toward a particular decision, ethical deliberation can proceed on its own without legal interference.

2. If the law does speak, does it state a permission or an imperative?

Sometimes, the law might appear to suggest a course of action that conflicts with normative ethical standards but in reality, only sets forth a permission that cannot result in legal reprisal. When this occurs, ethical deliberation can also proceed without fear of legal interference. For example, the legal principle that veterinarians may generally choose whom they shall serve states a permission and not an imperative. It says that veterinarians *may*, if they like, turn away whatever cases they wish to decline, but *need not* do so if this is their choice. On the other hand, many laws (for example, those prohibiting routine treatment of designated species of wildlife) set forth imperatives—requirements or prohibitions—the violation of which can result in criminal or civil liability.

3. If the law states an imperative, does it conflict with the requirements of normative ethics?

The fact that there is a law requiring or forbidding a veterinarian to undertake some course of action does not, of course, mean there must be a conflict between this law and the correct standards of morality. Indeed, in the great majority of cases one can expect no conflict whatsoever, and one can proceed with moral deliberation without having to balance the demands of ethics against those of the law.

4. If the law states an imperative and does conflict with the standards of normative ethics, what are the potential costs of violating the law, and how strong are the moral arguments in favor of violating the legal requirements?

Among the relevant considerations here are the likelihood that the law will be enforced, the severity of any potential punishment if it is enforced, the possible wider effects of disobeying the law whether or not it is enforced, and the strength of the moral arguments against the law. If, for example, there is a moral obligation of great importance which is opposed by a law that is never enforced and the violation of which is unlikely to have wider, bad effects, there may well be a strong argument in favor of ignoring the law.

5. Does the rationale for a law affecting a decision in veterinary practice suggest factors one should want to consider in determining the morally best course of action?

Because laws are often responses to ethical and social problems,[4] examining the purpose of a law can reveal considerations that are important to even a purely ethical discussion, considerations one might ignore had one not asked why this law exists in the first place. For example, the legal rule that veterinarians may choose who they serve expresses the ethical principle that people should generally be free to decide with whom they will enter into economic, professional, and personal relations. This is an important moral principle that must be taken into account in considering, for example, when veterinarians might be obligated to accept patients or to offer low or no cost services to needy clients.

~ EXAMPLES OF POTENTIAL CONFLICTS BETWEEN ETHICS AND THE LAW

There are many ethical issues arising in veterinary practice that compel one to ask what, if anything, the law says one should or should not do. There are also numerous circumstances in which a practitioner could argue that one should do what seems morally right, even when the law says otherwise.

The following cases present dilemmas between following the law and doing what (to some veterinarians at least) seems morally acceptable or obligatory. Do these situations affect one's approach to Case 4-1 and the general issue of whether or under what circumstances it is appropriate to do what is believed to be morally right rather than what is required by the law? All the cases should be considered. They are presented in an order and a manner to challenge one to clarify one's views about potential conflicts between legal and ethical requirements. Principles useful in approaching these cases are also developed later in this book. Here, two warnings are appropriate: (1) It is not always obvious whether a course of action that conflicts with legal requirements *is* morally acceptable; that one thinks one is acting rightly does not make it so. (2) The question whether it is morally acceptable to disobey even a bad law can also be a difficult one.

Case 4-2 A client refuses to authorize euthanasia for a terminally ill animal that is in great pain. The client insists the patient be kept alive as long as possible. You know it is unlawful to euthanize the animal without authorization but believe it is wrong to allow the patient to continue to suffer. The client probably can be convinced that the animal died on its own. Is it ethically acceptable to euthanize the animal? Is it not only ethically acceptable, but also ethically obligatory?

Case 4-3 The regulations of your state veterinary licensing board prohibit the use or dispensing of drugs after their labeled expiration date. You believe strongly that in many cases these dates are overly conservative and that no harm will be done by using certain "expired" drugs. You know that violations of state board regulations pertaining to competent practice are not only grounds for discipline by the board, but can be utilized as evidence in a lawsuit by a client if their violation has caused the patient or client injury or damage. Is it ethically acceptable for you to use a drug that is past its labeled expiration date but that you believe is still effective?

Case 4-4 A patient has died unexpectedly during surgery. You know that it is unlawful, without the owner's authorization, to perform a necropsy to determine the cause of death. The owner will never know that a necropsy has been done. You may learn something valuable from it, and it might provide information that could be useful in a potential malpractice lawsuit by the client. Must you ask for permission to do a necropsy and take the risk that the client will refuse? What should you do if you ask and the client does refuse? Is it appropriate to ask the client a question that might mean one thing to her but something else to you, such as "Shall I take care of everything, Mrs. Smith?"

Case 4-5 Veterinarians are required by law to truthfully inform clients of the availability of any procedure that ordinarily competent veterinarians would consider appropriate for a given condition. Such a procedure is chemotherapy for early stage lymphoma in cats. You have a cat with early stage lymphoma that is owned by clients of modest economic means. The procedure would cost them over $1,000, and if successful could bring the patient remission of the disease for several months, perhaps a year or more. The treatment can cause the patient uncomfortable side-

effects. Although legally obligated to inform the clients that their cat's lymphoma can be so treated, you are convinced that the patient and clients would all be better off if the animal is not given chemotherapy, but is either euthanized now or allowed to live until its quality of life deteriorates significantly. You know that the clients will opt for chemotherapy if informed of it. You know that that clients will opt for euthanasia or no treatment if you do not mention the chemotherapy alternative or greatly exaggerate the potential side effects for the patient. What should you tell the clients?

Case 4-6 You are presented with a healthy and well-behaved 1-year-old intact male Boston Terrier. The dog's owner informs you that he is moving to an apartment complex that does not accept pets. He wants you to put the dog to sleep. When you exhibit some discomfort at the request he tells you "Well, doctor, if you don't do it, I'll just let him loose on the street. It's your choice. And don't talk to me about adoption. I couldn't bear to have someone else own him." You accept the client's request and the fee for euthanasia. You know that you are now legally obligated to euthanize the dog. Your technician wants to give the dog to her sister, who lives several hundred miles away. She would provide the dog with a wonderful home, and the client would never know about it. What should you do?

∿ EFFECTS OF THE LAW ON OFFICIAL AND ADMINISTRATIVE ETHICAL STANDARDS

This chapter focuses on how the law affects normative ethical decision making, that is, the process of deciding how one ought to act. However, mention must be made here of the profound effects the law has upon official and administrative veterinary ethics.

As explained in Chapter 18, interpretations of the federal Constitution by the U.S. Supreme Court severely limit the ability of professional associations and state veterinary licensing boards to regulate advertising by practitioners. Chapters 9 and 19 discuss how laws prohibiting restraint of competition also restrict the authority of associations like the AVMA and to a lesser extent, state licensing boards to compel certain kinds of behavior. For reasons that will be explained later in detail, the legal restrictions placed on official veterinary ethics elevate the importance of normative veterinary ethics. Because veterinarians can no longer be compelled by their professional associations to engage in certain kinds of ethical conduct, it becomes even more important for them to decide individually how they ought to act. This, in turn, makes it important for veterinarians to consider legal requirements (such as those discussed in this chapter) which can affect their decisions about how they ought to act.

The relationship between the law and administrative ethics is substantially different from that between the law and official ethics. Constitutional and statutory guidelines do define and sometimes restrict the ability of administrative government bodies to dictate ethical standards for veterinarians. However, valid administrative ethical standards themselves have the force of law, because they are enforced by the government itself. Put another way, administrative ethical standards *are* the law. The importance and effect of these standards must then be factored into decision making, as must other kinds of laws, with one significant difference—veterinarians who disobey the legally enforceable administrative ethical standards of their state veterinary boards can face serious disciplinary action, including loss of their license to practice.

⮑ NORMATIVE VETERINARY ETHICS AND THE LAW: A TWO-WAY RELATIONSHIP
Legal Standards Can Affect Ethical Decisions

Ethics and the law affect each other. As we have already seen, legal standards can affect ethical decisions where veterinarians face moral issues, at least one approach to which is prohibited or required by law.

Ethical Standards Affect the Law

Ethics also affects the law. Because this is a text not in veterinary law but in veterinary ethics, how principles of normative ethics influence legal standards cannot be considered in detail. However, it is worth noting the good news which emerges from the fact that ethics influences the law—veterinarians who pay serious attention to professional ethics are well on their way to fulfilling legal requirements and are already protecting themselves against legal challenges.

Acting ethically can prevent lawsuits.

Veterinarians are rightly concerned about lawsuits charging them with malpractice or intentional wrongs. Courts and juries now award veterinary clients large sums of money. According to one report, "judgments, which once ran from $100-$1,000 in small animal practice, now go as high as $8,000 or $10,000 while awards for suits concerning horses or livestock commonly run to tens or even hundreds of thousands of dollars."[5] One lawsuit alleging a veterinarian's improper inspection of cattle for brucellosis resulted in a total payout by the AVMA Professional Liability Insurance Trust (PLIT) of $1.2 million.[6] When a practitioner's behavior has been especially bad, in many states, that practitioner may be forced to pay punitive damages, money intended not to compensate the client but to punish the veterinarian. Some courts are now willing to go beyond an animal's economic value or a client's economic losses and to consider the client's attachment to the patient in determining how much compensation clients may be awarded for veterinary malpractice on a companion animal.[7] Across the country, there are lawyers seeking to expand the grounds on which veterinarians can be sued.[8]

Between 1981 and 1983 the number of malpractice claims reported to the AVMA PLIT rose by 20%.[9] By 1985 there were approximately 6 claims annually for every 100 veterinarians.[10, 11] Between 1975 and 1985 the malpractice insurance premiums paid by large animal practitioners rose a staggering 875%, almost doubling in the last 2 years of this period alone.[12] Equine exclusive practitioners, who paid $445 for $1 million in coverage in 1985, found themselves paying $1,990 for the same coverage in 1988. By 1993 this coverage cost almost $2,200.

It would be incorrect to suppose that there is (at least at present) an uncontrollable "malpractice crisis" facing the profession. In fact, since the mid-1980s the rate of lawsuits against veterinarians appears to have stabilized,[13] and in 1994 the AVMA program announced substantial malpractice premium reductions.[14] Nevertheless, the dangers—to clients as well as veterinarians—of litigation are real. Like physicians, veterinarians may place greater emphasis upon defensive practice—more tests, written consent forms, witnesses to important conversations with clients, and attorneys to be consulted more frequently. The costs of such measures must be passed on to clients. An increasing number of animal owners may be unable to pay for veterinary services or may be forced to choose euthanasia as the only affordable alternative.

There is no doubt that a large proportion of litigation against veterinarians is attributable at least in part to the belief of some clients that their veterinarian has behaved unethically.

Thus the Tennessee Supreme Court decided to permit suits for intentional infliction of emotional distress against veterinarians who threaten to kill a pet unless the client pays the bill. The Court reached this conclusion in a case in which a client alleged that she brought her dog to the doctor after it had been hit by a car. The client claimed that she told the doctor she could not pay his $155 bill in full but was refused permission to pay in installments. According to the client, she was tormented by repeated telephone calls threatening that the hospital would "do away with" the dog as the doctor saw fit unless the bill was paid "in cash and in full." The Court agreed with the client that such conduct (if the client could prove it occurred) would have been "outrageous and extreme and is not tolerable in a civilized society."[15] In another case, a New York judge departed from precedent and awarded a client money for her emotional distress. The veterinarian had promised to deliver the body of her beloved dog to a pet cemetery for burial, but when the client and her sister arrived for the funeral, they found in the casket a dead cat.[16] It was the case of a dog severely burnt after being left on a heating pad, in the Court's words, "for a day and the better part of a second day with an absence of care or attention," in which a Florida court declared that veterinary clients can collect damages for their emotional distress where their animals are injured by negligence amounting to "great indifference."[17]

Heinous or grossly unethical behavior on the part of veterinarians is surely rare. However, it only takes one legal case—one outraged jury, judge, or appellate court—to break new legal ground and subject the entire profession to dramatically increased liability. Attorneys tell me that many clients who sue their veterinarians for malpractice are not bothered primarily by alleged incompetence. Rather, they feel more aggrieved by a fee perceived to be excessive, a doctor's failure to understand the importance they attach to an animal, or being treated like children who are incapable of making important decisions for themselves. Some observers believe that such criticisms of veterinarians are not uncommon.[18]

The medical profession understands the dangers of insensitivity to ethics. Its recent recurring malpractice crises cannot be explained by sudden outbreaks of physician incompetence, or by "lawyer greed." Attorneys do not prosecute lawsuits unless their clients want them to do so. Many people who years earlier would not have dreamed of suing a physician began to take their complaints to court, because they believed that they were being treated arrogantly, uncaringly, and unfairly. Today ethics has been brought into the medical school curriculum, hospital setting, and medical policy discussions—not only as a matter of morality, but also as a matter of self-protection. Veterinarians also may find that the most effective defense against litigation from clients and government is greater attention to ethics.

Legal requirements often mirror ethical standards.

For reasons I have explained in detail elsewhere,[4] studying and being sensitive to ethical standards can be an extremely effective tool to assure that one fulfills one's legal obligations. Many of the legal rules that courts, legislatures, and regulatory agencies have fashioned for veterinarians are motivated by fundamental ethical principles. Veterinarians who conduct themselves in ways that reflect acceptance of these principles will often find that they are following the law.

For example, as discussed in Chapters 7 and 18, veterinarians are prohibited by state practice acts and licensing boards from engaging in false, deceptive, or misleading advertising. Practitioners ought to know that this is the law. But if they operate with some very basic ethical principles that presuppose no knowledge of the law whatsoever—such as honesty and respect for clients—they *already* know that they should not tell falsehoods or attempt to deceive or mislead. Veterinarians are also required by many state licensing boards and principles of the law of contracts to respect the confidences of clients. But if they operate with some very basic ethical principles—such as honesty, respect for clients, and loyalty to clients—they *already* know that they should respect client confidences. Veterinarians are required to obtain an informed consent from a client before undertaking a procedure. But if they operate with some very basic ethical principles—such as respect and loyalty for clients, and compassion and sympathy toward patients—they know this *already*. Indeed, the most important legal principle of veterinary jurisprudence—the requirement that every doctor perform like any ordinarily competent, reasonable, and prudent veterinarian—follows from the basic *ethical* judgment of the law that animal owners are entitled to no less.

⟶ LEARNING ABOUT THE LAW

Although ethics is often a good guide to the law, it is sometimes necessary for veterinarians who face ethical issues to become familiar with legal principles affecting these issues. Some doctors may find this to be one too many burdens to bear and may be tempted to forsake the study of veterinary ethics. However, the law applies to veterinarians' professional activities whether they take veterinary ethics seriously. Therefore learning about the law is not an additional task imposed by ethics.

Knowing more precisely what the law says and how the law actually works (which are not always the same) can be important in approaching ethical problems. For example, in Case 4-6 one could consider what might actually happen if the client discovers the dog has not been euthanized. Is one's state licensing board likely to take disciplinary action, or a *severe* disciplinary action, in this case? Is the client likely to engage the services of a lawyer and sue for breach of contract or an intentional wrong if he learns that his dog was not killed as requested? If he can only recover the actual economic damage (the fee paid for euthanasia), a lawsuit will not be worth the time and legal fees. If this is a state that allows the awarding of punitive damages (money awarded not to compensate the plaintiff for actual loss but to punish the defendant), will the client be able to convince a jury that a veterinarian who ignored an agreement to kill a healthy (and adorable) Boston Terrier did something terrible that justifies punishment?

It is beyond the scope of this book to describe all laws relevant to veterinary ethics. As ethical issues are raised, certain laws important to the consideration of these issues will be discussed. Among the kinds of laws relevant to normative veterinary ethics are the following: (1) statutes enacted by federal and state legislatures (for example, the federal Animal Welfare Act and state cruelty to animals statutes); (2) general rules or particular determinations made by regulatory bodies (for example, the Animal and Plant Health Inspection Service of the U. S. Department of Agriculture and state veterinary licensing boards); and (3) common law principles of legal precedent developed by courts (for example, the rule that veterinarians are free to choose whom they shall serve).

REFERENCES

[1] *See,* Fur flies over ferret issue, *J Am Vet Med Assoc* 193:1028-1031, 1988.

[2] American Veterinary Medical Association: *Principles of Veterinary Medical Ethics,* 1993 Revision, "Emergency Service," *1994 AVMA Directory,* Schaumburg, IL, The Association, p 44.

[3] Plato: *Crito.* In Hamilton E, Cairns H, editors: Plato: *The Collected Dialogues,* Princeton, NJ, 1961, Princeton University Press, pp 27-39.

[4] Tannenbaum J: Ethics: The why and wherefore of veterinary law, *Vet Clin N Am: Sm Anim Pract* 23:921-935, 1993.

[5] Benson M: Malpractice suits on the rise, *DVM* 16(10):24, 1985.

[6] Dinsmore JR: Anatomy of AVMA's largest insurance malpractice claim, *J Am Vet Med Assoc* 188:26-27, 1986.

[7] *Jankoski v. Preiser Animal Hospital,* 510 N.E.2d 1084 (Ill. App. 1st Dist. 1987).

[8] Benson M: East Coast malpractice attorney rebuffs "quick buck" theory, *DVM* 16(10):30, 1985.

[9] Williams L: Malpractice suits escalating, *DVM* 14(10):1, 1983.

[10] Insurance note, *J Am Vet Med Assoc* 189:642, 1986 (reporting 7.01 claims per 100 participants in the AVMA insurance program in 1983, 6.03 per 100 in 1984, and 6.02 in 1985).

[11] Katz K: Letter dated March, 1988 to recent veterinary school graduates on behalf of the AVMA Professional Liability Insurance Trust (indicating a rate of 5.79 claims per 100 participants in 1987).

[12] 1985 AVMA activities summary, *J Am Vet Med Assoc* 188:347, 1986.

[13] Verdon D: Malpractice suits down; "threat" builds for DVMs, *DVM* 22(12):1, 1991 (reporting that 1 out of 16 veterinarians is sued each year).

[14] American Veterinary Medical Association: Trust chairman announces liability premium reductions, *AVMA Convention News,* San Francisco, July 10-11, 1994, The Association, pp 1-2 (announcing a $729 annual premium reduction for equine practitioners and average annual reductions of 23.7% for large animal practitioners, 18.1% for mixed animal practitioners, and 13.4% for small animal practitioners).

[15] *Lawrence v. Stanford,* 665 S.W.2d 927 (Tenn. 1983).

[16] *Corso v. Crawford Dog and Cat Hospital, Inc.,* 97 Misc.2d 530 (Civ. Ct., Queens Cty. 1979)(awarding plaintiff $700).

[17] *Knowles Animal Hospital, Inc. v. Wills,* 360 So.2d 37 (Fla. 3d DCA 1987)(holding the professional corporation, but not the practitioner-owner, liable for $1,000 compensatory and $12,000 punitive damages).

[18] Caras R: Public viewpoint of veterinary medicine, *J Vet Med Educ* 9:110-112, 1983.

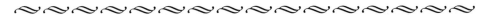

CHAPTER 5

Veterinary Ethics and Moral Theory

O ne remaining topic must be considered before the branches of veterinary ethics can be discussed in detail. This chapter examines several concepts and principles of philosophical moral theory essential to veterinary ethics.

Moral theory is a challenging field of study with its own professional practitioners, long history, specialized vocabulary, and competing points of view. This book cannot discuss all topics in moral theory relevant to veterinary ethics. Veterinarians need not (thank goodness!) become philosophers before they can study professional ethics. There is, however, much in moral philosophy of importance to veterinary medicine.

～ THREE APPROACHES TO NORMATIVE ETHICS

The history of ethics reveals many different kinds of ethical theories. However, there are three approaches to understanding how people ought to live and act that students of veterinary ethics will find useful to distinguish. These approaches are not mutually exclusive. Indeed, as shall become apparent, elements of each will play a role in any satisfactory account of descriptive, official, administrative, and normative veterinary ethics.

Virtue-oriented Ethical Theories

One approach to ethics concentrates on examining and promoting the moral virtues. A virtue is a personal character trait or disposition that manifests itself over a wide range of situations and that can be said to contribute to, or indeed be part of what is meant by, a good and moral life. Among the character traits that have been explored by virtue-oriented ethicists (who include the great philosophers Socrates and Aristotle) are honesty, kindness, generosity, courage, loyalty, modesty, moderation, compassion, and fairness.

A virtue-oriented approach to morality does not reject actions as irrelevant. Indeed, one could not speak of the virtues (or their opposite, the vices) apart from actions. One could not, for example, say that people are courageous unless, when faced with certain kinds of challenges, they act in certain ways. However, virtue-oriented theories are suspicious of attempts to formulate a set of rules or recipes for how people ought to behave in particular situations. People will only act well, according to virtue-based theories, if they *already* have those dispositions of character that are good and can be counted on over the long haul to motivate proper behavior. Virtue-oriented ethical approaches characteristically place a great deal of emphasis on education. They attempt to inculcate attitudes, feelings, and states of mind central to the virtuous dispositions.

Action-oriented Ethical Theories

In contrast, action-oriented ethical theories are less concerned about how we should be than about how we should act. While virtue-oriented approaches focus upon what it is to live a good and decent life, action-oriented theories ask what people ought to *do*. They tend to search for rules that can be applied to particular moral problems to determine the correct course of behavior. Action-oriented ethical theories tend to stress the concepts of duty and obligation.

Value-based Ethics

Some ethical theories propose basic values or "goods"—benefits, states of affairs, or ways of being that are valuable and to be sought after. Such goods can relate to individuals; the liberty to pursue one's goals is such a personal good. Fundamental values can also relate to groups of persons; the fair distribution of wealth is often proposed as an intrinsically valuable state of affairs pertaining to many people. Ethical theories in which discussion of goods are fundamental can vary widely. However, such theories tend to seek a hierarchy of goods, or a procedure for identifying and deciding among goods, that can be used to guide character and action. Goods proposed by value-oriented approaches are very general and relate to the most central aspects of life. One prominent philosopher, for example, bases a theory of justice on the free choice of "personal goods," which he characterizes as things people require for "the successful execution of a rational plan of life." Among these goods, he argues, are "liberty and opportunity, income and wealth, and above all self-respect."[1]

~ THE IMPORTANCE OF VIRTUES, ACTIONS, AND VALUES

Any satisfactory approach to normative veterinary ethics must give attention to virtues, actions, and values. For example, such virtues as honesty and compassion are clearly important in a veterinarian. Yet there are times when these virtues can lead to conflicting tendencies and when a practitioner will need a way of deciding between them. Thus it may be honest to tell a client who wants to know about his animal's prognosis the complete and unvarnished truth, but compassion may suggest giving a less truthful and less upsetting account. Here, it would seem, one needs some kind of rule for action to resolve the conflict or perhaps a theory of values that would suggest a proper approach. Likewise, views about the moral duties of veterinarians in certain kinds of situations will sometimes turn on very general principles concerning the value of animals and their value relative to humans.

~ ACTION-ORIENTED THEORIES: UTILITARIAN AND DEONTOLOGICAL

Philosophers distinguish between two fundamental kinds of action-oriented ethical theories: utilitarian and deontological.

Utilitarian (sometimes called "teleological" or "consequentialist") theories look to the consequences of actions or kinds of actions to determine whether they are right or wrong. These theories begin with a conception of what is good in itself and maintain that actions are right insofar, and only insofar, as they will in the future produce this good. Utilitarianism, although best viewed as an action-oriented theory, is in an important respect also a value-based approach. Utilitarianism postulates only one good (which utilitarians call "utility"), the more of which exists the better. Utilitarianism therefore concludes that people should maximize this good.

There have been a variety of utilitarian approaches based on different views of the "good" people ought to maximize. For some utilitarians, utility consists of pleasure in the sense of a primal feeling of contentment. Other utilitarians maintain that certain pleasures are better than others and that such "higher" pleasure is the good people should seek. Some utilitarians identify utility with happiness and others with the satisfaction of preferences. But for all utilitarians, it is the total quantity of this unitary good (however conceived) that determines one's moral obligations. Thus according to one prominent utilitarian, "the only reason for performing an action A rather than an alternative B is that doing A will make mankind (or, perhaps, all sentient beings) happier than will doing B."[2] In other words, a utilitarian asks us to sum up the consequences of each alternative act (or if the utilitarian is what is called a "rule-utilitarian," of each alternative general rule for behavior) and to choose that which, on balance, will produce no less good than any other.[3]

Deontological ethical theories, in contrast, maintain that there are some moral obligations which are independent of how much good (however defined) will be produced in the future. Deontologists can recognize that how much good one might produce is sometimes relevant to how one ought to act. However, a deontologist denies that future consequences are the *only* source of moral duties. As with utilitarianism, there have been many varieties of deontological approaches. Some deontologists, like the eighteenth century German philosopher Immanuel Kant, attempt to derive all moral obligation from a single principle or rule.[4] Others advocate a number of fundamental moral principles, (such as the duty to tell the truth and the duty to help others) each of which is generally obligatory but can be overridden in particular circumstances by one of its fellow fundamental principles.[5]

Protestant theologian Joseph Fletcher provides a famous example illustrating the difference between utilitarianism and deontology. He asks us to imagine that one has come upon a burning building, in which there are two people. The first is one's father. The second is "a medical genius who has discovered a cure for a common fatal disease."[6] One can rescue either the genius or the parent, but not both. Whom should one save?

For a utilitarian like Fletcher, who demands that we ask which of the alternatives would produce, on balance, the greatest good for the greatest number, the answer is obvious—the genius should be rescued. A deontologist, however, might maintain that there is a strong obligation to save one's parent in virtue of one's distinctive relationship with that person in the past—an obligation which must also be taken into account and exists independently of considerations of utility.

As will be seen when the subject of animal rights is considered (see Chapter 12), it is impossible to explore a number of major issues in veterinary ethics without understanding the difference between utilitarian and deontological approaches to these issues. Moreover, there are questions in veterinary ethics with solutions that depend in large measure on a utilitarian comparison of likely costs and benefits resulting from alternative actions. However, the overwhelming majority of people reject utilitarianism (even if they have never heard the term). Most people believe, for example, that promises generally ought to be kept not because or not only because doing so will cause more happiness than unhappiness, but because someone who makes a promise has *already* thereby obligated herself to keep it. Most people believe that it is generally wrong to lie, not because lying may create distrust and unhappiness in the future, but because there is something fundamentally disrespectful and dishonorable in telling falsehoods.

~ IDEALS AND FAILINGS

Utilitarians who seek to maximize good consequences also reject another notion most people find self-evident. To utilitarians, every alternative in every situation is either obligatory (if it produces no less utility than any other alternative) or prohibited (if it does not).

Most people, however, believe some actions are morally valuable and ought to be encouraged but are not obligatory. Failure to do them means that one has not acted as well as one might, but not that one has acted wrongly. For example, many people consider giving to charity when they do not have much money to spare a morally desirable thing to do but would not say that someone who fails to give under these circumstances has acted wrongly. Philosophers call such nonobligatory but desirable acts "supererogatory," a term that means "above and beyond the call of duty."

Just as most of us believe that there are supererogatory actions, we also believe that there are ways of behaving that are morally undesirable but at the same time cannot be said to be prohibited. Many would argue, for example, that people who abuse themselves with drugs are behaving in a morally unseemly and undesirable manner but are not morally prohibited from doing this so long as they harm only themselves.

Nonobligatory moral ideals and nonprohibited moral failings have played a major role in veterinary codes of ethics, as they have in the ethical codes of other professions. It has been a large part of official professional ethics to urge but not require adherence to certain ideals and to discourage but not prohibit the commission of certain disapproved actions.

~ ARE MORAL STANDARDS OBJECTIVELY RIGHT OR WRONG?

Sooner or later, in any discussion of ethics among veterinary students or practitioners, someone will voice the opinion that moral claims are really not objectively right or wrong but only express the personal preferences of those who make them. This opinion may take the form of what some philosophers call ethical skepticism, the view that no moral claim can be right or wrong. Or the troublemaker may be an adherent of ethical relativism, the view that each person's (or each society's) ethical opinions are as right and correct as any other.

Some veterinarians like others with scientific backgrounds are attracted to skepticism or relativism. Scientists are trained to demand that statements and theories be tested by empirical observation. And there can be no doubt that while one can, for example, determine with one's eyes whether a given disease involves certain physiological processes, there is nothing out there in the observable world that can be held up next to a moral claim to verify whether it is true or false. No photograph or videotape of an assault upon an elderly person itself demonstrates that such an action is wrong. The claim that such behavior is wrong is a proposition not about how the world *is* but how it *ought* to be.

If right and wrong were merely a matter of personal preference, then descriptive, administrative, and official veterinary ethics would still be possible—but highly unsatisfying. One need not believe in objective moral truth to discover what veterinarians actually believe is right and wrong or what moral views administrative bodies and professional veterinary associations impose on practitioners. However, most veterinarians want their actual moral attitudes to be morally correct. Most veterinarians think that the purpose of having administrative and official ethical standards is to encourage professional behavior that is really ethical, not just behavior that happens to fit the preferences of government administrators or professional associations. If skepticism or relativism were correct, normative veterinary ethics would be impossible, because there would be no objectively correct moral standards to discover.

The overwhelming majority of people reject skepticism and relativism. We believe that moral claims can indeed be right or wrong. It is, however, beyond the scope of this book to attempt a philosophical refutation of skepticism and relativism. Moreover, in my discussions with veterinary students and practitioners who do express these views, I have found almost invariably that any such refutation is unnecessary.

It has proven just as effective to point out that skepticism and relativism are abstract notions about the nature of ethics, not only which tend to be voiced in hypothetical discussions but also which virtually no one accepts in everyday life. When professed relativists for example, are confronted with a real challenge to their moral values, such as a burglary of their home or the mugging of an elderly relative, they will almost certainly protest that such actions are wrong and immoral. Relativists will not insist that the burglar or mugger is also right and that anyone who thinks otherwise, (including themselves) is just expressing a personal preference, which is as good as any other personal preference. Even in classroom discussions about hypothetical cases, skeptics or relativists soon find themselves talking like the rest of us. They insist that certain things are right and wrong. They do not claim that these things are right (for them) because they happen to prefer them but will ask others to prefer them *because* these things are right.

〜 DECIDING ISSUES IN NORMATIVE VETERINARY ETHICS

Granting that moral preferences and opinions can be correct or incorrect, how does one determine the correct approaches to moral issues in normative veterinary ethics?

This is the central question of normative veterinary ethics. It is also a question that cannot possibly be answered at the beginning of an exploration of veterinary ethics. Indeed, if normative veterinary ethics proves as complex and challenging as medical ethics, one might never have a complete answer, because there will always be new issues to resolve and new insights to attain.

Chapter 10 proposes a decision-making process for normative veterinary ethics structured around the interests of the three central protagonists in veterinary medicine: patients, clients, and veterinarians. This proposed structure is not intended to be a set of substantive ethical principles. It is a device, which together with the discussion of fundamental concepts in Part Two of this book, can be used to navigate through the often complex waters of normative veterinary ethics. The development of substantive normative standards for veterinarians and others who participate in providing medical care to animals is in its infancy. Stimulating such development is a major purpose of this book. However, even at this early point, several demands of any acceptable substantive approach to normative veterinary ethics can be reasonably made.

There must first be an interplay between our moral intuitions—on reflection, what people think is right or wrong about a particular alternative or moral position—and more general principles that can be used to justify and correct such intuitions. Mere intuitions are not enough. If all one could say is that some view is right because one feels that it is, there will be no objective standard or reasoning that can be measured against an intuition to justify it or to judge that it is correct or incorrect. This is why one is unhappy with the child who, when asked to explain the rock he just tossed through a neighbor's window, answers "Because!" One wants to know *why*; one wants a reason or justification.

On the other hand, general rules, principles, and theories must sometimes be tested against basic moral experiences and intuitions. Just as one would reject a scientific theory that implies the Earth is flat, because we all know it is not flat, so would one reject a moral theory that offends one's most basic views about right and wrong. This is why utilitarianism, which is intended as a general and complete theory to guide all our moral actions, is accepted by very few people; its recommendations contradict too many moral intuitions people know must be correct.

Recognizing this essential interplay between moral experience and moral theories, biomedical ethicists Tom L. Beauchamp and James F. Childress suggest five tests for judging whether approaches to determining correct moral behavior and attitude are acceptable. First, a proposed approach must be as clear as possible so that one can understand what it says and how it is supposed to be applied. Second, it should be internally consistent and coherent. Third, it should be as comprehensive as possible and should leave no major gaps or holes. Fourth, it should be as simple as possible; like a good scientific theory, it should have no more principles than necessary, and people should be able to apply it without confusion. Finally, a theory or general approach must be able to account for the whole range of moral experience, building on commonly accepted principles but also criticizing ordinary beliefs when this is appropriate. "A good theory consolidates and accounts for its data but need not mirror ordinary judgments; indeed, it should have the power to criticize defective judgments, no matter how widely accepted."[7]

These tests do not attempt to determine what is right and wrong in ethics generally or in normative veterinary ethics in particular. Moreover, at present, normative veterinary ethics is very far from anything like a general approach that can systematize all issues. However, the five tests are useful in reminding us that normative veterinary ethics should at least attempt to bring order to the moral issues facing veterinarians and must find reasoned arguments for ethical recommendations.

REFERENCES

[1]Rawls J: *A Theory of Justice*, Cambridge, MA, 1971, Harvard University Press, p 433.

[2]Smart JJC: *An Outline of a System of Utilitarian Ethics*. Reprinted in Smart JJC, Williams B: *Utilitarianism, For and Against*, Cambridge, UK, 1987, Cambridge University Press, p 30.

[3]The view that people should always choose an action that will produce no less good than any alternative is called "act-utilitarianism." Rule-utilitarianism has been proposed to avoid some of the counter-intuitive results of act-utilitarianism. For example, act-utilitarianism requires that people break any individual promise if doing so would produce more utility (pleasure, happiness, etc.) than would keeping it—an implication many people find unacceptable. A rule-utilitarian, however, can urge people to keep an individual promise even though breaking it would produce more good on the grounds that a following *general rule* requiring people to keep promises would produce more good than following a rule permitting people to break promises. Rule-utilitarianism is controversial. Some act-utilitarians claim it is incoherent; they point out that although rule-utilitarians advocate their the-

ory, because they are supposedly concerned with promoting good, at the same time, they settle for an approach that does not maximize good. See Smart JJC: *An Outline of a System of Utilitarian Ethics.* Reprinted in Smart JJC, Williams B: *Utilitarianism, For and Against,* Cambridge, UK, 1987, Cambridge University Press, p 5.

[4]According to Kant's famous "categorical imperative," one must always ask whether a proposed alternative is "universalizable," whether everyone could will the same principle. Thus for Kant, one must keep one's promises because "the universality of a law that everyone believing himself to be in need can make any promise he pleases with the intention of not keeping it would make promising, and the very purpose of promising, itself impossible, since no one would believe he was being promised anything, but would laugh at utterances of this kind as empty shams." Kant I: *Groundwork of the Metaphysic of Morals,* Paton HJ, translator: New York, 1964, Harper, Row, p 90. Kant's position is not utilitarian. His objection to the breaking of promises is not that it would lead to unhappiness but that it is inherently incoherent.

[5]*See,* for example, Ross WD: *The Right and the Good,* Oxford, 1930, Clarendon Press, p 21.

[6]Fletcher J: *Situation Ethics,* Philadelphia, 1966, Westminster Press, p 115.

[7]Beauchamp TL, Childress JF: *Principles of Biomedical Ethics,* ed 3, New York, 1989, Oxford University Press, pp 14-15.

CHAPTER 6

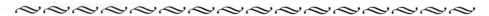

Descriptive Veterinary Ethics
Mapping the Profession's Moral Values

∾ EMPIRICAL AND INTROSPECTIVE DESCRIPTIVE VETERINARY ETHICS

Descriptive veterinary ethics is the study of the actual ethical views of veterinarians and veterinary students regarding professional behavior and attitudes.

One might be tempted to think that descriptive veterinary ethics should be considered a branch of social science. Thus conceived, descriptive ethics would base its conclusions about the attitudes of the profession on techniques used by social scientists, such as questionnaires presented to large numbers of persons or statistical analysis of reactions to hypothetical situations designed to elicit peoples' ethical attitudes.

There is, however, another way of approaching the examination of actual professional moral attitudes that is quite different from, and at least as valuable as, conducting scientific studies. Descriptive veterinary ethics can consist of an individual doctor or student seeking to understand his or her own professional moral values. Such an enterprise cannot proceed by empirical surveys or statistical analysis. It involves a process of *self-understanding* and evaluation. This kind of inquiry may sometimes involve asking the same questions a social scientist would put to large numbers of people. However, someone engaged in introspective understanding of his or her own professional moral values will often ask different questions from those raised by someone doing empirical research and will typically ask these questions for different reasons.

I shall call the scientific study of the professional moral attitudes of veterinarians (as well as those training to become veterinarians) *empirical descriptive veterinary ethics*. I shall call the personal description by any such person of his or her own professional moral values *introspective descriptive veterinary ethics*.

∾ GENERAL AND SPECIFIC ETHICAL ATTITUDES

Whether one is attempting to understand the ethical attitudes of oneself or of the profession, one must have a way of classifying or categorizing such attitudes.

Ethical attitudes can be classified according to their degree of generality or specificity. Some attitudes are extremely general as is; for example, the statement of the *Principles of Veterinary Medical Ethics* that "the responsibilities of the veterinary profession extend not only to the patient but also to society."[1] Very general attitudes can lie behind a wide range of different professional activities. Thus veterinarians who inspect meat, conduct spay and neuter clinics for local humane societies, or participate in biomedical research can all say legitimately that they are motivated at least in part by the desire to render service to society.

Ethical attitudes can also be extremely specific and assert detailed answers to very focused questions. An example of such an attitude is the statement of the *Principles* that it is "unethical and unprofessional for veterinarians to promote, sell, prescribe, or use any product the ingredient formula of which has not been revealed to them."[2]

Between general abstract ethical principles and very specific ethical opinions, there is a wide range of possible degrees of specificity.

Those engaged in empirical or introspective descriptive veterinary ethics must be careful to include in their descriptions a proper mix of general and specific attitudes. A useful account of professional attitudes cannot consist only of statements of very specific attitudes. Veterinarians face many situations about which they have specific moral views; a list of all such opinions (of a single practitioner much less of the entire profession) would be endless. Moreover, specific ethical attitudes are often generated by more general values that apply across a range of situations. It might not be inaccurate to say that Dr. Jones believes it is wrong to sell pet toys and that she believes it is wrong to run newspaper advertisements containing coupons entitling clients to discounted fees. However, both these ethical beliefs might better be seen as flowing from a more general view about what is appropriate behavior for a member of a healing profession (see Chapters 16 and 17).

On the other hand, one must also beware of classifying ethical attitudes in too general a manner. General attitudes can be consistent with quite different (and sometimes hostile) points of view. For example, two practitioners might agree that veterinarians should not be "overly competitive," but might disagree about whether operating low-overhead mobile clinics is being overly competitive. Likewise, we would not say enough about the ethical values of two veterinarians simply by describing both as devoted to rendering "service to society," if for one, such service means earning less than he might earn in private practice by working for the state public health department while for the other it means spending free time at local schools and community organizations speaking about pet care.

Because they can be so vague and often sound quite wonderful, very general statements of ethical values can also lull people into not thinking carefully about ethical issues and into not looking objectively at their own attitudes. Some of my students assert that a major attitude in their value system is a "love for animals." Yet many of these students support the euthanasia of stray animals in shelters, the culling of healthy but unproductive farm animals, and the use of animals in research. I am not saying that doing such things to animals is wrong, only that these practices do not reflect a blanket "love" for all animals. Professing a general "love for animals" may make one feel good. But it can also lead (especially in moments of warm-hearted exuberance about one's "love for animals") to a misunderstanding about one's real attitudes by obscuring the fact that one really does not believe all animals are entitled to protection and care properly described as love.

⁓ CENTRAL AND PERIPHERAL ETHICAL VALUES

Any useful description of one's own or of the profession's ethical attitudes must also recognize that some attitudes and values are more central—they are held more strongly and insisted on more firmly—than others.

Some attitudes are so central to a profession that they define that profession, in the sense that if these attitudes were abandoned, we would say it would be a different profession. For example, if the legal profession abandoned its deeply held view that it is right to try to convince judges and juries by argument and began using the old custom of trial by drowning (in which someone won a dispute if he survived being tied up and thrown into water), we would say that the legal profession as currently defined would have disappeared.

Other ethical attitudes, on the other hand, are less central to a profession. Thus some lawyers see criminals that they defend as victims of society, while other lawyers prosecute these same people believing that they are evil and ought to be punished. There are lawyers who like to sue big corporations because they view such businesses as greedy and immoral, while other lawyers are happy to represent them. All these (and many more) different ethical attitudes can be encompassed within the profession of law. Moreover, part of what differentiates, for example, a corporate lawyer from a public prosecutor is how they rank their values; for the latter, earning money is likely to be less important than service to society.

Like lawyers, veterinarians have some ethical attitudes that are more central and others that are less central to their profession. Like law, veterinary medicine contains within it subgroups and individual practitioners who rank certain values differently. It is surely impossible to be a *veterinarian* and not think it is important to protect patients from unnecessary suffering. On the other hand, some veterinarians and groups of veterinarians can have different ethical views and still remain within the profession. Veterinarians disagree about, for example, whether animals should be used to test cosmetics, whether it is ethical to crop dogs' ears or dock their tails so that they can meet breed standards, or whether it is morally appropriate to treat individual wild animals that are not members of endangered or threatened species.

∾ SELF- AND OTHER-REGARDING VALUES

Some philosophers maintain that ethics or morality relates only to behavior toward others. These philosophers assert that values or attitudes that pertain primarily to oneself (such as the value one places on art, contemplation, or research) are essentially esthetic or intellectual in nature and are not the concern of ethics. This distinction between the ethical and the personal or esthetic has been criticized by other philosophers who subscribe to the view that ethics must concern itself with the good life.[3] They argue that living the good life includes not only behaving well toward others but also behaving well toward oneself—acquiring knowledge about the world, enjoying art and music, appreciating nature, and so on. Therefore, these philosophers insist, ethics must consider values that relate to one's personality and personal lifestyle as well as to one's obligations toward others.

Whatever conclusion philosophers may reach about including self-regarding values in the study of ethics, descriptive veterinary ethics must concern itself with such values. Part of the purpose of descriptive veterinary ethics is to help practitioners appreciate what really underlies value judgments that they make in their professional lives so that they can understand what value issues are important to them and their profession and what solutions to these issues may be realistic. It is clear that personal attitudes do play an important role in the value judgments of many veterinarians. Some bovine practitioners, for example, tell me that they receive intense personal satisfaction from working outdoors with large animals, associating with farmers, and participating in a rural and agricultural lifestyle, and that these things are more important to them than a high standard of living. It is impossible to fully understand the value judgments such veterinarians make about how they ought to deal with clients and patients without understanding that they have these personal attitudes.

～ MAPPING THE VALUES OF VETERINARIANS

Descriptive veterinary ethics is in its infancy. Therefore any suggested way of studying the ethical attitudes of veterinarians will require revision and modification as we learn more about how to describe these attitudes.

Table 6-1 offers a schematic for describing the ethical values of practitioners and students. The table distinguishes several very general attitudes and several subcategories within these attitudes. For example, there are what can be called "self-oriented" attitudes of veterinarians and "society-oriented" attitudes. A doctor for whom self-oriented values are of great importance may choose a career in private practice, while another for whom society-oriented values are important may join government service. A veterinarian for whom profession-oriented values are important may become active in his state veterinary association; another, for whom scientific research is a consuming interest, may have little to do with other veterinarians. For one doctor, private practice may be the only possible vocation because he wants to help individual animals (a "patient-oriented" value); another may choose private practice because he wants to assist clients in achieving their desires regarding their animals (a "client-oriented" value). One veterinarian may be less interested in animals in the hospital or clinic setting than in promoting the welfare of animals in general (an "animal-oriented" value); while another may be engaged in the public health area protecting people from animal-transmitted diseases (a "society-oriented" value).

Within a general kind of value, there can be different and sometimes conflicting values. Among veterinarians legitimately described as patient-oriented, some may see the alleviation and prevention of animal suffering as an overriding goal and will have no problem with the slaughter of animals for food provided they do not suffer; other veterinarians may object to the termination of an animal's life for any reason other than benefiting that animal.

Many of the general and more specific values distinguished in Table 6-1 need not conflict with each other, may exist comfortably within the value structure of an individual practitioner, and indeed can be intimately connected. Thus a veterinarian may build a prosperous practice and join her state veterinary association, motivated to do both by an interest in monetary gain and a desire to be recognized as a valued member of the community. A veterinarian engaged in research may be committed to helping people as well as animals and may believe that the acquisition of knowledge about biological processes is valuable in its own right.

～ A DIVERSE PROFESSION

Doubtless many further subdivisions and refinements of the values listed in Table 6-1 are possible. However, the table and this brief discussion illustrate that veterinary medicine is an extraordinarily diverse profession, not only in terms of what its members

TABLE 6-1

Selected values in veterinary medicine

SELF-ORIENTED	ANIMAL-ORIENTED
• Monetary gain	• Protection of animal interests in general
• Personal satisfactions	• Protection of certain species/kinds of animals
• working outdoors	• Compassion for animals
• working indoors	**PROFESSION-ORIENTED**
• interacting with pet owners	• Enjoyment of professional associations/activities
• competitive lifestyle	• Protection of profession from external challenges
• participation in running a profitable practice	• Education of future professionals
• freedom from pressures of running a profitable	
practice	**KNOWLEDGE/SCIENCE/THEORY-ORIENTED**
• Recognition	• Scientific aspects of animals/animal disease
	• Scientific aspects of human disease
CLIENT-ORIENTED	• Promotion of basic animal research
• Promotion of clients' monetary gain	• Promotion of basic scientific research
• Promotion of clients' personal satisfaction	
	SOCIETY-ORIENTED
PATIENT-ORIENTED	• Public (human) health
• Alleviation of pain/suffering	• Individual human health and well-being
• Promotion of patient health	• Human-directed environmental concerns
• Preserving the lives of patients	• Human-directed industry/agriculture
	• Animal control

can do but also in virtue of their different ethical attitudes and priorities. Veterinarians traditionally have been associated with human as well as animal concerns. They have worked in areas ranging from agribusiness to biomedical research, to the pharmaceutical industry, to the military. The ethical "map" of veterinary medicine may well be more diverse and complex than that of human medicine or any of the other learned professions. Although all veterinarians share certain values, if descriptive veterinary ethics stops at such universal values, it will fail to describe accurately the attitudes either of the profession as a whole or of many of its members.

～ THE IMPORTANCE OF INTROSPECTIVE DESCRIPTIVE VETERINARY ETHICS
The Choice of a Professional or Practice Style

Because veterinary medicine can encompass such a diversity of ethical values and attitudes, it is extremely important for each practitioner and student to understand his or her own value structure. Failure to do so can have disastrous results.

For example, veterinary schools tend to encourage students who earn high grades to enter academic veterinary medicine. Because such a career is often perceived as the highest reward a veterinary school can bestow, the path to academic practice (including an internship, residency, board certification in a specialty, and veterinary school teaching) is seen by many students as the ideal in professional life.

Unfortunately, such a path involves values and attitudes that are not shared by all who are thrust toward it. Internships and residencies require long hours and intense competition for the smaller number of openings on each successive rung of the academic ladder. Those who make it into academic practice may find that because of the need to publish new research, they must ignore everyday kinds of cases and gravitate toward the unusual, the unexplained, or the "interesting." The academic veterinarian may sometimes be less concerned about assisting a particular animal than in learning about and ultimately being able to help larger numbers of animals. She may try a certain procedure on a research subject knowing that someone who wanted to do everything possible to help that particular animal might act differently.

Each year, embarking on the academic trail are veterinarians for whom enjoyment of leisure time is an important value, who abhor competition, who are so touched by the needs of each animal that they feel they must always do everything possible to help it, or who enjoy dealing with clients more than teaching students. Likewise, there are some academic veterinarians who yearn for the hubbub of private practice, and some doctors for whom the daily pressures of running a practice are intolerable and who would be happier and more productive in academic medicine.

Veterinarians whose temperaments and ethical values are not suited to the way they find themselves practicing may fail or if "successful," may be miserable for the rest of their lives. They may blame their misfortune on their area of practice or come to see it as morally wrong. They may think that they are somehow deficient. They may even abandon the practice of veterinary medicine.

We are not always able to choose the career or practice style we would prefer. Nevertheless, the profession and the schools can do a great deal more than they are now doing to help individual doctors and students to clarify their own values and to understand the values and attitudes of the various areas of veterinary medicine.

〜 THE IMPORTANCE OF EMPIRICAL DESCRIPTIVE VETERINARY ETHICS

Many issues in official, administrative, and normative veterinary ethics can be illuminated by empirical investigation of the actual views of practitioners or students. The following are only some of the things investigating the ethical values of such persons might reveal:

- What ethical issues are most troubling to the profession (or to different components of the profession) and therefore might require prompt discussion or resolution
- Whether an important ethical issue is appreciated as such by the profession and whether the profession might therefore require sensitization to the issue
- Whether an ethical problem important to the profession is appreciated sufficiently by clients or society and whether the profession should therefore educate them concerning its significance
- Whether an ethical issue assumed to be in need of urgent resolution is not sufficiently troubling to those affected to justify significant allocation of the profession's time and resources
- What proposed solutions to ethical issues are likely to be accepted by the profession and might therefore be attractive to authors of official or administrative ethical standards
- What ethical issues are likely to concern the profession in the future and which the profession might therefore want to consider before these issues become divisive

⌒ POTENTIAL BENEFITS AND PITFALLS IN EMPIRICAL VETERINARY ETHICS: A CASE STUDY

Moral psychologist Donnie Self and his colleagues have conducted a series of studies that mark the first published systematic research in empirical descriptive veterinary ethics.[4, 5, 6] Self's work is complex and challenging, and cannot be done full justice here. Nevertheless, it requires discussion in this textbook. The information presented in the papers may be significant in its own right. Moreover, Self's research utilizes assumptions and methodologies employed by prominent social scientists who have devised these methodologies as an approach to moral reasoning generally and independently of any interest in veterinary medicine. Self's studies are therefore useful in appreciating potential benefits and pitfalls of what may well become the leading approach to empirical descriptive veterinary ethics.

Structure of the Research

There has existed for several decades a field of empirical moral psychology that attempts to characterize and explain the development of peoples' moral attitudes and reasoning. This field stems largely from the research of Harvard psychologist Lawrence Kohlberg. Kohlberg claims to have found six stages or levels of moral reasoning through which people in all countries and cultures pass. These six stages mark a progression from making moral choices based on the dictates of authority figures, to making choices to satisfy one's own needs, to considering interpersonal relations in various ways, and finally, in the last stage, to "commitment to universal ethical principles of justice, equality, autonomy, and respect for the dignity of all human beings as individuals."[7] Kohlberg and others have developed interview techniques involving the presentation of moral dilemmas that, it is asserted, determine which of these various stages of "moral reasoning" people exemplify. Kohlberg's theory does not, it is claimed, focus on peoples' particular values or moral beliefs, but rather on more general patterns of justification given in ethical reasoning. As Self explains:

> According to the theory, people proceed through the 6 stages as they mature. The sequence is invariant, although the rate and end stage reached vary with the individual. Indeed, 20% of the adult population never get beyond stage 2.[8]

Kohlberg's views were challenged by one of his students, Carol Gilligan, who argued that Kohlberg's theory does not account for differences in ethical attitudes of males and females. Self's characterization of the difference between the Kohlberg and Gilligan approaches is significant for our discussion:

> In response to Kohlberg theory, which regards justice as the moral ideal, Gilligan formulated a moral development stage theory that treats care as the moral ideal. In Kohlberg model, what is morally right is defined by justice, fairness, and independent principle guidedness, whereas in Gilligan model, moral rightness is interpreted to mean care, relatedness, and refraining from doing harm or violence. Lacking comparable empirical support for her stage theory, Gilligan later moved away from the concept of moral stages. Rather, she began to emphasize the concept of moral orientation, or moral voice, for which she does have empirical evidence.[9]

According to Gilligan, these two moral "voices" of justice and care are related to gender. Gilligan is sometimes interpreted as characterizing the justice approach as male and the care approach as female. She insists that these associations are merely empirical: although both approaches are exhibited by males and females, as a group males exhibit justice orientation predominantly, and females exhibit care orientation predominantly.[10] Nevertheless, Gilligan maintains that the ethic of care illuminates distinctive ways in which *women* experience adult life.[11]

In their studies of veterinarians and veterinary students, Self and his colleagues attempt to apply both the Kohlberg and Gilligan models, utilizing the former to test for levels of development in moral reasoning and the latter to determine the occurrence of orientations of "justice" and "care."

Reported Results and Preliminary Comments

It must be emphasized again that Self's research and the work in moral psychology on which it is based raise more issues than can be addressed here.[12] There exists a vast literature in which the general theory of moral stages and the particular approaches of Kohlberg and Gilligan have been evaluated by social scientists, educators, and philosophers. There are, for example, psychologists who do not believe that people pass through Kohlberg's six stages, who reject his characterizations of moral stages through which people supposedly do pass, who reject Gilligan's distinction between two fundamental moral orientations, and who do not accept Gilligan's claim that males tend toward justice and women toward care. Kohlberg himself denies that there are two distinct moral orientations of justice and care, something Self accepts as fact.[13] Anyone who seeks to make short work of this literature risks falling into a maelstrom of objections from many who would assert that *their* views must also be considered.[14] At the same time, the general Kohlberg approach (with or without Gilligan's modifications) dominates the field of moral psychology and therefore can be expected to play a prominent role in empirical studies of the ethical attitudes of veterinarians.

Veterinary education and moral development

In one of Dr. Self's studies, 20 veterinary students at one veterinary college underwent the standard Kohlberg moral judgment interview in their first and last year of school. This sample represented 16% of the school's student body. The subjects were not chosen randomly, but were recruited as volunteers. The study concluded that "normally expected increases in [levels of] moral reasoning did not occur over the four years...suggesting that [the students'] veterinary medical educational experience somehow inhibited their moral reasoning ability rather than facilitated it."[15] "There is no reason to believe," the authors assert, that the "curricula and faculties of other veterinary colleges might exert a more positive influence on the moral development of their students" because "all veterinary students take similar subjects in about the same sequence, and frequently use the same textbooks or related teaching materials."[16] The authors believe their results "implicate qualities of the veterinary medical educational system"[14] as a whole. They assert that "the hierarchical, authoritarian structure of veterinary medical education, like education in human medicine, does not actively promote or encourage conflict about moral issues that is an important element in moral reasoning growth and development."[17]

These conclusions are not supported by the evidence on which they are based. The dilemmas presented to the students were not specifically tailored to issues in veterinary medicine. Therefore the research appears to rest on the assumption (which may be self-evident to supporters of Kohlberg but cannot be regarded as such by veterinarians or veterinary educators) that there is no difference in the moral reasoning of veterinary students relating to veterinary issues as distinguished from other matters. The study was done on only 20 volunteers with no evidence that they were representative of the student body of this school much less of other schools. Indeed, Self's paper concedes that this school did not have (as many do) formal ethics instruction. The authors' claim that veterinary education throughout the country is virtually identical is therefore incorrect, certainly with regard to ethics instruction. Nevertheless, they assert a lack of improvement in moral reasoning of veterinary students in general. The authors' general criticism of veterinary education as hierarchical, authoritarian, and uninterested in promoting cognitive conflict about moral issues is presented without any empirical evidence and is certainly not supported by this study of 20 students at one veterinary college. Indeed, a later survey conducted by Self and colleagues indicates that many veterinary schools offer serious ethics instruction.[18]

Orientations of justice and care in graduating veterinary school students

Another study of 10 male and 10 female students at the end of their final year of veterinary school applied an interview procedure developed by Gilligan to determine whether these students exhibited gender differences in their moral orientations. The participants were asked to report their own real-life ethical dilemmas. Some of the participants reported dilemmas that related to veterinary practice. This study too presents an unflattering picture of veterinary students. If, the authors assert, "the concept of justice is considered to exemplify the pinnacle or highest type of reasoning," the study reflects "poorly on veterinarians" because "less than half (45%) of [the subjects] relied predominantly on justice in resolving the conflicts, and even fewer (35%) actually aligned with or personally accepted and owned the justice orientation as their preferred mode of resolution of moral conflicts." On the other hand, "if the concept of care is regarded as representing the highest level of moral understanding," this too "reflects poorly on veterinarians" because "only 45% of them relied predominantly on care in resolving conflicts" and only 30% "actually aligned with care and personally owned a care orientation as their preferred mode of resolution of moral conflicts."[19]

Once again, these results do not say much (if they say anything at all) about veterinary students because of the small sample size, the fact that this was not a random sample of students even at this school, and the fact that exposure to ethics at this school was not representative of all schools or of veterinary education in general. Self's characterization of what reflects poorly on "veterinarians"—which is based entirely on data gained from *students*—appears to assume that the moral reasoning levels of veterinarians does not change after some time, a moderate time, or a long time practicing veterinary medicine. Self presents no evidence for this assumption, which is hardly self-evident.

However, the most puzzling conclusion of this study is its insistence, despite lack of clear evidence, that Gilligan's views concerning gender differences apply to veterinary students:

Although statistical analysis revealed no significant correlation between gender and moral orientation, these limited data appear to support Gilligan's claim that males are predominantly justice oriented and females are predominantly care oriented. On the basis of the data, justice orientation was exhibited 67% of the time by males and 33% of the time by females. Care orientation was exhibited 65% of the time by females and 44% of the time by males.[18]

If these data truly reveal *no* significant correlation between gender and moral orientation, then they do *not* support Gilligan's claim that there is such a difference. One is compelled to ask whether the Gilligan hypothesis is considered so obviously correct for human experience in general that its verification in the veterinary context requires less stringent proof than would ordinarily be required of empirical hypotheses. In any event, this paper does not indicate that there was an obvious or significant difference in moral orientation between even these 10 males and 10 females, much less male and female veterinary students or veterinarians. Interestingly, Self's earlier study of 20 first- and fourth-year veterinary students found that "gender differences were not evident between the subjects."[20]

Moral reasoning in small versus large animal practitioners

The tendency to find gender differences, even if the data do not clearly support such a conclusion, is illustrated by an earlier study in which Self surveyed 350 Texas veterinarians in large and small animal practice. This research was based on a questionnaire applying Kohlberg's theory of development. It found no significant statistical difference in the level of reasoning exhibited by large and small animal doctors. The authors found in the data "mild support" for the hypothesis that female veterinarians would use higher Kohlbergian levels than males.[21] However, the statistical variance between males and females on which this conclusion was based ($P=0.045$ where $P\leq0.05$ is the standard convention for statistical significance) can be characterized as minuscule at best.

General Requirements for Empirical Descriptive Ethics

As Self and his colleagues themselves maintain, more work is needed to refine and apply the Kohlberg and Gilligan methodologies in the veterinary context. If, for example, there really are important differences in the moral orientation of male and female veterinary students and practitioners, we ought to know what these are as the proportion of women in the profession increases. It is to be hoped that Self and others will continue this research so that its accuracy and relevance to veterinarians can be evaluated more adequately. Nevertheless, the work published to date suggests several important demands that students of veterinary ethics can rightly make of research in empirical descriptive veterinary ethics.

Conclusions must be proportional to supporting data.

Researchers must be careful to draw conclusions that are proportional to their data. Statements about veterinary students, male and female veterinary students, veterinary schools, veterinary education, and veterinarians must be based on adequately representative samples. Questions about how practitioners and veterinary students react to *veterinary* situations must figure predominantly in assessment of their ethical views relating to veterinary medicine in the absence of clear and convincing evidence that such an approach is unnecessary.

Researchers should entertain the possibility of aspects of ethical issues in veterinary medicine that involve distinctive moral concepts.

Because the Kohlberg and Gilligan theories play a prominent role in the science of moral psychology, it is understandable and of academic value that researchers attempt to assess the soundness of these theories in the veterinary context. However, one cannot but wonder whether either of these general approaches could possibly describe adequately the moral attitudes of veterinarians. Kohlberg's characterizations of justice relate to how people deal with other *people*, not animals.[22] Gilligan's characterization of the ethic of care is also made in terms of how *people* relate to each other.[23] Perhaps elements of "justice" and "care" could be applied to a medical profession whose patients are animals. However, it seems unlikely from the start that either of these concepts as defined by Kohlberg or Gilligan could encompass the activities of a profession only part of whose focus is on people. Interestingly, Self and his colleagues speculate that:

> ...there may be moral aspects other than justice and care that form the structure of moral reasoning in veterinarians... More than one third (35%) of the participants [in the study of graduating veterinary students] preferred other modes of resolution, which remain unidentified by the bipolar analysis of justice and care... Other possible moral considerations need to be identified, clarified, and researched thoroughly to account better for the moral reasoning and moral orientation of veterinarians. Among the possibilities that may be operative are benevolence, obedience to authority, professional honor, compassion, nurturance to animals, and duties to owners vs. animals.[24]

Surely, we already know that all of these attitudes (except, perhaps, obedience to authority) are not just *possible* operative ethical attitudes among veterinarians. They are *obviously* important attitudes among veterinarians. If the science of moral psychology does not know this—or more importantly, does not develop tools to analyze attitudes that might not fit nicely into Kohlberg's or Gilligan's categories—the career of empirical descriptive veterinary ethics might be short-lived indeed. If empirical investigation of the ethical attitudes of veterinarians is to have much value, it must concern itself at the very least with attitudes we know are important in veterinary medicine, such as those listed in Table 6-1.

Values cannot masquerade as fact or definitions of morality.

There is a basic methodological problem in the Kohlberg methodology regarding which normative veterinary ethics must be vigilant. Kohlberg's theory is laden with values. The theory maintains that certain kinds of moral reasoning are better than others. It also maintains that certain kinds of ethical choices (associated with "higher" levels of moral reasoning) are *better* than others. Thus Kohlberg's theory, as well as Gilligan's modifications of it, are more than descriptive accounts of how people engage in moral reasoning. Kohlberg and Gilligan believe that people *ought* to approach moral reasoning in certain ways.

The obvious normative character of the Kohlberg methodology can be seen in many of Self's characterizations of the methodology and its purported application to veterinarians. For example in a passage quoted earlier, Self states that people proceed through Kohlberg's six stages "as they mature." The sixth stage is a sign of true maturity, and clearly, it is *better* in Self's view to be mature than immature or more mature than less mature. This is why Self characterizes his finding that 20 veterinary students did not move toward higher Kohlbergian levels as evidence that there was "lack of moral reasoning growth." Thus he characterizes students whose levels moved in the opposite direction as having undergone "regression." There is undeniable normative content in the characterizations, also quoted earlier, of the Kohlberg concept of justice and the Gilligan ethic of care as proposed "moral ideals" and definitions of "moral rightness."

The danger of this value-laden approach for normative ethics, and for normative veterinary ethics in particular, can be seen from Self's and Kohlberg's characterizations of the final stage of moral reasoning. According to Self:

> Stage 6 involves commitment to universal ethical principles of justice, equality, autonomy, and respect for the dignity of all *human beings* as individuals; what is considered right is required by a personal commitment to these universal ethical principles.[25]

Kohlberg writes that in stage 6:

> Right is defined by the decision of conscience in accord with self-chosen *ethical principles* appealing to logical comprehensiveness, universality, and consistency, These principles are abstract and ethical (the Golden Rule, the categorical imperative); they are not concrete moral rules like the Ten Commandments. At heart, these are universal principles of *justice*, of the *reciprocity* and *equality* of human *rights*, and of respect for the dignity of human beings as *individual persons*.[26]

It is interesting to learn that the Ten Commandments, (and indeed any concrete moral rules) represent a less "mature" approach to morality. More important for our purposes, Kohlberg's stage 6 includes respect for the dignity of human beings but does not include (at least explicitly) respect for, or indeed *any* attitude toward, *animals*. This is not surprising because Kohlberg bases his concept of justice largely on the views of philosopher John Rawls.[27] Rawls bases just rules and a just society on what a group of adult humans in an ideal contractual process would agree would be good for them. As has been noted by several of Rawls' critics, animals cannot participate in such a process; Rawls does not explicitly accord their interests significant value, aside from asserting that they ought not to be treated cruelly.[28] Other Kohlbergian stages also appear to have a human bias. As characterized by Self, stage 5 involves a level of moral reasoning:

> ...emphasizing individual rights such as life and liberty but endorsing a social contract that protects all *people's* rights with a contractual commitment freely entered upon to serve the greatest good for the greatest number; what is considered right is what is rationally calculated to be for the best welfare of all *humankind*.[29]

Here also animals are not mentioned. Moreover, not only does Kohlberg's theory apparently relegate utilitarianism (see Chapter 5) to a less mature level of reasoning,[25] it mischaracterizes the theory. Utilitarians do not believe in moral rights, they do not base moral rules on a social contract. Most utilitarians, recognizing that animals also feel pain, do not restrict their moral calculations to what benefits *human* welfare. Whatever else one might say about utilitarianism, at least it explicitly demands that we include in moral deliberation the effects of our behavior on animal suffering.[30]

The objection that Kohlbergian theory prescribes moral values in the guise of a descriptive theory of development is not new, and Kohlberg responds to it.[31] He concedes that although his six stages have a normative content—people in stage 6 are viewed as morally advanced over people in lower stages—but maintains that the normative aspect of the stages does not result from independent substantive value judgments. Rather, Kohlberg claims, stage 6 reasoning represents what the term "morality" *means*. It is not until people reach stage 6 that they are making what people would call fully "moral" decisions. According to Kohlberg, each of the stages represents an approach (logically implied by the stage below it) that approaches closer toward the truly moral point of view of stage 6. If stage 6 reasoning is associated with certain views about right and wrong, it is because such views are part of what it means to engage in "moral" reasoning or to assume a "moral point of view" properly described.

Unfortunately, Kohlberg's stage 6 does not merely reflect what people mean by moral reasoning or decisionmaking. As philosopher William Alston observes, there is vigorous disagreement among philosophers about what is meant by "moral" or "ethical" reasoning.[32] Many philosophers would reject Kohlberg's contention that reasoning that exemplifies something other than stage 6 cannot be morally correct because it is not strictly speaking, moral at all. Utilitarianism provides a convincing counter example to Kohlberg's definition of morality. Utilitarians may or may not espouse incorrect moral views, but these views are surely *moral* in nature. It is routine to refer to utilitarianism, or any number of theories Kohlberg places in inferior stages, as fully ethical or moral theories.

The fact that Kohlberg is wrong about what constitutes moral reasoning is also demonstrated by his apparent restriction of his definition of "morality" to how human beings deal with each other. It may be morally correct or incorrect to think people have direct duties to animals, that we should take the interests of animals seriously or that animal pain and distress limit what people may do to animals. However, such judgments are, clearly, moral in nature. Those of us who believe that animals also count may be mistaken. But we are certainly entitled to object if told that our contentions are not ethical or moral or that we do not exhibit a sufficiently mature level of moral reasoning.

As Alston comments, although Kohlberg's theory might be valuable as a tool for describing ethical attitudes, he has simply pulled "a moral theory out of a hat." He chooses one of definition of the "moral," but:

> ...fails to do anything by way of showing that this is more than a choice of what seems congenial and interesting to him. That is quite acceptable if it is just a matter of carving out a subject for empirical research...But if he wants to use the developmental approximations to the purely moral in his sense a basis for pronouncements about how people *ought* to reason in their action-guiding deliberations, that is another matter.[32]

Even if some people do move during their lives toward certain kinds of moral reasoning or certain substantive ethical views, this does not render such reasoning or views *better* than others—any more than the fact that people "progress" toward old age and death makes these states better and more desirable than what precedes them. If, for example, there are distinct moral orientations of "justice" and "care" and if male veterinarians exhibit the former and female veterinarians the latter, this would not render either orientation more or less correct than the other. Indeed, we might find that either or both are ethically questionable and should therefore be discouraged. If a "justice" orientation involved overvaluing the interests of veterinary clients at the expense of patients, and if a "care" orientation involved the overvaluing of patients at the expense of clients, we would probably want to encourage veterinarians and veterinary students to move away from both "justice" and "care." Insofar as any moral "stages," "orientations," or "voices" really exist,* and insofar as each might involve general or specific ethical positions, these positions must still be assessed for their correctness.

～ DESCRIPTIVE VERSUS NORMATIVE VETERINARY ETHICS

Ethical views about how animals or people ought to be treated must be established by the only means we have to establish them: *argument* aimed at evaluating whether these views are *correct*. Whether it is ethically acceptable to administer pain-killing drugs to race horses prior to competition, to euthanize healthy, well-behaved pets on demand, or to encourage a client to authorize a potentially stressful and costly chemotherapy for an elderly animal cannot possibly be determined by examining the moral "stages" or "voices" of veterinarians. One must examine closely what will happen to the animals, to clients, and others affected by a veterinarian's behavior. One must then ask what *ought* to be done.

The development of empirical veterinary ethics should be encouraged because it can be important to understand how and why people reach their ethical views. For example, if there are different general moral orientations among veterinarians, we ought to know about it. Such knowledge might enable us to craft more ethically appropriate ways of dealing with animals and clients, or to structure discussions that may more effectively assist veterinarians to determine how they should act. However, such a process would not involve merely acknowledging that there might be different patterns of moral reasoning or views about proper behavior. It would involve comparing such patterns or views against what one would determine—independently and through moral argument—are appropriate ethical standards.

In sum, empirical science will never replace ethical argument about the correctness of moral positions. Descriptive veterinary ethics cannot substitute for normative veterinary ethics.

---

*The reader may detect my skepticism about claims that male and female veterinary students and veterinarians have different moral orientations. As of this writing, I have taught ethics to almost 1,000 veterinary students, the majority of whom have been women. This teaching has not been based on limited interviews or presentation of hypothetical dilemmas—but on repeated and protracted interaction, focused on ethical issues in veterinary medicine, and involving oral and written responses to vigorous interrogation. I am also married to a veterinarian. I have not noticed any differences in general moral orientation or specific ethical views between male students as a group and female students as a group. I do believe that my students today are somewhat more concerned about animal welfare and the interests of patients than were students of a decade ago, but this change appears to have occurred generally, irrespective of gender.

REFERENCES

[1] American Veterinary Medical Association: *Principles of Veterinary Medical Ethics*, 1993 Revision "Guidelines for Professional Behavior," paragraph 10, *1994 AVMA Directory*, Schaumburg, IL, The Association, p 42.

[2] American Veterinary Medical Association: *Principles of Veterinary Medical Ethics*, 1993 Revision, "Secret Remedies," *1994 AVMA Directory*, Schaumburg, IL, The Association, p 44.

[3] *See*, for example, MacIntyre A: *After Virtue*, ed 2, South Bend, IN, 1984, University of Notre Dame Press, pp 154-155.

[4] Self DJ, Safford SK, Shelton GC: Comparison of the general moral reasoning of small animal veterinarians vs large animal veterinarians; *J Am Vet Med Assoc* 193:1509-1512, 1988, hereinafter referred to as *Self, Comparison of general moral reasoning*. To facilitate presentation, the discussion speaks of Dr. Self to refer to him and his coworkers.

[5] Self DJ and others: Study of the influence of veterinary medical education on the moral development of veterinary students, *J Am Vet Med Assoc* 198:782-787, 1991, hereinafter referred to as *Self, Study of the influence of veterinary education*.

[6] Self DJ and others: Moral orientations of justice and care among veterinarians entering veterinary practice, *J Am Vet Med Assoc* 199:569-572, 1991, hereinafter referred to as *Self, Moral orientations of justice and care*.

[7] *Self, Study of the influence of veterinary education*: 783.

[8] *Self, Comparison of general moral reasoning*: 1511.

[9] *Self, Moral orientations of justice and care*: 569.

[10] Gilligan C: *In a Different Voice*, Cambridge, MA, 1982, Harvard University Press.

[11] *Id*, p 173.

[12] For example, this chapter focuses on critical methodological principles that relate specifically to descriptive and normative ethics and does not attempt to question factual contentions of Kohlberg, Gilligan, or Self. For the purposes of discussion, I accept as accurate Self's contentions regarding the distribution of Kohlberg's stages of moral reasoning and of orientations of "justice" and "care." My aim is to inquire what can be concluded if Self's factual contentions are correct. A more complete discussion might question from a more purely empirical standpoint some of the Kohlberg and Gilligan techniques or Self's utilization of these techniques. For example, Self reports that to eliminate problems of "inter-rater reliability" all the transcripts of the interviews of the veterinary students who participated in the study of moral orientations of justice and care were interpreted by a single reader. *Self, Moral orientations of justice and care*: 570. It can be asked whether, especially in such an early study of the applicability of Gilligan's techniques to veterinary students, there should have been more than one person evaluating the student interviews. Substantial agreement among several readers would show that the reported findings were not dependent on the tendencies or preferences of any single evaluator. Disagreement among readers might raise questions about the findings reported by Self or, perhaps, the soundness of the underlying approach.

[13] Kohlberg L, Levine C, Hewer A: *Moral Stages: A Current Formulation and a Response to Critics*, Basel, Switzerland, 1983, Karger, p 139 (stating that "we do not believe there exist two distinct or polar orientations or two tracks in the ontogenesis of moral stage structures" and that "it remains for Gilligan and her colleagues...to demonstrate the progressive movement, invariant sequence, structured wholeness, and the relationships of thought to action for her orientation in a manner similar to the way Kohlberg has demonstrated such ontogenetic characteristics for the justice orientation").

[14] For interesting discussions supporting and criticizing Kohlberg and Gilligan, *see*, Munsey B, editor: *Moral Development, Moral Education, and Kohlberg*, Birmingham, AL, 1980, Religious Education Press; Larrabee MJ, editor: *An ethic of care*, New York, 1993, Routledge.

[15] *Self, Study of the influence of veterinary education*: 782.

[16] *Self, Study of the influence of veterinary education*: 785.

[17] *Self, Study of the influence of veterinary education*: 783.

[18] Self DJ, Pierce AB, Shadduck JA: A survey of the teaching of ethics in veterinary education, *J Am Vet Med Assoc* 204:944-945, 1994.

[19] *Self, Moral orientations of justice and care*: 571.

[20] *Self, Study of the influence of veterinary education*: 784.

[21] *Self, Comparison of general moral reasoning*: 1511.

[22] Kohlberg offers several different characterizations of stage 6, all of which refer to one's views of the status and value of other people. In one essay, for example, he describes the principles endorsed in stage 6 as (1) "universal principles of justice, of the reciprocity and equality of human rights, and of respect for the dignity of human beings as individual persons." Kohlberg L: From is to ought: How to commit the naturalistic fallacy and get away with it in the study of moral development. In Mischel T: *Cognitive Development and Epistemology*, New York, 1971, Academic Press, p 165; (2) "the principle of respect for personality" (*Id*, p 208); (3) the principle that "'*persons are of unconditional value*,' translatable into the Kantian principle 'act so as to treat each person as an end, not as a means" (*Id*, p 210); and (4) the principle of "individual *justice*, 'the right of every person to an *equal* consideration of his *claims* in every situation, not just those codified into law." (*Id*, p 210)

[23]"For women, the integration of rights and responsibilities takes place through an understanding of the psychological logic of relationships. This understanding tempers the self-destructive potential of a self-critical morality by asserting the need of all *persons* for care." Gilligan C: *In a Different Voice*, Cambridge, MA, 1982, Harvard University Press, p 100, emphasis supplied.

[24]*Self, Moral orientations of justice and care*: 572.

[25]*Self, Comparison of general moral reasoning*: 1511, emphasis supplied.

[26]Kohlberg L: From is to ought: How to commit the naturalistic fallacy and get away with it in the study of moral development. In Mischel T: *Cognitive Development and Epistemology*, New York, 1971, Academic Press, p 165, emphases in the original.

[27]Kohlberg L, Levine C, Hewer A: *Moral Stages: A Current Formulation and a Response to Critics*, Basel, Switzerland, 1983, Karger, pp 87-90.

[28]Regan T: *The Case for Animal Rights*, Berkeley, 1983, University of California Press, pp 163-174. As Regan notes, Rawls' principles might be consistent with the inclusion of animals in the moral domain, if the people in Rawls "original position" are supposed to imagine how they would want to be treated if they lived on the earth as animals. However, Rawls does not appear to have intended such imaginings.

[29]*Self, Comparison of general moral reasoning*: 1511, emphasis supplied.

[30]Bentham J: *The Principles of Morals and Legislation*, chap. XVII, Sec. I., 1789, New York, 1948, Hafner, p 311 (stating that "The question is not, Can they [animals] reason? nor Can they *talk*? but, *Can they suffer?*"). Although Kohlberg classifies rule-utilitarianism as a stage 5 view, he relegates Jeremy Bentham to stage 2, which sees right action as "that which instrumentally satisfies one's own needs and occasionally the needs of others. Human relations are viewed in terms like those of the market place." Kohlberg L: From is to ought: How to commit the naturalistic fallacy and get away with it in the study of moral development. In Mischel T: *Cognitive Development and Epistemology*, New York, 1971, Academic Press, pp 164, 208, and 222. In fact, a central tenet of Bentham's philosophy, and of utilitarianism in general, is that any other person's happiness or unhappiness is worthy of no more consideration than one's own.

[31]Kohlberg L: From is to ought: How to commit the naturalistic fallacy and get away with it in the study of moral development. In Mischel T: *Cognitive Development and Epistemology*, New York, 1971, Academic Press, pp 213-226.

[32]Alston WP: Comments on Kohlberg's "From is to ought." In Mischel T: *Cognitive Development and Epistemology*, New York, 1971, Academic Press, pp 276-277.

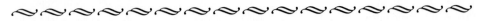

CHAPTER 7

Administrative Veterinary Ethics

The Governmental Application of Moral Standards

*A*dministrative veterinary ethics is the process of the application of ethical standards to veterinarians by administrative governmental bodies. It is important to recognize administrative veterinary ethics as a separate branch of veterinary ethics. Almost every aspect of veterinary practice can be affected by administrative ethical standards. Moreover, because administrative agencies are branches of government, they can use the substantial force of the law to compel adherence to these standards. In recent years, government bodies, such as state boards of registration, have exhibited a marked increase in activity in the regulation of physicians and attorneys. If this trend extends to veterinarians, administrative veterinary ethics may become a major concern of all practitioners.

~ THE NATURE AND FUNCTIONS OF ADMINISTRATIVE GOVERNMENT AGENCIES

An administrative agency can be defined as "a governmental authority, other than a court and a legislative body, which affects the rights of private parties through either adjudication, rule making, investigating, prosecuting, negotiating, settling, or informally acting."[1] Administrative agencies can consist of varying numbers of persons (including one). They can have various names, none of which need carry any special significance in defining their activities.

It is not the courts or legislatures but administrative agencies that perform the overwhelming majority of governmental functions. From the U. S. Department of Agriculture (USDA) to state departments of public health, from the Food and Drug Administration (FDA) to the National Institutes of Health, from the Federal Bureau of Investigation to county district attorneys offices, from the Internal Revenue Service to municipal zoning boards, administrative agencies affect virtually every aspect of the lives of everyone.

Administrative bodies exist because there is too much for legislative and executive officeholders to do by themselves and because certain areas of government require expertise such officeholders do not possess. No administrative agency is entirely free to do what it wants. All branches of government are subject to federal or state constitutional limitations. Statutes usually define the functions and proper activities of an agency; decisions that violate these boundaries or that are in error can often be appealed in the courts. Administrative bodies differ widely in the amount of independence they possess. Sometimes, as in the case of the Federal Trade Commission or state boards of veterinary medicine, agencies are relatively independent; their members are appointed for fixed terms, and they can sometimes adopt policies or make decisions that the current legislature, President, or Governor may oppose. Sometimes, as in the case of the USDA or state departments of agriculture, agencies are subdivisions of a branch of government (usually, the executive); such agencies often take orders directly from, or are ultimately accountable to, an elected official.

Although the powers of administrative bodies differ, many perform the following kinds of functions:

- Enforcement of specific standards or requirements contained in a statute
- Interpretation of statutory provisions
- Writing regulations to assist them in carrying out their functions
- Granting licenses or permissions based on statutory standards or their own regulations
- Investigation of suspected violations of statutory or regulatory standards
- Determination in adjudicatory proceedings conducted by themselves (and not the courts) whether violations have occurred
- Imposition of penalties on those found to be in violation
- Referral of matters to another government agency for criminal or civil action
- Issuing of specific rulings or opinions that determine whether a certain kind of activity or a specific person is in compliance with the agency's standards
- Engaging in a wide range of informal actions not ordinarily subject to public scrutiny or court review, including pressuring those under their jurisdiction to meet their standards, assisting parties privately, publicizing standards and policies, negotiating agreements and settlements, and deciding whether to investigate, negotiate, or prosecute

✧ ADMINISTRATIVE AGENCIES AND ETHICAL STANDARDS

Administrative agencies impose or apply ethical standards in several ways. First, they may apply statutes or regulations that are purely ethical in nature. For example, many veterinary practice acts direct state boards of veterinary medicine to grant licenses only to people with good moral character and permit the boards to discipline licensed practitioners who engage in fraud or false and misleading advertising. Such standards are purely ethical in the sense that they need not relate to a doctor's competence or technical ability to practice veterinary medicine.

Second, administrative agencies sometimes make decisions applying ethical as well as technical standards. The USDA's regulations pursuant to the Animal Welfare Act governing the housing and care of laboratory animals draw heavily on the Department's scientific knowledge about the needs of different laboratory species and the nature of laboratory facilities. However, the underlying aim of these regulations is to assure due regard for the animals' welfare. This is an ethical goal that is applied in light of technical knowledge to generate what are hoped are morally appropriate standards. Likewise, when the FDA proposes policies governing the use of drugs in food animals, it must consider empirical data about the effects and elimination times of these drugs in light of ethical concerns — including how the public's moral and legal right to safe food should be balanced against the need of farmers and veterinarians to earn a living. It is sometimes easy to forget the extent to which administrative bodies are motivated by ethical concerns. The rules they adopt can be technical in appearance and do not always make explicit reference to the underlying ethical motivation. As they do their jobs, the meat inspector, customs agent, racing commission veterinarian, or state health department toxicologist may not be engaging in ethical deliberation. Nevertheless, many of the technical standards they apply have resulted from decisions that certain interests ought to be protected and that certain kinds of behavior (such as selling adulterated meat or overworking race horses) are morally unacceptable.

Finally, ethical considerations can play an important role in an administrative body's exercise of what lawyers call its "discretionary power," its ability to make decisions (such as whom to investigate or prosecute and when not to investigate, negotiate, or prosecute) that are generally not open to challenge by the public or the courts. A state veterinary licensing board, for example, may decide to give friendly and private guidance to practitioners who have committed acts of incompetence if these doctors exhibit an appropriate attitude of remorse. On the other hand, the board may suspend the license of other veterinarians who have done the same things but are disrespectful and unrepentant. One cannot overestimate the extent to which administrative bodies are sometimes affected in their discretionary decisions by perceptions of whether they are dealing with a morally good person who merits sympathy or with a morally bad one who deserves punishment.

～ THE RANGE OF ADMINISTRATIVE VETERINARY ETHICAL STANDARDS

It is beyond the scope of this book to discuss all administrative agencies that apply ethical standards to veterinarians. Subsequent chapters consider the ethical activity of several of the more visible agencies. Table 7-1 lists some of the administrative bodies that impose ethical standards upon veterinarians. The table is illustrative only. It does not list all ethical issues relating to veterinarians in which administrative agencies are involved, all administrative bodies applying ethical standards to veterinarians, or indeed all the areas of ethical involvement of the listed agencies.

～ ADMINISTRATIVE ETHICS ON THE FRONT LINE: THE STATE VETERINARY LICENSING BOARDS

By far the most important source of administrative veterinary ethical judgments are the state veterinary licensing boards. These boards, unlike other administrative bodies that regulate veterinarians, deal exclusively with providers of veterinary services and their relations with patients, clients, and the public. Moreover, the boards have at their disposal many more rules that are purely ethical in nature than do other kinds of administrative agencies whose activities affect veterinarians.

The Veterinary Licensing Boards

The law begins with the principle that veterinary practice is not a right but a privilege, and that the state (not the federal) government has the responsibility to decide upon whom to confer this privilege. Each state makes this decision by means of a statute (usually called the veterinary practice act) which sets forth the legislature's deci-

TABLE 7-1
❧

Ethical areas of concern of administrative agencies other than the state veterinary licensing boards

AREA OF CONCERN	FEDERAL AGENCIES	STATE AND LOCAL AGENCIES
Animal diseases, protection of animals from contagious	USDA	State departments of agriculture, public health
Animal food products, protection of public from impure and asulterated	FDA	State departments of agriculture, public health
Competition among doctors, assurance of fair	Federal Trade Comission (FTC); Department of Justice	State attorneys general
Controlled substances, use by veterinarians	Drug Enforcement Administration; Department of Justice	State public health departments, district attorneys, and attorneys general
Cruelty to animals (general)		District attorneys; Special animal protection agencies
Deceptive commercial and trade practices by veterinarians	FTC	State attorneys general
Discrimination against employees on the basis of race, religion, age, sex, disability	Equal Opportunity Employment Commission	State and local antidiscrimination agencies
Drugs, use of by veterinarians	FDA	
Food animals, humane slaughter of	USDA	State agriculture departments
Insecticides, and pesticides, use by veterinarians	Environmental Protection Agency	
Laboratory animal welfare	USDA (Animal and Plant Health Inspection Service [APHIS]); FDA; National Institutes of Health (NIH); Public Health Service	State public health departments (in some states)
Meat and poultry, protection of public from impure	USDA (Food Safety and Inspection Service)	State meat inspection agencies
Marine mammals, protection of those in captivity	USDA (APHIS)	
Pets, commercial raising and transportation of	USDA (APHIS)	State animal protection agencies (in some states)
Racing animals, regulation of drug use in and conditions of		State racing commissions
Safety of veterinary premises for the public		Local building, fire, and health departments
Safety of working conditions for veterinary employees	Occupational Safety and Health Administration	State departments of labor, occupational safety, public health
Show horses, protection of from certain inhumane practices	USDA (APHIS)	
Unfair labor practices	Department of Labor; National Labor Relations Board	State labor departments
Wildlife, protection of, veterinary care by private doctors	Department of Interior (Fish and Wildlife Service)	State departments of fisheries and wildlife
Veterinary facilities, proper location and use of		Local zoning boards and planning commissions
Zoonoses	Department of Health and Human Services (Centers for Disease Control; NIH), USDA	State and local public health departments

sions about who will be permitted to practice veterinary medicine and under what conditions. The veterinary practice act creates an administrative agency (usually called the "board of registration" or the "board of examiners") that grants licenses to practice and has the authority to supervise the activities of licensees and to discipline them for failure to meet required standards. Typically, many of these standards are specified in the practice act. Often, boards enforce standards they write themselves, pursuant to their authority to make rules and regulations.

There are significant differences among the veterinary boards. The veterinary practice act of each state is different. A standard imposed in one state may not exist in another. In some jurisdictions, the legislature has placed all its requirements (both technical and ethical) in the veterinary practice act; other states have statutes and regulations governing all licensed professionals that apply standards to veterinarians in addition to those found in the veterinary practice act. In some states the board itself disciplines practitioners; in others the board makes a disciplinary recommendation, which is reviewed and can be modified by a supervisory administrative agency. The procedures used in investigating and adjudicating cases differ from state to state. Some boards have nonveterinarian members, and among those with public members, some have a larger number of public members than others. The boards also vary widely in how actively they make regulations, investigate licensees, and impose supervision or punishment for technical or ethical infractions.

Ethical Standards of the Veterinary Boards

The following are some of the more common ethical standards contained in the veterinary practice acts and regulations of the states. The typical practice act and associated regulations contain several of the kinds of provisions listed below. The precise wording of these standards can vary from state to state.*

Good moral character

Many states permit licensing only of persons of good moral character, although in recent years several states have removed this requirement from their practice acts. Many practice acts that do include good moral character as a prerequisite for licensure do not define or characterize good moral character and appear to leave it to the board to decide who might and who might not have such character. At least one state requires good moral character "as it relates to the functions and duties of a licensed veterinarian."[2] However, there usually is no such restriction. Some practice acts list absence of good moral character among the grounds for disciplining present licensees, while the statutes of other states specify that new applicants can be denied a license if they lack good moral character. It seems clear, however, that if a board can deny a new license because of bad moral character, it can revoke or suspend an already existing license for the same reason.[3]

---

*The following discussion lists practice act provisions as they are typically phrased. References in brackets are to states that have the listed provisions though not necessarily in these words. State listings are illustrative only; when a state is listed, there may be other states with the same or similar provisions. State references are given only for provisions that are unusual or must be distinguished carefully from other provisions listed. References to states are not given for provisions that are shared by many states. Veterinary practice acts and associated regulations are subject to revision. In recent years the practice acts of several states have been substantially rewritten, and some contain a "sunset" provision that mandates their expiration and revision at a specified future date. Readers should therefore consult their practice act and regulations for the precise wording of the standards currently applicable in their jurisdictions.

The theory behind the good moral character requirement—and of many ethical standards applied by state veterinary boards—is that society has a right to expect its veterinarians to be more than technically proficient. Veterinarians must also be good and decent people. They must be worthy of the trust placed in them by clients, and they must be sensitive to the great power they exercise over the health and lives of patients.

Conviction of a felony or of a crime involving moral turpitude

The underlying rationale for these disciplinary grounds is that a conviction of a felony or of a crime involving moral turpitude can itself provide evidence of bad moral character and lack of trustworthiness.

In most jurisdictions, a felony is any crime punishable by more than 1 year imprisonment. A judgment based upon a guilty plea is a conviction, and a person can be convicted of a felony even if he in fact serves less than 1 year in jail or is ordered to pay a fine instead of being incarcerated. The reason that moral turpitude is not added as an extra requirement to felonies is that the law tends to consider a felony conviction as itself evidence of bad moral character.

A crime involving moral turpitude is one that by its very nature always reflects bad moral character. Sometimes, this definition leads to odd results. For example, in one California court case, a chiropractor had been charged with owning and operating a house of prostitution but pleaded guilty only to the lesser charge of willfully residing in a house of ill repute. The court ruled that he could not be disciplined by the board of chiropractic for conviction of a crime involving moral turpitude, because he was only convicted of *living* in a house of ill repute, and a chiropractor could conceivably live in such a place and not contribute other than peripherally to the enterprise of prostitution.[4] Among the crimes generally regarded as involving moral turpitude are theft, fraud, tax evasion, homicide, violent crimes, indecent exposure,[5] and, increasingly, crimes involving abuse of alcoholic beverages or drugs.[6]

Conviction of a crime directly relating to the practice of veterinary medicine or the ability to practice veterinary medicine [CA, FL, IN][7]

Some states permit the board to discipline a practitioner who has been convicted of any crime (felony or misdemeanor) provided the crime related directly to the practice of veterinary medicine or is evidence of a lack of ability to practice veterinary medicine. Generally, practice acts with such a provision appear to allow the state board to determine whether an act that led to a criminal conviction relates to veterinary practice. The Florida practice act specifies that "any crime which demonstrates a lack of regard for animal life relates to the practice of veterinary medicine."[7] In fact, a provision permitting discipline for a crime related to practice or one's ability to practice probably could be applied to a conviction for *any* serious crime, and certainly does not require a board to find that a criminal conviction is evidence of technical incompetence. As one court has observed, any crime that reflects poorly on a practitioner's honesty, truthfulness, and good reputation is a crime related to the practice of veterinary medicine. For veterinarians not only take possession of and promise to protect the valued property of others— they also engage to help beings that are "often as deeply revered as members of the family."[8] The Supreme Judicial Court of Massachusetts, upholding the revocation of the license of a physician who had been convicted of illegal possession of unregistered submachine guns, stated that any crime which is evidence of bad moral character or "undermines public confidence in the integrity of the profession" calls into question a doctor's "ability to practice."[9] This Court endorsed the traditional legal doctrine that:

> Mere intellectual power and scientific achievement without uprightness of character may be more harmful than ignorance. Highly trained intelligence combined with disregard of the fundamental virtues is a menace.[10]

The great majority of criminal offenses involve dishonesty or disrespect for the rights of others, traits a board could easily find inconsistent with the high moral standards essential to veterinary practice.

Conviction of any crime [MA, NY][11]

Some states permit the board to discipline a veterinarian on the grounds that he or she has been convicted of committing *any* crime, whether or not the crime is a felony or misdemeanor, involves moral turpitude, or relates to veterinary practice. Courts have upheld such provisions as a legitimate exercise of a state's strong interest in licensing only those with high moral character.[12]

Conviction of violation of federal or state drug laws

Although such crimes are almost always felonies, crimes of moral turpitude, or crimes evidencing an inability to practice veterinary medicine, many state practice acts make specific reference to drug offenses. Again, there is usually no requirement that the act giving rise to the drug conviction have been related to the licensee's ability to practice competently. In one case, the license of a California veterinarian was revoked in part because of his conviction of conspiracy to smuggle 12,000 pounds of marijuana into the country. The court reviewing the board's action stated that this act "would constitute a crime involving moral turpitude as far as a veterinarian is concerned."[13] Veterinarians should not be misled into thinking that conviction of only "serious" infractions of drug laws will endanger their licenses. Because of the special trust the law places on veterinarians regarding possession and dispensing of controlled substances, any conviction relating to misuse of such drugs is likely—and rightly—to result in discipline by one's state board.

Chronic inebriety or habitual use of or addiction to drugs

Drug use or dependency that interferes with one's ability to practice competently

The practice acts of some states[14] specify as a ground for discipline inebriety or drug use that has affected the veterinarian's ability to practice competently. However, many states do not impose such a restriction; they permit the board to suspend or revoke a license simply on the grounds that the practitioner is chronically affected by alcohol or drugs. A very strong argument can be made in favor of this stricter standard. Although it may be possible for some veterinarians who are impaired by alcohol or other drugs to guarantee that they will not be affected when they are providing professional services, for some practitioners, surely, the effects of drug use cannot be extinguished the moment one enters one's place of employment. In any event, the state licensing board's primary function is not to protect veterinarians but to safeguard the public and its animals. Given this function, it seems reasonable to err, if at all, on the side of keeping alcohol- or drug-impaired practitioners away from clients and animals until they are fully rehabilitated.

Traditionally, alcoholic- or drug-dependent practitioners were considered fundamentally bad, people of obviously deficient moral character. As a growing number of states adopt or endorse formal programs to rehabilitate alcoholic- or drug-impaired veterinarians, it can be argued that inebriety and drug dependency are coming to be viewed by practice acts as signs of medical illness rather than of moral badness. However, even where such programs exist, boards are still permitted a good deal of ethical deliberation. Impaired veterinarians can engage in outright immoral behavior. They can resort to illicit or illegal means to support their dependency. They can stubbornly deny their impairment and recklessly subject clients and animals to inferior services. Thus even where a board can divert impaired practitioners into a rehabilitation program, it usually still has the discretion to decide that they have acted so immorally that they merit punishment instead of or in addition to rehabilitation. Moreover, even where a board suspends or revokes the license of an impaired practitioner and considers her to be ill rather than evil, the board is still applying the fundamental *ethical* principle that underlies the inebriety and drug dependency standard—the public has the right to a veterinarian whose ability to function in a competent and trustworthy manner is beyond question.

Use of false, misleading, or deceptive advertising

Although the First Amendment of the U. S. Constitution prohibits the government from banning advertising by professionals, administrative bodies are authorized to protect the public against such abuses as false, deceptive, or misleading advertising by professionals.[15] Whether a board can constitutionally discipline a veterinarian for such things as "sensational or flamboyant"[16] advertising or "demonstrations, dramatizations, or other portrayals of professional practice on radio or television"[17] remains to be decided by the courts.

Conviction of cruelty to animals
Cruelty to animals [ID, IN, ME][18]
Conviction of cruelty or cruelty [NC][19]

Although the practice acts of some states mention cruelty to animals as a ground for discipline, the statutes of many others specify that the veterinarian must have been convicted of the crime of cruelty. Convictions of state cruelty-to-animal statutes are rare. All criminal convictions require proof beyond a reasonable doubt and adherence to strict rules of evidence and court procedure. Moreover, animal cruelty cases are seldom a high priority in overburdened prosecutors' offices. States that include cruelty to animals or patients as grounds for discipline permit the board itself to make an administrative determination of whether a practitioner has engaged in such behavior.

The employment of fraud, misrepresentation, or deception in obtaining a license
Fraud or dishonesty in the application of or reporting of any test for disease in animals
Fraudulent issuance or use of any health certificate, vaccination, test chart, or blank forms used in the practice of veterinary medicine to prevent the dissemination of animal disease, transportation of diseased animals, or the sale of inedible products of animal origin for human consumption [CO][20]
Misrepresentation in the inspection of food for human consumption [CO][21]
Fraud, deception, misrepresentation, dishonest or illegal practices in or connected with the practice of veterinary medicine [CO][22]
Failure to conduct one's practice on the highest plane of honesty, integrity, and fair dealing with clients in time and services rendered, and in the amount charged for services, facilities, appliances, and drugs [TX, WA][23]
Using the term "specialist" or an equivalent without being board-certified

Using the term "specialist" or an equivalent without being certified with the state board as a specialist [OH][24]

Provisions prohibiting deliberate fraud and misrepresentation have long been present in veterinary practice acts. The problem of fraudulent issuance of health and transportation documents is mentioned more fully in Chapter 23. Some veterinarians caught issuing fraudulent documents have been given temporary suspensions (usually a few months in duration) of their federal accreditation. A state veterinary board however, can temporarily—or permanently—remove one's ability to practice. A state board can do this either by relying on an administrative determination of fraud by the USDA or by making its own determination that there has been fraud or misrepresentation. Likewise, the profession's concern about practitioners who are not board-certified in a recognized specialty but call themselves "specialists"[25] could be addressed quickly and decisively by boards authorized to discipline doctors for misrepresentation.

Permitting, aiding, or abetting an unlicensed person to perform activities requiring a license

Permitting another to use one's license for the purpose of treating or offering to treat sick, injured, or afflicted animals [CO][26]

Knowingly maintaining a professional connection or association with any person who is in violation of provisions of the practice act or regulations of the board [FL][27]

There have been a number of court decisions upholding board discipline of doctors who have aided or abetted unlicensed persons to engage in the practice of veterinary medicine.[28]

Guaranteeing a cure or result

Violating the professional confidences of a client

Exercising undue influence on the patient or client, including the promotion of the sale of services, goods, appliances, or drugs in such a manner as to exploit the patient or client for the financial gain of the practitioner or of a third party [NY][29]

Paying or receiving kickbacks, rebates, bonuses, or other remuneration for receiving a patient or client or for referring a patient or client to another provider of veterinary services or goods

Attempting to restrict competition in the field of veterinary medicine other than for the protection of the public [FL][30]

These standards are intended to curtail unfair or anticompetitive business practices in which practitioners promote their own interests at the expense of individual clients, the public at large, or other veterinarians. Especially noteworthy is the prohibition, contained in many practice acts or regulations, against receiving or paying commissions, rebates, or kickbacks. Such a prohibition does not require a showing that a kickback influenced the judgment or choice of treatment of the doctor making or receiving it.

Engaging in lewd or immoral conduct in connection with the provision of veterinary services [AK, IN][31]

This provision appears intended to permit discipline for immoral behavior that does not necessarily reflect an inability to practice competently but nevertheless occurs during the providing of veterinary services. It can be argued that restriction of discipline to lewd or immoral conduct during professional activities protects practitioners against questionable objections to their personality, character, or lifestyle. On the other hand, restricting discipline to lewd or immoral behavior during the providing of veterinary services might sometimes subject clients to unfair risks by preventing board action until an egregious act has actually taken place during a practitioner's interactions with clients.

Disciplinary action taken in another state for a reason specified in this state's practice act or regulations as grounds for discipline

Failing to inform the board of disciplinary action taken against one by the licensing board of another state

At the time of this writing, the National Association of Veterinary State Boards was attempting to institute a national registry to collect information about disciplinary actions taken by all the state boards. Such a clearinghouse of data would enable each board to determine whether any of its licensees or applicants for a new license has already been disciplined in another state. Without such a registry, it is extremely difficult for a board to know about disciplinary action taken against a licensee in another state. There have been a number of instances in which veterinarians disciplined in one state have simply moved to another jurisdiction.[32] A specific requirement in a practice act or board regulations requiring disclosure of disciplinary action in another jurisdiction cannot itself guarantee that a licensee will make such disclosure. However, this requirement provides unassailable grounds for discipline if a board does discover that a licensee was disciplined elsewhere and failed to make this fact known.

Unprofessional conduct

Professional misconduct

Conduct reflecting unfavorably on the profession of veterinary medicine

These are the most general standards that can be applied by the boards. In some states, the practice act or regulations list kinds of conduct considered to be unprofessional. (Typically, these lists include such things as making fraudulent statements in an application for a license and false, deceptive advertising.) However, many practice acts provide no definition or examples of unprofessional conduct, misconduct, or conduct reflecting unfavorably on the profession. In these states, the board must decide either on a case-by-case basis or after promulgation of its own regulations what constitutes such conduct. Even practice acts that do provide examples of unprofessional conduct usually do not preclude the board from including other, unlisted kinds of behavior.

The courts have held that the phrases "unprofessional conduct," "professional misconduct," or "conduct reflecting unfavorably on the profession of veterinary medicine" are not impermissibly vague and can be used by the boards to discipline licensees.[33] These phrases can encompass behavior that the profession considers technically incompetent or ethically unacceptable.[34] As one court stated, unprofessional conduct "of necessity involve(s) conduct in the common judgment dishonorable;" moreover, a profession "so long established and regulated" as veterinary medicine has developed a storehouse of shared judgments about what is professionally dishonorable.[35]

A prohibition against unprofessional conduct permits a board to discipline a veterinarian for something that may not fall within the strict letter of a practice act provision or regulation but is nevertheless fundamentally incompatible with honorable practice. For example, cruelty to a patient is obviously unprofessional conduct for a veterinarian. Therefore it is clear that a board could revoke or suspend a practitioner's license for engaging in behavior the board determines was cruel or inhumane to a patient, even if the practice act lists *conviction* of cruelty to animals as a ground for discipline. Likewise, even if a practice act does not explicitly mention charging clients for services not actually rendered, putting undue pressure on clients to agree to certain procedures, or fraudulent completion of health certificates, as grounds for discipline, a board could clearly find such conduct—and many other kinds of behavior as well—fundamentally unprofessional.

Several states have incorporated the AVMA *Principles of Veterinary Medical Ethics* into their definitions of professional conduct.[36] An argument can be made in favor of this approach. As is explained in Chapter 9, the *Principles* reflect the profession's fundamental judgments about what it finds "in the common judgment dishonorable." A board that adopts the *Principles* can quickly have at its disposal, and in the hands of all doctors in the state, a lengthy and familiar set of ethical guidelines.

However, there are two strong arguments against wholesale incorporation of the *Principles* into state board definitions of professional conduct. First, as discussed in Chapter 9, the *Principles* are a text of *official* veterinary ethics. Among the most important functions of official veterinary ethics is promotion and protection of the *profession.* In contrast, the primary function of the state boards, and indeed all administrative veterinary ethical activity, is protection of the *public* and its *animals.*

Second, the constitutions of most states prohibit administrative agencies from delegating their responsibilities to others. It can be argued that adoption of the entire *Principles* by a state board would violate its obligation to determine on its own what constitutes professional or ethical conduct. This argument seems reasonable in light of the fact that official ethical standards tend by their nature to concentrate on the interests of members of the profession rather than on the public.

The state boards need not be prohibited from consulting the *Principles* as one source of standards of professional conduct, provided the boards exercise discretion and incorporate rules that truly protect the interests of the public and its animals.

⟨⟩ ASSESSING THE ACTIVITY OF STATE BOARDS IN APPLYING ETHICAL STANDARDS

It is virtually impossible at the present time to obtain an accurate general picture of how actively state boards are applying ethical standards. Although the laws of most states declare disciplinary decisions of licensing boards to be a matter of public record, very few veterinary licensing boards take it upon themselves to disclose, publish, or disseminate facts regarding disciplinary actions. It can be time-consuming, difficult, and costly to petition a state board for such information, even if one is entitled to it.

The California Board of Examiners in Veterinary Medicine is a notable exception to the apparent reluctance of some boards to publicize information regarding the discipline of licensees. The Board publishes a newsletter that details specific information about disciplined practitioners, including their name, address, the behavior forming the basis of the Board's action, and the disciplinary action taken. For example, one issue of this newsletter[37] reports the permanent revocation of the licenses of two doctors and the placing of a third on 5 years' probation. All three practitioners engaged in behavior that violated the Board's ethical standards. The doctor placed on probation deceived another doctor by falsifying a patient's biopsy report and not disclosing that he had performed surgery to remove a sponge from the animal's abdomen; this doctor also fraudulently and deceptively altered the medical records of another animal and performed several surgeries without knowledge or consent of their owners. One of the doctors whose license was revoked had been charged not only with various acts of negligence but also with employing fraud, misrepresentation, and deception in obtaining a practice permit. The second doctor whose license was revoked prescribed medication to employees and fabricated medical records. This same issue of the newsletter contains other advice of an ethical nature, including a discussion of the necessity of a veterinarian-client-patient relationship in renewing prescriptions used routinely by patients over a long period of time, and information about a new state law prohibiting licensing boards from renewing licenses of those in arrears of child or spousal support. Also included are a list of drugs most commonly abused by veterinarians and a discussion of how the state's prohibition against offering or receiving a rebate or commission for a referral prevents licensees from participating in a veterinary referral service.

I have been told by members of several state boards that they would like to follow the California Board's approach but lack sufficient staff or budget. The Board's newsletter is, I submit, a model to which all boards should aspire. It is impossible for veterinarians themselves to periodically request information about disciplinary and regulatory issues from their respective state board and then disseminate this information to colleagues in a manner that assures its accuracy. Such a process must be conducted by the boards themselves. They know best what they are doing and how they interpret their regulations. I know many veterinarians who have never read the veterinary practice act of their own state. Many veterinarians are unfamiliar with their board's technical and ethical regulations. Many do not know what kinds of complaints the board has been addressing. Many are ignorant of new statutory or regulatory provisions that can impose significant requirements. This is not the fault of doctors alone. Most have more than enough to do already. For the protection of clients, patients, and practitioners, the licensing boards must engage in serious and when necessary, repeated education of licensees regarding technical and ethical standards.

It is to be hoped that as more attention is paid by the profession and the public to veterinary ethics, ways will be found to determine accurately what all the licensing boards are doing in the ethical arena. Such information is necessary to be able to assess the effectiveness of administrative veterinary ethics in maintaining standards of professionalism in ways that are fair to patients, clients, and veterinarians.

∼ ADVANTAGES OF ADMINISTRATIVE APPLICATION OF ETHICAL STANDARDS

There are many potential advantages of the administrative application of ethical standards. It is usually much easier for a client to make a complaint of an ethical nature to an administrative agency than in a court of law. Veterinarians cannot be sued merely because they have acted unethically or unprofessionally; their actions must also have resulted in some compensable injury or damage to the client. Even where a client could prove such damage, it may cost more to prosecute the case than could be won in a trial. In contrast, administrative agencies typically permit a simple written complaint or telephone call to initiate an investigation, the costs of which are then borne by the agency.

Court trials and appeals can also stretch on for years, leaving both accused and accuser on tenterhooks. Most administrative agencies are not encumbered by rigid court procedures or rules of evidence and can resolve complaints and disputes relatively quickly. To the veterinarian, an administrative agency can also provide an audience that is more sensitive to the realities of veterinary practice than a civil court jury. Veterinary boards are composed largely (and in some states entirely) of veterinarians. Such people may be able quickly to see through unjust complaints. An administrative agency may also be able to settle a dispute or remedy a problem with a minimum of publicity.

Of course, the most significant potential advantage of the administrative application of ethical standards is that administrative bodies can compel adherence to moral norms. The AVMA or a state veterinary association for example, can suspend or revoke the membership of doctors who behave unethically. However, a veterinary board can suspend or revoke a doctor's license to practice or impose a wide spectrum of other incentives, ranging from censure to continuing supervision to (in some states) a fine.

⮠ PROBLEMS IN THE ADMINISTRATIVE APPLICATION OF ETHICAL STANDARDS

Unfortunately, some of the advantages of administrative application of ethical standards pose potential problems as well. In states in which people can complain against veterinarians with minimal trouble and expense, practitioners may find themselves easily exposed to frivolous or malicious complaints. Rigid rules of court procedure and evidence can sometimes delay discovery of the truth or resolution of a complaint. But these rules also protect the accused against allegations that cannot be substantiated or against accusers who cannot be cross-examined. The ability of a government agency to bear the costs of its investigation may assist complaining clients. However, this can be a disaster to a veterinarian, whose malpractice insurance does not cover legal fees for representation before an administrative agency or court appeals of its decision.

Application of ethical standards by the veterinary boards can pose special problems. A board's power to take away the ability to earn a living in one's chosen profession is frightening enough. However in addition, the boards can do this by appealing to a number of standards that are exceptionally vague or that might appear to give them virtually unbridled discretion to apply their own moral values.

What, after all, *is* bad moral character or unprofessional conduct? People differ about these things. Some may find bad moral character in a veterinarian who demonstrates against nuclear power by trespassing on the property of a nuclear plant, while others may see the same behavior as a brave moral act. For some, homosexuality is a vice utterly inconsistent with good moral character, while for others, it is a disease, and for still others, it is merely a different lifestyle. (Several jurisdictions now prohibit discrimination by government agencies against persons on the basis of sexual orientation; such a prohibition would presumably prevent a state board from denying the license to practice or disciplining a licensee on the grounds of sexual orientation alone.) Opinions about good moral character and professional conduct also change over time. In the 1950s several physicians had their licenses suspended by their medical board after they were found in contempt of Congress for refusing to cooperate with the House Committee on Un-American Activities.[38] Such disciplinary action would be highly unlikely today.

Veterinarians accused of bad moral character or unprofessional conduct or threatened with revocation of their license on the grounds that they have been convicted of a felony, a crime involving moral turpitude, or any crime may wonder whether they are being subjected to standards that simply reflect the moral tastes of their place and time.

∾ A TASK FOR ADMINISTRATIVE VETERINARY ETHICS

The answer to these potential difficulties is not for administrative agencies to turn their backs on ethics and to restrict themselves to issues of technical competence. The public has a moral and legal right not only to technically proficient veterinarians but also to doctors who are honest, trustworthy, and compassionate. The public and its animals must rely on some government intervention to promote these ideals. Good moral character and professional conduct are not irrelevant or outdated concepts because there have been some disagreements about how these concepts should be applied. Many of the ethical standards enforced by administrative bodies, such as prohibitions against theft, fraud, and illegal use of dangerous drugs, are unambiguous and clearly legitimate.

The study of current and proposed administrative ethical standards may help government bodies to articulate moral standards that reflect the legitimate interests of the public and its animals without infringing unduly upon veterinarians' personal values and lifestyles.

REFERENCES

[1] Davis KC: *Administrative Law Text*, ed 3, St. Paul, MN, 1972, West, p 1.
[2] UTAH CODE ANN. 58-28-4(1).
[3] *Raymond* v. *Board of Registration in Medicine*. 443 N.E.2d 391 (Mass. 1982).
[4] *Cartwright* v. *Board of Chiropractic Examiners*. 548 P.2d 1134 (Cal. 1976).
[5] Annot., 12 ALR3d 1213 (1967).
[6] Annot., 93 ALR2d 1398 (1964).
[7] CAL. BUS. & PROF. CODE 4883(a) (West 1994); FLA. STAT. ANN. 474.214(1)(c) (West 1994); IND. CODE ANN. 25-1-9-4(2) (Burns 1991).
[8] *Thorpe* v. *Board of Examiners in Veterinary Medicine*. 163 Cal.Rptr. 382, 385 (Cal. App. 1980).
[9] *Raymond* v. *Board of Registration in Medicine*. 443 N.E.2d 391, 395 (Mass. 1982).
[10] *Id*, at 394, quoting *Lawrence* v. *Board of Registration in Medicine*. 132 N.E. 174 (Mass. 1921).
[11] *Raymond* v. *Board of Registration in Medicine*. 443 N.E.2d 391 (Mass. 1982); N.Y. EDUC. LAW 6509(5)(a) (McKinney 1985).
[12] *See*, for example, *Barsky* v. *Board of Regents of the University of New York*. 11 N.E.2d 222, 226 (N.Y. 1953), *aff'd* 347 U.S. 442, 452 (1954); *Matter of Erdman* v. *Board of Regents of the State of New York*. 24 A.D.2d 698 (3d Dept. 1965); *Raymond* v. *Board of Registration in Medicine*. 443 N.E.2d 391 (Mass. 1982).
[13] *Thorpe* v. *Board of Board of Examiners in Veterinary Medicine*, 163 Cal.Rptr. 382, 385 (1980).
[14] For example, ALASKA STAT. 08.98.235(7)(B) (1991); ILL. ANN. STAT. ch. 225, 115/25.1.J (Smith-Hurd 1994).
[15] *Bates* v. *State Bar of Arizona*. 433 U.S. 350 (1977).
[16] Rules of The New York State Board of Regents Relating to Definitions of Unprofessional Conduct. 8 NYCRR 29.1(b)(12)(i)(a) (1981).
[17] *Id*, 29.1(12)(iv).
[18] IDAHO CODE 54-2113(12) (1993); IND. CODE ANN. 25-1-9-6 (Burns 1991); ME. REV. STAT. Ann. tit. 32, 4864(9) (1988).
[19] N.C. *Gen.* STAT. 187.8(c)(12) 1993.
[20] COLO. REV. STAT. 12-64-111(f) (1990).
[21] COLO. REV. STAT. 12-64-111(e) (1993).
[22] COLO. REV. STAT. 12-64-111(d) (1990).
[23] TEX. ADMIN. CODE tit. 22, 573.24; WASH. ADMIN. CODE R. 246-933-080 (1992).
[24] OHIO REV. CODE ANN. 4741.22(U) (Baldwin 1994).
[25] *See*, American Veterinary Medical Association: *Principles of Veterinary Medical Ethics*, 1993 Revision, "Guidelines for Use of Specialty Titles," *1994 AVMA Directory*, Schaumburg, IL, The Association, pp 86-87.
[26] COLO. REV. STAT. 12-64-111(s) (1990).

[27]FLA. STAT. ANN. 474.214(k) (West 1994).

[28]*See,* for example, *In re Walker's License,* 300 N.W. 800 (Minn. 1941); Hannah H: Professional association with unlicensed persons, *J Am Vet Med Assoc* 189:510-511, 1986.

[29]Rules of The New York State Board of Regents Relating to Definitions of Unprofessional Conduct. 8 NYCRR 29.1(b)(2) (1981).

[30]FLA. STAT. ANN. 474.214(n) (West 1994).

[31]ALASKA STAT. 08.98.235(8) (1991); IND. CODE ANN. 25-1-9-4(a)(5) (Burns 1991).

[32]Bixler T: Association creates registry, *DVM* 24(4):1, 1993..

[33]For example, *Hand* v. *Board of Examiners in Veterinary Medicine,* 136 Cal. Rptr. 187 (Cal. App. 1977); *Megdal* v. *Oregon State Board of Dental Examiners,* 586 P.2d 816 (Or. App. 1978); *Matter of Bell* v. *Board of Regents,* 65 N.E.2d 184 (N.Y. 1946).

[34]*Fitzgerald* v. *Board of Registration in Veterinary Medicine,* 507 N.E.2d 712 (Mass. 1987); *Willoughby* v. *Veterinary Examiners,* 82 N.M. 443 (1971).

[35]*In re Walker's License,* 300 N.W. 800 at 802 (Minn. 1941).

[36]For example, 49 PA. ADMIN. CODE 31.21(c) (Shepard's 1994).

[37]California Board of Examiners in Veterinary Medicine: *News and Views,* Summer 1993, the Board.

[38]*Barsky et al.* v. *Board of Regents of The University of New York.* 111 N.E.2d 222 (N.Y. 1953).

CHAPTER 8

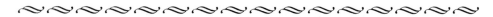

The Nature and Functions of Official Veterinary Ethics

Official veterinary ethics is the process of the articulation and application of ethical standards for veterinarians by the organized profession. Official veterinary ethics is a rich and complex enterprise. This chapter presents an overview of its structure, functions, and substantive standards. Chapter 9 considers the two core texts of official veterinary ethics: the Veterinarian's Oath and the *Principles of Veterinary Medical Ethics.*

∼ OFFICIAL PROFESSIONAL ETHICS

It is no accident that professions, such as veterinary medicine, law, and medicine, have developed procedures by which members articulate and enforce ethical standards for themselves. The process of self-imposed regulation, both ethical and technical, distinguishes what we call the learned professions from occupations. Engineers or business executives may learn their trade at an accredited school, may be regulated by governmental bodies, and may join associations that promote their interests. But their training and supervision differ markedly from that of the veterinarian, lawyer, or physician. The latter attended a school, the curriculum of which must meet the expectations of their respective organized professions and indeed are unlikely to be approved by licensing authorities unless they meet these expectations. Although professionals must be licensed to practice and are regulated by governmental bodies, these bodies give great deference to what the organized professions deem to be appropriate behavior— from the choice of acceptable schools and training programs, to the standards of competence expected of practitioners, to the values that define acceptable professional behavior.

Most importantly, fields traditionally recognized as professions have a long history of officially agreeing upon ethical codes that express their most central moral ideals. They have invested these codes with dignity and importance by creating and enforcing them much like the law creates and enforces—code standards are adopted by formal vote of representatives of the profession, and they are applied by quasijudicial bodies that resemble courts of law. The ethical self-regulation of a profession like veterinary medicine is so central to the definition of an individual as a veterinarian that even practitioners who do not choose to belong to the AVMA will have great difficulty convincing a court of law or administrative government body that the official ethical standards do not apply to them.

⮑ WHAT OFFICIAL VETERINARY ETHICS IS NOT

Although official veterinary ethics by its very nature involves veterinarians deciding upon and applying ethical standards for veterinarians, there are several things official ethics does not entail.

First, an official decision that some kind of behavior is right or wrong does not make that conduct right or wrong. Veterinarians, like other people, can be mistaken in their moral judgments and therefore can be mistaken in their official ethical pronouncements.

Second, neither veterinarians nor the public need view the official ethical apparatus as the sole or final judge of ethical issues involving practitioners. Administrative bodies, for example, must come to their own conclusions about the propriety of certain kinds of behavior by veterinarians. Veterinarians can also regard official standards as open to debate in forums in which veterinarians do not control the outcome. However, such discussions cannot be considered part of the process of official veterinary ethics, although changes in official standards made by veterinarians motivated by discussion with nonveterinarians will be part of official professional ethics.

Third, although decisions regarding official ethics are controlled by veterinarians, there is nothing that prevents nonveterinarians from observing or participating in the process of developing and applying official standards. Ethicists, lawyers, and members of the public and other learned professions can be consulted about (and might even be given limited voting power regarding) official norms.

⮑ WHO NEEDS OFFICIAL VETERINARY ETHICS?

Because official standards need not coincide with moral truth, several philosophers have questioned the wisdom of allowing the professions to engage in official ethics. Medical ethicist Robert Veatch, for example, concludes that official professional ethics "can have *no* ethical bite."[1] "The fact that a professional or his or her group believes that a confidence should be kept, a patient killed, or an advertisement proscribed cannot definitively resolve the issue of whether each of these acts is ethically or legally right."[2] Veatch finds it "strange that lay people and professionals alike assume that it is correct for professions to form their own codes of ethics and then adjudicate ethical disputes arising out of the application of these codes."[3] Issues of professional ethics, Veatch insists, should be the business not only of professionals but also of the clients they serve and indeed of anyone who is affected by their actions.

Veatch is surely correct that official decisions cannot be the sole means of resolving ethical questions regarding professionals. It is also possible that, in the past, some people in the professions and the public have granted official ethics too much authority. However, official ethics still has a useful role in addressing ethical concerns.

One important benefit of official ethics is its ability to address moral issues effectively and efficiently. Neither government nor the populace has the time or resources constantly to monitor the ethical values of any of the professions. The public may take an interest in certain flashy issues (such as animal experimentation). But its attention to such matters can be fleeting, and it may never focus sustained attention on some of the less conspicuous ethical issues arising from everyday professional practice.

Official veterinary ethics offers an apparatus that is continuously in place raising questions and suggesting solutions. Sometimes, this apparatus can effectively compel adherence to ethical norms without expenditure of resources by government or by disgruntled clients or members of the public. If government and the public like what they see, they can leave the process of official ethics alone. If society has questions about the official ethical positions of the profession, it can ask the profession to justify its standards. By demanding reasons or justifications from the profession as a whole, the public can expect informed and carefully presented responses prepared with the resources available to the official apparatus.

The following are just two examples that illustrate the value of official veterinary ethics.

In 1977 the U. S. Supreme Court ruled that professionals have a constitutionally protected right to advertise.[4] The Court also stated that certain kinds of inappropriate advertising could be prohibited by government or the professions. However, the Court deliberately refrained from defining or listing all kinds of advertising that could be proscribed, leaving suggestions for new legal standards to future cases and emerging attitudes. Like other professions, veterinary medicine had to reconsider many of its previous disapprovals of advertising and had to search for new ethical rules that would meet yet undefined constitutional requirements. By allowing veterinary medicine to discover new advertising standards, the law gained several benefits. First, it could count on the official apparatus to assure that the old blanket prohibitions against advertising were not enforced. Second, the law could call on the official apparatus to do something courts are rarely good at, the process of changing entrenched values and nurturing over time new attitudes consistent with new freedoms. Finally, the law could ask the profession to begin looking for ethical standards that reflect not only the legal right to advertise but also specific ethical needs and concerns of veterinarians. In the years since the decision permitting professional advertising, this process of probing the limits of professionally acceptable marketing by the official ethical apparatus has continued. Should the courts need to decide how far the profession can go in limiting professional marketing, they will have at their disposal, to assist them, a substantial body of official ethical deliberations, contained both in the Advertising section of the *Principles of Veterinary Medical Ethics* and in the pronouncements of the AVMA Judicial Council.

A second valuable use of official veterinary ethics involves its ability to resolve disputes before they result in lawsuits or government action. As noted in Chapter 4, malpractice lawsuits against veterinarians are sometimes brought because clients believe their veterinarian has acted unethically. By settling some of these complaints, state ethics and grievance committees and the AVMA Judicial Council can spare veterinarians and clients unnecessary and costly litigation. Resolution of ethical issues by the official professional apparatus can sometimes also make intervention by the state veterinary licensing board unnecessary.

In addition to its ability to address moral disputes, official ethics plays a crucial role in binding together veterinarians as a unified profession that can speak forcefully to both members and the public. This cohesiveness enables the profession to improve the competence of practitioners by helping it promote strong veterinary school curricula, effective continuing education programs, dissemination of knowledge, and veterinary research. As part of the cement that strengthens the profession, official veterinary ethics contributes to better services for patients and clients.

∽ THE STRUCTURE OF OFFICIAL VETERINARY ETHICS
Component Organizations of Official Ethics

Because the profession articulates and applies standards of official ethics, only groups that are part of the organized profession can be considered components of official ethics. There can be no disagreement that the AVMA and the state and local veterinary medical associations recognized by the AVMA are part of the structure of official veterinary ethics. All these organizations are considered by the great majority of veterinarians not as limited groups seeking to promote some kind of viewpoint or platform but as elements of a national apparatus that in its totality, speaks for the profession. Moreover, the AVMA and state and local associations all subscribe to a universal code of ethics for all American practitioners, the AVMA *Principles of Veterinary Medical Ethics.*

It is clearly a task for the profession itself to decide what groups will be considered part of its official apparatus for the purposes of articulating ethical standards. This process is an ongoing one—a group that today might not be considered part of the apparatus or on the borderline, might tomorrow be recognized as part of it. For the purposes of this discussion, I want to suggest that at the very least, any association with representation in the AVMA House of Delegates be considered a component of the organized profession and therefore capable of taking part in official veterinary ethics. Such representation is a sign that an organization is considered a part of the organic whole of the profession.*

The fact that an organization can qualify as a proponent of official ethical standards does not mean it is or should be active in the ethical area. Moreover, that an organization is not part of the official apparatus does not mean the profession should ignore its views in formulating official norms.

The American Veterinary Medical Association

The *Principles of Veterinary Medical Ethics* state that "[q]uestions of ethical and professional behavior on the part of a veterinarian should be considered and dealt with first by the local associations' ethics or grievance committees. Members of such committees are familiar with local customs and circumstances and are in a position to confer with all parties concerned."[5]

Although ethical issues usually can be handled most effectively at the local level, the AVMA remains the foundation for all of official veterinary ethics. When local, state, or practice associations discipline a practitioner or take a position on an ethical issue, they apply the AVMA *Principles* and other official AVMA ethical pronouncements. (The *Principles* themselves urge component associations to adopt the *Principles* "or a similar code"[6]; because there is no other such code, it is not surprising that the *Principles* are followed.) Component associations also look to the national standards, because these organizations are represented in the AVMA House of Delegates and

---

*Article VI, Section 1 of the AVMA Bylaws provides criteria for representation in the House of Delegates. By 1994 the following practice associations were included: the American Animal Hospital Association (AAHA); the American Associations of Avian Pathologists, Bovine Practitioners, Equine Practitioners, Feline Practitioners, Food Hygiene Veterinarians, Industrial Veterinarians, Small Ruminant Practitioners, Swine Practitioners, and Veterinary Clinicians; the American Society of Laboratory Animal Practitioners; the Association of Avian Veterinarians; the National Association of Federal Veterinarians; and the Society for Theriogenology. All state veterinary medical associations (VMAs) are represented in the House of Delegates.

therefore play a role in the adoption of these standards. Finally, the AVMA Judicial Council is very much a general reviewing body on issues of veterinary ethics throughout the profession. The Council hears cases referred by constituent associations; it is asked to provide definitive opinions about the appropriateness of certain kinds of behavior; and it is charged with preparation of annotations and amendments to the universally-adopted *Principles.*

The Judicial Council is the chief regulatory arm of the AVMA regarding official ethics. It consists of five active members elected by the House of Delegates and has "jurisdiction on all questions of veterinary medical ethics."[7] The Council can investigate complaints of an ethical nature by itself or can request the AVMA President to appoint "investigating juries" to which it can refer complaints or evidence "of unethical conduct, which in its judgment, are of a serious and substantial nature."[8] Such juries can then file complaints under the formal Rules of Disciplinary Procedures of the AVMA.[9] These set forth procedures by which the Council hears and adjudicates complaints. The General Appellate Procedures of the AVMA contain rules for reconsideration of an adjudication by the Judicial Council and appeal to the AVMA Board of Governors.[10]

The Council can make five kinds of adjudication: acquittal, censure, probation, suspension, or expulsion from the AVMA. However, the Council is not restricted to the explicit provisions of the *Principles of Veterinary Medical Ethics* or of other official AVMA ethical pronouncements. It may also discipline a member who has been convicted of a "felony or a crime involving moral turpitude" or who has been "guilty of other behavior detrimental to the profession of veterinary medicine."[11]

The notion of being "detrimental" to the profession is vague and could conceivably be used in ways some might find arbitrary. Nevertheless, this provision is an important tool for the advancement of official veterinary ethics. It allows the Council to explore and define new standards much as courts do, by responding on a case-by-case basis to situations that may not be covered by existing rules.

The Council makes its views known to the profession in regular reports in the *Journal of the American Veterinary Medical Association.* These reports provide the best evidence of what ethical issues the organized profession finds most pressing and how official norms are likely to develop. They show that for several years the major concern of official ethics has remained the proper limits of advertising, promotion, and marketing.[12] In 1993 the Council took a number of important actions,[13] including the following: (1) revising the section of the *Principles* dealing with "Commissions, Rebates, and Influences on Judgment" to prohibit kickbacks for referrals to nonveterinarian providers of services; (2) concluding that a coupon rebate program of two pharmaceutical companies would place participating veterinarians in conflict with the *Principles*; (3) proposal of an official policy to track felony convictions of members so that convicted felons would not only be expelled from the AVMA but would be denied membership after any such conviction; (4) advising a veterinary hospital and several practitioners that to advertise or represent themselves as specialists, the *Principles* require that each be a diplomate of an approved specialty board; (5) advising a veterinary school facility that one of its advertisements was misleading; and (6) requesting each state and allied association to establish an ethics and grievance committee if it did not yet have one in place.

State and Local Veterinary Medical Associations

There are many state and local VMAs, and not all VMAs report their activities as comprehensively as does the AVMA. It is therefore difficult to offer general characterizations regarding their activity in addressing ethical concerns. However, based on frequent contacts with members of state and local VMAs in various regions of the country and on events reported in the press, I believe I can report with confidence an emerging trend in official ethics at the state and local levels.

Most state and many regional or local VMAs have ethics and grievance committees, as recommended by the AVMA. However, many of these committees are reluctant to hold formal proceedings to adjudicate complaints of an ethical nature against a member. Moreover, few members of VMAs are eager to file a formal complaint of an ethical nature against a member. There appear to be two reasons for this reluctance, both of which are justified. First, many VMAs are aware of investigations or threatened prosecutions of veterinary associations by the Federal Trade Commission for restraint of trade (see Chapter 19). Fearful of the expense and potential consequences of FTC action, a number of VMAs will not do anything that could be interpreted as an attempt to hinder the activities of any doctor. Second, many VMAs and individual members who would like their ethics and grievance committee to consider a complaint of an ethical nature against a member are fearful of being sued by that practitioner for defamation of character. Although some veterinary malpractice policies cover defamation, knowledge of this fact does not appear to increase the palatability of being a defendant in a defamation case. The high cost or lack of availability of association liability insurance can dampen any initial enthusiasm of an ethics and grievance committee to investigate an ethical complaint.

Although many VMAs seem unwilling to discipline (or to threaten discipline of) individual members, several have taken a course that may be both safer and more effective. They are addressing their ethical concerns to government agencies: legislatures, administrative agencies (such as state licensing boards), and the courts. In short, VMAs are taking their ethical concerns public, sometimes with remarkable effectiveness. The following are but a few representative examples.

In 1990 the California VMA persuaded that state's Governor to veto a bill which would have allowed any layperson to remove tartar from above an animal's gum line; the CVMA persisted in opposing this bill when it was introduced again the following year. The Georgia state legislature passed an amendment to the veterinary practice act submitted by the Georgia VMA specifically including dentistry within the definition of the practice of veterinary medicine thereby prohibiting unlicensed practitioners from performing dental procedures on animals.[14] In response to the sale of pet vaccination kits to the general public by a chain of pharmacies, the Maryland VMA supported legislation to prohibit over-the-counter or mail-order sales of syringes and needles.[15] In 1993 the New Jersey VMA brought to the attention of a city health officer and the state veterinary licensing board the activities of a vaccination clinic to be conducted in a retail pet "superstore." This led to the temporary suspension of the clinic pending the receipt of an appropriate waste disposal permit. The state board required that the clinic comply with regulations applicable to all mobile facilities in the state and that it employ area veterinarians to whom clients could have access should problems develop.[16,17] The Pennsylvania VMA and three local associations joined in a lawsuit seeking to prohibit a mobile vaccination clinic from conducting business at pet stores, schools, and munici-pal buildings on the grounds that the ownership of the operation by persons who were not licensed veterinarians violated state board regulations.[18] The Massachusetts VMA submitted a bill to its state legislature that would prevent anyone from suing a veteri-narian who in good faith reports a case of suspected animal abuse to an appropriate enforcement authority. The California VMA successfully opposed a bill that would place a special tax on dog food to construct and operate government-owned spay and neuter facilities.[19] The Minnesota VMA objected to a pet food tax on the grounds that it would cost consumers more than they would benefit from the small, partial subsidy for spays and neuters to which the tax was to be applied.[20]

Addressing ethical concerns to governmental bodies generally avoids the possibility of lawsuits for defamation of character. The law affords people a privilege against such lawsuits when they petition their government for relief, if they utilize appropriate gov-ernment mechanisms and make their case in good faith. Addressing ethical concerns to the government can also be more effective than instituting investigations against indi-vidual association members, because government action can affect larger groups of people and is not, like the jurisdiction of a VMA ethics and grievance committee, restricted to members of the VMA.

The apparent trend toward open airing of ethical concerns by state and local VMAs is also exemplified by the extent to which some associations have become involved in public education and public health campaigns. The Massachusetts VMA, for example, conducts forums and makes members available to the news media to educate people about the dangers of the animal rabies epizootic in the region. Several VMAs utilize open discussion to address ethical issues by placing sessions on ethical issues or holding entire continuing education meetings on such matters as practitioner advertising, criti-cism of colleagues, animal welfare, and ethical issues in animal research. In New York, the Westchester-Rockland County VMA devotes a portion of each issue of its newslet-ter to ethical questions and member responses. Several VMAs have standing animal welfare committees and others utilize their ethics and grievance committee to report periodically to the membership about recurring ethical issues.

The enthusiasm with which VMAs appear to be embracing the consideration of ethical issues may play an important role in motivating all veterinarians to make atten-tion to ethics an essential part of their professional activity.

Practice Associations

Associations defined by the nature of the practices of their members rather than geographical location can bring especially valuable points of view to the articulation of official standards. The interests of these organizations transcend regional issues but are at the same time more focused than those of the AVMA. Practice associations can artic-ulate their own ethical rules, which can differ from the ethical standards of other asso-ciations or the AVMA itself. For example, AAHA adopted a policy permitting the dis-play of nonprofessional products in waiting rooms, although such behavior was pro-hibited at the time by the AVMA *Principles.* In 1993 AAHA's Animal Welfare Committee formulated its own policy (similar to a 1976 AVMA policy) recommending that ear cropping be removed from dog breed standards because of the procedure's sur-gical and anesthetic risks.[21] The American Association of Equine Practitioners (AAEP) also has a standing animal welfare committee, which, like the AAHA committee, conducts an animal welfare session at each of the association's annual national meetings. The AAEP has been active in addressing concerns raised about the treatment of racehorses. It has issued policies or recommendations on, for example, proper veterinary examination for pre-race soundness[22] and the use of corticosteroids[23] prior to racing.

～ OVERVIEW OF THE SUBSTANTIVE STANDARDS OF OFFICIAL VETERINARY ETHICS

Like standards of administrative ethics, statements of official veterinary ethics vary in the manner in which they express moral values. Some official standards are purely ethical, in the sense that they are restricted to judgments about what is obligatory or ideal; the Veterinarian's Oath and *Principles of Veterinary Medical Ethics* are examples of such official standards. Some official texts offer statements about scientific or medical matters together with ethical judgments relating to these matters. The AVMA Positions on Animal Welfare[24] contains provisions (for example, those dealing with animal agriculture, and veal calf care and production) that set forth factual contentions as well as ethical judgments. Still other statements of official veterinary ethics are largely scientific or medical in nature but can still be classified as expressions of official ethics because their underlying motivation is moral in nature. The *Report of the AVMA Panel on Euthanasia*[25] a scientific discussion based on the ethical judgment that animals to be killed must be euthanized humanely, is an example of this kind of approach.

The following are the most important substantive standards of official veterinary ethics.

The Veterinarian's Oath

The Veterinarian's Oath expresses the most general values of the profession. Professional oaths are not intended to provide a decision procedure for the solution of all ethical issues. They are offered to inspire in practitioners a sensitivity to core values and goals.

The Principles of Veterinary Medical Ethics

This is the definitive statement of the profession's official ethical standards. Like the codes of other professions, the *Principles* are an amalgam of general ideals and specific requirements and prohibitions.

Adjudications, Advisory Opinions, and Statements of Official Judicial Bodies

The AVMA Judicial Council and state and local VMA ethics and grievance committees apply official ethical standards to particular cases. These judicial bodies make different kinds of judgments that take on independent significance in the enunciation of official standards.

An adjudication is an official response to an actual complaint against a member of the professional association. Adjudications are often accompanied by an expression of a general principle justifying the decision. When reports of adjudications are disseminated to the profession, they can serve as general warnings about, or approvals of, the kinds of behavior involved in the particular case. An advisory opinion is a pronouncement by a judicial body, not part of an adjudication of an actual complaint, regarding a matter about which ethical guidance has been requested. Advisory opinions can be prompted by the request of a practitioner or association about the appropriateness of some activity in which they would like to engage. An advisory opinion can also be sought after some conduct has occurred, but it is raised hypothetically to the judicial body with the hope of bringing a practitioner into line before a formal complaint must be brought. Advisory opinions can apply to individual practitioners or to general kinds of behavior. Like adjudications, advisory opinions can put practitioners on notice about what the judicial body is likely to do if confronted with a certain kind of situation. A judicial body can also issue statements at its own instigation expressing its concern about certain kinds of behavior that have come to its attention.

Reports and Statements of Delegated Bodies

Veterinary associations, such as the AVMA, also have standing councils or committees and specially designated bodies or panels that issue statements and recommendations of an ethical nature. Because these bodies can be delegated the responsibility to issue such statements by the association, their opinions represent the views of a portion of the official organizational apparatus. Statements of delegated bodies can be proposed to the representative body for inclusion in the ethical code or an official policy statement. One of the most important standing committees of official veterinary ethics is the AVMA Animal Welfare Committee, comprised of members representing various kinds of practice. This committee proposes statements for inclusion in the AVMA's official policies. One of the most important special bodies of official veterinary ethics is the AVMA Panel on Euthanasia, which is appointed periodically to survey and recommend humane methods of euthanasia for various species and kinds of animals. The guidelines contained in the Panel's *Report of the AVMA Panel on Euthanasia* are expected to be followed by members of the AVMA and are also required to be used in research facilities that come under the jurisdiction of the federal Animal Welfare Act.

Official Policies, Positions, Statements, and Guidelines

Veterinary associations can also adopt ethical views directed at a wide range of practice or social issues. These official views can take different forms, such as general policies that express abstract ideals, more specific positions on various kinds of issues, statements directed at a particular problem or question, and rules or guidelines to be applied by practitioners in certain situations.

The AVMA has a set of policies, positions, statements, and guidelines that provide supplementation to the *Principles of Veterinary Medical Ethics* and stand in their own right as important standards of official veterinary ethics. Some of these texts enunciate recommendations that practitioners are strongly urged to follow; others contain definitive prohibitions that can be applied in official disciplinary proceedings.

In recent years, most debates regarding what official ethical views should be endorsed by the profession have not centered around the Veterinarian's Oath or the *Principles.* Those who wish to reaffirm, amplify, or change official ethical standards have instead turned to the process by which the AVMA generates official policy statements on ethical issues.

Table 8-1 lists the major official ethical statements of the AVMA. These statements occupy several dozen pages of the annual *AVMA Directory.* In their totality, they are

TABLE 8-1
⮂

Major ethical policies and positions of the AVMA

OFFICIAL POLICY	DATE OF ADOPTION OR LAST REVISION
Animal Welfare*	
Protocol for the Tattoo Identification of Dogs and Cats that Have Been Spayed or Neutered	1980
Guidelines for Horseshow Veterinarians	1982
Memorandum of Understanding for Humane Organizations and Veterinarians	1982
Guidelines for Veterinary Associations and Veterinarians Working with Humane Organizations	1983
Guidelines for Veterinarians Participating in Ovariohysterectomy-Orchiectomy Clinics	1984
Guidelines on Emergency Veterinary Service	1988
Wild Animals as Pets	1990
Positions on Animal Welfare	1993
AVMA Policy on Animal Welfare and Animal Rights	
Companion Animals, Horses, and Wildlife	
Use of Animals in Research and Teaching	
Animal Agriculture	
AVMA Guide for Veal Calf Care and Production	
Position on Controlled Substances	1993
Position on Early-age Spay/Neuter of Dogs and Cats	1994
Position on Ferrets	1994
Client/Consumer Protection	
Protocol for the Tattoo Identification for Dogs and Cats that have been Spayed or Neutered	1980
Guidelines for Horseshow Veterinarians	1982
Guidelines on Pet Health Insurance and Other 3rd Party Animal Health Plans	1985
Guidelines on Emergency Veterinary Service	1988
Guidelines for the Naming of Veterinary Facilities	1988
Position on Drug Use in Show Animals	1990
Prescription Writing	1993
Guidelines for Use of Specialty Titles	1993
Guidelines for Veterinary Prescription Drugs	1994
Guidelines on Surgery for the Correction of an Injury	1994
Position on Ferrets	1994
Public Health and Safety	
Position on Presigned Health Certificates	1974
Position on Use of Sodium Pentobarbital by Lay Persons	1981
Dangerous Animal Legislation	1988
Guidelines on Management of Clinical Listeroisis	1988
Wild Animals as Pets	1990
Position of the AVMA's Professional Liability Insurance Trust on Vaccination of "Wolf Hybrids"	1992
Recommended Minimal Standards of Performance for Practicing Veterinarians Who Offer Milk Quality Control Programs	1992
Model Rabies Control Ordinance	1993
Position on Controlled Substances	1993
Position on Pasteurization of All Milk	1993
Position on Ferrets	1994

*Official policies that address more than one kind of concern are listed in additional categories. This table reflects policies as of the 1994 meeting of the House of Delegates.

TABLE 8-1 CONT'D

Major ethical policies and positions of the AVMA

OFFICIAL POLICY	DATE OF ADOPTION OR LAST REVISION
Professional Regulation and Improvement	
Guidelines for Horseshow Veterinarians	1982
Memorandum of Understanding for Humane Organizations and Veterinarians	1982
Statement on Continuing Education in Bovine Mastitis	1982
Guidelines for Veterinary Associations and Veterinarians Working with Humane Organizations	1983
Model Program to Assist Chemically Impaired Veterinarians, Veterinary Students, Animal Technicians and Their Families	1985
Embryo Transfer and the Practice of Veterinary Medicine	1986
Guidelines on Alternate Therapies	1988
Guidelines for the Naming of Veterinary Facilities	1988
Guidelines for Use of Volunteers in Veterinary Practice	1988
Guidelines for Referrals	1990
Peer Review Procedures Manual	1990
AVMA Strategic Plan	1991
Position on Embryo Transplant Procedures	1991
Guidelines for Hazards in the Workplace	1992
Guidelines for Veterinary Practice Facilities	1992
Model Veterinary Practice Act	1992
Position on Animal Dentistry	1992
Prescription Writing	1993
Guidelines for Use of Special Titles	1993
Guidelines for Veterinary Prescription Drugs	1994
Model Policy on Harassment	1994

many times lengthier than the *Principles*, and they are growing longer. The table also indicates that the pace of adoption of official ethical policies appears to be accelerating. Most of the policies are of recent adoption, and each succeeding year tends to see additional ethical policy statements. While the *Principles* are viewed by the AVMA much as the U.S. legal system views a constitution—a fundamental statement of values that should not be changed—the process of adopting ethical policies seems to be regarded as akin to legislation. Like a legislature, the AVMA House of Delegates is open each year for the business of voting on proposed rules. A body whose function is to consider proposed policies is probably destined to keep adding to the number of policies it approves.

Moreover, the process by which ethical statements are proposed and considered can be heated and exciting. Sometimes, an ethical statement will be drafted by an AVMA standing committee and approved without much comment in the House of Delegates. However, those who seek approval of an official ethical policy can also petition the House of Delegates to consider the policy directly in the form of a resolution. This can lead to vigorous debate of a sort that rarely arises regarding suggested revisions to the *Principles of Veterinary Medical Ethics*. For example, for years the statement in the AVMA's Positions on Animal Welfare had said that steeljaw leghold traps are "considered by many to be inhumane," insisted that such traps "may be used legitimately in some aspects of wildlife management and predator and pest control by reasonable and informed trappers," but added that use of these traps "should be discouraged as soon as acceptable alternatives become available." In 1993 a resolution was submitted to the House declaring that the AVMA opposes the use of these traps, whether padded or unpadded, as cruel. The AVMA Executive Board recommended disapproval of the resolution on the grounds that the word "cruel" was not helpful but proposed its own statement that "the AVMA considers the steel-jaw leghold trap to be inhumane." The resulting debate in the House was vigorous. Impassioned arguments in favor and against the existing and proposed policies were made by several delegates. In the end, the old policy was overturned and the characterization of the traps as "inhumane" was adopted.[26]

This example also illustrates an important difference between provisions in the *Principles* and official ethical pronouncements approved by the AVMA House of Delegates. For reasons that will be explained more fully in Chapter 9, statements do not appear in the *Principles* unless they are acceptable to virtually all veterinarians. In this sense, the code can be said to be backward-looking; it tends to follow what the profession has already accepted. In contrast, the new statement on leghold traps is controversial. Some veterinarians do not like it. Nevertheless, the adoption of the policy on traps probably indicates that the sentiments of most doctors have changed. The policy was adopted in part to encourage others to change their minds as well. At the time they are adopted, official ethical policies therefore tend to reflect how the profession is developing and the ethical issues the profession's leaders believe will occupy center stage in the future.

Many veterinarians appear to be unfamiliar with the official AVMA ethical policies, positions, statements, and guidelines. This is unfortunate, because these texts contain much of substance and value and much that can stimulate discussion and debate.

REFERENCES

[1]Veatch RM: *A Theory of Medical Ethics*, New York, 1981, Basic Books, p 97, emphasis added.
[2]*Id*, p 110.
[3]*Id*, p 100.
[4]*Bates* v. *State Bar of Arizona*, 433 U.S. 350 (1977).
[5]American Veterinary Medical Association: *Principles of Veterinary Medical Ethics*, 1993 Revision, "Relationships of Local, State, and National Associations on Matters of Ethics," *1994 AVMA Directory*, Schaumburg, IL, The Association, p 42.
[6]American Veterinary Medical Association: *Principles of Veterinary Medical Ethics*, 1993 Revision, "General Concepts," *1994 AVMA Directory*, Schaumburg, IL, The Association, p 42.
[7]American Veterinary Medical Association: AVMA Bylaws, Art V. Sec. 2(b)(ii), *1994 AVMA Directory*, Schaumburg, IL, The Association, p 34.
[8]American Veterinary Medical Association: AVMA Bylaws, Art. V. Sec. 2(b)(iv), *1994 AVMA Directory*, Schaumburg, IL, The Association, p 34.
[9]American Veterinary Medical Association: Rules of Disciplinary Procedures of the AVMA, 1990 Revision, *1994 AVMA Directory*, Schaumburg, IL, The Association, p 47.
[10]American Veterinary Medical Association: General Appellate Procedures of the American Veterinary Medical Association, *1994 AVMA Directory*, Schaumburg, IL, The Association, pp 48-49.
[11]American Veterinary Medical Association: AVMA Bylaws, Art. I. Sec. 8, *1994 AVMA Directory*, Schaumburg, IL, The Association, p 31.
[12]For examples of the Judicial Council's historical focus on such issues, *see*, for example, Specialist designation a Judicial Council concern, *J Am Vet Med Assoc* 181:859, 1982; Council proposes "Principle" revisions, *J Am Vet Med Assoc* 184:913, 1984; Judicial Council looks at discount advertising, *J Am Vet Med Assoc* 189:10, 1986.
[13]1993 AVMA activities summary: Judicial Council, *J Am Vet Med Assoc* 204:586-588, 1994.
[14]Amid controversy, Calif., Ga., say "no" to lay dentists, *DVM* 22(6):4, 1991.

[15]Miller J: OTC sale of syringes unleashes explosive confrontation between DVMs, supermarket chain, *DVM* 22(12):8, 1991.

[16]New Jersey DVMs help stall Petco vaccination clinic, *DVM* 24(12):4, 1993.

[17]Stultz TB: Pet vaccine company battles it out with New Jersey veterinary board, *DVM* 25(5):4, 1994.

[18]Pennsylvania files suit, *J Am Vet Med Assoc* 202:1796, 1993.

[19]CVMA boasts success in legislative effort, *DVM* 23(8):3, 1992.

[20]Verdon DR: Minn. proposes pet food tax to curb overpopulation, *DVM* 22(6):4, 1991.

[21]Suttell RD: Ear cropping debate continues to simmer, *DVM* 24(8)9, 1993.

[22]Bixler T: AAEP committee writes guidelines concerning pre-race inspections, *DVM* 24(2):1, 1993.

[23]Verdon DR: AAEP takes stand on steroid use; racing federation sits on position, *DVM* 22(4):1, 1991.

[24]American Veterinary Medical Association: Positions on Animal Welfare, *1994 AVMA Directory*, Schaumburg, IL, The Association, pp 56-59.

[25]*1993 Report of the AVMA Panel on Euthanasia*, *J Am Vet Med Assoc* 202:232-233, 1993.

[26]House tightens grip on leghold trap, *J Am Vet Med Assoc* 203:594, 1993.

CHAPTER 9

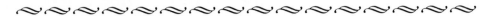

Oath and Principles

*T*wo documents of official veterinary ethics, the Veterinarian's Oath and the *Principles of Veterinary Medical Ethics* are of paramount importance to the profession and require separate discussion.

∾ THE VETERINARIAN'S OATH

In 1969 the AVMA House of Delegates adopted the Veterinarian's Oath. It reads as follows:

Being admitted to the profession of veterinary medicine,
    I solemnly swear to use my scientific knowledge and skills for the benefit of society through the protection of animal health, the relief of animal suffering, the conservation of livestock resources, the promotion of public health, and the advancement of medical knowledge.
    I will practice my profession conscientiously, with dignity, and in keeping with the principles of veterinary medical ethics.
    I accept as a lifelong obligation the continual improvement of my professional knowledge and competence.

Importance of the Oath

Although the Oath is not cited as frequently in print as, and is considerably shorter than, the *Principles of Veterinary Medical Ethics*, its importance should not be underestimated. The Veterinarian's Oath is intended to be for veterinarians what the Hippocratic Oath has for centuries represented to physicians—a statement of the highest ideals and most central values of the profession, made at the time when a person graduates from being a student to becoming a member of the profession.

The fact that the Oath is usually taken when the doctorate is conferred, before one has received a license to practice, is of great significance. Entry to the "practice" of veterinary medicine, as this is defined by the law, is controlled by government. In contrast, the Oath reflects the view of the profession that it has the right to admit persons to its ranks prior to, or indeed irrespective of, governmental permission to practice in the legal sense. This is not just an assertion of authority. It is a statement that however important it might be for individual veterinarians or the profession in general, practice in the legal sense is only one possible manifestation, or use, of one's professional status.

Five Pillars of Professionalism: Science, Ethics, Society, Animal Health, and Self-Improvement

Despite its brevity, the Oath identifies five distinct foundations of professionalism in which veterinarians can take pride.

The Oath begins by specifying scientific knowledge as the means through which the aims of veterinary medicine are to be attained. The Oath thus defines the veterinarian as more than a craftsman who possesses certain mechanical or technical skills. It commits each veterinarian to the study of science. The Oath also links the profession to biomedical research aimed at the advancement of veterinary knowledge and techniques.

Also identified as a foundation of professionalism is attention to ethics in the form of conscientiousness, dignity, and adherence to the *Principles of Veterinary Medical Ethics.*

Society—that is, people—is given a prominent place in the Oath. Indeed, the benefit of society is identified as the aim of all the activities enumerated in the Oath's second paragraph. Societal interests are also alluded to implicitly in the Oath's references to the conservation of livestock resources, public health, and medical knowledge.

Not surprisingly, the protection of animal health and the prevention of animal suffering are also included as central goals of the profession.

Finally, the Oath concludes with a pledge to engage in self-improvement and in knowledge and technical competence.

Criticisms of the Oath

In evaluating the Veterinarian's Oath, one must keep in mind what one can expect of a professional oath. Philosopher Bernard Rollin has complained that unless the aims of the Oath's second paragraph are:

> ...elaborated and rank ordered, these values are clearly incompatible. For example, the advancement of knowledge is often at odds with the relief of animal suffering. Clearly much fleshing-out through dialogue is required to make the oath more than a pious but vacuous statement of good intentions.[1]

Rollin is correct in asserting that the Oath would be empty and useless unless it serves as a stimulus for further reflection and consideration. At the same time, it cannot be the purpose of a professional oath itself to provide a detailed elaboration or ordering of fundamental values. A professional oath must be sufficiently brief to fulfill its ceremonial role of inducting doctors into the profession, and of calling to their attention the fundamental values of their new profession during this commencement. Moreover, fundamental values can, by their very nature, point toward different approaches in particular situations. For example, the statement of the *Declaration of Independence of the United States of America*, that all people have the inalienable right to "life, liberty, and the pursuit of happiness" is far from vacuous, even though the defense of liberty sometimes requires the sacrifice of life, or because too much liberty can lead to unhappiness.

Rollin observes that the advancement of knowledge, or the promotion of public health, can sometimes conflict with the maximization of animal welfare. This is not a defect in the Veterinarian's Oath. It is an inescapable fact that must be faced by the profession, which serves both human and animal interests. As is noted throughout this book, human and animal interests sometimes conflict. Indeed such conflict is one of the central challenges faced by veterinary ethics. Nothing in the Veterinarian's Oath prevents the profession from providing further elaboration about how the Oath's five central concerns might be ranked or applied in particular kinds of situations. Nevertheless the present Oath does raise several questions.

To whom is the Oath taken?

First, it is unclear to whom one is swearing when one takes the Oath—to oneself, one's fellow veterinarians, clients, the public, or some combination of these. To whom the Oath is taken can make a significant difference. If one is swearing just to one's colleagues, one is not thereby giving clients or society the right to complain about violations of the Oath. On the other hand, if the Oath is a promise to more than just veterinarians, it would be more than a text of official veterinary ethics and would permit nonveterinarians to appeal to the Oath in ethical discussions not controlled by the profession.

Should more than conscientiousness, dignity, and adherence to the *Principles* be included in the oath's ethical concerns?

Conscientiousness and dignity are clearly appropriate virtues for a veterinarian. It is also understandable that a document of official veterinary ethics like the Oath should mention adherence to the leading text of official ethics, the AVMA *Principles*, even though doctors might on occasion differ with the code as a matter of conscience. As we shall see, the *Principles* cannot be expected to contain the final word on ethical issues. Indeed, the code has changed as veterinarians have changed their ethical views. Because a professional oath proclaims the most central aspirations of the profession, one might therefore ask whether the Veterinarian's Oath ought to imply something that is clearly the desire of all veterinarians—that the *Principles* not only be followed but that they also be continually improved in light of the requirements of morality.

Does the Oath give sufficient attention to animals?

Veterinary medicine is a diverse profession, in which one can use one's attainments in the service of human beings as well as (or instead of) animals. Yet, the present Oath does not place caring for animals on the same level as service to people. All the enumerated aims of the Oath's second paragraph, including the protection of animal health and the relief of animal suffering, are stated as means toward the benefit of society, which by definition includes only people. The focus on people is reinforced by the references to conservation of livestock, public health, and medical knowledge.

I have found considerable hostility to the Oath among some of my veterinary students because of its identification of society as the beneficiary of *all* of veterinary medicine. (Some students are so offended by this statement that they refuse to utter the Oath at graduation.) One need not believe that animals are as important as people or that veterinarians should favor the interests of patients over those of clients, to assert that at the very least, caring for animals is as worthy a general goal for veterinarians as service to society. Any oath that fails to recognize this will fail to reflect the attitudes of many veterinarians.

Why is conservation of livestock singled out for special consideration?

Although veterinarians deal with many different kinds of animals, only one kind of animal is mentioned explicitly in the Oath. Perhaps continuing to include the conservation of livestock resources in the Oath is intended to make clear the profession's commitment to farm animals and farm animal practice in the face of attacks on meat production by animal rights activists. However if this is the intention, it can be argued that the Oath should also pledge the profession to the conservation of laboratory animal resources, which are also extremely important to society and are if anything, even more a target of activist attacks than animal agriculture. Dr. Michael Fox, who notes the increasing appreciation by the profession of wild animals and the environment, argues that the Oath should be amended to exhort the "conservation of livestock *and wildlife* resources."[2] The problem with Fox's suggestion is not that the conservation of wildlife is unimportant to veterinarians, but that once one begins to include certain kinds of animals in the Oath, a strong argument can be made for including still other kinds of animals. Thus in light of attacks by some animal rights advocates on the breeding and keeping of companion animals (see Chapter 21), it could be argued that the Oath should also commit the profession to the preservation of companion animals and the human-companion animal bond. Still other kinds of animal uses, such as the use of horses for racing and riding, and the keeping of animals in zoos, might strike many veterinarians as sufficiently important for inclusion in the Oath.

An Oath that commits the profession in general terms to benefiting both society and animals need not single out any specific kind or use of animals. Omitting the conservation of livestock resources from the Oath would not signal an abandonment by the profession of animal agriculture or farm animal welfare, nor would it constitute a slight to farm animal veterinarians. Indeed, an Oath that speaks generally and inclusively about "animals" would underscore even more emphatically the profession's commitment to *all* appropriate uses of animals.

Revising the Oath

The task of revising a professional oath must be approached with caution and sensitivity. An oath will lose credibility with members of the profession and the public if it is changed often. A profession's fundamental values—its core ethical ideals—do not change quickly. Frequent or drastic changes would lead to questions about whether an oath does express the profession's fundamental ethical beliefs or, perhaps, whether the profession is unable to decide what its central beliefs are. Moreover, suggested revisions in a profession's oath must accurately reflect the actual ideals of the vast majority of members of the profession. Otherwise, it cannot be accepted by those who are called upon to swear allegiance to its ideals.

A lesson in how not to suggest changes in the Veterinarian's Oath has been provided by the Association of Veterinarians for Animal Rights (AVAR), which submitted a new oath to the AVMA in 1993. Titled "Contemporary Veterinarian's Oath," this revision would have veterinarians swear to use their scientific knowledge and skills:

> …to protect the health and well-being of all nonhuman animals, to relieve pain and suffering in
> nonhuman animals, to strengthen the understanding of the inherent needs and interests of all
> nonhuman animals, and to promote the preservation of wildlife and their natural environment.[3]

This revision was quickly rejected by the AVMA, as it should have been. Aside from the fact that its title appears to imply that the current Oath is out-of-date—a claim that is false—the AVAR proposal removed all the provisions of the Oath that identify human interests as a legitimate aim of the profession. The promotion of human as well as animal interests will always be a major focus of veterinary medicine, as it should be. Suggested revisions of the Veterinarian's Oath will not be useful if they depart markedly from the profession's values, serve as a means of criticizing the profession, or are intended to cause heated debate. Such suggestions will never be adopted, because they misunderstand the function of a professional oath.

The Oath has not been modified since its creation over a quarter century ago. To reflect more accurately the attitudes of the profession, a fine-tuning would now be appropriate. The following modest revisions are suggested to stimulate discussion among veterinarians about possible modifications of the present Oath. This revised oath preserves the character and strengths of the current text while addressing the questions raised above. Its major feature is giving increased prominence to animals, animal welfare, and veterinary (as distinguished from medical) knowledge. It also makes clear, as the present text does not, that one is swearing to uphold the values of the entire Oath and not just its second paragraph:

> Being admitted to the profession of veterinary medicine, I solemnly swear to my fellow veterinarians, to my future clients, and to society.
>
> That I shall use my scientific knowledge and skills for the benefit of society, the protection of animal health and welfare, the relief of animal suffering, the promotion of public health, and the advancement of veterinary and medical knowledge;
>
> That I will practice my profession conscientiously, with dignity, and in keeping with the *Principles of Veterinary Medical Ethics*; and
>
> That I accept as a lifelong obligation the continual improvement of my professional knowledge and competence and of the moral values of myself and my profession.

～ THE PRINCIPLES OF VETERINARY MEDICAL ETHICS

The *Principles* is a lengthy document. It is therefore generally advisable to evaluate its provisions when considering the ethical issues these provisions address. However, several things that can be said of the code as a whole that aid in one's approach to it.

The Nature of a Professional Code

In considering the *Principles*, one must keep in mind what a professional code is and what is reasonable to expect of it.

Official standards reflect agreement and compromise.

One important difference between the standards of normative ethics (see Chapters 2 and 10) and those of an official ethical code is that the latter derive from agreement among the members of the profession. Therefore while normative ethics is a process of discovery of right and wrong, the fashioning of official ethical standards is often akin to politics. Typically, proponents of differing viewpoints will express their desires regarding an ethical principle, and through a process of negotiation and compromise, a standard will be hammered out.

Because official ethical standards often reflect compromise among competing points of view, it is to be expected that they will not always embody the complete truth about a moral issue. Like politicians, veterinarians engaged in the formulation of a proposed official ethical standard must recognize that they might sometimes have to settle for less than what they believe is morally right to get the best official ethical standard they can achieve. They might have to give a little on one proposed ethical standard to prevail on another.

Official codes tend to stress obviously correct positions and to accommodate competing points of view.

Because official codes are adopted by professions for all of their members, code standards must enunciate positions with which the great majority of members are comfortable. Thus codes, such as the AVMA *Principles*, are replete with statements that are obviously correct or that "split it down the middle" between opposing approaches. For example, there can be no argument with the statement: "no member shall willfully place professional knowledge, attainments or services at the disposal of any lay body...for the purpose of encouraging unqualified groups or individuals to diagnose and prescribe for the ailments and diseases of animals."[4] And the *Principles* resolve differences about whether all veterinarians must offer emergency service with a compromise: although "every practitioner has a moral and ethical responsibility" to provide such service, this responsibility can be fulfilled by joining "with colleagues in the area to see that emergency services are provided consistent with the needs of the locality."[5]

Official codes tend to avoid controversial or divisive issues.

The need for general acceptance of official ethical standards also tends to filter out of a professional code statements or references to issues that a significant portion of the profession finds divisive. For example, there probably are too many veterinarians who are seriously troubled, or undecided, about the usefulness of the concept of animal rights to permit the *Principles* to safely refer to this concept in the very near future (see Chapter 12). This does not mean that the profession must discourage vigorous discussion of such issues among members, but only that it might not be prepared to express positions regarding these issues in its official code.

Official codes contain ambiguities and generalities.

Another way official codes accommodate differing viewpoints is by building into their pronouncements enough ambiguity and generality to permit practitioners with varying viewpoints to live with the final result. This is especially important in a profession like veterinary medicine, which encompasses great diversity in values and practice styles. A good example of an abstract statement that can embrace different viewpoints is the declaration of the *Principles* that veterinarians "should seek for themselves and their profession the respect of their colleagues, their clients, and the public through courteous verbal interchange, considerate treatment, professional appearances, professionally acceptable procedures, and the utilization of current professional and scientific knowledge."[6] As discussed in Chapters 18 and 19, there is disagreement in the profession about whether certain kinds of promotional and business activities are consistent with a professional image and do foster respect among clients and the public. The general statement regarding professionalism allows these debates to continue while at the same time asserting the profession's general belief in the importance of professionalism.

Code standards change slowly.

It is also more difficult for a professional association like the AVMA to change its ethical code than it is for a legislature to amend or repeal a statute. Official ethical codes are presented both to members and the world as statements of the profession's fundamental values. If these codes were to change drastically from year to year or even from decade to decade, members of the profession and the public might justifiably wonder whether the profession has very many central moral values. This is why a code like the *Principles* can contain some standards that a good number of practitioners oppose and why a standard that no longer reflects shared values might not be swept away until long after it has ceased to seem reasonable to the majority.

Official codes reflect attitudes and concerns of their times.

Because official ethical codes are written by and for professionals, they tend to reflect what is bothering these persons. There is no better way of appreciating how a profession's values have changed than to read its successive codes of ethics. In 1867, when the United States Veterinary Medical Association's first *Code of Ethics* was written, veterinarians were not yet required to be licensed. They were struggling to separate themselves in the public's mind from charlatans without legitimate scientific training. This early code therefore prohibited the advertising of "secret medicines" as well as "specific medicines, specific plans of treatment, advertising through the medium of posters, illuminated bills, newspaper puffs, etc."[7] By 1940 veterinarians had established themselves in the public's view as true professionals and were more concerned about competition from within the profession. The *Code* of that year devoted more than half its length to advertising. It denounced all advertising as "unethical and unprofessional." It specifically banned, among other things, calling oneself a specialist in a public directory and the "distribution of cards or circulars by mail or otherwise reminding clients that the time is at hand for rendering certain services (vaccinations, worm-parasite treatment *et al.*)."[8]

Another provision that speaks volumes about changes in the profession's attitudes was the requirement, enunciated in the 1928 *Code of Ethics*, that members of the AVMA "are expected to conduct themselves at all times as professional gentlemen."[9] This was changed in 1940 to demand "conduct characterizing the personal behavior of a gentleman,"[10] language that remained in the *Principles* until 1983.

∽ THE LANDMARK 1989 REVISION OF THE *PRINCIPLES*

In 1989 the AVMA House of Delegates approved a major revision of the *Principles*. This revision embodied significant changes in both the organization and the substantive provisions of the code. It is important to understand the history of 1989 Revision because many of the changes made in the code were not voluntary. What happened to the *Principles* in 1989 also illustrates the limitations of official veterinary ethics in a legal system that seeks to protect free competition among businesspeople and professionals.

The Proposed 1988 Revision and the Federal Trade Commission Inquiry

In 1986 the AVMA Judicial Council decided to undertake a review of the *Principles* to improve the organization of the document and to clarify certain ambiguous or problematic sections.[11] This effort culminated in the preparation of a new version of the code, to which I shall refer as the "proposed 1988 Revision." The proposed 1988 Revision left virtually all the existing substantive provisions of the code in place. Significant substantive additions (which are discussed later) included a statement describing veterinarians as "colleagues rather than competitors," a provision on assisting chemically dependent practitioners, and a guideline advising doctors to consider the welfare of their patients more important than personal advantage or pecuniary gain. However, the major changes of this Revision were structural rather than substantive. Redundant statements were removed, and the entire document was reorganized to make clear which provisions were intended to enunciate very general ideals and which to provide specific obligations or prohibitions.

The document was to be voted on by the House of Delegates at the AVMA's annual convention in 1988. Shortly before the Revision was to be considered by the House, the AVMA received an inquiry from the Federal Trade Commission (FTC) regarding the code of ethics. The FTC requested information about 52 points in the *Principles* that, according to the FTC, could be in violation of federal antitrust laws prohibiting professional associations like the AVMA from restraining competition by members. The Judicial Council informed the House of Delegates that any action on the new Revision would be inappropriate until the AVMA had the opportunity to respond to the FTC's questions. No action was taken on the proposed 1988 Revision, and the pre-1988 code was left in place pending the outcome of the FTC inquiry.

After negotiations with the FTC, in 1989 the AVMA Executive Board presented to the House yet another Revision of the *Principles*. This 1989 version incorporated the organizational changes of the 1988 Revision. However, the 1989 Revision made many changes in the code's substantive provisions. A great many sections or statements, which had been in the *Principles* prior to 1989 and would have been preserved by the proposed 1988 Revision, were simply removed. A few additions that would have been made by the proposed 1988 Revision were not included in the 1989 code. The only significant additions made by the 1989 Revision had already been suggested by the proposed 1988 Revision.

In proposing the new version, the AVMA Executive Board accepted a number of suggestions made by the FTC. However, the Board rejected some proposals of its own attorney and approved several guidelines it conceded could be contested by the FTC.[12] At the AVMA Annual Meeting in 1989, the House of Delegates approved the new revision. It was not challenged by the FTC. Clearly, the 1989 Revision will likely remain the basis of the *Principles* for many years to come.

Table 9-1 summarizes what happened to the code as a result of the FTC inquiry. Several of the changes are discussed below and in subsequent chapters. It is immediately apparent from the table the extent to which provisions were removed from the document and the extent to which the changes resulted from the FTC inquiry.

Anticompetitive provisions

As Chapter 19 explains in greater detail, the FTC enforces federal antitrust laws that prohibit businesspeople and professionals from restraining others from competing in the marketplace. The *legal* rules the FTC applies should not be confused with normative *ethical* standards. The fact that the law prevents the AVMA from restraining certain kinds of competition does not mean these kinds of competition are ethically

TABLE 9-1

Major substantive changes made by the
1989 Revision of the *Principles of Veterinary Medical Ethics*

Removed from the *Principles* by the 1989 Revision*

- Three references to the Golden Rule.
- Disapproval of "aggressiveness and promotional tendencies" and the statement that those with such qualities would "probably have the same difficulty" under a more specific ethical code than the *Principles*.
- Prohibition against guaranteeing a cure.
- Inclusion in the kinds of false, deceptive, or misleading statements specified as impermissible by the Advertising Regulations, any statement or claim that "contains a prediction of future success or guarantees that satisfaction of a cure will result from the performance of professional services."
- Prohibition against advertising relating to professional fees, other than a statement of the fee for a specific professional service or a statement of the range of fees for specifically described services.†
- Prohibition against advertising fees without "reasonable disclosure of all relevant variables and considerations affecting the fees," such as the necessity for additional professional services.†
- Prohibition against advertising discounts and discounted fees.
- Prohibition against written solicitation of specific individuals "provided it does not exert undue influence, pressure for immediate response, intimidation, or overreaching."
- Unqualified prohibition against participating in fee splitting and rebating, or accepting or paying a fee in connection with referrals.
- Unqualified prohibition against soliciting or accepting a commission, rebate, or kickback in connection with or referral of a client to nonveterinarian purveyors of merchandise or services.‡
- Statement that the display and sale of nonveterinary products is "undesirable," but is "permissible if such nonprofessional products are generally unavailable or are difficult to obtain in the general vicinity of the client being served."
- Prohibition against participation by veterinarians in "coupon redemption schemes" on the grounds that participation many be regarded as an endorsement of or testimonial for a commercial product.
- Provision on "Press Relations," permitting members to write articles for local press regarding contagious or other important diseases and their prevention and treatment, "provided the motive is a bona fide attempt to protect the health and welfare of animals and the public, rather than personal gain."
- Provision on "Boarding Kennels" permitting veterinarians to own a commercial boarding kennel but stating that it "should not be operated under the veterinarian's name, and the telephone number should be separate from that used by the veterinarian in the conduct of the hospital."†
- Prohibition against members using "any degree or title granted by an institution declared unworthy by contemporary institutions of its class."
- Prohibition against public display of continuing education course certificates or diplomas, on the grounds that such documents "might lead the public to infer that the veterinarian to whom they are issued is a specialist in the specific subject matter."†
- Requirement that a "veterinarian who does not own or operate a cemetery or crematorium as a separate business but does provide such service on request should in no way announce or advertise the service."
- Statement referring to "problems that have arisen when specialists go into communities to conduct diagnostic clinics under sponsorship of breed associations, sometimes with animosity developing between the specialists and local veterinary practitioners" and requirement that such clinics be jointly sponsored by a breed association and a local veterinary association.
- Statement that to "criticize or disparage another veterinarian's service to a client is unethical."

*Except where noted, all the provisions in this category were also included in the proposed 1988 Revision of the *Principles*.
†This provision was eliminated in the proposed 1988 Revision and was therefore not suggested for inclusion in the 1989 Revision.
‡This provision was reversed in the 1993 Revision, which reinstated the prohibition of kickbacks from nonveterinarians.

TABLE 9-1 CONT'D

Major substantive changes made by the
1989 Revision of the *Principles of Veterinary Medical Ethics*

Included in the proposed 1988 Revision but omitted from the 1989 Code
- Declaration that veterinarians "should consider themselves as colleagues rather than competitors."
- Statement that "a veterinarian has an obligation to charge fees to allow him to remain financially viable and professionally competent."
- Statement that the "advertising of services for senior citizens in 'Silver' or 'Golden' pages of telephone directories is permissible provided that the advertisement itself does not include any reference to a discounted price."

Added to the 1989 Revision§
- Statement, in the introductory "Guidelines for Professional Behavior," that "in their relations with others, veterinarians should speak and act on the basis of honesty and fairness."‖
- Statement, in the "Guidelines for Professional Behavior," that "Veterinarians should consider first the welfare of the patient for the purpose of relieving suffering and disability while causing a minimum of pain or fright. Benefit to the patient should transcend personal advantage or monetary gain in decisions concerning therapy."
- Definition of the veterinarian-client-patient relationship.
- Provision on "Drug, Chemical, and Alcohol Abuse" advising veterinarians impaired by such substances to seek assistance from qualified sources, and recommending colleagues to encourage such individuals to seek assistance.

§Except where noted, all the provisions in this category were included *verbatim* in the proposed 1988 Revision of the *Principles*, and therefore did not result from the FTC inquiry.
‖In the 1988 proposed Revision, this statement reads as follows: "In their relations with others, veterinarians should speak and act on the basis of honesty, fairness, and the Golden Rule (generally interpreted to mean treating others as one would be treated by others). Veterinarians should consider themselves as colleagues rather than competitors."

appropriate. For example, I argue in Chapter 17 that the sale of nonmedical products, such as nonprescription foods, pet toys, and pet clothing, is inappropriate from an ethical standpoint because such activity will diminish the image of the veterinary profession and its long-term ability to inspire trust among clients. If this argument is correct, individual veterinarians and practices can—and should—decide for themselves not to sell nonmedical products. However, it is also clear that it would violate the antitrust laws for the AVMA (or any group of two or more veterinarians) to prevent, or agree to try to prevent, another doctor or practice from selling such products. For the antitrust laws prohibit professional associations from attempting to restrain business practices that are lawful, and it is lawful for veterinarians to sell nonmedical products.*

*To be sure, the power of the AVMA actually to compel behavior is extremely limited. Veterinarians disciplined or threatened with discipline by the AVMA for violating the *Principles* can simply resign their membership, and continue the offending behavior. Nevertheless, because of the attractiveness and importance of membership in the AVMA to veterinarians, the *Principles* do have potential to exert sufficient influence on members to come within the scope of federal antitrust laws.

This point is so vitally important, it bears repeating. Legal prohibitions against attempts to restrain trade mean that the AVMA and groups of veterinarians cannot attempt to prohibit or cannot discourage any practitioner from engaging in a lawful business activity, such as the sale of nonmedical products, distribution of discount coupons for veterinary services, advertising, and solicitation. But absent any specific legal directive (say, by one's state veterinary licensing board), no individual veterinarian or practice is *required* by law to engage in such business activities. Individual doctors or practices can legally—and as I argue in this book should sometimes morally—decide on their own not to engage in these activities.

Certain statements of the *Principles* did violate the antitrust laws. For example, the pre-1989 code allowed the sale of nonprofessional products but only if such products were unavailable or difficult to obtain in the general vicinity of a client's residence. Because such items are available in most communities at ordinary commercial establishments, this provision was intended to discourage the sale of nonmedical products by the great majority of veterinarians.

Other provisions of the pre-1989 code that could have had the effect of restraining lawful competition were the prohibition against participating in programs in which clients redeem coupons from pet product companies for a fee reduction; the prohibition against advertising reduced or discounted fees; the provision permitting doctors to write articles for local newspapers on animal disease provided the motivation was not personal gain; the prohibition against operating a boarding kennel under the veterinarian's name and using the same telephone number for both the practice and kennel; and the prohibition against advertising a cemetery or crematorium that one does not own or operate as a business separate from one's practice.

In response to the FTC inquiry, all these provisions were removed from the *Principles*.

Criticizing colleagues

The 1989 Revision also toned down substantially several sections of the code relating to criticism of fellow veterinarians. These sections could have been interpreted as intended to prevent a veterinarian from revealing to clients truthful information about other doctors that clients might want to make informed decisions. For example, the old code stated that no member of the AVMA "shall belittle or injure the professional standing of another member of the profession or unnecessarily condemn the character of that person's professional acts."[13] This prohibition could have prevented a veterinarian from making a negative statement about another veterinarian, even if true. The 1989 and subsequent Revisions state that no member of the AVMA "shall belittle or injure the professional standing of another member of the profession or unnecessarily condemn the character of that person's professional acts in such a manner as to be false or misleading."[14] The old code stated that when a veterinarian is called into consultation by a colleague, the consulting doctor shall handle all "findings and discussions with the client. . .in such a manner as to avoid criticism of the attending veterinarian by the client."[15] In the 1989 and subsequent Revisions, this became a requirement that "findings and discussions with the client shall be handled in such a manner as to avoid criticism of the attending veterinarian by the consultant or the client, if that criticism is false or misleading."[16] The pre-

1989 code stated, without qualification or exception, that "to criticize or disparage another veterinarian's service to a client is unethical."[17] This statement was removed by the 1989 Revision.

The qualification that criticisms of colleagues are prohibited if they are false or misleading stems from the decision of the Supreme Court of the United States (see Chapter 18) that professional associations and state licensing boards may ban false, deceptive, or misleading statements. By adding this qualification, the *Principles* reasserted the profession's interest in restraining unfair criticism of doctors by colleagues, but in a manner immune from objections even by the Federal Trade Commission.

Competition and the Golden Rule

One of the most interesting developments relating to the 1989 Revision involved the Golden Rule.*

For decades, the *Principles* had not only cited the Golden Rule in support of key provisions of the code but proclaimed the Golden Rule as the foundation of veterinary professional ethics. For example, the first substantive section of the pre-1989 code stated that:

> The *Principles of Veterinary Medical Ethics* are purposely constructed in a general and broad manner, but veterinarians who accept the Golden Rule as a guide for general conduct and make a reasonable effort to abide by the *Principles of Veterinary Medical Ethics* in professional life will have little difficulty with ethics. Those whose aggressiveness and promotional tendencies cause them to run afoul of the *Principles* would probably have the same difficulty under more specific rules.[18]

The code then mentioned the Golden Rule three more times, twice in statements reiterating the fundamental nature of the Golden Rule, and once in support of the statement that it is unethical to criticize or disparage another veterinarian's service to a client. The proposed 1988 Revision would have preserved these references to the Golden Rule, including the paragraph quoted above. However, the 1988 Revision added yet another reminder that, in the view of the AVMA, veterinarians who obeyed the Golden Rule would exercise restraint in competing with fellow practitioners. The new "Guidelines for Professional Behavior" in the proposed 1988 code began with the declaration that:

> In their relations with others, veterinarians should speak and act on the basis of honesty, fairness, and the Golden Rule (generally interpreted to mean treating others as one would be treated by others). Veterinarians should consider themselves as colleagues rather than competitors.[19]

The distinction between being a "colleague" and a "competitor" appeared to link the Golden Rule, and indeed the entire *Principles*, to a condemnation of not only overly aggressive competition but also of competition itself.

The repeated connections made by the pre-1989 code between the Golden Rule and disapprovals of competition and criticizing colleagues could give the impression that the Golden Rule was intended at least in part to prevent veterinarians from competing against their colleagues. This was how the FTC saw the code's use of the Golden

---

*The Golden Rule is usually phrased "Do unto others as you would have them do unto you." It derives from Matthew 7:12, "Whatsoever ye would that men should do to you, do ye even so unto them."

Rule, and not without some justification. The problem, however, was not the Golden Rule. The problem was that in places the *Principles* seemed to adopt a special, and too limited, interpretation of the Golden Rule. As employed in parts of the pre-1989 code, the Golden Rule appeared not to counsel a veterinarian to treat other *people* as one would want to be treated by them, but rather to treat other *veterinarians* as one would want to be treated by *them*. Only on such an interpretation could the Golden Rule be interpreted to imply that a veterinarian should *never* criticize a colleague's performance to a client or that a veterinarian should avoid "promotional tendencies." Many veterinarians would probably not want to be criticized in front of a client by another doctor, and would prefer that colleagues who compete with them not engage in overly aggressive promotion. In contrast, if the Golden Rule were meant to counsel a veterinarian to treat all people—including clients—as one would want to be treated by them, the Golden Rule would have quite different implications. The Golden Rule would sometimes require a doctor to tell a client that a colleague made a mistake, because one might under certain circumstances want to know this if one were a *client*. Likewise if the Golden Rule applied to all people, veterinarians might, at least under certain circumstances, engage in healthy competition with colleagues because *clients* might sometimes want the benefits of such competition, including expanded services and lower fees. In its response to the FTC, the AVMA recast the code's references to the Golden Rule. The 1989 Revision omitted the statement that those "whose aggressiveness and promotional tendencies cause them to run afoul of the *Principles*" would not benefit from a more specific code. The assertion of the proposed 1988 Revision that veterinarians are colleagues rather than competitors was dropped. The number of references in the *Principles* to the Golden Rule was reduced from four to one, and although the Golden Rule remains a foundation of professional ethics it is not linked to the subject of competition. The first substantive section of the code now declares that

> The *Principles of Veterinary Medical Ethics* are purposely constructed in a general and broad manner, but veterinarians who accept the Golden Rule as a guide for general conduct and make a reasonable effort to abide by the *Principles of Veterinary Medical Ethics* in professional life will have little difficulty with ethics.[20]

Did the 1989 Revision go too far?

It is difficult to fault the AVMA Executive Board for its handling of the FTC inquiry. Had the FTC rejected the 1989 Revision, the AVMA could have faced protracted and costly litigation. The entire apparatus of official veterinary ethics might have had to be temporarily suspended in anticipation of final court action. Because litigation is sometimes unpredictable, there is no telling what would have remained of the code in the end. The AVMA removed from the *Principles* provisions that could have been employed to restrain trade, even if doing so was not always intended or even likely. Also excised from the code were statements (such as the condemnation of "aggressiveness") that although probably not sufficiently concrete to allow the prohibition of specific behavior, could be interpreted as presenting an anticompetitive flavor or tone. On matters it believed are essential to the profession's values, the AVMA wisely made its case. Still prominent in the code are the Golden Rule, and many sections that advise veterinarians to take seriously the interests of patients and clients. As will be discussed, the *Principles* still provide much valuable advice regarding a broad range of ethical issues.

Nevertheless, in certain respects the 1989 Revision went too far. Several important changes in the code do not appear to have been required by antitrust laws. These new provisions are not only questionable from an ethical standpoint, but do not accord with ethical rules applied by many state veterinary licensing boards. Veterinarians must therefore understand that they can get themselves in serious trouble with some state licensing boards if they simply follow the *Principles.*

Guarantees of cures or results

Many state veterinary licensing boards specifically prohibit licensees from guaranteeing a cure or result. Such a prohibition accords with the ruling of the U.S. Supreme Court allowing state licensing boards and professional associations, such as the AVMA, to prohibit false, deceptive, or misleading claims. Promising or guaranteeing a cure or result is inherently false, deceptive, and misleading. Because of the variability of medical conditions and the unpredictability of a patient's progress, the courts have uniformly held that competent practice does not of itself include success. To guarantee that a treatment or procedure will succeed is to overstep the bounds of expected competence. Guaranteeing results takes advantage of clients, and prevents them from making informed choices and decisions, by presenting an enticement that no doctor can truthfully present. Guaranteeing results is also unfair to honest practitioners who would never promise or guarantee success.

The pre-1989 code had a separate section prohibiting guarantees of cures or results. The code also listed in the Advertising Regulations as an example of false, deceptive, or misleading advertising any statement or claim that "contains a prediction of future success or guarantees that satisfaction or a cure will result from the performance of professional services." The 1989 Revision contains no explicit reference to, or prohibition of, statements promising success or guaranteeing results.

Kickbacks and rebates

Many state boards also prohibit a veterinarian from offering or taking a kickback, rebate, or commission in return for a referral to another practitioner. As is discussed in Chapter 20, such behavior violates the obligation of loyalty veterinarians have to clients. Clients assume that their veterinarian will suggest a referral to another practitioner because this will benefit the animal, and not to make money for himself. The official ethical codes of other healing professions unequivocally and unconditionally condemn kickbacks or fee splitting in return for referrals.[21]

The pre-1989 *Principles* declared that it is "unethical for a veterinarian to participate in fee splitting and rebating and to accept or pay a fee in connection with referrals."[22] The old code also prohibited a veterinarian from soliciting or receiving a "commission, rebate, or kickback" from a nonveterinarian in connection with a recommendation or referral of a client to a purveyor of nonprofessional products or services, such as dog food, cremation or burial services, insurance, or livestock supplies.[23] The 1989 Revision retracted the prohibition on fee splitting, stating instead that "it is unethical for a veterinarian to participate in fee splitting and rebating or to accept a fee in connection with referrals, *without informing the client of the arrangement.*"[24] The prohibition against kickbacks from nonveterinarians was also changed. It was now "inconsistent with the *Principles of Veterinary Medical Ethics* for veterinarians to enter an agreement whereby, through the commissions or rebates, *judgment or choice of treatment would be influenced* by considerations other than the needs of the patient, welfare of the client, or safety of the public."[25]

The notion that a doctor may receive or offer a kickback in return for a referral provided the client is informed of the arrangement is unacceptable. First, even if the client is told, the possibility remains that monetary considerations are motivating the making of a referral, or of a referral to a particular doctor. Moreover, informing a client of a kickback need not of itself extinguish any temptation on the referring doctor's part to be influenced by the arrangement. Clients may just tend to trust a representation by a veterinarian that, of course, the fee splitting had nothing to do with the referral, even if that representation is false.

Kickbacks are a seedy business. They have no place in professional life. The *Principles* should not tolerate kickbacks under any circumstances. Interestingly, in 1993 the *Principles* were amended to remove the qualified permission of kickbacks from nonveterinarians. As of that date, the code stated that:

> It is inconsistent with the *Principles of Veterinary Medical Ethics* for veterinarians to enter an agreement whereby they stand to profit through referring clients to other providers of services or products. The veterinarian should not jeopardize client trust by accepting rebates or commissions for referring clients to other providers.
>
> The choices of animal care should not be influenced by considerations other than the needs of the patient, welfare of the client, and safety of the public.[26]

This provision recognizes correctly that kickbacks present an inherent influence on judgment. Unfortunately, the code left in place the section allowing veterinarians to offer and receive kickbacks from other veterinarians. Ironically, the *Principles* now provide clients greater protection when nonveterinarians are involved in kickbacks than when *veterinarians* "stand to profit" from referrals to colleagues.

Miscellaneous deceptive acts

The 1989 Revision also removed, unnecessarily, specific prohibitions against certain kinds of behavior that are clearly false, deceptive, or misleading. The old code explicitly banned advertising of fees that do not indicate whether additional fees might be required for further necessary related services. The pre-1989 code also explicitly targeted advertisements using "unqualified use of terms such as '$20 and up' or '$20 to 30'" on the grounds that such statements did not reasonably disclose variables that would be relevant in determining the actual fee in an individual case.[27] Also removed from the code (as a result of the 1988 proposed Revision and not the FTC inquiry) was the display of continuing education certificates or diplomas on the grounds that these might lead the public to conclude that a veterinarian displaying such documents is a specialist in these areas.[28]

It could be argued that all such behavior is encompassed by the present code's broad prohibition of false, deceptive, or misleading claims. However, the *Principles* can usefully mention specific kinds of deceptive behavior capable of misleading the public and being unfair to reputable doctors.

～ GENERAL FEATURES OF THE CODE

It is much easier to point out the relatively few problems in a lengthy document like the *Principles* than it is to discuss its many strong points. To place in proper perspective criticisms of the code that are to follow in this and subsequent chapters, I want to state at the outset my view that the *Principles* is in general a sound code that compares very favorably with the official codes of other professions. But nothing is perfect. It is the task of the scholar to note problems and areas for improvement.

A Useful Structure

As a result of the proposed 1988 revision, the *Principles* now has an extremely helpful structure that makes clear what its various provisions are intended to do and allows for flexibility in adding general provisions or specific rules as the need arises. The code begins with two statements of very general ideals, in sections titled "Attitude and Intent" and "General Concepts." The former section specifies the Golden Rule and the code itself as the foundations of professional ethics. The latter section calls for the study, application, and improvement of professional ethics by individual doctors, state associations, and the veterinary schools. There then follows the core of the document, the 10 "Guidelines for Professional Behavior." These statements specify the code's most fundamental rules. Following the Guidelines are the longest part of the *Principles*, the "Explanatory Notes." These contain more specific interpretations of the 10 basic guidelines, as well as several general rules for decisionmaking. The Explanatory Notes also set forth concrete obligations and prohibitions that can be used as grounds for disciplining members. As the AVMA perceives specific problems that need addressing in the code, appropriate additions or amendments can be made in the Explanatory Notes, without necessitating changes in the more fundamental statements of values of the Guidelines for Professional Behavior.

Ideals and Obligations

The following are among the code's many strong points. The *Principles* recognize that a comprehensive code must not only lay down specific obligations and prohibitions, but must also identify very general values and virtues without which the promotion of ethical behavior is impossible. The document acknowledges that it cannot dictate answers for the entire field of veterinary medicine and that professional life is too complex to formulate one's moral duties into a hard and fast "set of rules."[29] Among the general values identified by the code are service to society,[30] improvement in professional knowledge and skill,[31] protection of the public and the profession against those deficient in moral character or professional competence,[32] and the prevention and relief of animal suffering.[33] The *Principles* also demand such virtues as honesty in dealing with clients and the public,[34] truthfulness in promoting one's own name or practice,[35] diligence in attending to patients,[36] and respect for the privacy and confidences of clients.[37]

Many of the specific obligations or prohibitions of the code are beyond dispute. For example, the prohibition against choosing a method of treatment based on the pecuniary gain of the practitioner rather than the needs of the patient,[38] is intended to assure that veterinarians work in the first instance for patients and clients. The requirement that client confidences be respected also protects clients against unscrupulous behavior. The *Principles* contain the recommendation that the code itself be "subjected to review with the object of clarification of any obscure parts and the amendment of any inadequate or inappropriate items."[39]

Problems in the Code

Even when the *Principles* are considered in light of what one can reasonably expect of an official code, several general deficiencies detract from their effectiveness.

Excessive reliance on the Golden Rule

The first substantive section of the code still states, as it did in previous revisions, that "veterinarians who accept the Golden Rule as a guide for general conduct and make a reasonable effort to abide by the *Principles.* . .in professional life will have little difficulty with ethics."[40] As discussed throughout this text, there are many situations in which veterinarians will find the Golden Rule an essential guide for behavior. Certainly how one deals with clients—how one sympathizes, for example, with their emotional and economic problems in caring for their animals—will often be improved by asking how one would want to be treated if one were a client. Moreover, the presentation of the Golden Rule in the *Principles* has been improved. The Golden Rule is not linked to professional self-protection and now seems to apply to clients as well as veterinarians. Nevertheless, the *Principles* still overemphasize the usefulness of the Golden Rule as a guide for ethical behavior. This is so not because the Golden Rule is a bad standard for considering how one ought to treat other people but because the Golden Rule is a standard for considering how one ought to treat other *people*. The Golden Rule asks us to treat other people as we would want to be treated by them. It does not refer explicitly or implicitly to animals. It does not ask us to consider how we would want to be treated if we were animals in general or veterinary patients in particular.* The Golden Rule has an important but limited function in veterinary professional ethics, because many questions in veterinary ethics relate to how animals should be treated.

Missing subjects

Although the code addresses many questions of great importance to the profession, there are conspicuous gaps in its coverage. Most of the provisions of the code that attempt to provide specific guidance concern problems faced by private practitioners who are in economic competition with each other. The code offers no explicit, detailed provisions regarding the welfare of farm, laboratory, or industrial animals, even though official veterinary ethics has labored long and hard on these issues and has produced

---

*Some have suggested that the Golden Rule ought to include reference to animals, but this is not the Golden Rule as enunciated in the *Bible* and cited in the *Principles*. Moreover, it is often far from clear how one would go about trying to imagine how one would want to be treated if one were an animal. For example, would it really help in determining whether to euthanize a terminally ill animal in great pain to ask how one would like to be treated if one were that animal and the animal were the veterinarian? The point of the Golden Rule is to ask us to imagine how one would think and react if one were to be treated by someone as we propose to treat that person. This exercise presupposes that all parties that can be affected by a given course of action can understand how it is to be treated as the other would treat him. How can one even begin to imagine how a veterinary patient would react if it were a veterinarian? Does it even make sense to attribute to an animal patient the kinds of wants and interests that are normally taken into consideration in applying the Golden Rule to others?

other documents that discuss them. In contrast, the American Medical Association *Principles of Medical Ethics* contain lengthy discussions of the obligations of physicians regarding research subjects and industrial practice.[41]

The *Principles* also do not address the ethical obligations of practitioners regarding veterinarians, technicians, and other support personnel in their employ (see Chapter 24).

Although the profession has paid considerable attention to the human-companion animal bond, there is missing from the *Principles* explicit reference to this concept or to many of the important ethical issues it raises. For example, although many veterinarians believe that the euthanasia of companion animals poses some of the most difficult moral issues they face in practice, the word "euthanasia" does not appear in the code.

Animals and veterinary ethics

The 1989 Revision added to the code an important provision that reflects the profession's increasing concern in promoting the interests of its patients. The "Guidelines for Professional Behavior" now state that:

> Veterinarians should consider first the welfare of the patient for the purpose of relieving suffering and disability while causing a minimum of pain or fright. Benefit to the patient should transcend personal advantage or monetary gain in decisions concerning therapy.[42]

This statement reflects the growing interest of the profession in the scientific study of animal pain and the development of effective means of relieving pain in a wide range of veterinary patients.[43] The statement also challenges veterinarians to consider making economic sacrifices when doing so would benefit a patient. Veterinarians are faced frequently with situations in which clients cannot afford to pay either for treatment or the most effective treatment available. As argued in Chapter 20, veterinarians do not have a general moral obligation to assist clients in need. However, there are cases in which it can be argued that a practitioner should either reduce a fee or the burden of the fee.

Despite this section and others in the *Principles* directed to the promotion of the interests of patients, the code appears reluctant to grant something that every veterinarian believes—veterinarians have moral obligations relating to their animal patients as well as to people. In some of its most fundamental and central statements of its values, the *Principles* omit any reference to animals as objects of concern for official veterinary ethics. The code fails to mention animals when it states that "(p)rofessional life is too complex to classify one's duties and obligations to clients, colleagues, and fellow citizens into a set of rules."[29] (This statement appears to imply that moral obligations and ideals regarding animals are not part of a veterinarian's "professional life.") Likewise, there is no mention of animals in the declaration that the *Principles* are "standards by which an individual may determine the propriety of conduct in relationships with clients, colleagues, and with the public."[44] (This statement appears to imply that the code is not intended to contain standards by which a practitioner may determine the propriety of conduct in relation to patients.) Presumably, the absence of a reference to animals in these pronouncements does not reflect the view that to establish itself as a "real" profession, veterinary medicine must emphasize its ethical obligations to people. The fact that the profession has such obligations is obvious. However, the fact that veterinarians deal with and have many moral obligations and ideals regarding animals is not an unfortunate accident. Nor is it something about which any veterinarian should feel guilty or embarrassed.

The easiness of veterinary ethics

Finally, the code makes a significant mistake when it declares that veterinarians who accept the Golden Rule as a guide for general conduct and make a reasonable effort to abide by the *Principles* "will have little difficulty with ethics." This statement is false, and not just because the Golden Rule cannot encompass all of veterinary ethics or because the code itself does not provide definitive guidance on all ethical issues. As discussed earlier, no official ethical code can provide complete and satisfactory direction regarding all the moral questions that confront members of a profession. More importantly, veterinary ethics cannot be made easy by any single moral principle or official ethical document. Veterinary ethics is inherently and unavoidably difficult. Veterinarians face many difficult ethical problems, some of which stem at least in part from deep and difficult philosophical, religious, and ethical notions about the value of animals and the legitimacy of their interests. In stating that veterinarians will be able to have "little difficulty with ethics" the *Principles* diminish the seriousness and importance of the entire subject.

It would not be difficult for the code to discuss or to give greater emphasis to animal welfare, employer-employee relations, the human-companion animal bond, and the status of animals as objects of direct concern of official veterinary ethics. Where questions (for example, those concerning euthanasia) are especially difficult, the code need not attempt to settle them definitively but could highlight the profession's interest in them. However, if the *Principles* are to stand as a definitive statement of the profession's values, its focus must be expanded, so that it will speak to all areas of major concern to veterinarians.

~ THE LIMITATIONS OF OFFICIAL VETERINARY ETHICS

Veterinarians should be proud of their Oath and *Principles,* and the official ethical apparatus of which these texts are a part. Clearly, professional behavior has been improved and will continue to be improved by official veterinary ethics.

However, we are now in a position to better appreciate why official veterinary ethics can be only a part of the total ethical commitment and activity of veterinarians.

Because of their need to speak for the entire profession on many issues whose solution is not obvious, the Oath and *Principles* contain some provisions that do not answer questions, but rather identify important ethical concerns and channel further discussion and debate. These texts do not, and they probably cannot, determine when it is morally appropriate to euthanize a terminally ill animal, how far veterinarians should go in attempting to offer reduced fees to needy clients, what veterinarians should do about clients who abuse their animals, or to what extent race horses may be given drugs to improve their performance. To answer these and many other questions, veterinarians must supplement the guidance of official standards with objective *Principles* of morality—with normative veterinary ethics.

Insofar as official veterinary ethics attempts to regulate rather than just to suggest or exhort, it must comport with legal standards that restrict the effects professional associations may have upon competition and commerce. Normative veterinary ethics encounters no such restrictions. Its function is only to question, discuss, discover, suggest, and where possible, exhort.

Finally, because official ethics is controlled by the profession, the process by which it answers ethical questions does not include equal input from nonveterinarians. This can sometimes lead to conclusions that do not adequately take into account the interests of patients, clients, or society. In striving fervently to protect its members, any profession can lose sight of the legitimate interests of others. To the norms of official ethics there must be added a healthy dose of normative veterinary ethics in which, the legitimate interests of all affected by veterinarians must be given due regard.

REFERENCES

[1] Rollin BE: Updating veterinary medical ethics, *J Am Vet Med Assoc* 173:1017, 1978.

[2] Fox MW: *Inhumane Society*, New York, 1990, St. Martin's Press, p 205, emphases in original.

[3] AVMA rejects new veterinary oath, *AVAR Directions*, Fall 1993, p 4.

[4] American Veterinary Medical Association: *Principles of Veterinary Medical Ethics*, 1993 Revision, "Alliance with Unqualified Persons," *1994 AVMA Directory*, Schaumburg, IL, The Association, p 44.

[5] American Veterinary Medical Association: *Principles of Veterinary Medical Ethics*, 1993 Revision, "Emergency Service," *1994 AVMA Directory*, Schaumburg, IL, The Association, p 44.

[6] American Veterinary Medical Association: *Principles of Veterinary Medical Ethics*, 1993 Revision, "Guidelines for Professional Behavior," paragraph 4, Schaumburg, IL, The Association, p 42.

[7] USVMA Proceedings, 4th Annual Meeting, New York, September 3, 1867, *USVMA Minutes Book*, pp 42-47. Quoted in Miller EB: History and evolution of the AVMA veterinary medical Code of Ethics, 1867-1940, *Calif Vet* 39:18, 1985.

[8] *Code of Ethics of the American Veterinary Medical Association, J Am Vet Med Assoc* 96:92-93, 1940.

[9] American Veterinary Medical Association: *AVMA Membership Directory, 1928-1929, Constitution and By-Laws*, Detroit, 1928, The Association, p 70. Reprinted in Miller EB: History and evolution of the AVMA Veterinary Medical Code of Ethics, 1867-1940, *Calif Vet* 39:19-20, 1985.

[10] *Code of Ethics of the American Veterinary Medical Association, J Am Vet Med Assoc* 96:92, 1940.

[11] Discount advertising and waiting-room displays reviewed by Judicial Council, *J Am Vet Med Assoc* 189:1408, 1986.

[12] Memorandum of the AVMA Executive Board to the Judicial Council, March 17, 1989.

[13] American Veterinary Medical Association: *Principles of Veterinary Medical Ethics*, 1987 Revision, "Deportment," *1988 AVMA Directory*, Schaumburg, IL, The Association, p 474.

[14] American Veterinary Medical Association: *Principles of Veterinary Medical Ethics*, 1993 Revision, "Guidelines for Professional Behavior," paragraph 5, *1994 AVMA Directory*, Schaumburg, IL, The Association, p 42.

[15] American Veterinary Medical Association: *Principles of Veterinary Medical Ethics*, 1987 Revision, "Consultations," *1988 AVMA Directory*, Schaumburg, IL, The Association, p 475.

[16] American Veterinary Medical Association: *Principles of Veterinary Medical Ethics*, 1993 Revision, "Referrals, Consultations, and Relationships with Clients," Schaumburg, IL, The Association, p 43.

[17] American Veterinary Medical Association: *Principles of Veterinary Medical Ethics*, 1987 Revision, "Professional Relationships with New Clients," *1988 AVMA Directory*, Schaumburg, IL, The Association, p 477.

[18] American Veterinary Medical Association: *Principles of Veterinary Medical Ethics*, 1987 Revision, "It's Attitude That Counts," *1988 AVMA Directory*, Schaumburg, IL, The Association, p 474.

[19] American Veterinary Medical Association: *Principles of Veterinary Medical Ethics*, Proposed 1988 Revision, "Guidelines for Professional Behavior," paragraph 1, AVMA 1988 Annual Convention Delegates' Agenda, Schaumburg, IL, The Association, p 17f.

[20] American Veterinary Medical Association: *Principles of Veterinary Medical Ethics*, 1993 Revision, "Attitude and Intent," *1994 AVMA Directory*, Schaumburg, IL, The Association, p 42.

[21] American Medical Association: *Principles of Medical Ethics and Current Opinions of the Council on Ethical and Judicial Affairs—1989*, paragraph 6.02, "Fee Splitting." In Gorlin RA, editor: *Codes of Professional Responsibility*, ed 2, Washington, DC, 1990, Bureau of National Affairs, p 211; American Dental Association: *Principles of Ethics and Code of Professional Conduct*, Paragraph 1-I, "Rebates and Split Fees." In Gorlin, *supra*, p 163; American Psychiatric Association: *Principles of Medical Ethics with Annotations Especially Applicable to Psychiatry*, Section 2, paragraph 7. In Gorlin, *supra*, p 241.

[22] American Veterinary Medical Association: *Principles of Veterinary Medical Ethics*, 1987 Revision, "Fees for Service," *1988 AVMA Directory*, Schaumburg, IL, The Association, p 475.

[23] American Veterinary Medical Association: *Principles of Veterinary Medical Ethics*, 1987 Revision, "Commissions, Rebates, or Kickbacks," *1988 AVMA Directory*, Schaumburg, IL, The Association, p 475.

[24] *See*, American Veterinary Medical Association: *Principles of Veterinary Medical Ethics*, 1993 Revision, "Fees for Service," *1994 AVMA Directory*, Schaumburg, IL, The Association, p 43, emphases added.

[25] *See*, American Veterinary Medical Association: *Principles of Veterinary Medical Ethics*, 1990 Revision, *1993 AVMA Directory*, Schaumburg, IL, The Association, p 44.

[26] American Veterinary Medical Association: *Principles of Veterinary Medical Ethics*, 1993 Revision, "Fees for Service," *1994 AVMA Directory*, Schaumburg, IL, The Association, p 43.

[27] American Veterinary Medical Association: *Principles of Veterinary Medical Ethics*, 1987 Revision, "Advertising Regulations," *1988 AVMA Directory*, Schaumburg, IL, The Association, p 476.

[28] American Veterinary Medical Association: *Principles of Veterinary Medical Ethics*, 1987 Revision, "Certificates or Diplomas, Continuing Education, Display of," *1988 AVMA Directory*, Schaumburg IL, The Association, p 477.

[29] American Veterinary Medical Association: *Principles of Veterinary Medical Ethics*, 1993 Revision, "Attitude and Intent," *1994 AVMA Directory*, Schaumburg, IL, The Association, p 42.

[30] American Veterinary Medical Association: *Principles of Veterinary Medical Ethics*, 1993 Revision, "Guidelines for Professional Behavior," paragraph 10, *1994 AVMA Directory*, Schaumburg, IL, The Association, p 42.

[31] American Veterinary Medical Association: *Principles of Veterinary Medical Ethics*, 1993 Revision, "Guidelines for Professional Behavior," paragraph 7, *1994 AVMA Directory*, Schaumburg, IL, The Association, p 42.

[32] American Veterinary Medical Association: *Principles of Veterinary Medical Ethics*, 1993 Revision, "Guidelines for Professional Behavior," paragraph 9, *1994 AVMA Directory*, Schaumburg, IL, The Association, p 42.

[33] American Veterinary Medical Association: *Principles of Veterinary Medical Ethics*, 1993 Revision, "Guidelines for Professional Behavior," paragraph 2, *1994 AVMA Directory*, Schaumburg, IL, The Association, p 42.

[34] American Veterinary Medical Association: *Principles of Veterinary Medical Ethics*, 1993 Revision, "Frauds," *1994 AVMA Directory*, Schaumburg, IL, The Association, p 44; "Advertising," pp 42-43.

[35] American Veterinary Medical Association: *Principles of Veterinary Medical Ethics*, 1993 Revision, "Advertising," *1994 AVMA Directory*, Schaumburg, IL, The Association, pp 42-43.

[36] American Veterinary Medical Association: *Principles of Veterinary Medical Ethics*, 1993 Revision, "Guidelines for Professional Behavior," paragraph 6, *1994 AVMA Directory*, Schaumburg, IL, The Association, p 42.

[37] American Veterinary Medical Association: *Principles of Veterinary Medical Ethics*, 1993 Revision, "Confidentiality," *1994 AVMA Directory*, Schaumburg, IL, The Association, p 44.

[38] American Veterinary Medical Association: *Principles of Veterinary Medical Ethics*, 1993 Revision, "Therapy, Determination of," *1994 AVMA Directory*, Schaumburg, IL, The Association, p 44.

[39] American Veterinary Medical Association: *Principles of Veterinary Medical Ethics*, 1993 Revision, "General Concepts," *1994 AVMA Directory*, Schaumburg, IL, The Association, p 42.

[40] American Veterinary Medical Association: *Principles of Veterinary Medical Ethics*, 1993 Revision, "Attitude and Intent," *1994 AVMA Directory*, Schaumburg, IL, The Association, p 42.

[41] American Veterinary Medical Association: *Principles of Medical Ethics and Current Opinions of the Council on Ethical and Judicial Affairs—1989.* In Gorlin RA, editor: *Codes of Professional Responsibility*, ed 2, Washington, DC, 1990, Bureau of National Affairs, pp 194-198, and 210.

[42] American Veterinary Medical Association: *Principles of Veterinary Medical Ethics*, 1993 Revision, "Guidelines for Professional Behavior," paragraph 2, *1994 AVMA Directory*, Schaumburg, IL, The Association, p 42.

[43] *See*, for example, AVMA Panel report and Colloquium on the recognition and alleviation of animal pain and distress, *J Am Vet Med Assoc* 191:1186-1296, 1987.

[44] American Veterinary Medical Association: *Principles of Veterinary Medical Ethics*, 1993 Revision, "General Concepts," *1994 AVMA Directory*, Schaumburg, IL, The Association, p 42.

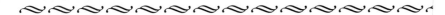

How to Approach Problems in Normative Veterinary Ethics

Normative veterinary ethics is the branch of veterinary ethics that attempts to discover correct moral norms for veterinary practice.

Normative veterinary ethics is the most important branch of veterinary ethics. When veterinarians ask the question "What should I do?", they usually want to know what is morally right for them to do. They are not interested in what they or other practitioners think ought to be done (descriptive veterinary ethics) or what is considered appropriate by a government body (administrative veterinary ethics) or the organized profession (official veterinary ethics). Understanding these things can be relevant to a determination of what is right or in making a decision about how one should act. However, there is no necessary correspondence between one's own ethical standards or those of other veterinarians, government bodies, the profession's official ethical apparatus—and the requirements or ideals of morality.

Government bodies and professional organizations should also regard normative veterinary ethics as fundamental. Government and the organized profession should also want their ethical standards to be correct. They too must be prepared to compare their ethical judgments against objective principles of morality.

∽ REALISTIC AIMS OF CONTEMPORARY NORMATIVE VETERINARY ETHICS

Like other branches of ethics that attempt to determine what is morally correct in an area of human endeavor, normative veterinary ethics seeks a general and systematic account of moral issues (see Chapter 5). Such an account would include a survey of the virtues one should expect in veterinarians. It would identify the general values the profession should embrace and explore how these values can help to solve particular issues. Normative veterinary ethics would also attempt to formulate a set of principles veterinarians can use in guiding responses to moral questions about how they ought to act.

Normative veterinary ethics is today very far from such a comprehensive approach. The literature of normative veterinary ethics is tiny compared to that of normative medical or legal ethics. There must be more articles and books, more ethics scholars active in the veterinary schools, and more practitioners participating in ethical discussion before normative veterinary ethics can collect enough perspectives and proposed conclusions to produce a comprehensive body of knowledge.

Because of the present rudimentary state of normative veterinary ethics, no one is in a position to offer definitive answers to all of its most important problems. Nor does this book attempt to do so. Rather, it is the purpose of the remainder of this volume to survey many of the critical issues facing normative veterinary ethics, and to provide a structure one can use to elaborate one's own thinking about these issues. Along the way, I offer some of my own conclusions about how some of these ethical questions ought to be answered to stimulate discussion and debate.

∾ THREE FUNDAMENTAL ISSUES OF NORMATIVE VETERINARY ETHICS

Normative veterinary ethics faces three fundamental issues in examining veterinary practice.

What Questions Should Be Asked?

Normative veterinary ethics must first determine when to ask questions and what sorts of questions to ask. Clearly, if there is an ethical problem one does not see in a situation or if one asks the wrong questions about a perceived problem, one will not do justice to the situation.

For example, I once visited animal quarters maintained by a respected laboratory animal veterinarian. The facility housed several dogs. They appeared clean and healthy and were receiving excellent veterinary care. However, the pens in which the dogs were kept contained only food, water, and bedding. I asked the veterinarian what he thought about supplying chew toys to make the animals' lives more enjoyable. He responded by raising clearly relevant questions regarding whether such toys would be economically feasible and would frustrate the purposes of the experiment. But the veterinarian (to his own surprise) had never thought of asking any of these questions because he had never considered the issue of supplying toys to laboratory dogs.

On the other hand, one must avoid asking too many questions, lest one invent ethical issues where they do not exist. I sometimes sneak into situations I discuss with my veterinary students problems that raise medical cases in which ethical questioning should be delayed pending medical analysis. I ask, for example, what the students would do about a client who wants her animal euthanized because it is urinating all over the house. When presented with this situation in a medicine course, students invariably focus first on possible medical causes of the problem. However, when they are "doing ethics," more than a few will ask *immediately* whether the owner has mistreated the animal or failed in his moral duties to train it properly. This is, of course, a poor response. It illustrates an important point: *asking ethical questions before one practices competent veterinary medicine is bad veterinary medicine as well as bad ethics.*

Certain questions must be addressed by normative veterinary ethics because they are matters of controversy among veterinarians or the public. However, one's judgment about whether some questions are worth asking can depend on one's ethical views. Some veterinarians may believe that inquiring about toys for laboratory dogs is foolish because in their view, one does not have an obligation to make such animals happy but only to prevent their experiencing unnecessary pain (see Chapter 11). It is clear, therefore, that among the issues normative veterinary ethics must consider is what questions are worth raising in the first place.

What Is the Best Approach to These Questions?

A second fundamental task of normative veterinary ethics is quite obviously attempting to determine what the best approach to a situation would be.

Who Should Make the Decision?

Normative ethics has a third concern quite different from discovering the best approach—the issue of who should have the authority to make a decision regarding a problem. Assuming for the purposes of argument that the dogs discussed earlier ought to have been given toys, it would not follow that I had any moral right to make the decision whether to give them toys. Indeed I did not have such authority, because neither the dogs, the animal quarters, or the experiments of which the animals were a part were mine. Although it may sometimes be obvious who has the moral right to make a decision regarding an ethical issue, this can be a matter of disagreement. For example, some veterinarians believe that they have the right and indeed the obligation to make important decisions for a client by assuring that a client agrees to what they have already decided ought to be done. Others (including myself) would argue that in all but the most extreme cases, the client and not the veterinarian has the moral right to make the decision, even if the client might make a morally incorrect decision.

One could consider the issue of who should have the authority to make a decision as part of the question of what the best approach would be. The point of separating these questions is to call attention to the fact that the question of who ought to make a decision is frequently an important one. The answer to this question can depend on factors other than what is beneficial to the patient, client, veterinarian, or society.

⮜ THE IMPORTANCE OF POLICIES IN ETHICAL DECISIONS

The consideration of hypothetical ethics cases or individual real-life moral dilemmas can obscure an important fact about normative ethical decisions. Sometimes, one's most important ethical choices are not directed at particular cases or problems. It is sometimes necessary to decide whether to have in place for oneself or one's practice a general policy or set of policies to handle recurring issues.*

By a "policy" I do not mean a written statement, posted on a wall or handed to all doctors, support staff, or clients—although in some hospitals such ways of distributing policies might sometimes be useful. Nor is a policy an approach that necessarily precludes exceptions or on-the-spot discretion by whoever must make an ethical decision. A "policy" as I understand the term is an approach that is to be applied to all one's actions if one is a sole practitioner, or to the actions of all doctors and employees in one's practice. A policy seeks to formulate a consistent response to a certain kind of problem or situation. The fundamental ethical and practice management aim of policies is to treat like cases similarly.

Many kinds of ethical problems in veterinary practice call for the formulation and enforcement of general policies. Consideration of one example must suffice here. As discussed in Chapters 20 and 22, veterinarians sometimes face the difficult problem of

---

*I am indebted to Dr. John Saidla of Cornell University for an appreciation of the importance of policies in approaching ethical issues.

clients whose animal can be helped but who cannot afford their fees. Some veterinarians tell me that in such cases they sometimes reduce their fees, agree to special payment arrangements, or in extreme cases provide services free of charge. Several larger animal hospitals and veterinary school facilities have a separate fund to which the public contributes and is used to assist needy clients. In speaking with doctors and hospital administrators who do attempt to subsidize the cost of veterinary care for such clients, I have been shocked that some do not have *general policies* regarding how such cases should be handled. What sorts of medical problems justify subsidization or fee reduction? (For example, will the hospital subsidize only treatments that can cure patients? To what extent will chronic care be subsidized?) What sorts of patients will be assisted ? (For example, will younger animals be favored over older?) What kinds of clients will be helped? (For example, will dedicated clients, or those for whom an animal is of great emotional or economic importance, be favored? Is it relevant whether a veterinarian is dealing with a new client or an established one with whom there has been a long professional relationship?) If a certain amount of money will completely cure several animals of minor ailments that are not life-threatening and one patient with a serious potentially lethal condition, to which will the hospital allocate scarce funds or uncompensated time? How needy must clients be to receive assistance, and how strong a showing of need should one require? Then there is the most important question of all—can the facility afford to subsidize services for certain clients, and if so, what limitations must be placed on such assistance so that the hospital remains financially profitable?

Clinicians at such hospitals will sometimes decide to take something off the customary fee or apply budgeted moneys or uncompensated services based on a "gut feeling" about the patient or client. At one veterinary hospital with a fund to assist needy clients, the application of such gut feelings has two inevitable results: (1) Animals and clients with similar medical and financial problems are treated differently by different clinicians, who have different gut feelings about the necessity for financial assistance. (2) The fund runs out of money well before the end of each fiscal year, making it impossible to help some animals unfortunate to have gotten sick late in the year. One veterinarian who does not have such a fund but tries to "budget" a certain amount of free services for needier clients reported to me a similar experience. After providing fee assistance several times, he determines that he cannot do more until he has generated sufficient revenue to allow some assistance to begin again. He concedes that some animals and clients he cannot afford to help at a given time may be more worthy of assistance than others he has already helped, but these clients and patients just happen to appear at the wrong time.

These examples demonstrate how the lack of a general and consistent policy can create ethical problems. First, some animals and clients that, given the willingness and ability of a hospital to provide financial assistance, ought to receive such assistance are not receiving it. Second, animals and clients that are less deserving of assistance are receiving it and animals and clients that are more deserving are not. Third, there can be fundamental unfairness in not treating like cases alike. Assuming again that a practice provides assistance to needy clients (and I am *not* arguing here, nor do I think, that every practice should), it can be wrong to deny one client and animal assistance when another client and animal in virtually identical circumstances receives it.

Policies, then, can assist a doctor or practice to act ethically. They can also help a hospital present to the public a consistent practice philosophy. This is good both from ethical and practice management standpoints. Hospitals with a consistent approach to certain kinds of issues make it easier for clients to choose a veterinarian, because clients will know what kind of services and general approaches they are likely to receive. Policies can also make for better relations among doctors and support staff. If all doctors in a practice know, for example, in what kinds of cases financial assistance may be contemplated, disagreement, inefficiency, and economic problems for the practice can be avoided.

The following are among the kinds of issues regarding which ethical policies can be useful:

- Determining whether, and under what conditions, to provide financial breaks or assistance for clients
- Whether the practice will euthanize healthy, well-behaved animals on client request, and if not, what steps, if any, the practice will take regarding such animals, such as transporting them to a shelter or attempting to adopt them out (see Chapter 21)
- Whether or under what circumstances the practice will perform procedures such as ear-cropping and tail-docking of dogs and declawing of cats (see Chapter 21)
- Whether the practice will engage in the sale of nonmedical products and services (see Chapter 17)
- Determining under what circumstances the practice will provide clients and patients services that are in scarce supply, such as blood transfusions or space in the intensive care unit (see Chapter 22)
- Determining how to respond to cases of client neglect or abuse of patients (see Chapter 21)
- How to deal with stray or owner-absent animals needing immediate care and brought into the practice by Good Samaritans (see Chapter 20)

Potential problems in formulating and applying policies should not be minimized. Policies do not always have their intended effect. It may sometimes be impossible to assure that all similar cases are treated alike. For example, at some point a fund or amount of budgeted services for needier clients may simply run dry. Some deserving animals or clients may have to do without, not because there is no policy but because there is no more money. It is not always easy to decide what is a morally appropriate approach for a given practice, especially if its doctors disagree about what kinds of approaches should be applied consistently. There can be issues about who in the practice should have the final say about certain kinds of situations, and whether and how much flexibility to allow each doctor. Some practices may find it appropriate to allow individual doctors to adopt their own, differing policies regarding certain kinds of medical or management issues. However, the formulation of ethical policies must be an important part of one's total approach to professional decisionmaking.

⁓ IDENTIFYING AND WEIGHING LEGITIMATE INTERESTS: A BATTLE PLAN FOR NORMATIVE VETERINARY ETHICS

As the eighteenth-century Scottish philosopher David Hume observed,[1] if people could always have whatever they wanted or needed, and if no one ever offended the wants and needs of anyone else, justice would be a superfluous concept. In a land of milk and honey, where riches could be had for the taking, it would be a waste of time to discuss what kinds of wages would be fair to pay employees or what kinds of distribution of wealth are just. No one would bother with these questions because they would have no complaints and no need for guidance about such matters. If people always treated each other and all other sentient creatures with saintly perfection, and if no one ever showed disrespect for, took advantage of, thieved from, assaulted, or violated the rights of anyone else, no one would be concerned about how people ought or ought not to behave. Everyone would just be happy and would behave well, automatically.

In veterinary medicine also, ethics is important largely because those who participate in or are affected by veterinary practice are not all perfectly situated and do not all have the same wants and interests. Veterinarians are concerned about how far they may go in promoting their practices, because many doctors are not doing as well as they desire and because many members of the profession believe that certain marketing techniques may harm the profession and ultimately, the interests of both clients and patients. Likewise, euthanasia would not be an issue for normative veterinary ethics if everyone felt comfortable about or behaved properly regarding the killing of veterinary patients.

It would be a mistake to think that all ethical issues involve conflicts of interests or desires or that those that do all require lengthy and acrimonious battles before a resolutions can be achieved. Patients, clients, and practitioners often have the same interests. Sometimes, their differing interests can argue for the same course of action.

Nevertheless, my experience discussing moral issues with veterinary students and practitioners has led me to conclude that the best way of making progress in normative veterinary ethics is to ask, at least initially, about differences in interests and about potential conflicts among these interests. Such an approach moves one quickly to the heart of the most important ethical issues facing the profession.

The following list of questions sets forth my proposed approach to normative veterinary ethics. It is offered not just as a framework for the remainder of this volume. It is presented as a tool that veterinary students, veterinarians, and others can use to structure their thinking about ethical issues in veterinary medicine.

This decision procedure results from years of teaching and speaking with many hundreds of veterinary students, veterinarians, veterinary technicians, clients, scientists, and educators about ethical issues in veterinary practice. It is not a substitute for the kinds of background information this book presents about ethical concepts and issues—background without which discussion of ethical questions can quickly degenerate into a venting of one's "gut feelings." However, I have found that even those who are just beginning a serious consideration of veterinary ethics can proceed much more quickly to intelligent and more satisfying discussions if they structure their thinking using this procedure. In short, it appears to work.

∽ A GENERAL APPROACH TO ETHICAL ISSUES IN VETERINARY MEDICINE

In determining what questions should be considered, the best approach to these questions, and who ought to have the authority to make a decision regarding them, one should routinely ask the following:

(1) What are the parties participating in, or potentially affected by, a problem or some aspect of veterinary practice?

In answering this question, consider whether any or all of the following should be included as relevant parties:

(a) any particular animal or animals directly involved in or affected by the situation or issue;

(b) other animals that could be affected by what might be done in the situation under consideration;

(c) any particular client or clients directly involved in or affected by the situation or issue;

(d) other actual or potential clients of this or other veterinarians who could be affected by what might be done in the situation under consideration;

(e) members of the public and society at large;

(f) the particular veterinarian or veterinarians directly involved in or affected by the situation under consideration;

(g) other veterinarians and the profession at large; and

(h) other actual or potential participants in the provision of veterinary services, including employees of the veterinarian under consideration, employees of other veterinarians, and veterinary students.

(2) What are the legitimate interests of these parties?

(3) How should these interests be weighed, balanced, or reconciled?

In considering how these interests ought to be weighed relative to each other, one should ask the following questions:

(a) What are the possible alternatives that reasonably can be considered, and what are the potential advantages and disadvantages of these alternatives to the relevant parties? Is it advisable to have a general practice policy for considering or dealing with this kind of situation?

(b) Does the law (including the pronouncements of the state board of veterinary medicine and other administrative bodies) attempt to choose an alternative or channel one's thinking toward or away from certain alternatives? How much weight should one give to any such legal guidance?

(c) Do standards of official veterinary ethics require that a certain approach be taken, or suggest ethical ideals useful in determining how one might act? If official norms do require some approach, how strongly should such requirements count in deciding what one ought to do?

(4) To what extent can one derive from one's response to the problem or issue, principles concerning virtues, values, and action-oriented rules for veterinarians that might contribute to a systematic approach to normative veterinary ethics?

ᵔᵕ EXPLAINING THE APPROACH

It will be the task of the remainder of this book to demonstrate the usefulness of this suggested approach to ethical issues. However, it is important that certain features of the approach be understood from the outset.

A Rough and Ready Battle Plan

First, the approach does not present an exhaustive list of all questions to be asked when considering ethical issues in veterinary medicine. There are many interesting and important issues in veterinary ethics, and one could make a strong case for including questions regarding any number of them in a general approach. One could, for example, argue that the approach should ask more specifically about factors relevant in weighing the interests of veterinary employees, veterinary students, or female practitioners. Nor does the approach specify all the possible ways of further refining and inquiring about those matters that are listed. Indeed, even the entries on my list of parties the interests of which should be routinely considered are capable of considerable refinement. For example, one could further divide the category of "other animals" that could be affected into (1) other animals owned by a particular client; (2) other animals owned by all of one's other clients; (3) all other animals owned by clients of other practitioners; (4) all other animals located in one's geographic region; (5) all nonowned wild animals; and (6) animals used in research and industry. Sometimes, as we shall see, several of these categories are among those one will want to consider in approaching an ethical problem.

Clearly, the success of any approach to ethical issues will turn on the ability of those using it to make further refinements and to ask additional questions when these are required by the issues at hand. Indeed, it is the purpose of my suggested approach to stimulate such refinement and questions. However, I have found that too long and complex an outline of questions tends to get put on the shelf and does not get used by students and practitioners looking for a manageable way of attacking ethical problems.

The Difficulty of the Questions

Because the approach is designed to elicit important questions and many important questions in normative veterinary ethics raise difficult and controversial issues, the approach will sometimes stimulate many more questions than it answers. For example, balancing the interests of an animal patient against those of its human owner is not always a routine exercise. One will sometimes first have to address the ethical question of what *ought to* be recognized as a legitimate interest of the animal. This in turn will often raise the issue of whether the animal may have a moral right to be treated or not treated in a certain way, or whether utilitarian considerations ought to apply.

The task of weighing legitimate interests is complicated not only by the fact that the interests of different parties can conflict. There can also be conflicts in the interests of each of the parties, the resolution of which itself can involve difficult moral issues. For example, I argue in Chapter 17 that among the potentially conflicting interests of veterinarians can be (1) their self-interest in increasing the profits of their practices and (2) their interest in belonging to a profession that is included among the healing arts. I argue that the merchandising of nonprofessional goods and services may in the short run promote the former interest for some doctors but ultimately will injure the latter interest for the profession as a whole. However, as we shall see, one cannot resolve this conflict merely by attempting to balance against each other only these interests of practitioners. One must also weigh these potentially conflicting interests against the interest that clients have in obtaining products and services at a reasonable price and the effect that furthering this interest will have upon the interest of patients in receiving services clients can afford.

Elaboration of Basic Concepts

The importance of several of the questions in my suggested approach has already been demonstrated. We have seen that an ethical problem may have more alternative solutions than may at first meet the eye (see Chapter 1); how the law sometimes attempts to choose among the alternatives and how one might assign a proper weight to such a choice (see Chapter 4); how administrative governmental bodies can impose their ethical judgments upon veterinarians (see Chapter 7); and how official ethical standards can apply to moral issues (see Chapters 8 and 9).

However, several general concepts and issues require further elaboration before the approach can be applied in earnest. Chapter 11 discusses factors relevant in determining the interests of veterinary patients. Chapter 12 focuses on one such factor, the concept of animal rights. Chapter 13 considers the most important patient-oriented ethical concept, animal welfare. Chapter 14 develops principles regarding the legitimate interests of veterinary clients. Chapter 15 defines and asks pointed questions about the human-companion animal bond. Chapter 16 discusses the legitimate interests of veterinarians and presents four models of veterinary practice currently struggling for the hearts and minds of doctors.

These are not the only concepts or concerns one will need in approaching issues in normative veterinary ethics. However, they will aid considerably in identifying and weighing the legitimate interests of the three most frequent participants in the arena of veterinary ethics —patients, clients, and veterinarians.

After establishing general principles regarding the legitimate interests of patients, clients, and veterinarians, the text turns to ethical issues in which the interests of these parties, and sometimes of others as well, come into play.

REFERENCE

[1]Hume D: *Treatise of Human Nature*, Sec II. In Aiken HD, editor: *Hume's Moral and Political Philosophy*, New York, 1966, Hafner, p 63.

PART TWO

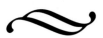

Fundamental Concepts

CHAPTER 11

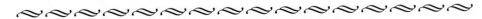

The Interests of Animals

*T*here are, surely, few people who do not think that animals have interests. Few veterinarians would have difficulty concluding that it is in the interest of a dog or cat in severe pain and near death from terminal cancer to put the poor animal out of its misery. Nor are judgments about what is good or bad for an animal patient reserved for situations in which one must contemplate ending its life. Veterinarians act in the interests of their patients every day—by assisting them in giving birth and being born, by vaccinating them against disease, by treating and repairing them when they become ill or injured, and by helping them to live long and happy lives through preventive medicine and good nutrition.

The issue faced by normative veterinary ethics is not establishing that animals have interests, but determining what interests they have and how strong these interests are. About this question there is considerable disagreement, among veterinarians and the public at large.

∼ THE ANTI-CRUELTY POSITION: FREEDOM FROM PAIN OR SUFFERING

According to one view, which I shall call the *anti-cruelty position*, the only very strong interest animals possess is an interest in not experiencing pain or suffering, or, if they must undergo some pain or suffering in their use by people, in not experiencing unnecessary pain or suffering.

This is probably still the predominant view regarding animals in American society today. It is found in numerous laws, and in the thinking of many in the veterinary and scientific communities. For example, the anti-cruelty to animals statutes of the various states do not require that people be good or kind to certain animals, but only that they not be cruel to them. (One cannot be prosecuted for failing to make one's dog happy by not playing with it or loving it as much as one might.) Moreover, according these laws, merely killing an animal or using it for food, fiber, draught, or innumerable other purposes cannot of itself constitute cruelty.* One must also have done such things in a manner causing the animal unjustifiable or unnecessary pain or discomfort. U.S. laws also require the "humane" slaughter of food animals, by which is meant killing them with a minimum of pain or discomfort.

Likewise, the great majority of animal researchers believe that their primary moral obligation is to protect their animals from unnecessary pain.[1] Many researchers also

---

*There are laws prohibiting the killing of other peoples' animals, but these typically are not anti-cruelty laws. It should also be noted that although in many jurisdictions the crime of "cruelty" to animals once required a malicious intent to harm an animal or taking pleasure in doing so, today in the great majority of states there is no such requirement. It is sufficient that one cause an animal unnecessary or unjustifiable pain.

believe that there is no moral issue in using an animal in an experiment if it is anesthetized prior to the beginning of the protocol and is never permitted to regain consciousness. For in such circumstances the animal will experience no pain whatever.[2]

In the food animal area, also, the anti-cruelty view holds sway. According to several leading livestock scientists "it is in the best interest of the American livestock producer to optimize the living conditions or environment of farm animals."[3] However, by "optimization" or animal "welfare" is not meant maximization of goods or positive states enjoyed by such animals, but "the absence of an excessive amount of stress."[4] Identification of "welfare" and "well-being" with lack of stress or negative states is also to be found in that standard reference, the *Merck Manual*. Its discussion of these concepts recommends that "from a practical stand" the veterinarian ask the following question: "Do the methods of handling, housing, and general management adopted by this owner/operator impose the least amount of distress (negative side of stress) on animals of this age, weight, stage of development, etc."[5]

In prohibiting "unnecessary" pain or suffering, the anti-cruelty position presupposes the legitimacy of certain human endeavors. By "unnecessary" pain the anti-cruelty position means pain that is not required for some legitimate human use of animals. No amount of pain or discomfort is strictly speaking "necessary" for any animal that is used by people. It is not, for example, absolutely required that people use animals for food or in research; animals are so used because people decide to use them in these ways. From the point of view of the anti-cruelty position as it is applied in American society, pain or discomfort undergone by food or research animals would be "necessary" if it is required for the use of the animal as food or in a scientifically defensible experiment. Both of these kinds of animal use are considered acceptable. On the other hand, if some amount of animal pain is required for a human endeavor that is thought to be illegitimate (for example, organized dog fighting or experiments with utterly no scientific justification), using animals in such endeavors will be judged to inflict "unnecessary" pain and will therefore be categorized as "cruel" or "inhumane."

The anti-cruelty position does permit one to take into account the amount of animal pain caused by a certain kind of animal use in determining whether that use is a legitimate one and the pain is therefore "necessary." But quite often, adherents of the anti-cruelty position will begin with the acceptance of a certain animal use as legitimate and then require that it be conducted so as to cause no pain or no more pain than "necessary."

The anti-cruelty position also permits one to view animals as having interests other than being free from pain or unnecessary pain. However, the anti-cruelty position does not consider such other interests to be very strong.

Thus a veterinarian who subscribes to the anti-cruelty position can give as one of her reasons for treating a dog or cat that treatment will assure the animal a better life. She can agree that these patients have an interest not just in being free from pain but in being positively healthy and happy. However, she will see no ethical problem in euthanizing the same animals when asked to do so, as long as they will not suffer in the process. She may, in short, believe it would be a moral ideal, something to strive for, that clients not have their healthy animals killed. But she will view an animal's interest in living or living a healthy and happy life as so weak that it is easily outweighed by the client's desire to be rid of it. She will believe that her overriding ethical obligation is to make sure that the animal will not experience any unnecessary suffering.

⮵ THE PARTIAL BREAKDOWN OF THE ANTI-CRUELTY POSITION

It seems fair to say that as a general position regarding the interests of all animals, the anti-cruelty position is no longer accepted by many people. An increasing number of people appears to be adopting the view that at least some animals are morally entitled not just to freedom from pain or unnecessary suffering but to certain positive benefits, even if providing these benefits entails considerable expense or inconvenience for people. There are veterinarians who will not painlessly kill an animal simply because the client wants to be rid of it, but will insist at the very least that it be taken to a shelter for possible adoption. These practitioners may not believe that such animals have an unqualified right to live, but they do believe that it is wrong not to try to give some animals a second chance. Every companion animal doctor has clients who view their animal as a member of the family, and entitled to the best veterinary care money can buy, even if such care is much more expensive than a painless death. In the area of animal research as well, some animals are coming to be seen as having interests over and above being free from pain or discomfort. The federal Animal Welfare Act requires that primates used in research be afforded "a physical environment adequate to promote [their] psychological well-being."[6] Some thinkers in the area of farm animal welfare too advocate not only the minimization of negative mental states but also the promotion of positive well-being.[7]

The beliefs of society or of the veterinary profession regarding the legitimate interests of animals are not in total disarray. Nevertheless, it is equally true that there is not a universal consensus about the interests of all animals, on which one could comfortably rely in weighing the interests of animals. There is, surely, enough disagreement to compel those who accept the anti-cruelty position, as well as those who reject it, to say something in defense of their positions.

⮵ THE INADEQUACY OF THE ANTI-CRUELTY POSITION

The decision procedure for approaching issues in normative veterinary ethics suggested in Chapter 10 is intended to facilitate discussion of moral issues and not to dictate solutions. Nevertheless, I would argue that as an exhaustive account of the interests of all animals, the anti-cruelty position is obviously incorrect.

The easiest place to find counterexamples to the anti-cruelty position is in the relationship between people and animals which is now termed the "human-companion animal bond." More about the nature of this bond is discussed in Chapter 15. For now it can be said that this relationship brings great benefits to a central aspect of the lives of human and animal alike. We may not always be able to say that an animal in such a relationship is able to "give of itself" with the "expectation" that it will receive something in response. However, we can certainly say that what such an animal gives can often make it enormously disrespectful, ungrateful, and wrong to treat it as having no more than an interest in avoiding pain or discomfort.

My late Yorkshire Terrier may not have known he did me a favor when he greeted me joyously at the door or when we played fetch with his little toys. Yet great favors and pleasures he bestowed nevertheless. In light of the many benefits I received from him over the years, I was surely obligated to attend to many of his interests. He was entitled to attention, the opportunity for exercise, and good nutrition so that he could have his happiness too. He deserved to be taken to the veterinarian regularly, not just so that he could be free of pain but also so that he could continue to enjoy his own pleasures. None of this meant that I had to bankrupt myself to meet his needs or that his interests usually took precedence over my own—although they sometimes did! But it did mean that I was obligated to treat him as having legitimate interests that went beyond freedom from discomfort and that sometimes outweighed my desires or predilections.

What I have said about my dog is no different from what many people would say about their animals. However, once one begins to view certain animals as having legitimate interests beyond freedom from pain or discomfort, one is forced to draw some lines. There are limits to such interests. There are many times when human interests do outweigh those of animals. Moreover, it is not the case that all animals have the same legitimate interests or have them to the same degree. Once we admit that some animals sometimes have interests above and beyond freedom from pain we must be prepared to justify our decisions about when this is the case and when it is not. To assist in this process, normative veterinary ethics must utilize principles regarding the nature and weight of animal interests.

∼ RELEVANT FACTORS IN IDENTIFYING AND WEIGHING LEGITIMATE INTERESTS OF ANIMALS

The following are suggested as very general factors to be taken into account in weighing the interests of animals. Although all these factors seem intuitively relevant to weighing animal interests, many require further elaboration and research. It is, for example, easy—and surely correct—to say that an animal's capacity to experience stress is relevant to determining its interests. But how animal stress is to be defined, measured, and compared is a matter that could require many decades of solid investigation.

Capacity to Experience Pain, Suffering, Stress, and Other Forms of Discomfort

Although some animals may sometimes have interests beyond freedom from pain or discomfort, the capacity of an animal to experience what we would call unpleasant or negative psychological states remains a crucial factor in determining the nature and weight of its interests. Although pain and other negative states can be beneficial in assuring an animal's health or safety and are undoubtedly products of natural selection, all other things being equal it is better not to feel pain (or another negative state such as distress or discomfort) than to feel it. Moreover, intense or long-lasting pain is worse than weak or fleeting pain. Therefore it seems intuitively clear that the interest an animal has in not suffering pain, or a certain kind of negative psychological state, is greater the more intensely and the longer it can experience that negative state. And it has a greater interest in not experiencing a severe negative state than a mild one, and in not experiencing a long negative state than a short one.

Amount and duration, however, are not the only factors. Certain negative psychological states carry extra weight. For example, when one feels a sharp pain, that is bad. But if one also feels anxiety and fear about the pain—if one worries about it, contemplates its potential effects, and then troubles about whether more is on the way—one will feel worse than if one just felt the pain alone. Such anxiety and fear can be so intense that they can not only continue after the pain has disappeared but can be more unpleasant than the pain ever was.

To the extent that an animal can feel not only pain but also stress, fear, and anxiety, its interest in avoiding a situation might be greater than the interest of another animal that might only feel pain in the same situation. Veterinarians and animal owners all know a common example of this distinction. A dog or cat may be up and about hours after surgery. If a person has a similar operation, the agony can last for weeks or months. It is possible that human pain receptors are more sensitive and that the person is really feeling more pain than the animal. However, it seems just as likely that what makes the human's condition worse is the fact that he feels terrible in many ways *about* the pain. This process itself can call attention to the pain, make it worse, and make it last longer.

Capacity to Experience Pleasure and Other Positive Mental States

If it can be in the interest of certain animals to be spared pain or discomfort, it may also be in their interest to experience pleasure or other positive mental states. Research indicates that there are "reward circuits" in the brains of both human beings and animals.[8] These pathways could have evolved as a mechanism for reinforcing behaviors that promote the survival of the individual and the species; they may also play a fundamental role in the human appreciation of beauty and the desire to learn. If animals have such reward circuits some may have the capacity to experience some of the "higher" pleasures. We may well decide upon reflection that animals, or some animals, have a much stronger interest in avoiding pain than in experiencing pleasure. Thus animal pleasures might not weigh heavily against human needs. However, if some animals do have an interest in experiencing pleasure, we also might be able to determine that they have a greater interest in experiencing a more intense pleasure than mild pleasure and in experiencing a long positive mental state than a short one.

Intelligence

One factor that surely counts in influencing the weight of an animal's interests is its intelligence. Most people feel more uncomfortable about subjecting chimpanzees to invasive laboratory experiments than rats because the former are able to perceive and react to their surroundings in a far more complex and innovative way. Likewise, one reason there is such intense interest in protecting whales is that, although we may have little idea of what is going through the minds of these creatures, we do know that they are enormously intelligent.

In many cases, intelligence may increase the weight of an animal's interests because it leads to or makes possible something else of value. Dogs, cats, and certain primates can interact and form bonds with people, in part because they are intelligent. Another result or aspect of intelligence that itself may have value is self-awareness, the ability to reflect upon or understand what is happening to one. Likewise, the capacity to experience certain painful or pleasurable states seems linked to intelligence; for example, the cat that appears to take great pleasure in attempting to bat an errant insect with its paws is able to have such experiences because it is capable of sophisticated awareness and interpretation.

Although intelligence can lead to other things of value, it is itself valuable. We regard the retarded human as unlucky (but not without great worth) because we view being able to perceive and react to the world in certain ways preferable to not having such capacities. Likewise we view chimpanzees' extraordinary intelligence itself a lucky and precious condition, in part because it enables these animals to take in more of the world than can a laboratory rodent or even the family dog.

Capacity to Experience or Exhibit Valuable Emotions and Character Traits

Another feature of some animals that increases their value in our eyes is their ability to experience emotions or to have traits of character that we value in our fellow humans. We admire a dog that loves its owner and praise it for being loyal and obedient. On the other hand, a dog that is vicious, nasty, and selfish may be valued less—so much so, that an owner of such an animal will sometimes appear justified in not expending the time or resources to assist its interests as one might want him to expend upon a loving and friendly animal. It may seem unfair to favor some animals and disfavor others because of traits for which they may not be responsible. But we also favor nice and disfavor disagreeable people even though we may not be able to say that they somehow decided to be so. Just as friendliness in people is better than viciousness and belligerence, so can it be in animals, and so can it make a difference in our judgments about how strongly we ought to value their interests.

Self-Awareness

One feature of most human beings that appears to give them greater value than many animals is the fact that we possess self-awareness. Not only do we experience certain things, but we are also aware that it is ourselves who are experiencing them, and we are aware of ourselves as beings distinct from others. It can be worse to do something to a being that possesses such self-awareness than to one that does not. While beings that do and those that do not possess self-awareness may both be able to experience pleasure, only those with self-awareness can anticipate experiencing pleasure and can feel further pleasure at the anticipation of experiencing pleasure. Similarly, while beings that do and those that do not have self-awareness may feel pain, only the former can feel anxiety or fear at the prospect that they will feel pain, can be ashamed of fearing the experience of pain, and so on. Self-awareness is also related to autonomy, the capacity to decide on one's own that one will make decisions and long-term plans and to work to put these decisions into effect.

There is some evidence that certain animals may possess self-awareness to a limited degree. Primate psychologist Gordon Gallup has demonstrated that chimpanzees, and orangutans, but not gorillas or monkeys, are capable of looking into a mirror and recognizing that is themselves they are seeing. Gallup argues that the former animals have a sense of self.[9] Chimpanzees deceive each other, a kind of behavior that requires them to impute some thought or self-awareness to other beings.[10] Dolphins may display reciprocal altruism not related to kinship.[11] Elephants appear to demonstrate elaborate grieving behaviors on the death of other elephants.[12] These behaviors indicate that certain animals do sometimes exhibit some degree of self-awareness and should be accorded a higher moral status than other animals.

Interaction with Human Beings

As noted above, we do think that certain animals are owed greater consideration because of their interactions with human beings. Thus even if a pig and the family dog have comparable mental abilities, we often believe we owe something to the dog because of what it has done for us and what we have already done for it. It is not irrational and unjustifiable to single out for special treatment certain beings with which one has interacted even though there may be others that, in the abstract, may seem as worthy. Most people believe that they have greater obligations to members of their own families than to strangers. They believe this not just because of blood lineage (some people are, of course, adopted) but because they think they owe more to those they have known, interacted with, and loved than to strangers.

An Animal's Nature

Rollin argues that animals have a biologically determined nature (he uses the Greek word "*telos*") which they have an interest in satisfying and which is therefore entitled to respect.[13] As Rollin points out, it seems plausible to say that it is in the interest of a dog with an innate need for vigorous activity, to be given opportunities for exercise. Likewise, as argued in Chapter 21, it is wrong to "de-bark" some pet dogs because this takes away from these animals an important part of their "dogness," an essential part of what it is for them to be a *dog*.

The notion that an animal's "nature" contributes to its legitimate interests is intuitively appealing, but requires considerable refinement and discussion. Do we think animals possess an interest in having parts of their "nature" respected simply because frustrating their natures causes them discomfort or prevents them from experiencing pleasures they might otherwise experience—or because there is something inherently wrong in violating their *telos*? Do some animals (predators, such as wolves, for example) have natures that do not entitle them to as much respect as other animals which happen to have more benign natures? Are certain features of an animal's nature more important to it or (not necessarily the same thing) worthy of greater respect than other features? What is the relevance of the fact that certain animals have been given inborn "natures" by humans to make them more amenable to certain human uses?

Utilitarian Considerations

As is explained in Chapter 5, utilitarianism maintains that the right action (or general rule for action) is one that will in the future produce no less benefit to all affected than any other action (or rule). Utilitarianism is unsatisfactory as an exhaustive normative theory because people do not believe that the only consideration in determining the morality of an action or practice is the amount of benefit or detriment that action or practice will produce in the future.

Nevertheless, comparing the resultant benefits and detriments of alternative actions is sometimes relevant in determining what one ought to do, and such considerations often play a role in deciding our moral obligations regarding animals. We often apply utilitarian considerations to a single animal, for example, when we conclude that we ought to euthanize a terminally ill patient because ending its life will prevent it from suffering unnecessary pain. (To be sure, one can also argue that such an animal has a right not to be kept in pain.) Utilitarian arguments are also applied from animal to animal. Thus we sometimes justify experimentation on selected animals to develop and test veterinary drugs on the grounds that causing some pain or discomfort to these animals will produce great benefits for other animals on which these drugs will be used.

Utilitarian considerations are also applied from animals to humans. The argument that animal experimentation is justified by resultant benefits to people, or that farrowing crates ought to be designed so as to maximize productivity while at the same time minimizing pain or discomfort to the animals, are utilitarian arguments.

~ HUMAN PRIORITY

I have identified several considerations that appear to be legitimate in identifying and weighing animal interests. However, it is one thing to maintain that an animal may have a legitimate interest and quite another to conclude that this interest ought to be given priority over the interests of people or other animals in a given set of circumstances. In the area of normative veterinary ethics, recognition of this distinction is extremely important because animal interests—as indisputably present as they may be—are often less weighty than and must often give way in particular circumstances to human interests.

In applying any palatable approach to veterinary ethics, therefore, one will often find oneself appealing to the principle that the interests of a particular person or of people in general are so much more important than those of some animal or animals, that the animals' interests must give way partially or entirely.

It is beyond the scope of this book to offer a complete justification for the widely held belief that human interests are generally entitled to greater weight than animal interests. In recent years, some philosophers have claimed that there are no morally relevant differences between humans and many animals or that the differences are often far less widespread or important than many have supposed them to be.[14] Some of these discussions are sophisticated and challenging and cannot be done justice here. Nevertheless, any discussion of normative veterinary ethics cannot ignore completely certain arguments challenging the view that human beings are superior in moral value and status to animals.

The Argument from Animal Mental Complexity

One argument which is supposed to show that some animal interests are as important as human interests recognizes the relevance of mental sophistication to the weight of human or animal interests. However, according to this argument, many animals are in fact as mentally sophisticated as most human beings, at least in respects relevant to assessing their moral value. It is concluded that human and nonhuman animals have equally weighty interests in such things as living, not being eaten or experimented on, and in not being used as a means toward any one else's ends.

One proponent of such an argument is philosopher Tom Regan. He asserts that:

> ...perception, memory, desire, belief, self-consciousness, intention, a sense of the future—these are among the leading attributes of the mental life of normal mammalian animals aged one or more. Add to this list the not unimportant categories of emotion (e.g., fear or hatred) and sentience, understood as the capacity to experience pleasure or pain, and we begin to approach a fair rendering of the mental life of these animals.[15]

Regan does not indicate why he thinks all "normal" mammals have such mental complexity after they reach 1 year of age. Nor does he provide credible evidence for his contention that a laboratory hamster, for example, can be self-conscious in the same way that a human being is, has a sense of the future, or can be said to experience not just pain but such sophisticated emotions as hatred (which requires not just a negative feeling, but such a feeling directed at someone or something that one identifies as the hated object).

One should not ignore behavioral or biochemical evidence of the mental attributes of any animal. However, it is just not the case that a hamster, cow, horse, dog, or even a chimpanzee, is capable of all the same kinds of pleasures and pains, thoughts and decisions, and autonomous life as an adult human being of average mental ability. Regan's blanket generalizations are incompatible with the kind of ethical approach to animals we surely need—one that is willing to look carefully and scientifically at what animals really are and what they can do, and one that takes into account the enormous variety among animal species and individual animals of the same species.

The Argument from Genetic Similarity

An argument that has been raised by some people interested in protecting the great apes (chimpanzees, gorillas, and orangutans) appeals to the genetic similarity of these species and human beings. This similarity, it has been argued, requires that the great apes be given the same rights as human children and mentally impaired adults, and be included with humans in a "community of equals."[16] Animal welfare scientist Andrew Rowan characterizes the appeal to genetic similarity as follows:

> Darwin provided a logical explanation of the similarities with his theory of evolution that indicated a common ancestry for humans and apes. Now, molecular dating has validated Darwin and puts the common ancestor at around seven million years ago, a very short time when considering the time-span of life on earth. DNA studies show that humans share 98.4% of their DNA with the two living species of chimpanzees. Gorilla DNA differs from human and chimpanzee DNA by about 2.3%, which means that the chimpanzee's closest relative is not the gorilla, but the human.[17]

Rowan observes that this argument is not welcomed by some animal activists, who see the inclusion of the great apes within a circle of special concern as an exclusion of most other animal species. More importantly, the argument from genetic similarity is just not convincing. Imagine there are two beakers each filled with an equal volume of liquid. The first beaker contains only distilled water. The second contains distilled water and a deadly poison amounting to 1.6% in weight or volume (for the purposes of this example it matters not which). This is enough poison to make it lethal to drink the contents of the second beaker. Is there a significant difference between the beakers? There certainly would be to someone who had to drink the contents of one of them. Further, suppose that the poison in the second beaker will degenerate and become harmless, but that this process will take 7 million years. Is this a significant time? It certainly would be to someone who had to drink from this beaker. Indeed, although 7 million years may be insignificant from the perspective of the history of life on earth, such a time span constitutes an eternity to almost anything individual humans, nations, cultures, or humankind in general would contemplate. Most of us would be inclined to say that it took a very long time indeed for humans and chimpanzees to evolve from our common ancestors, that is, enough time to weaken considerably any claim that we ought to include them in a "community of equals," because they are really our "close" relatives.

The point of this example is not to assert that humans are good and apes somehow evil or poisonous, but rather to suggest that percentage differences in our genetic material, or the time it may have taken humans and apes to evolve from any common ancestor, are themselves of no moral significance. Whether a small (or large) percentage difference (of genetic material or anything else) carries any weight depends on the larger nature of one's enterprise and the considerations relevant to that enterprise. That chimpanzees differ from humans in "only" 1.6% of their DNA does not make them as sophisticated mentally or behaviorally as the human being of average, or even far below average, intelligence. Nor would those of us who believe we ought to treat chimpanzees or other primates much better than we treat, say rats or mice, recant our views, if scientists learned that they were mistaken and that the genetic difference between humans and the great apes exceeded 10%, 20%, or 50%—or, indeed, is significantly less than 1.6%. Some animals, such as whales, undoubtedly have much less genetic material in common with humans than chimpanzees do with humans but nevertheless seem worthy of special consideration because of their apparent mental complexity and sophistication.

The kind of treatment chimpanzees, gorillas, orangutans, and other animals as well, deserve depends on the kinds of factors relating to mentality, emotion, and behavior discussed above. As philosopher James Rachels observes, the genetic similarity between great apes and humans may be important, not because this similarity is of independent moral significance, but because it makes physically possible kinds of mentality and behavior that are of moral significance.[18]

The Argument from Deficient Humans

Perhaps the argument raised most frequently in favor of equal consideration for people and animals proceeds from the fact that there are many human beings, including young infants, the severely mentally retarded, and deeply senile, whom most people regard as having very strong moral rights. Included among these rights are the right not to have their lives terminated just because they are not mentally sophisticated and the right not to be used in biomedical research. According to the argument from deficient humans, there are many animals that are at least as sophisticated mentally as these deficient humans. Therefore it is concluded, if deficient people have the moral right not to be eaten or experimented on without their consent, so do these animals.[19]

There are many things wrong with this argument. It is far from clear that it even makes sense to say that a human being has the same mental level as, say, a bat or hamster, because if he did, he might not be a human being but a bat or a hamster.[20] Nor does the argument from deficient humans take into account crucially important differences between many deficient humans and animals that often give the former greater moral value than selected animals. The infant who is now mentally unsophisticated is *potentially* a human adult of great mental sophistication, while the laboratory hamster will never reach such a level. Moreover, many deficient human beings have become so only *after* a long and productive life and are, we want to say, entitled to certain respect and care from their relatives and society, in part because of what they have given to others.

However, even if we set aside the past and futures of certain deficient humans, we can still see that there are important morally relevant differences between animals and deficient humans which show there is something special about being a deficient human. These differences reinforce rather than undercut most peoples' basic moral belief that human beings are more valuable than animals.

The Relevance of Being a *Deficient* Human

One clear difference between all deficient humans as we have been speaking of them and, for example, all normal laboratory hamsters, is that the former are all deficient while the latter are not.

Because deficient humans fall short of what normal humans can experience and do, we are inclined to feel sorry for them (although many live happy or productive lives and all are entitled to the utmost respect and regard). We would certainly say the following about human beings who have the mental capacity of a hamster.

- They are *disabled* in virtue of their having restricted capabilities.
- They *suffer* from a disability. (We would say this even if they are not suffering because of their disability.)
- They have been *harmed or injured.*
- They have already been subjected a great evil or *misfortune.*
- Their impairment is a *tragedy.*

None of these things would be said of the normal laboratory hamster, and several things follow from this fact.

First, in experimenting on a deficient human one would be making him worse off than one would be making a hamster of (let us suppose) equal mental abilities on which the same experiment would be conducted. For if we suppose that both deficient human and hamster would be treated equally (confined in the same way, caused the same amount of pain, etc.), the experiment will nevertheless bring the deficient human to a level far beneath the level of a non-deficient human than the hamster will be brought beneath the level of a normal hamster. Even before the experiment, the deficient human with the mental life of a hamster is enormously disabled, harmed, and tragic. (Remember, we are speaking here of a human with the mental capacity of a *hamster.*) During and after the experiment, he may become even more so. The hamster, on the other hand, begins as a normal, nonharmed, noninjured, nontragic hamster. It can be harmed by the experiment, of course. But treating it and the deficient human equally will probably never render it worse off than the deficient human.

Put another way, in determining the extent of an injury or harm to a being, one must take into account more than the quantity or quality of unpleasant sensations it may experience. One must consider what it means that *such* a being is having these experiences.

It does not follow that we can experiment freely on hamsters or other animals or use them in any way we please. Nevertheless, where the total of harm or injury suffered by potential subjects of an experiment is a relevant consideration in determining which subjects to use, this consideration will argue much more strongly in favor of using an animal, the normal mental state of which might be equal at best to that of a deficient human, than using a deficient human.

There are other reasons the enormous degree of a deficient human's disability can weigh more strongly against using him in experiments than against using, say, a hamster. We feel a reluctance to harm someone who has suffered a great injury unless there is a very strong reason to do so. Other things being equal, it is wrong to hurt someone when he is down. Because deficient humans are already gravely disabled, subjecting them to further deprivation is like beating the fallen; it just is not fair to hurt them more. I suggest that one reason we feel less reluctant to experiment on hamsters is that they are not already deprived. Indeed many laboratory animals have safer, more comfortable lives than they would experience in the wild.

Also, when faced with the necessity of choosing which of a number of persons must suffer some deprivation or harm (as, for example, where budget cuts make it necessary to deprive some students of low-interest loans), justice sometimes requires that those who are already deprived suffer less of the necessary burden than those for whom the new deprivation will be less of an injury. And this can be so even where none of those affected are responsible for their condition or for the need to impose a burden upon anyone. Thus aside from our obligation to avoid inflicting harm on already disabled humans, where an experiment or some use of a living creature is appropriate (and when this is the case, will admittedly sometimes be in need of discussion), justice will almost always require doing it on a normal animal first, and if at all possible, instead of, on a disabled human.

～ LIMITATIONS ON HUMAN PRIORITY

In short, weighing animal interests will often involve recognizing the priority of human interests. However, animal interests do count. Sometimes, these interests can prohibit a human activity entirely. Sometimes, animal interests create significant limitations on what people may morally do to animals. The strength of animal interests is reflected in the concept of animal rights, which is the subject of the next chapter.

REFERENCES

[1]Loew FM: Alleviation of pain: The researcher's obligation, *Lab Anim* 9:36-38, 1981.

[2]Hewitt HB: The use of animals in experimental cancer research. In Sperlinger D, editor: *Animals in Research,* Chichester, UK, 1981, John Wiley & Sons, p 170 (stating that the "painless taking of animal life" is not an immoral act; and that "I should be more upset by my having caused one animal to suffer by my neglect or ineptitude than I should be by my administering euthanasia to 50 animals at the termination of an experiment in which none had been caused suffering").

[3]Friend TH, Dellmeier GR: *Applied Animal Euthenics Program,* Mk. II, College Station, Texas, undated, published privately, p 3.

[4]*Id*,7.

[5]Fraser CM, editor: *The Merck Veterinary Manual,* ed 7, "Animal Welfare," Rahway, NJ, 1991, Merck, pp 928-929.

[67] U.S.C.A. § 2143(a)(2)(B). But note that for animals in general, the Secretary of Agriculture is directed to promulgate regulations "to ensure that animal pain and distress are minimized." § 2143(a)(3)(A).

[7]Fox MW: *Farm Animals: Husbandry, Behavior, and Veterinary Practice,* Baltimore, 1984, University Park Press, p 205.

[8]Wise RA: Catecholamine theories of reward: A critical review, *Brain Res* 152:215-247, 1978; Prado-Alcala R, Streather A, Wise RA: Brain stimulation reward and dopamine terminal fields. II. Septal and cortical fields, *Brain Res* 301:209-219, 1984.

[9]Gallup GG: Toward a comparative psychology of mind. In Mellgren RL: *Animal Cognition and Behavior,* Amsterdam, 1983, North Holland, pp 473-510.

[10]Premack D, Woodruff G: Does the chimpanzee have a theory of mind? *Behav Brain Sci* 4:515-526, 1981; Woodruff G, Premack D: Intentional communication in the chimpanzee: the development of deception, *Cognition* 7:333-362, 1979.

[11]Connor RC, Norris KS: Are dolphins reciprocal altruists? *Am Naturalist* 119:358-374, 1982.

[12] Douglas-Hamilton I, Douglas-Hamilton O: *Among the Elephants,* New York, 1975, Viking Press.

[13]Rollin BE: *Animal Rights and Human Morality,* Buffalo, 1981, Prometheus Books, pp 54-57.

[14]For an impressive argument for the latter contention, see Rachels J:*Created from Animals: The Moral Implications of Darwinism,* Oxford, 1990, Oxford University Press.

[15]Regan T: *The Case for Animal Rights,* Berkeley, 1983, University of California Press, p 81.

[16]Cavalieri P, Singer P, editors: *The Great Ape Project*, New York, 1994, St. Martin's Press. Although all the contributors to this volume contend that the great apes and humans be included in such a "community of equals," some do not appeal to the argument from genetic similarity in support of this demand.

[17]Rowan A: The great ape project, *Tufts University School of Veterinary Medicine Animal Policy Report* 8:4, 1994.

[18]Rachels J: Why Darwinians should support equal treatment for other apes. In Cavalieri P, Singer P, editors: *The Great Ape Project*, New York, 1994, St. Martin's Press, p 156.

[19]For an exhaustive account of several forms of this kind of argument and a defense of one of them, *see*, Regan T: An examination and defense of one argument concerning animal rights. In Regan T: *All That Dwell Therein*. Berkeley, 1982, University of California Press, pp 113-147.

[20]Nagel T: What is it like to be a bat? *Philos Rev* 83:435-450, 1974.

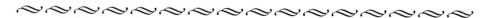

CHAPTER 12

Animal Rights

*T*he subject of animal rights has caused considerable disquiet and discomfort among veterinarians. Some see in animal rights yet an additional challenge to the economic viability of the profession.[1] For others, the concept of animal rights poses a danger to the natural order, science, and progress.[2] Many veterinarians find animal rights so antithetical to the aims and values of the profession that they prefer not to speak of animal "rights" at all.[3-7] One astute observer has remarked that the battle over animal rights has caught veterinarians in a "crossfire"[8]—a metaphor that might suggest to some that veterinarians are doomed, and to others that the profession must make a quick retreat from the entire controversy.

Much of this unhappiness is justified. There is, in fact, a great deal in the animal rights movement that is morally repugnant and deeply subversive of the interests of veterinarians, their patients, and clients.

This chapter argues that a proper response to the animal rights *movement* is not abandonment of animal *rights*.

～ WHAT IS A "RIGHT?"

There is disagreement among philosophers about the nature of rights, about who or what does or does not have certain rights, and why.[9] For the purposes of this discussion, however, there are several things one can say are true of rights.

There Is a Difference between Moral and Legal Rights.

Some moral rights (for example, the right of parents to respect from their children) are not enforced by the law. And the law can enforce as a right (for example, the right to own slaves in the Confederacy) practices that violate moral rights. Legal rights can be a matter of political decision: if the government decrees that something is a right and backs its decision with the force of law, then it is a legal right. On the other hand, although decisions of individuals or groups of people often are relevant to determining their moral rights, something does not become a moral right simply because the majority, or anyone for that matter, decides that it is. Thus when one asks whether animals "have rights," it is important to keep in mind whether one is talking about moral or legal rights, or both.

Moral and Legal Rights Mark Out Very Strong Claims.

When people say that someone has a moral right to some kind of treatment they are saying something much stronger than that it is right to treat him in this way. For example, it may be the right thing for you to give to a charity when a solicitor appears at your door. But this does not mean that the charity has a *right* to your money. Moral rights mark out claims that ordinarily do not require another's permission to be respected and that cannot be overridden merely because overriding them would, on balance, produce more benefit than detriment to all affected.[10] For example, because a person ordinarily has the right to use her car as she likes, she may quite properly drive to a basketball game and pass in good conscience a stranger who might better use the car to support his family—even though lending the car to the stranger might on balance produce more happiness to all affected. This does not mean that considerations of the general happiness or welfare, or others' rights can never override a right. In a snowstorm, for example, when private use of cars might endanger the lives of others and prevent cleaning the road, one's right to use one's automobile may properly be overridden, in favor of the greater good of the greater number. However, part of the point of saying it is a person's moral right to use one's property as one wants is to say that one should not ordinarily be prevented from using it as one likes, and that this liberty can be overridden, if at all, only for extremely grave and important reasons.[11]

Philosopher Joel Feinberg explains why rights are so valuable. Rights stem from basic interests of right-holders. We do not say, for example, that a child has a moral and legal right not to be abused by its parents because the next-door neighbors might be offended by the sounds of the regular thrashings, or because regular beatings of the child might make its parents worse people. Rather, we say that the child has a right not to be abused because the abuse is something that is a wrong to the *child* and gives rise to a moral and legal claim that can be raised *in the child's behalf*, and for *its* sake. This is why, as Feinberg observes, a right is:

> ...an extremely valuable possession, neither dependent on or derivative from the compassionate feelings, propriety, conscientiousness, or sense of *noblesse oblige* of others. It is a claim against another party in no way dependent on the love of the other party or the loveableness of its possessor. Hence, wicked, wretched, and odious human beings maintain certain rights against others, and the duties of others based on those rights are incumbent even on those who hate the claimant, and hate with good reason. A right is a matter of justice, and justice, while perhaps no more valuable than love, sympathy, and compassion, is nevertheless a moral notion distinct from them.[12]

Moral and Legal Rights Presuppose That Holders of Rights Have Interests.

Another essential feature of "rights" (both moral and legal) follows from the fact that a right is a claim that can be made either directly by a right-holder in its own behalf, or on behalf of a right-holder like a child who may be incapable of understanding and asserting its rights for itself. Rights can be possessed only by beings that have interests. For it is impossible to make a claim on behalf of someone or some being unless that person or being is capable of being benefited, unless that being has a good or "sake" of its own. I have a right to free speech because this is a good for *me*. A child who is not old or mature enough to understand its right not to be abused still has such a right because not being abused is a *good* for *it*, not being abused is in *its* interests, and its interest in not being abused is so strong that the law will allow someone to step in and claim its right not to be abused in *its* behalf. However, as Feinberg observes, "a being without interests has no 'behalf' to act in, and no 'sake' to act for."[13] This is why it makes no sense to ascribe rights to inanimate objects, such as buildings, statues, rocks, or rivers. One cannot act in behalf of such things (although it may be ethically wrong and legally prohibited to do certain things to them) because they are incapable of having a good of their own. They cannot have a good of their own because they are not the sorts of things that can have interests.

～ THE DISTINCTIVENESS OF ANIMAL RIGHTS

To say that animals have moral rights is to make a distinctive kind of assertion which is different from the statement that people have moral obligations regarding animals. Those who argue that human beings should not abuse animals because this would lead to mistreatment of our fellow human beings,[14] or who assert that animals may be used in scientific experiments only if doing so will produce greater benefits for people than harm to the animals,[15] do not base their arguments on the claim that animals have rights. Thus Peter Singer, the author of *Animal Liberation*,[16] opposes the use of animals for food and in research. However, he does so solely on the grounds that these practices cause more pain and harm than benefits to all those animals and human beings affected. Although his book is commonly misinterpreted as "the definitive text of the animal rights movement,"[3] he is a utilitarian and does not believe there are any moral rights, either for animals or people.[17]

To say that animals have moral rights is to mean that they have some inherent worth independent of the value we human beings place on them. It is also to say that animals sometimes have interests that must be respected, even if failing to respect these interests would result in more pleasure for people than pain for the animals.

～ WHY MANY PEOPLE BELIEVE THAT ANIMALS HAVE MORAL RIGHTS

Clearly, many people believe that some animals have some moral rights—even if some of these people do not use the word "rights." For example, many people find organized dog fighting morally unacceptable. They would find it so even if the aggregate of pleasure brought to those who enjoy such events outweighs the aggregate of pain suffered by the combatants. What is wrong with dog fighting is that, irrespective of the total resulting benefits and detriments, it is unfair to the animals to subject them to such treatment. Dogs count for something in their own right, and they count enough to make dog fighting a cruelty, a moral offense, to them. Like human infants or incompetents whose moral rights can be abridged even though they may be unable to articulate a complaint, these animals have a moral claim against society (which members of society can make in their behalf) not to use them in certain ways. However, to say these things is precisely to ascribe a moral right to these animals—the right not to be used in fights for the pleasure or monetary gain of people. There is nothing radical or earth-shattering in such an ascription. It does not of itself commit one to such demands of the animal rights movement as the abolition of horse and dog racing, meat-eating, or animal experimentation.

There are numerous other moral rights many people believe animals have. Most people reject unnecessary infliction of pain on laboratory animals, or painful slaughter of livestock, or neglect and mistreatment of household pets. When people reject these things they do not appeal merely to some utilitarian calculation of pain versus benefits. They say these things are immoral, because they are gravely unfair and a serious wrong to the animals, and a serious violation of their most basic interests.

Because many animals do count for something in their own right and proper treatment of animals cannot always be reduced to comparison of resultant benefits and detriments, one should not abandon the notion of animal rights when thinking about how one may morally interact with animals. People might, I suppose, try to speak only of animal "welfare," if they included in the concept of animal welfare the presence of some moral claims of animals not reducible to utilitarian calculation. But if one is willing to do this, why should one not use the term "rights," which already exists in our moral vocabulary and which appropriately captures one consideration most people want to endorse?

Surely, refusing to use the term "rights" will not cause extremists to change their views or forsake their demands. More importantly, there is a danger that those who refuse to use the term "rights" may abandon the legitimate and important idea the term denotes. Suppose people decided to continue to believe in certain human rights, such as the right not to be forced to turn one's property over to others, but for some reason, decided to abandon the term "rights" and to speak only about human "welfare." One could say that a component of human welfare is not being forced to turn one's property over to others. However, people surely would soon be drawn to the major thrust of the concept of human welfare, which is what is good for particular humans or humanity in general. Then, people would be drawn to the question of whether it is good for them to decide on their own how to use their property, and then to arguments about the legitimacy of someone else's deciding how people should use their own property. These may well be legitimate issues. But they are not the same issues raised by the claim that people have a right to their property. This latter claim asserts that under normal circumstances one should just be left alone to use his property as one likes, and that others generally have a duty to refrain from asking whether such use should be curtailed because one's own or others' welfare would be furthered.

Of course, there are important differences between human rights and animal rights. Many human moral rights derive from the ability of normal human adults to make deliberate decisions and life choices. Few, if any, nonhuman animals are autonomous in the same way. Nevertheless, the concept of animal rights suggests that there are some ways of treating animals that are beyond the moral pale because of basic interests some animals have. One may want to argue about the nature, extent, and foundations of inviolable areas. However, one risks aborting such necessary arguments altogether if one jettisons entirely the concept around which these issues turn, the concept of moral rights.

Interestingly, strong proof of the attractiveness of the concept of animal rights can be found in some statements by veterinarians, scientists, and physicians that animals do *not* have rights. Some of these people demand the humane use of animals but also seek to separate themselves from extremists who identify the concept of animal rights with the position that animals should never be used by humans for our own ends. Some of these supporters of humane animal use will then argue that animals have moral rights as I have analyzed this concept while at the same time rejecting the *word* "rights." For example, the World Veterinary Association (WVA) has adopted an animal welfare policy, which includes the following statement:

> We do not accept the view that animals have specialized rights as an entity on their own. We believe that animals can benefit more from the point of view that man is responsible for the provision of animal welfare, rather than from the view which promotes animal rights alone.[18]

This looks like a decisive rejection of animal rights. However, the WVA policy statement proceeds, in a section titled "Freedoms of Animals," to insist that animals have exceedingly strong moral claims against people who use them:

> It is recognized that certain provisions of care are essential to welfare in the form of five freedoms. Modified from various sources in applied ethology, these can be stated as follows:
>   i. freedom from hunger and thirst
>   ii. freedom from physical discomfort and pain
>   iii. freedom from injury and disease
>   iv. freedom from fear and distress
>   v. freedom to conform to essential behavior patterns.[18]

This is a statement of animal *rights* in the sense I have been expounding. The WVA statement is not, surely, intended to prohibit people from ever allowing animals to experience the enumerated ills, for this would amount to a prohibition, for example, of animal research. The WVA's attribution of these "freedoms" seems to say that animals, in virtue of their biological nature, have certain basic needs and interests, and that they have a very strong moral claim against people who wish to use them in certain ways not to subject them to such negative conditions in the absence of compelling justification. Thus interpreted, these statements of animal "freedoms" are demands for animal rights, which are based on considerations of animal welfare.

Does it matter whether we call some of the moral claims of animals "rights," "freedoms," or something else—as long as we accept the ethical principle that some animals have some fundamental interests of their own that are entitled to great weight in our moral deliberations? Perhaps not. But it hardly seems to foster clarity of thought and consistency of action to reject a word and adhere to an idea for which this word stands.

～ FAULTY OBJECTIONS TO ANIMAL RIGHTS

There is no shortage in the philosophical and veterinary literature of arguments against ascribing moral or legal rights to animals. It is impossible to consider all these arguments here. However, some of these objections to animal rights require discussion, because they are raised frequently.

1. A number of philosophers object to the ascription of moral or legal rights to animals on the grounds that animals cannot understand or claim these rights in the same way adult human beings can.[19] This objection is sometimes based on the observation that animals are not autonomous moral agents who are full-fledged members of a moral community and who can be held responsible for their actions or hold others responsible.[20] According to philosopher Alan R. White, rights by their very nature are things that "can be claimed, demanded, asserted, insisted on, secured, waived, or surrendered." Because animals cannot engage in such activities, White concludes, they are conceptually incapable of possessing moral or legal rights.[21]

The problem with this objection to animal rights is that it would also deny moral and legal rights to others who obviously have them. Infants, many children, and severely mentally deficient human beings have moral and legal rights. It is, for example, a violation of their moral and legal rights that they be neglected or abused by their parents or those entrusted with their care. Yet these people are unable to understand that they have moral and legal rights. They are not autonomous beings who can claim rights or who can be said to participate in a "moral community." Such abilities or attributes therefore cannot be essential to the possession of "rights" as this term is used in morality or law.

An analysis of "rights," which requires right-holders to be able to understand and claim rights, misses much of the point of rights-language. The concept of rights undoubtedly arose within communities of adult, autonomous people who could voice moral or legal claims against each other. However, the concept of rights has long had another important function. Rights protect not only those who are able to claim them. Rights protect the miserable, the weak, the downtrodden, and those who are prevented from obtaining their due because they are *not* included as members of the larger "moral community." In what sense would slaves in pre-Civil War America or Jews in the Nazi empire have been called members of the moral community? They could "claim" their rights in the sense of mouthing such claims. But who in positions of power would listen to these claims, much less respect them? Their claims fell on deaf ears. These people were excluded from the community of *effective* claimers. However, their moral rights were surely violated.

It is difficult to understand how the mere ability some such downtrodden people might have had to intellectualize their rights—to understand them and to utter them—transformed their moral interests into rights. The ability to intellectualize and utter their interests certainly did not render the seriousness of the wrongs done to them any more serious. It is, I submit, impossible to reconcile the indisputable importance of rights with the view that what makes an interest into a right is the mere fact that the right holder can understand and utter a claim of rights. This ability can mean too little to constitute the crucial, necessary component of having a *right.* If one were to attend to the history of the concept of rights one would find not just autonomous people who boldly and articulately claimed their rights. One would also find people who could *not* make such claims, and others who took it upon themselves to speak in their behalf. One would find the powerless and the voiceless, and people who sought to help and protect them.

In sum, "rights" are not restricted to claims that can be made by those who are intelligent, articulate, or strong enough to make them.

2. Another objection to animal rights links the ascription of rights to animals to a patent absurdity. It is said that if animals had rights, they would have the right not to be attacked or preyed on by other animals, which is clearly not the case because many animals, especially in the wild, have little regard for other animals.[22]

However, the concept of animal rights does not imply that animals have rights against other animals. If animals have rights, they have rights against some *people.* Animals cannot have rights against other animals because such other animals are not capable of recognizing and acting upon rights. That a right-holder does not have rights against those who cannot understand and recognize rights is not something true of animal right-holders alone. Imagine an unfortunate situation in which one severely deranged and irrational patient in a mental institution who cannot control his behavior (John) has beaten another patient (Don). Neither John nor Don, let us suppose, knows what a right is, or is capable of thinking about, much less articulating, what either one is owed morally or legally. It would make no sense to accuse John of violating Don's right not to be beaten. (Imagine a relative of Don's confronting John and accusing him of "violating Don's rights" as John looks at the accuser without any understanding of what is being said to him.) John cannot be said to have had an obligation not to hit Don because, as I have supposed, John is completely unable to control his behavior, to understand what it is to act rightly or wrongly, or to conform his behavior to any standards of right or wrong. We could, and probably would, say that Don had a right not to be beaten. But we would say that Don had such a right against the hospital's administration. They can be blamed morally and sued legally for what happened to Don. They have a legal and moral obligation not to permit one patient to be beaten by another, and they can understand and act on this obligation.

It *would* be absurd to accuse a cat that eats a bird of violating the bird's rights. However, it would be no less absurd to accuse John of violating Don's rights. It hardly follows that John and Don do not have moral and legal rights. Animals, like some humans, cannot violate rights. Animals, like some humans who cannot violate rights, can nevertheless have rights against people who are capable of violating their rights.

3. An argument against animal rights, which appears with some frequency in the veterinary literature, maintains that rights are "a human creation," from which it is supposed to follow that there are only human rights.[23] This statement can be interpreted in different ways, none of which counts against animal rights.

Perhaps the contention that rights are "human" creations is supposed to mean that rights-language is a feature of human language. This is true, but it would not follow that rights-language can only be applied to humans, any more than it would follow from the fact that pain-language or physiology-language is part of human language that such language can only be applied correctly to human beings.

Perhaps the contention that rights are human creations means that rights-language would not have arisen without, and still functions predominantly among, humans who are physically and mentally capable of having obligations and asserting moral claims. This also is true, but it does not follow that rights-language is inappropriately applied to some animals in some circumstances. Very few people would deny that some animals can experience pain and other unpleasant sensations. However, it is surely the case that pain-language, in all its complexity, arose and still functions predominantly in human communities among people who communicate and make requests of each other in ways animals cannot. Surely, much of the point of our pain-language is to complain about pain and seek help from others to alleviate it. If people could not or did not bother to seek help about pain we probably would just scream, moan, or grunt on feeling pain. Instead, we have words that describe the location, duration, severity, and often the quite precise experiential characteristics of pain and other unpleasant sensations, so that we can tell others about this pain. Yet we still apply some of this same language to animals, because given what these terms mean, they are applied *correctly* to animals.

4. Finally, it is said that ascribing moral or legal rights to animals is objectionable because it implies unacceptable ethical positions, such as the immorality of eating meat or using animals in research. This objection to animal rights is also incorrect, for reasons that will be explained in greater detail below. Here, it can be said that there is nothing in the ascription of moral or legal rights to animals that implies animals cannot be used in various ways by people, ways that can sometimes include killing them. To say that some animals have some moral or legal claims against us that are of compelling (though not necessarily conclusive) strength is not to say anything about what these claims are.

⁓ ANIMAL RIGHTS VERSUS THE ANIMAL RIGHTS MOVEMENT

In thinking about animal rights, one must be careful to distinguish between the concept of animal rights and what has come to be known as "the animal rights movement." Confusion between the two has led many who in fact believe that animals have rights to reject the word "rights." This is precisely what some members of this so-called animal rights movement want.

What Is the Animal Rights Movement?

Whether one classifies a certain group or thinker as a member of the animal rights movement can depend on one's point of view. For example, the International Society for Animal Rights, an opponent of animal research, applies the term "regulationist" to all who would permit any use of animals in research.[24, 25] On the other hand, some use the words "rightist"[26] or "antivivisectionist"[27-29] to refer to people who question a good deal of animal experimentation, even if they endorse much animal research. There is also controversy within what most thoughtful people would call "the" animal rights movement.

Granting the impossibility of defining the animal rights movement in a way that will satisfy everyone, I want to suggest that one view as members or sympathizers of "the movement" those who subscribe to at least all the following positions: (1) The vast majority of mammals (and certainly typical companion, farm, and laboratory mammals) not only have moral rights, but also have some of the same moral rights as human beings. (2) Such animals have these rights at least in part because they have many of the same mental capabilities and activities as people. (3) Just as one would be violating a person's rights if one were to eat him or use him in research without his consent, or use him merely as a means to one's own ends, so does doing these things to most mammals violate their moral rights. (4) The law should enforce such moral rights by, among other things, allowing these animals to sue in their own behalf, just as children and other human incompetents can have lawsuits brought in their behalf by legal representatives.

I believe this definition reflects how most participants and observers conceive of the movement and allows for important internal theoretical and practical controversies within its ranks. (For example, as I have defined it, membership in the animal rights movement does not entail approval of illegal acts, even if some members of the movement do engage in such tactics.) Among the members of the animal rights movement so defined must be counted the Animal Legal Defense Fund, the Animal Liberation Front, the Coalition to End Animal Suffering in Experiments, the International Society for Animal Rights, People for the Ethical Treatment of Animals, and the Association of Veterinarians for Animal Rights.

Of course, veterinarians must not restrict their attention to the animal rights movement. Other persons and organizations sometimes level sharp criticisms at veterinarians and, indeed, occasionally ally themselves with the animal rights movement.

However, if one lumps everyone who challenges—for whatever reason and to whatever extent—currently accepted animal uses under the banner of "the animal rights movement," one distorts reality, and makes it more difficult to respond adequately to these challenges.

Three Myths of the Animal Rights Movement
"One must choose between animal rights and animal welfare."

Some leaders of the animal rights movement insist that only the movement is entitled to advocate animal rights and that anyone who thinks animals may be used for food, clothing, in sport, or in research must talk only of animal "welfare," "humane treatment," or "animal protection."[24, 25] Quite a few veterinarians have accepted this supposed inconsistency between animal rights and animal welfare.[3-6] Dr. Robert M. Miller, for example, writes that he is "opposed to the concept of animals having inherent rights...[b]ecause, if we accept the premise that animals have such rights as the right to be 'free' and to live 'natural' lives, then almost every utilization mankind makes of animals must be considered immoral."[5] However, the concept of animal rights does not entail any such particular claims about what moral rights animals might have. Nor is there any inconsistency in advocating animal welfare, or animal protection, or humane treatment, and some animal rights.

I believe the animal rights movement dearly wants veterinarians to accept its claim to exclusive use of the concept of rights. As one philosopher observes, today "rights are the principal currency of moral, political, and legal dispute."[30] If the animal rights movement can get veterinarians to refuse to talk about rights at all—even if veterinarians would in the end want to maintain that animals have limited moral rights—they could be separated from the mainstream of ethical and political debate. The animal rights movement wants to convince society that many in the veterinary community are mired in inadequate concepts and ways of thinking. This was precisely the claim made by some[31] when in 1983 the AVMA Animal Welfare Committee stated that "the AVMA believes that use of the term 'animal rights' has to do with personal philosophical values and therefore recommends that the term 'animal rights' not be used and encourages the profession to focus its attention on the welfare and humane treatment of animals."[32]

There also is a danger that acceptance of this imaginary inconsistency between animal welfare and animal rights will lead some who would prefer to take a more moderate position into the camp of the animal rights movement. For if a veterinarian wants to maintain that some animals have rights, and if he believes that to advocate animal rights at all he must agree with the claims of the animal rights movement, his only choice, it would seem, is to join the movement. If the animal rights movement can (somehow) convince a veterinarian that it is wrong to use animals for human ends, that is one thing. But no one should embrace such a view merely because one believes that animals have moral rights.

"Animals do not yet have legal rights."

According to animal rights activists[33, 34] something cannot have a legal right unless it has what lawyers call "standing" to sue, which means it can sue in its own name or have someone appointed by a court to sue in its behalf and can recover money damages or other relief directly for its own benefit. Animal rights activists note that children and human incompetents can have such standing because lawsuits can sometimes be brought for (and thus legally by) them for their own benefit. However, civil lawsuits cannot be instituted in the same way for an animal, and cannot result in that animal's receiving money or other relief from someone who harms it. According to animal rights activists, even anti-cruelty to animals statutes do not give animals any legal rights. For such laws empower a public authority to bring legal action and do not provide for the appointment of a representative or guardian to further the interests of a particular animal or animals.

The claim that animals now have no legal rights and that legal standing is necessary for their having rights is important to the animal rights movement. The movement will not rest on moral persuasion but seeks to use the law to force people to behave according to many of its precepts. The movement knows that our society tends to enforce fundamental moral rights as legal rights. Therefore if it can establish that legal rights imply legal standing, it can try to move people from the eminently reasonable claim that animals have some fundamental moral rights, to the conclusion that animals should be treated by the law as legal persons, with standing to sue in their own behalf.

In fact, the American legal system affords many rights the possessors of which do not have standing to enforce. For example, generally only a government authority, and not a private citizen, can sue to abate a nuisance (such as a polluting factory) that affects the public at large.[35] Yet most lawyers and laymen would say that individual members of the public have a legal right not to be harmed by such a nuisance. Nor would one say that people could not have a legal right to be free from crimes if the only redress from such offenses were the criminal justice system, which in fact gives public prosecutors, and not the victim of a crime, standing to sue, and which typically does not grant compensation to the victim.

As for animals, Joel Feinberg states that "there is no reason to deny that animals have general legal rights to noncruel treatment derived from statutes to protect them."[36] Feinberg explains that a being or entity can have a legal right if the law permits someone (such as a public authority) to make enforceable claims in its interest. While conceding that animal protection statutes can be we ', and poor in legal rights for animals, Feinberg recognizes that this need not be so. example, Feinberg notes that the British Cruelty to Animals Act confers on animals "the right to 'complete anesthesia' before being used in 'any experiment calculated to give pain,' and can give rise to a "criminal prosecution for violation of [a laboratory] rat's legal rights."[36] There is a long history, much of it predating the activity of contemporary animal use abolitionists, of lawyers and judges speaking openly and without embarrassment of the legal rights of animals. For example, in 1897 the Louisiana Supreme Court declared that:

> The [cruelty] statute relating to animals is based on "the theory, unknown to the common law, that animals have rights which, like those of human beings, are to be protected. A horse, under its master's hands, stands in the relation of the master analogous to that of the child to the parent."[37]

The following year the Mississippi Supreme Court, explaining cruelty to animals laws generally, reiterated that:

The common law recognized no rights in [domestic animals] and punished no cruelty to them, except in so far as it affected the rights of individuals to such property. [Cruelty] statutes remedy this defect, and exhibit the spirit of that divine law which is so mindful of dumb brutes as to teach and command, not to muzzle the ox when he treadeth on the corn; not to plow with an ox and an ass together; not to take the bird that sitteth on its young or its eggs; and not to seethe a kid in its mother's milk. To disregard the rights and feelings of equals, is unjust and ungenerous, but to willfully or wantonly injure or oppress the weak and helpless, is mean and cowardly.[38]

There are many more recent examples of statements by legal scholars and philosophers that current laws afford some legal rights to animals.[39]

If one believes, as many people surely do, that animals should have some legal rights, one is not thereby committed to the demand of the animal rights movement that animals should be given legal standing to sue their owners, their veterinarians, or other people for money or other kinds of relief. The concept of legal rights for animals, like the concept of moral rights for animals, does not entail the platform of the animal rights movement.

"The animal rights movement is good for veterinarians."

Although they condemn much in veterinary practice as immoral, some leaders of the animal rights movement argue that veterinarians should join their cause.[40, 41]

The myth that the animal rights movement will benefit veterinary medicine, unlike the first two myths I have discussed, has not yet gained much acceptance among veterinarians. However, this myth is worth addressing. If they become increasingly familiar fixtures in veterinary publications and gatherings, animal rights movement members might not appear so worrisome. More importantly, some are seeking to play a major role in the teaching of ethics to veterinary students.

According to the animal rights movement, it is immoral to use animals as tools in the service of human ends. It would seem that horse racing must stop, as must commercial raising of animals for fiber, dairy products, or eggs. Using animals for draft and other work would have to end, and it would appear that people who have horses largely for the pleasure of riding or showing them also violate the precepts of the animal rights movement. Thus gone forever would be a significant portion of today's veterinary profession, including food and fiber and laboratory animal practitioners, and the great majority of equine practitioners. Moreover, the death of these fields would probably spell doom for most veterinarians who could survive, in theory, the demands of the animal rights movement. For the profession as a whole rests on an economic base supported in significant measure by those who now require farm, sports, or laboratory animal practitioners. Without this base, it seems highly unlikely that there could exist many schools to train veterinarians or pharmaceutical and supply companies to provide them with necessary goods and services.

Similarly, given the acceptance of such a position, even companion animal practice would not long survive the animal rights movement. Many things people now do to companion animals, and that generate veterinary revenue, such as breeding and showing them largely for human comfort, convenience, and enjoyment, would have to stop. Indeed, it is not clear that the animal rights movement can countenance very much human keeping of companion animals. Much of what people with these animals, including housetraining or restraining them, or using them for companionship or protection, is done at least in part for human purposes. Some in the movement believe that the number of people permitted to have companion animals should be sharply curtailed. Reduction in the number of animal owners would directly reduce the number of potential veterinary clients. Also, allowing animals to sue their owners and veterinarians would make animal ownership and veterinary services less attractive to owners and practitioners, who would face expensive and upsetting lawsuits. Permitting greatly increased awards against veterinarians in malpractice suits, another demand of some in the animal rights movement, could make veterinary care still more expensive and might reduce the market for veterinarians.

Of course, the termination of animal research conducted for the benefit of other animals would prevent the development of many new veterinary drugs, vaccines, and techniques. This would curtail the potential growth of veterinary services. Just one new kind of disease or scourge that might be controllable with animal research could wipe out most of the patients for which the veterinarians in the animal rights movement's ideal world are supposed to care. Indeed the movement seems logically committed to the view that people should stop using on animals any drugs or techniques that have already resulted from animal research. For this too would be no less a utilization of benefits obtained in violation of animals' rights. This alone would decimate the population of companion animals, and veterinarians, in very short order.

The fact that something is good or bad for business does not make it right or wrong. It is also a rare profession indeed that does everything perfectly. Doubtless many in the animal rights movement sincerely believe that their program would benefit veterinarians. However, the animal rights movement is engaging in fantasy when it proclaims its devotion to animals and veterinarians, and puts forth a program that could in fact destroy both.

~ SIGNS OF CHANGE

As noted previously, in 1983 the AVMA adopted an official policy recommending "that the term 'animal rights' not be used" and encouraging the profession to "focus its attention on the welfare and humane use of animals."[32] This statement reflected a view still endorsed by many veterinarians—that the espousal of animal rights entails the abolition of the human use of animals.

In 1990 the AVMA issued a new policy regarding animal rights. The AVMA now states that:

> Animal welfare and animal rights are not synonymous terms. The AVMA wholeheartedly endorses and adopts promotion of animal welfare as official policy; however, the AVMA does not endorse the philosophical views and personal values of animal rights advocates when they are incompatible with the responsible use of animals for human purposes, such as food, fiber, companionship, recreation and research conducted for the benefit of both humans and animals.[42]

This new policy marked an important change. The AVMA no longer rejects the term "animal rights" but only rejects views that equate animal rights with the abolition of human use of animals. In crafting the new policy, the AVMA Animal Welfare Committee was aware of philosophical arguments in favor of limited rights for animals. The Committee also heard from some of its own members who reported that some clients believe their animals have the right to good veterinary care. These members were not about to inform clients that veterinarians insisted otherwise (Dr. Charles Sedgwick, AVMA Animal Welfare Committee Member: Personal communication). Indeed, one survey has found that most Americans believe animals have rights, and also support the use of animals for a wide range of purposes, including biomedical research.[43]

The change in the AVMA policy was wise. Neither philosophers nor veterinarians can dictate how people use language, however much some might want to do so. The AVMA is sensitive to the fact that there is ongoing debate about animal rights among philosophers and members of the public. Retaining the old policy that condemned animal rights could have committed the profession to a losing, entirely unnecessary, and ultimately embarrassing battle.

Most importantly, those of us who believe in animal rights *and* the humane use of animals by people must try to prevent the concept of animal rights from becoming the exclusive property of animal use abolitionists. We cannot afford to lose the participation of veterinarians who, in fact, believe that animals have rights but have been frightened away from using the word "rights." The word will endure, irrespective of protestations by veterinarians. The task ahead is to assure the consistency of animal rights with responsible uses of animals.

∼ WHAT MORAL RIGHTS DO ANIMALS HAVE?

One task of contemporary normative veterinary ethics is to articulate to society and government why the animal rights movement cannot be permitted to have its way. This task, I have suggested, will be made more difficult than it really is if one accepts the claims of the animal rights movement that moral rights for animals entail abolition of human use of animals, that legal rights for animals entail treating animals as legal persons, and that the animal rights movement is good for veterinarians and veterinary science.

However, normative ethics cannot rest content with confronting the animal rights movement. Moral questions regarding animal rights will remain long after the animal rights movement falls victim to its own overblown and unacceptable demands. It is far more important to investigate when animals do have moral rights, how strong these rights are, and when these rights must give way to legitimate interests of people and other animals. This task cannot be accomplished at the beginning of one's study of normative veterinary ethics, but must proceed by careful analysis of particular issues and situations. I offer the following suggestions and warnings regarding such an endeavor.

1. **Not every interest translates into a moral right.** A right reflects an interest that is so strong it generally must be respected even though others' interests or the promotion of utility would suffer by respecting it. A "right" which can be overridden as a matter of course is not properly spoken of as a right at all. Thus, I would be inclined to say that a laboratory dog may have an interest in having toys for amusement and that this interest is sometimes sufficiently strong to require that such toys be provided. However, it is quite another thing to assert that such animals have the right to these things, because there are many considerations that can often argue against respecting the interest.

2. **Moral rights can be outweighed by the interests or rights of others.** That one might be reluctant to respect a proposed right in all situations does not mean one should refuse to recognize it as a right. For example, it seems plausible to say that a veterinary patient has the right to receive nursing and medical care appropriate to

its condition. However, many veterinary hospitals cannot afford to remain staffed in the evenings, and it is sometimes impossible for clients to place an animal in a facility that can provide around-the-clock care. In some cases, it seems correct to say that an animal's interest in receiving appropriate nursing care must be overridden by the veterinarian's interests in maintaining his practice and in a client's ability to afford veterinary care.

3. Rights can be negative or positive. Philosophers sometimes distinguish between negative rights, rights not to be treated in certain ways, and positive rights, rights to certain kinds of treatment, goods, or benefits. It is sometimes possible to rephrase a negative right as a positive right, and *vice versa*. For example, one often can speak interchangeably of the right of animals not to be treated inhumanely and their right to humane treatment. Nevertheless, the distinction between negative and positive rights is important for animal and veterinary ethics. Because of the predominance of the anti-cruelty position (see Chapter 11), many people believe animals have far more negative rights, rights not to be treated in certain ways, than they have rights to positive benefits. If the anti-cruelty position continues to lose ground as an exhaustive account of our obligations to animals, we can expect more people to assert positive moral rights for animals, and indeed to verbalize some rights traditionally phrased in the negative (such as the right not to be treated inhumanely) as positive rights.

4. Rights can be general or specific. In examining particular situations, one must sometimes be prepared to identify quite specific rights. I shall argue, for example, that terminally ill patients in great and unrelievable pain have the right to a quick and painless death. On the other hand, one might say that this specific right is an example of a more general right of patients to be treated with compassion.

5. Very general statements of rights tend to raise more issues than they answer or are so obviously plausible that they do not assist in answering difficult moral questions. This does not make such statements worthless, but one must not think that they provide more guidance than they really do. For example, it seems reasonable to attribute to animals a very general right to be treated humanely, in the sense of not being caused unnecessary or unjustifiable pain or suffering. The problem, of course, is that this statement is acceptable to almost everyone, precisely because it does not attempt to address the enormously difficult question of what does constitute sufficient justification for animal pain or suffering.

Small animal practitioner and commentator Dr. Jacob Antelyes offers a plausible list of moral rights of veterinary patients.[44] He urges five basic rights for all patients: (1) respect (the right to "dignified nursing care and medical attention, delivered with decency and sincerity"); (2) privacy (the right "to be housed separately in well-lit and properly ventilated quarters" and not to experience "stress created by the presence of other animals or unessential people"); (3) purposeful death (the right "not to suffer frivolous pain or gratuitous death for the purposes of entertainment and amusement"); (4) unavoidable pain (the right "to prompt relief of pain by the most effective mode possible") and (5) food and water (the right "to receive food and water appropriate for its medical condition").

One might question certain of Antelyes' characterizations of these rights. For example, it is not clear why a right not to suffer pain for frivolous purposes belongs under the general right to a purposeful death, and Antelyes provides no argument for his apparent contention that any pain inflicted for the purposes of human entertainment is frivolous. But a belief in the five very general rights he identifies surely belongs in some form in the value system of every veterinarian.

Nevertheless, the rights identified by Dr. Antelyes are so obviously plausible that they do not provide much assistance in answering the most difficult questions facing contemporary normative ethics. It is doubtful whether there are many veterinarians who deprive sick animals of adequate housing, food, and water, and who tolerate harsh or inattentive treatment of patients. If some veterinarians allow such things, it is not a difficult matter to show they are acting wrongly.

The difficult issues lie elsewhere. When might an animal have the right to be a veterinary patient in the first place? When may any such right give way to a client's economic or psychological problems in treating or keeping the animal? How much economic sacrifice does a patient's right to adequate and competent care require of its owner or of a veterinarian who might have difficulty offering the owner reduced fees? What kind of death is sufficiently purposeful and pain sufficiently justifiable so that it does not violate a patient's rights? To what extent does a patient's right to respectful care place constraints on what a doctor should agree to do at the client's request? (Does it, for example, prohibit such practices as ear cropping and "de-barking" of pet dogs?)

Normative veterinary ethics should seek characterizations of animal rights that can be useful in addressing these and other issues.

REFERENCES

1Schiller BJ: Letter, *J Am Vet Med Assoc* 183:748, 1983.
2Jacobs FS: A perspective on animal rights and domestic animals, *J Am Vet Med Assoc* 184:1344-1345, 1984.
3Tillman PC, Brooks DL: Animal welfare, animal rights, and human responsibilities, *Calif Vet* 37:33, 1983.
4Held JR: Letter, *J Am Vet Med Assoc* 182:855, 1983.
5Miller RM: Animal welfare-Yes! Humane laws-Sure! Animal rights-No! *Calif Vet* 37:21, 1983.
6Grady AW, Tambrallo L, and others: Animal rights jeopardize animal welfare,*Vet Econ* June 1989:122.
7Smith SJ, Hendee WR: Animals in research, *JAMA* 259:2007, 1988.
8Armistead WW: Public health responsibilities of veterinary medicine, *J Am Vet Med Assoc* 187:1110, 1985.
9*See*, for example, Lyons D, editor: *Rights*, Belmont, CA, 1979, Wadsworth.
10Dworkin R: Taking rights seriously. In Dworkin R: *Taking Rights Seriously*, Cambridge, 1978, Harvard University Press, pp 184-205.
11Some philosophers maintain that "rights" are so strong they can never be overridden. On this view, if someone has a *right* to something, he can never be denied it; his right can never give way either to a right possessed by someone else or to considerations of the greater good; and one person's rights cannot be stronger and therefore entitled to greater weight than another person's conflicting rights. *See*, for example, Feinberg J: The nature and value of rights. In Lyons D, editor: *Rights*, Belmont, CA, 1979, Wadsworth, pp 78-91. Such assertions are counterintuitive. We do speak, for example, of the right to free speech, and say that this is a right even if it must sometimes be overridden by other persons' rights or needs. Interestingly, Feinberg argues that animals have rights even in this strong sense, among them the right not to be treated cruelly. Feinberg J: Human duties and animal rights. In Morris RK, Fox MW, editors: *The Fifth Day: Animal Rights and Human Ethics*, Washington, DC, 1978, Acropolis Books, pp 45-69.
12Feinberg J: Human duties and animal rights. In Morris RK, Fox MW, editors: *The Fifth Day: Animal Rights and Human Ethics*, Washington, DC, 1978, Acropolis Books, p 47.
13Feinberg J: The rights of animals and unborn generations. In Feinberg J: *Rights, Justice, and the Bounds of Liberty*, Princeton, 1980, Princeton University Press, p 167.
14Kant I: *Lectures on Ethics*, Infield L, translator, New York, 1963, Harper & Row, p 239.
15Seligman MEP: *Helplessness*, San Francisco, 1975, Freeman, p xi.
16Singer P: *Animal Liberation*, New York, 1975, The New York Review of Books, Inc.
17Singer P: The parable of the fox and the unliberated animals, *Ethics* 88:122, 1978.
18World Veterinary Association establishes animal welfare policy, *Synapse* 22(4):2, 1989.

[19]The 1991 Report of the National Academy of Sciences Committee on the Use of Animals in Research asserts that "most ethicists...generally ascribe rights only to members of species that are capable of applying mutually accepted ethical principles to specific situations. Animals are not capable of forming or belonging to such societies. In this light, they cannot be ascribed rights." *Science, Medicine, and Animals*, Washington, DC, 1991, National Academy Press, p 17. This assertion about ethicists is made without supporting evidence and is incorrect. Although philosophical issues are not settled by majority vote, in recent years the number of philosophers who ascribe rights to animals has grown markedly and may well exceed the number who do not. A reader of the National Academy of Sciences Committee report who is unfamiliar with the growing philosophical literature regarding animal rights would think, erroneously, that whether animals have rights is a settled issue among ethicists. For philosophical arguments against animal rights, see, in addition to sources already cited in this chapter: Carruthers P: *The Animals Issue: Moral Theory in Practice*, Cambridge, UK, 1992, Cambridge University Press; Cohen C: The case for the use of animals in biomedical research, *N Eng J Med* 315:866, 1986; Frey RG: *Interests and Rights*, Oxford, 1980, Clarendon Press; McCloskey HJ: Moral rights and animals, *Inquiry* 22:23-54, 1979; and Passmore J: *Man's Responsibility for Nature*, Scribner's, 1974. For philosophical arguments supporting various characterizations of animal rights, *see*, in addition to sources already cited in this chapter: Cavalieri P, Singer P, editors: *The Great Ape Project*, New York, 1994, St. Martin's Press; Clark SRL: *The Nature of the Beast*, Oxford, 1982, Oxford University Press; Rachels J: *Created from Animals: The Moral Implications of Darwinism*, Oxford, 1990, Oxford University Press; Regan T: *The Case for Animal Rights*, Berkeley, 1983, University of California Press; Rollin BE: *Animal Rights and Human Morality*. Buffalo, 1981, Prometheus Books; Sapontzis SF: *Morals, Reason, and Animals*, Philadelphia, 1987, Temple University Press; and Warren MA: The rights of the nonhuman world. In Elliot R, Gare A, editors: *Environmental Philosophy*, University Park, PA, 1983, Pennsylvania State University Press, pp 109-134. For a discussion which denies animals have a moral right not to be killed but suggests that animals might have a right not to be caused pain by people who use them, *see* Thomson JJ: *The Realm of Rights*, Cambridge, MA, 1990, Harvard University Press, pp 42 and 292-293.

[20]Gray JC: *The Nature and Sources of the Law*, ed 2, Boston, 1963, Beacon Press, 1963.

[21]White AR: *Rights*, Oxford, 1984, Oxford University Press, p 90.

[22]For example, Ritchie D: *Natural Rights*, London, 1984, Allen & Unwin. In Regan T, Singer P, editors: *Animal Rights and Human Obligations*, ed 1, Englewood Cliffs, NJ, 1976, Prentice Hall, pp 182-183.

[23]McLaughlin RM: Letter, *J Am Vet Med Assoc* 196:11, 1990. *See also*, Jacobs F: A perspective on animal rights and domestic animals, *J Am Vet Med Assoc* 184:1345-1346, 1984.

[24]Jones H: Animal Rights: A view and comment, *Soc Anim Rights Rep* October 1981:3.

[25]Holzer H: Editor's comment, *Anim Rights Law Rep* April 1983:15.

[26]Visscher MB: Animal rights and alternative methods, *The Pharos* Fall 1979:11-19.

[27]Visscher MB: The newer antivivisectionists, *Proc Am Phil Soc* 116:157-162, 1972.

[28]Caplan A: Beastly conduct: Ethical issues in animal experimentation. In Sechzer JE, editor: *The Role of Animals in Biomedical Research*, *Ann NY Acad Sci* 1983:159-160.

[29]Miller NE: Value and ethics of research on animals, *Lab Prim News* 22:1-10, 1984.

[30]Lyons D: Introduction. In Lyons D, editor: *Rights*, Belmont, CA, 1979, Wadsworth, 1979, p 1.

[31] For example, Wolff NR: Letter, *J Am Vet Med Assoc* 183:36, 1983.

[32]Guiding principles and the term "animal rights," *J Am Vet Med Assoc* 182:769, 1983.

[33]Regan T: Animals and the law. In Regan T: *All That Dwell Therein*, Berkeley, 1982, University of California Press, pp 156-157.

[34]Tischler JS: Rights for nonhuman animals: A guardianship model for dogs and cats, *San Diego Law Rev* 14:484-506, 1977.

[35]Prosser W: *Handbook of the Law of Torts*, ed 4, St. Paul, MN, 1971, West, p 586.

[36]Feinberg J: Human Duties and Animal Rights. In Morris RK, Fox MW, editors: *The Fifth Day: Animal Rights and Human Ethics*, Washington, DC, 1978, Acropolis Books, p 57.

[37]*State v. Karstendiek*, 22 So. 845 (La. 1897), quoting *Bishop St. Cr.* 1101 *et seq.*

[38]*Stephens v. State*, 3 So. 458 (Miss. 1898).

[39]*See*, for example, in addition to Feinberg *supra*, Lamont WD: *Principles of Moral Judgment*, Oxford, 1946, Clarendon Press, pp 83-85; Friend C: Animal cruelty laws: The case for reform, *Univ Richmond Law Rev* 8:223-224, 1974 (endorsing the statement of *Stephens v.*State that cruelty laws afford legal rights to animals; Varner GE: Do species have standing? *Environ Ethics* 9:66-67, 1987 (distinguishing between a *de jure* legal right for animals, which is obtained when the stated purpose of a law is to benefit animals for their own sake, and a *de facto* legal right for animals, which exists when a law in fact functions to protect animals even if this is not its stated purpose); Leavitt ES: *Animals and Their Legal Rights*, ed 4, Washington, DC, 1990, Animal Welfare Institute (the classic comprehensive survey of the history and coverage of American cruelty to animals statutes).

[40]Regan T: *The Case For Animal Rights*, Berkeley, 1983, University of California Press, p 390.

[41]Tischler JS: Veterinarians: The sleeping beauties of the animal rights movement, *Calif Vet* 37:27-28, 1983.

[42]Animal welfare/animal rights, *J Am Vet Med Assoc* 197:311, 1990.

[43]For example, Are laboratory animals treated humanely? *Associated Press*, October 28, 1985 (NEXIS, Current library), cited in Garvin LT: Constitutional limits on the regulation of laboratory animal research, *Yale Law J* 98:388, 1988 (poll showing that 76% of Americans believe that animals have rights, 81% think it is necessary to use animals in some applied medical research, and 42% of those who believe that animals have rights think that their use in research violates these rights).

[44]Antelyes J: Animal rights in perspective, *J Am Vet Med Assoc* 189:757-759, 1986.

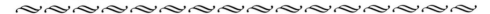

CHAPTER 13

What is Animal Welfare?

*A*lthough there is controversy about whether animals have moral or legal rights, clearly, it makes perfect sense to say that various conditions are (or are not) conducive to their welfare. Indeed, many people whose professional activities involve animals consider their most important ethical obligation to be the promotion of animal welfare.

This chapter considers fundamental issues relating to animal welfare, including the definition of the term, and attempts by some investigators to separate the scientific study of animal welfare from ethical decisions about how animals ought to be treated. Subsequent chapters discuss specific issues relating to welfare in various aspects of veterinary practice.

∼ COMMON MISCONCEPTIONS ABOUT ANIMAL WELFARE
Polar Definitions: Welfare versus Rights

It is useful to examine the concept of animal welfare after some consideration of animal rights (see Chapter 12). For many people not only view animal welfare as an alternative to animal rights, but they also *define* "welfare" (at least in part) by contrasting it with rights.

The following statements are typical of definitions of animal welfare in terms of its supposed polar opposite of animal rights. According to several laboratory animal veterinarians:

> Animal welfare is the foundation of veterinary science. As pet owners, practitioners, and the stewards of all animals, we [veterinarians] are instilled with the value of animal health and obligated to uphold the principles of animal welfare…Those who raise the banner for animal rights proclaim an equivalent moral value for humans and animals.[1]

A frequently cited discussion of controversies relating to animal experimentation distinguishes animal welfare from animal rights by appealing to diametrically opposed positions regarding the use of animals in research: approval and complete rejection.

> Most individuals who are concerned with the use of animals in biomedical research can be divided into two general categories: (1) those concerned with *animal welfare* who are not opposed to biomedical research but want assurance that animals are treated as humanely as possible…and (2) those concerned with *animal rights* who take a more radical position and totally oppose the use of animals in biomedical research.[2]

The 1990 American Veterinary Medical Association official "Policy on Animal Welfare and Animal Rights" also defines animal welfare by distinguishing welfare from rights.

Animal welfare is a human responsibility that encompasses all aspects of animal well-being, including proper housing, management, nutrition, disease prevention and treatment, responsible care, humane handling, and, when necessary, humane euthanasia.

Animal rights is a philosophical view and personal value characterized by statements by various animal rights groups. Animal welfare and animal rights are not synonymous terms. The AVMA wholeheartedly endorses and adopts promotion of animal welfare as official policy; however, the AVMA does not endorse the philosophical views and personal values of animal rights advocates when they are incompatible with the responsible use of animals for human purposes, such as food, fiber, companionship, recreation and research conducted for the benefit of both humans and animals.[3]

Problems in Welfare versus Rights Definitions
A different sense of "welfare"

These quotations illustrate several problems in attempts to define animal welfare by contrasting it with animal rights.

There are important differences between what is conducive to human and animal welfare. Education, for example, is important in the promotion of human welfare because without education, people cannot earn a living or appreciate their world. Education is not conducive to animal welfare because animals cannot be "educated" in any appropriate sense of the term. Nevertheless, what is meant by "welfare" is presumably the same whether one is speaking about human or animal welfare. Otherwise, it would not make sense to contrast *human* with *animal* welfare. The contrast depends on using the term "welfare" in one sense and *then* distinguishing between what contributes to or more specifically constitutes the welfare of humans and animals. Indeed, it would be inappropriate to use the term "welfare" to apply to animals if one employed this term in a different sense than one applied it to people. One should then not speak about animal "welfare" but about animal something-else.

Although there remains disagreement about whether animals have moral or legal rights, any definition of the term "welfare" that precludes the simultaneous ascription of welfare and rights to animals employs the term in a different sense than that in which it is ordinarily employed. Speakers of English (and of other languages with equivalent terms) see no inconsistency between talking about the welfare of people and the rights of these same people. Indeed, we sometimes say that people have a moral or legal *right* to certain conditions conducive to their *welfare*. For example, all civilized countries give children the right to a publicly financed education, in order to further these persons' welfare.

Restriction of "welfare" to certain positions regarding appropriate uses of animals

A second problem in definitions of animal welfare that contain a contrast with animal rights is that they typically include within the definition of welfare approval of certain uses of animals. An assertion that animals have "welfare," it is commonly maintained, includes support for the use of animals in biomedical research, and for food, fiber, companionship, and entertainment.

As is argued in Chapter 12, the concept of animal rights is not inconsistent with the use of animals for such purposes. One can say, I argue, that animals do not have a right to life and that people may utilize them for food and in research—but that when they are so used, they have a right not to be treated inhumanely or to be caused unnecessary pain. Nor does the concept of animal rights imply that animals and humans are of equal importance. Therefore definitions of animal welfare err from the start when they contrast animal welfare and animal rights, and consider the latter to imply the immorality of the human use of animals.

Linking animal welfare, by definition, to approval of certain uses of animals has an even more significant defect. As this chapter maintains, there is an ethical component in the concept of animal welfare. Nevertheless, it is often possible and important to separate the issue of what constitutes animal welfare from the question of what it is appropriate to do to animals. Put another way, we often want to ask whether, or to what extent, we are morally obligated to respect, protect, or promote the welfare of any given animal. For example, it is certainly not conducive to a research animal's welfare to subject it to intense and long-lasting pain. However, it is a separate issue whether it is right or wrong to subject an animal to such pain in a particular experiment. It might be acceptable to cause an animal intense and long-lasting pain to test a promising pain-killing drug to be used in cancer patients. It might be inappropriate to cause the same animal the same kind of pain to test the safety of a new shampoo.

Definitions that link animal welfare to positions regarding appropriate uses of animals muddy the distinction between what constitutes an animal's welfare and the separate issue of whether it is ethically appropriate to use this animal in certain ways. By building support for very broad positions regarding animal use into what is meant by animal welfare itself, these definitions can make it impossible to assess various kinds of animal use on the basis of their effects on welfare. Some people believe it is an unacceptable compromise of animal welfare to test cosmetics in the eyes of rabbits, to subject food-producing animals to intensive production methods that deprive them of a range of normal behaviors, or to use horses and dogs in competition racing. Whether or not these positions are morally correct they are surely coherent. One understands what they mean, whether or not one agrees with them. However, if by animal "welfare" we mean, at least in part, approval of (for example) the use of animals in research or for food or entertainment, it would be self-contradictory to assert that considerations of animal welfare argue against any such uses of animals.

It is unscientific and intellectually suspect to begin one's approach to animal welfare with the view that whole categories of animal use are so obviously acceptable that we shall build approval of them into the very definition of welfare. One must allow at least for the *possibility* that scientific evidence about what certain practices do to animals can indicate that some of these practices are not conducive to animal welfare or result in enough compromise of welfare to render them inappropriate.

Assertion that "welfare" is value-free

Paradoxically, having included value judgments regarding acceptable uses of animals in the very meaning of the term, proposed definitions of "welfare" which include a distinction between animal welfare and animal rights, also tend to proclaim themselves to be completely value-free. Welfare, it is asserted, is a scientific concept, and the study of animal welfare is a purely factual enterprise. In contrast, it is said, statements about animal "rights" involve value judgments and therefore cannot be evaluated by strictly scientific evidence. The view that animal welfare does not include reference to ethical values is so important that it requires detailed consideration.

⟋ THE PURE SCIENCE MODEL OF ANIMAL WELFARE
The Model Defined

I call the view that animal welfare investigation can be separated from ethics and values the "pure science" model of animal welfare. This model is accepted by many veterinarians and animal welfare scientists.[4]

The pure science model does not deny that the underlying motivation for investigating animal welfare can be the ethical principle that people should pay due regard to animal welfare. Rather, the model asserts that once one begins to study welfare scientifically, one need not consider or take any positions with respect to ethical issues. According to the model, one need not make any value judgments in studying animal welfare because welfare is a state or condition that is experienced or undergone by an animal itself. Determining whether an animal is living in conditions that are conducive to its welfare is thus like discovering whether it can see. In determining whether an animal can see, one engages in empirical observation of the animal. One would not ask whether the world would be a better place if this animal could see or whether human beings have a moral obligation to assure that animals like this retain their ability to see. These might be important questions, but they are different from the question of whether an animal can see. According to proponents of the pure science model, asking when people ought to afford conditions conducive to animal welfare is an important question. But this is a different question from asking whether animals are living in conditions conducive to their welfare. The latter issue is purely factual, and addressing it does not involve making value judgments.

The pure science model does not imply that it is always easy to determine what conditions are conducive to animal welfare. Most investigators agree that the presence of stress, for example, is relevant to animal welfare, but there are disagreements about how to determine whether "stress" is present in animals, and even about the meaning of the term itself. There are vigorous debates among proponents of the pure science model about what factors (for example, absence of pain or suffering, absence of stress-related chemicals, reproductive success, absence of disease, choice of various stimuli) should be included among components of animal welfare. However, adherents of the pure science model all insist that deciding what conditions are relevant to animal welfare and determining whether such states are present, is a purely factual, descriptive task that does not involve making value judgments.

Nor does the pure science model imply that animal welfare is a simple, indivisible quality that is or is not present in its entirety at any given time. Animal welfare scientists commonly speak of varying degrees or levels of animal welfare, ranging from conditions so minimally beneficial that they barely qualify as being conducive to animal welfare, to conditions that approach or constitute optimal welfare.[5] Proponents of the pure science model concede that it is a matter for ethical discussion to determine what level of welfare is morally appropriate. Nevertheless, they maintain that determining the level of animal welfare is an entirely empirical undertaking devoid of value judgments, just as determining the level of acuity of an animal's eyesight does not involve making value judgments.

The official AVMA "Policy on Animal Welfare and Animal Rights," quoted above, reflects the pure science view of welfare. Moreover, included in the preface to the entire set of AVMA positions on animal welfare is a further reminder that while "rights" involve philosophical views and personal values, welfare is purely factual and scientific. The AVMA's positions on welfare "deal primarily with the scientific aspects of the medical well-being of animals. It is also recognized that all veterinarians have ethical, philosophical, and moral values that must be considered as positions are developed."[6] In other words, characterizations of animal welfare derive from scientific investigation. To these descriptions there may have to be added ethical positions about how one should or should not approach animal welfare, but these latter kinds of views are different from characterizations of welfare itself.

Professors Fraser and Broom offer a clear statement of the pure science model in their treatise on farm animal welfare:

> The assessment of welfare can be carried out in an objective way which is quite independent of any moral considerations. Mortality rate, reproductive success, extent of adrenal activity, amount of abnormal behavior, severity of injury, degree of immunosuppression, or level of disease can all be measured...In addition to measurements of poor welfare, it is possible to investigate the preferences of animals and the value which they place on various resources or other aspects of their environment. Such studies and a wide range of work on the basic biology of animals give information about the biological needs of animals...When scientific evaluation of welfare has been carried out, there remains the moral question of how poor welfare should be before it is regarded as unacceptable. This is an issue where the farmer, the veterinary surgeon, the welfare research worker, or the member of the public are equally entitled to have an opinion.[7]

Regarding ethical issues, the authors believe, everyone is entitled to an opinion because these are essentially matters of attitudes and values and no one possesses special expertise in matters of values. In contrast, animal welfare is the special province of scientists because this is an area that restricts itself to the scientific observation and measurement of facts. The pure science model postulates an inseparable theoretical gap between animal welfare science (a realm of facts) and animal welfare ethics (a realm of values). According to the model, those who are engaged in welfare science cannot be engaged simultaneously in welfare ethics; the latter involves a qualitatively different activity, the expression of moral judgments.

Attractiveness of the Pure Science Model

The pure science model is understandably attractive to veterinarians and animal welfare scientists. Although most people believe they have a moral obligation not to subject animals to miserable conditions, there is nothing approaching unanimity regarding what conditions of welfare are morally acceptable. Sometimes, controversies about what is morally owed to animals can be difficult and unpleasant. If the pure science model is correct, animal welfare investigators can go about their business unaffected by such ethical and political debates. They need not attempt to decide difficult moral issues when society may not be prepared to resolve them. Their investigations will be driven not by public demand or by the passing moral preferences of the day, but by scientific considerations of what is known and what needs to be learned. Animal welfare researchers will provide a storehouse of objective factual information, which will be available when the public and government are ready to decide how much or what sort of animal welfare should be provided. Animal welfare research can, in short, be kept where any branch of science is "supposed" to belong, safely in the field or laboratory and away from messy and perhaps unresolvable ethical controversies.

The pure science model also appeals to the (surely admirable) tendency of veterinarians and scientists not to make proclamations on matters about which they have no special expertise. Veterinarians and animal scientists do have special knowledge about the biological characteristics of animals. They do not speak with special knowledge or wisdom about ethics. At the same time, the pure science model gives veterinarians and animal welfare scientists a special status. As scientists, they clearly are entitled to speak on matters relating to welfare. Layman, however, are not scientists and thus according to the model are not "equally entitled to have an opinion."

Cracks in the Pure Science Model
Which animals' welfare?

Problems in the pure science model appear quickly when one examines how animal welfare is really investigated.

The first question that must be asked by anyone interested in understanding animal welfare is which animals' welfare will be the focus of one's concern. Very few people are interested in the welfare of all animals. The choice of which animals' welfare is worth understanding reflects value judgments about which animals *ought* to be protected or helped.

For example, there exist in most cities large numbers of rats, which can be quite dangerous to people and other animals. Few but the hardiest animal activists would suggest that we should worry about these animals' general welfare. There has been no call for scientific studies to determine what conditions would be conducive to these rats' welfare, so that they can be exterminated in accordance with minimal violation of their welfare, or so that some of them can be relocated to environs satisfactory to rat welfare.

There is little if any interest in these animals' welfare because it is generally believed that they are owed very little. In fact, most people believe that we ought to try to kill as many of them as possible. This is not to say that we have absolutely no ethical obligations regarding these animals. People do, I would maintain, have a minimal obligation not to cause the rats they kill more pain than is necessary to get the job done in a successful and cost-effective manner. However, this is quite different from saying that one should be concerned about their *welfare*. When we speak of the "welfare" of an animal we refer to conditions that go beyond what is minimally obligatory. As is explained below, whatever else we mean by the term, "welfare" refers to a state that includes some measure of a successful life. Most of us do not speak about the welfare of urban rats because we do not believe that we owe them this much.

Scientists, like laymen, usually take an interest in an animal's welfare only if they believe that its welfare *ought* to be respected to some extent. There are, to my knowledge, no scientists undertaking studies of the welfare of urban rats, vampire bats, tsetse flies, and man-eating sharks. Some scientists investigate the behavior of these animals and may be interested in what conditions are conducive to their thriving. However, researchers who might proclaim an interest in these animals' welfare would probably be considered odd, or worse.

Some people may have forgotten that the decision about what animals' welfare to study is in part an ethical one because there is widespread consensus about the moral appropriateness of protecting the welfare of many kinds of animals. Indeed, there is such wide-ranging concern that species we humans use for our own purposes be treated properly that it might seem obvious that the study of "animal welfare," in general, is a worthy undertaking. However, not so long ago there was little general regard for animal welfare. Prior to 1800, well before the advent of anti-cruelty to animals statutes in England and the United States, farm animals were routinely tortured, neglected, and subjected to the most miserable conditions.[8] Before the passage of the first federal Animal Welfare Act in 1966, many experimental animals were treated abysmally.[9] People who worked at these times for the study and promotion of farm or laboratory animal welfare were viewed as moral crusaders, by themselves and their opponents.

How much welfare?

Even after animal welfare scientists make ethical decisions concerning which animals' welfare is worth studying, they must face another difficult ethical task: they must decide how much welfare is worth studying.

It is generally agreed that animal welfare is often a matter of degree. For example, a pig farmer can use various kinds of outdoor husbandry techniques. Or, if he uses an indoor confinement system, he can (among other things) use floors constructed of and covered by various materials, provide various amounts of space to his animals, keep the facilities at various temperatures and levels of lighting, and provide the animals a range of different possible activities. Some of these conditions may provide what could be called minimal welfare, some might yield a higher level of welfare, and some might provide conditions that approach or constitute what could be called optimal welfare.

Let us suppose for the moment that the concept of "minimal animal welfare" is a purely scientific one, i.e., that one can determine whether minimal animal welfare is present without making an ethical judgment. It nevertheless is an undeniably ethical decision what level of welfare ought to be provided to various kinds of animals. Thus if providing a certain high level of welfare would be so costly that it would bankrupt farmers, many people would agree that affording this level of welfare is not morally obligatory—provided that at least a satisfactory level of welfare is maintained. Sometimes it can be argued that an animal's interests are not sufficiently weighty to require even a minimal cost. For example, sows and their piglets appear to enjoy looking at and attempting to manipulate objects suspended above them, and Curtis suggests that providing such objects can raise these animals' level of welfare.[10] However, some producers will argue that pigs do not have a very strong need for such visual stimulation because they can get along nicely without it. From this some might conclude that it is not morally obligatory for a producer to incur even a modest expense or effort to provide such visual stimulation.

Although Fraser and Broom concede that deciding what level of welfare ought to be provided is an ethical issue, they insist that animal welfare science can study such levels without resorting to values.[7] However, no successful animal welfare investigator could long do this. Imagine a researcher who proposes to study the levels of welfare experienced by swine in various conditions of housing. To explore the "upper" levels of welfare, she wants to investigate situations in which sows and their piglets receive luxurious care. She proposes that several buildings be constructed to house the animals. One building will house one sow and her piglets, a second, two sows and their piglets, a third, three sows and their piglets, and so on. Each set of animals will be attended around the clock by researchers who will simulate farm workers; the number of work-ers in attendance at all times will vary from one to six. These workers will make sure that temperature and lighting are continuously adjusted in various ways and will attempt to provide frequent stimulating human-animal contact. The workers will attempt several different farrowing techniques. For example, while sows now typically are not exercised during their no-more-than-14-day stay in farrowing crates,[11] these workers will periodically try to remove the piglets from around the crate, help the sow to exercise, place her back in the crate, and return the piglets.

I could go on, but my aim is to imagine our scientist proposing to investigate con-ditions that are incompatible with successful economic production and thus would never be adopted. I suggest that no animal welfare investigator would propose such studies. This is so not because welfare investigators are only interested in scientifically determining various levels of welfare, for if this were really their only interest they might study conditions that had no possibility of being adopted. Investigators would not propose such studies because doing so would be pointless, and animal welfare sci-entists make the *value judgment* that it is not appropriate to conduct pointless investi-gations. Such studies also would not be undertaken because few people believe that producers have a moral obligation to provide such upper levels of welfare if (let us sup-pose) doing so would make the entire production process economically unfeasible.

Many of Fraser and Broom's own discussions illustrate that when investigators are not engaged in theoretical discussions about the value-free "objectivity" of animal wel-fare science, they frequently engage in moral judgments about what levels of welfare might be obligatory—in their choice of research questions and in their recommenda-tions regarding the treatment of animals. For example, the authors state that in a far-rowing crate, the sow:

> …is very restricted in her movements…and she cannot move much toward the piglets. Hence it would seem to be a rather frustrating situation for the sow. Before farrowing, sows will build large nests if they are given the opportunity and there are indications that the inability to build a nest is frustrating for the sow…Overall the widely used farrowing crate is easy to manage but is far from ideal for the sow. Although it is better for the piglet than a farrowing pen of similar size with no crate in it, a large amount of space and deep straw would seem to be better still. Research on alternative farrowing accommodation is being carried out but much more work is needed in this area.[12]

Assume for the sake of discussion that when the authors say the farrowing crate is far from "ideal" for the sow and that it would be "better" for piglets to have more space and deep straw they are making purely factual judgments about relative levels of wel-fare. It is nevertheless clear that they also believe that, if possible, alternative farrowing accommodations which would provide better welfare for sows and piglets ought to be used. There is a value judgment here, namely that a higher level of welfare *ought* to be found and implemented if possible.

Throughout the discussions of animal welfare investigators, one finds the identifi-cation of issues or "problems" and the suggestion of solutions that are based on researchers' perceptions about whether animals are being treated as they *ought* to be treated.[13] Researchers commonly evaluate practices on the grounds that welfare conditions are morally intolerable or acceptable. And when they do so, they rarely claim that they are speaking only as ordinary citizens, not as scientists.

⮠ ETHICAL COMPONENTS OF WELFARE

At this point a proponent of the pure science model may assert that there is still a large area for scientific study devoid of value judgments, namely welfare itself and its varying levels or degrees. Even if, it might be maintained, many of the questions addressed by animal welfare science are motivated by ethical concerns, once these concerns indicate that the welfare of certain animals and certain levels of welfare should be studied, investigation will be solely into matters of fact, observation, and measurement. For example, once it is decided on ethical grounds that the welfare of pigs should be studied, and that pigs should be provided conditions that do not cause them to suffer but at the same time do not bankrupt producers, scientists can study pig welfare in this range without reference to values. Society can then determine how much or what level of welfare it wants to provide.

This position too is untenable, because the very concept of animal welfare—what ordinary people as well as scientists mean by the term—includes an ethical component.

Welfare and What is Good for One

We can see this by examining how the term "welfare" is applied to human beings. "Welfare" refers in part to a state that is good for the person about whose welfare one is speaking. This is why we can talk of sacrificing the welfare of an individual for the good of others. When we speak in this way we recognize that "welfare" refers in part what is good for the individual, to what is conducive to his or her success in some sense. To sacrifice one's own welfare for another's good is to make some compromise in what is good for one.

That an individual's welfare has something to do with its "success" may have led some animal welfare scientists to suppose that one can find and measure animal welfare without making value judgments. For there is a sense of "success" in which whether an animal is successful does not seem to have anything to do with values. Consider our city-dwelling rat. If this animal is fat, energetic, and free of disease it is in some sense being "successful" functioning as a rat. We can say that the rat is being successful and still say at the same time that it would be morally appropriate for people to kill it. Therefore it might appear that one can judge whether it is living in conditions conducive to its "welfare" without making any value judgments about what is good or bad or about how people ought to act. Moreover, because such rats can appear to have more or less success in prospering, proponents of the pure science model may suppose that characterizing the degree of this success (the level of "welfare") involves no moral judgments.

However, the concept of welfare is not synonymous with being successful in a way that makes no reference to values. This can be appreciated by considering the nineteenth-century English philosopher John Stuart Mill's famous statement about human happiness and welfare. "It is better," he wrote, "to be a human being dissatisfied, than a pig satisfied; better to be Socrates dissatisfied than a fool satisfied."[14] Mill reminds us that there is a fundamental difference between welfare and contentment. An individual's welfare sometimes involves loss of contentment, satisfaction, or feelings of well-being. Thus it is better to become educated and to learn about the world—even though doing so may be difficult and even if some of the knowledge one obtains makes one dissatisfied, impatient, angry, or sad.

As Mill recognized, most people believe that the uneducated (but contented) person experiences a lower level of welfare because we regard such a person as occupying "a lower grade of existence."[14] Not lower in a biological sense, for a fool need be biologically no less successful than an educated person; both may be physically vigorous and healthy. People think that the educated person attains a higher level of welfare because it is *better*—it is morally preferable, to be an educated person than a contented fool. There is a sense in which we can regard such a person as living a more "successful" life than the fool, but in this sense, being more successful is living closer to how one *ought* to live, not simply living with one's biological needs or drives satisfied.

Welfare and Death

The fact there is an ethical component in the concept of welfare can also be appreciated by considering the following question: Does killing an animal harm or affect its welfare, even if this killing involves no pain, distress, or discomfort for the animal?

Most, if not all, people believe that death is inimical to human welfare. We think this not just because living is necessary for experiencing welfare, but also because we value human life as a good. Death frustrates human welfare because it takes away the most precious gift one can have—life—and all that living can bring.

With respect to animals, however, many people deny that death is inimical to, frustrates, or indeed has any relevance to welfare. Fraser and Broom, for example, state that:

> If an animal is suddenly shot, with no previous warning that this might happen, and it dies instantaneously, then there is a moral question about whether such killing should occur but there is no welfare problem. If an animal dies slowly with much pain, or is wounded by a shot which results in pain and difficulties in normal living, then its welfare is poor…If animals are kept in order that they will eventually be eaten, their welfare could be good throughout their lives even up to the point of slaughter.[15]

Although this statement is supposed to show that "welfare" does not presuppose value judgments, it demonstrates the opposite. Why would we say that a genocidal maniac negatively affects human welfare even if he kills his human victims immediately, without warning or pain? Because we believe that the taking of innocent human life is evil and because we value the lives that would be taken. What is the difference between such human beings who would be killed and animals that are killed instantaneously and painlessly? The difference, clearly, is that many people (including Fraser and Broom) do not regard the taking of animal life as itself an evil and do not regard life as something that is morally owed to animals.

However, people who object to the killing of animals even when this might be done painlessly, *do* believe that such killing is inimical to animal welfare, precisely because they consider the taking of animal life under these circumstances morally wrong. Philosopher Tom Regan maintains that even the painless killing of animals for food or in experimentation harms their welfare because, in his view, such animals have an interest in living that ought to be respected. For Regan, the farmer or experimenter who kills an animal, even painlessly, oversteps the boundary of animal welfare:

Death is the ultimate, the irreversible harm because death is the ultimate, the irreversible loss, foreclosing every opportunity to find satisfaction. This is true whether death is slow and agonizing or quick and painless. Though there are some fates worse than death, an untimely death is not in the interests of its victims, whether human or animal, independently of whether they understand their own mortality, and thus independently of whether they themselves have a desire to continue to live.[16]

My point is not that Fraser and Broom are incorrect in thinking that it is sometimes morally permissible to kill animals. Rather, their characterization of the relevance of death to animal welfare rests on a value judgment that might appear so obvious and self evident to them that they do not recognize it as a value judgment. Fraser and Broom appear to endorse the anti-cruelty position, the view that one's major moral obligation to animals is not to cause them unnecessary pain or suffering (see Chapter 11). However popular this view may be among animal welfare scientists and the public, it is an expression of values nonetheless.

Value-laden Definitions of "Animal Welfare"
A Tower of Babel?

Perhaps the most persuasive proof that claims about welfare involve value judgments can be found in the definitions of animal welfare offered by welfare investigators themselves.

The following are some of the definitions that have been proposed or endorsed by prominent animal welfare scientists. Such definitions are often set forth as truisms, with little supporting argument. These definitions typically occur at or near the beginning of discussions. Claims are then made about whether a given practice promotes "welfare" as already defined. The term "welfare," it has been claimed, refers to:

- "a state of complete mental and physical health where the animal is in complete harmony with its environment"[17]
- "a condition of physical and physiological harmony in the animal itself and of the animal with its environment. The indications of well-being are good health and behavior which is entirely normal."[18]
- "the degree to which [animals] can adapt without suffering to environments designated by man"[19]
- absence of "methods for handling and management [that] are so extreme as to induce stress or its overt symptoms, distress, on animals. Stress is understood to mean extensive physiological and behavioral disturbance in the animal resulting from noxious environmental factors."[20]
- absence of "suffering"[21]
- "mental well-being," which is identified with the absence of "suffering."[22] Suffering is defined as "a wide range of unpleasant emotional states" including "fear, pain, frustration and exhaustion" and other mental states "such as those caused by loss of social companions."[23]
- "both the physical and mental well-being of the animal"[24]
- "freedom from pain and suffering." "Pain" is defined as "aversive stimulation of the central nervous system (CNS) originating from the damage of tissues, and, or organs either by disease, injury or functional disorder." "Suffering" is defined as "aversive stimulation of the CNS originating from behavioral and physiological conflicts with the environment."[25]

- "well-being," characterized as the fulfillment of "needs"[26]
- an animal's "state as regards its attempts to cope with its environment."[27] The level or degree of welfare is seen as the degree of success achieved by the animal in coping "with difficult conditions."[28]
- "Welfare is not health…it is not *being* ill that reduces welfare but *feeling* ill."[29]
- The above view is "simplistic and inappropriate…[because] an animal is in a state of poor welfare *only* when physiological systems are disturbed to the point that survival or reproduction are impaired."[30]
- "When the biological cost of a management practice exceeds a level of acceptable risk, then we can state that the animal's well-being (and thus welfare) is at significant risk…"[31] Biological cost is understood as the "diversion of biological resources away from normal nonstress functions." [32] Accordingly, the best indicators of lack of welfare are often not the actual disturbance of physiological systems but "prepathological states…[in which] the opportunity exists for pathologies to develop."[32]

One fact is apparent from just these definitions: animal welfare science has a serious problem that derives, at least in part, from differences in what is understood by the term "welfare." Different investigators sometimes reach different conclusions about whether certain conditions promote or inhibit welfare not because (or not just because) these investigators disagree about the facts—but because they begin with a different idea of *what* they are seeking to discover facts *about*.

The definitions quoted above differ significantly, and several are incompatible with others. For example, while the "absence of suffering" connotes only the absence of certain very unpleasant experiences, the term "well-being" as it is ordinarily used refers to the presence of positive sensations, feelings, or experiences. Likewise, animals that might experience some degree of "welfare" because they are not subjected to treatment that is so extreme as to induce stress, might nevertheless not be experiencing welfare (or might be experiencing a much lower level of welfare) under a definition that identifies welfare with a state in which an animal is both physically and mentally "in harmony" with its environment. Similarly, an investigator who defines "welfare" in terms of the degree of successful coping with adverse conditions might differ with one who defines "welfare" as well-being and is therefore prepared to compare levels of welfare in various situations some of which could not be called "adverse."

The last three definitions quoted above illustrate starkly how different views regarding the relevance of health and illness to the definition of "welfare" could lead to different factual conclusions about whether animals are experiencing welfare. The first of these definitions rejects health as an essential feature of welfare, and regards both health and illness relevant to welfare only if they result in an animal's feeling good or bad. The second of these definitions restricts poor "welfare" to conditions in which animals are actually ill, or are at least experiencing disruptions of normal physiological or reproductive processes. The last of the definitions defines "welfare" so that describing (and improving) welfare includes attention to prepathological states that need not be associated with current bad feelings or disturbances of physiological processes. Proponents of these three definitions could well look at the same animal and agree about what that animal is experiencing. However, they might disagree about whether it is experiencing a state of welfare, a high or low level of welfare, or conditions that in the long or short term are likely to be conducive or inimical to its welfare. Likewise, two investigators might agree that a veal calf confined in a crate and fed a low-iron liquid diet is not experiencing pain or distress. One, who defines welfare as the absence of suffering will conclude that there is no compromise of the animal's welfare. The other, who defines welfare as a state of complete mental and physical health and who also views the ability to move, groom, and socialize as aspects of an animal's mental health, will probably consider the situation to be inconsistent with welfare.

Why so many definitions of animal welfare?

Some of the differences among the various definitions of "animal welfare" may derive from different views about what animals actually experience or about what it is possible to measure in them. Nevertheless, it is clear that all the definitions have an ethical component. Someone who believes that welfare is the absence of suffering takes the position that what constitutes an acceptable kind of life for an animal is one without suffering. Someone who believes that this is not sufficient for welfare believes that animals are owed more. Someone who defines welfare as the ability of animals to adapt without suffering to environments "designated by man"[19] will assume the propriety of many kinds of animal care methods (provided they can be accomplished without suffering). In contrast, someone who defines welfare in terms of the satisfaction of needs may insist that one start with the animals' needs first and adapt environments to them—on the grounds that *this* is the morally correct approach.

Because so many animal welfare scientists appear to accept the pure science model of welfare, few investigators will admit that built into their definitions of welfare are value judgments regarding how animals ought to be treated. Gary Moberg (whose definition is the last of those quoted above) is refreshingly explicit about the ethical component of his definition. Moberg concedes that "each of us defines animal welfare with reference to our perceptions of the ideal relationship between humans and animals." He believes that his own definition promotes what he finds ethically appropriate: "a strategy that establishes guidelines for animal welfare that not only protects animals but also permits sufficient latitude to set realistic, workable conditions for the production and use of domestic animals."[33]

There are many different definitions of "animal welfare" at least in part because there are many different possible views about what people are ethically obligated to do, or not to do, to animals.

∾ THE MISCHIEF OF THE PURE SCIENCE MODEL

Those who maintain that their conceptions of "welfare" are value-free do not err in employing definitions of welfare that incorporate values. For, I have argued, it is impossible to use the term "welfare" without committing oneself to certain ethical judgments. The denial that values are being endorsed does, however, lead to serious methodological problems.

First, because those who accept the pure science model do not recognize that they are making value judgments, they do not recognize certain important ethical issues as meriting discussion. For example, someone who defines welfare in terms of the fulfillment of needs will not recognize as independently relevant to welfare the fulfillment of what might better be termed "wants"—desires or preferences the fulfillment of which might give satisfaction or pleasure but the denial or frustration of which might not have adverse or unpleasant physiological or behavioral effects. Because they assume that what we owe animals is the fulfillment of certain "needs," such investigators may not take seriously the ethical issue of whether people sometimes have a moral obligation to allow animals to do what they want.

Second, adoption of the pure science model leads to the foreclosing of potentially significant scientific questions. Dawkins' studies of animal preference illustrate how this can happen. Dawkins found that hens prefer an outside run to a battery cage, although hens raised in a battery cage take some time to express this preference.[34] Other work has shown that laying hens prefer floors of fine-gauge hexagonal mesh to heavy rectangular mesh;[35] that pigs prefer light to darkness and will turn on lights at night;[36] and that gilts prefer an earth floor over a pen adjacent to another pig but prefer being next to another gilt over straw or wood shavings.[37] Although such results suggest that animals can sometimes be made happier by being allowed to choose part of their environments, Dawkins sees a serious limitation in viewing preference as evidence of welfare:

> Now the obvious rejoinder to the finding that hens prefer being outside in a run to being inside in a battery cage is that this does not tell us anything about whether they suffer in battery cages. A gourmet might prefer caviar to smoked salmon, but it would be difficult to argue that he would suffer if he had to make do with smoked salmon. This is another way of saying that preference by itself is not an indicator of suffering. To show that a preference does indicate suffering in the less preferred environment, we have to find out not merely what the preference is, but how strong it is. If it were shown that hens would do literally anything to get out of a battery cage and that their preference for the run was so strong that it overruled everything else, then it might be possible to conclude that they suffered in cages.[38]

Dawkins is a proponent of the definition of welfare as the "absence of suffering,"[39] a definition based on a value judgment that people ought not to permit animals they use to suffer. This definition not only leads Dawkins to ignore the possibility of considering whether farmers sometimes ought to allow animals to express their preferences even if doing so is not necessary for the alleviation or prevention of suffering. But the definition also leads her to dismiss as irrelevant to welfare, studies that would not show how animals would "do literally anything" to express their preferences. For she appears to think (mistakenly, I would argue) that extremely strong preferences indicate only flight from suffering and not impetus toward pleasure. In any event, she rules out a whole line of inquiry relevant to the view that animals ought sometimes be allowed to express their preferences irrespective of whether this would affect their level or degree of suffering. For, someone might argue, even if certain conditions preferred by farm animals were analogous to unnecessary but nevertheless, pleasurable Epicurean delights, might it not sometimes still be incumbent on farmers to provide them with such conditions—simply because these conditions make the animals happier? Might not this added happiness or pleasure heighten the level of their welfare?

There is no purely factual justification for the contention that preference is relevant only when it provides evidence of *suffering*. Rather, Dawkins appeals to unspoken value judgments that do not include the principle that animals are sometimes owed not just freedom from suffering but positive pleasures.

Another problem Dawkins finds in preference testing is that:

...animals do not always choose what is best for their own long-term physical well-being...there is probably some connection between what animals choose on the one hand and what is best for their survival and reproduction on the other. The connection is not, however, a hard and fast one. Animals do not always choose what is best for them...Domestic cattle...[s]ometimes eat poisonous plants or bloat themselves with clover. Animals such as pigs and rats have a strong liking for saccharine, and yet it has no food value. We can add other examples from everyday experience; people choose to smoke and do other things which may damage their health in the long run.[40]

Here, welfare appears to be identified with physical health in the long run (perhaps because Dawkins thinks that the absence of such health is associated with suffering). Dawkins seems to find inimical to welfare behavior that either frustrates such health (for example, consuming poison) or does not further it (for example, consuming non-nutritive saccharine).

Dawkins is correct that free choice can be injurious to welfare because people and animals can make poor choices. However, the connections between choice and welfare are not done justice by the statement that choice and welfare sometimes conflict. Sometimes, we regard the ability to choose what one wants and the pleasure brought by such choices as a fundamental feature of welfare, even if what is chosen might not turn out to be optimal for physical health. For example, most of us would regard our welfare to be diminished if we were forced to eat only healthful foods or to exercise instead of enjoying certain sedentary pleasures, even if it could be demonstrated that our "health in the long run" might be damaged somewhat. Moreover, we do not regard as inimical to welfare a whole range of nonbeneficial activities, such as the consumption of pleasurable but nonnutritive foods. Indeed, most people would say that their welfare would be diminished if they were not permitted to choose such harmless pleasures.

We include within human welfare the freedom to enjoy some harmful and some harmless pleasures because we regard a life with such freedoms and pleasures *better* than a life without them. Is it self-evident that this cannot sometimes be true with regard to animals? Some people maintain that it is better, and therefore conducive to welfare, for wild animals not to be kept in captivity even if keeping them in captivity provides them longer lives and protects them from predation and disease.[41] It can also be argued that animals in the wild may experience pleasures greater than those they will experience in captivity, or that living in the wild accords with their inborn natures.[42] Nor is it patently ridiculous to argue that pigs and other farm animals might live a better life if they could enjoy certain pleasures that did not result in their living an optimally healthy life, or even in their producing the amount and quality of foodstuffs farmers desire.

People who think that animal welfare is served by sometimes allowing animals to do what they want might be making incorrect value judgments. However, it hardly seems fair to dismiss their value judgments simply by proclaiming a definition of welfare that incorporates a contrary value judgment. The only way to determine which of such value judgments is preferable is to approach them as value judgments and to assess them accordingly.

∾ SHOULD THE CONCEPT OF WELFARE BE ABANDONED?

Dr. Michael Fox suggests that because the concept of animal "welfare" has become entwined in ethical arguments relating to the proper treatment of animals, the concept is now a burden to veterinarians and scientists. According to Fox, some veterinarians and ethologists are already "tending to avoid the term and advocacy of animal welfare in favor of advocating animal health and well-being (well-being implying provision of an environment and standards of care and husbandry that cause minimal stress and distress and satisfy the animal's basic behavioral and social requirements)." Unlike welfare, "animal health and well-being can be objectively and scientifically determined, thus providing a basis for evaluating the humaneness of how animals are treated." By avoiding talk of welfare, veterinarians will not have to "stand in judgment of how society uses animals." The profession will be able to "focus objectively on areas of animal use wherein improvements in health and overall well-being are clearly needed."[43]

Fox's proposed solution for the "problem" of value-laden discussions of animal welfare cannot work. First, as philosopher Bernard Rollin demonstrates, what counts as "health" or "disease" in both human and veterinary medicine includes reference to the values of those who determine that a physical or mental state or condition is to be considered healthy or diseased.[44] For example, societies that prize heaviness do not classify obesity as a disease, while in the United States obesity is seen not just as contributing to illness, but as an illness in itself. Likewise, animals used in agriculture are frequently not considered ill even though they may be experiencing some distress if these animals are producing as expected. In contrast, the owners of companion animals with similar distress will rush their animals to a veterinarian for treatment because these people find such distress unacceptable. Thus Dr. Fox's recommendation that we replace the term "welfare" with the notion of "health" will not eliminate value judgments.

The same thing is true of the term "well-being," which, like the words "health" or "welfare" incorporate values. Dr. Fox says that the advocacy of "well-being" will help the veterinary profession "best serve society and its animal constituency."[43] Thus the promotion of well-being is a moral imperative, something that is owed to the animals. By including satisfaction of "the animal's basic behavioral and social needs" in his definition of well-being, Fox is saying that the kind of life some animals are owed is one in which these needs are fulfilled.

Suppose someone objects that animals are not owed such a life. Fox cannot respond that animals just are owed "well-being" as he defines it. For even if Fox's opponent accepted his definition of well-being, the opponent could still reject the claim that animals are entitled to well-being in this sense. Fox must offer—and in fact he does offer[45]—ethical arguments to demonstrate that what he deems to be basic behavioral and social needs ought to be fulfilled. Fox's importation of his own ethical views into his definition of "well-being" is no different from the importation of ethical views into definitions of animal *welfare*. His discussion provides further proof that veterinarians, welfare scientists, and members of the public want a term that refers to what is good for an animal in the sense of what would provide it with the life we ordinarily ought to permit or encourage it to live. In sum, the idea or concept of animal welfare has such potent moral force that if it somehow did not exist, it would soon be invented.

～ GETTING DOWN TO BUSINESS WITHOUT DEFINITIONS OF "ANIMAL WELFARE"

As the philosopher Ludwig Wittgenstein observed, many people have assumed that it is impossible to talk about something unless one has a proper definition of the word which stands for that thing, and that a proper definition must consist of a list of conditions that are necessary and sufficient for the correct application of the defined word. Wittgenstein demonstrates that these assumptions are incorrect.[46] Many terms are too complex and are used in too many different contexts to allow such definitions, or indeed precise definitions of any kind. Many of our most important concepts can be compared to a rope. A rope consists of many individual strands that are woven together, but no one of which runs through the entire rope and is either a necessary or sufficient part of it. Yet the rope can be recognizable, strong, and useful. Wittgenstein uses the term "game" to illustrate his critically important observation. We can identify various activities as games, and we can describe games and express our views and preferences about games or kinds of games. However, it is impossible to find a single feature that is either necessary or sufficient for all "games." We can, of course, focus on aspects that appear to be central to many games, or to certain kinds of games—such as the presence of more than one player, winning and losing, keeping score, and rules of play. But one can always find games that do not exemplify one or more of these features.

Many leading animal welfare scientists appear to believe that they cannot proceed without a precise definition of "welfare."[47] There are at least three reasons to be skeptical of this position.

First, the term "welfare" has been in use for centuries and in many different contexts (animal as well as human). Like the term "game," we might *expect* "welfare" to resist easy or rigorous definition.

Second, as we have seen, "animal welfare" refers in part to what is regarded as good for animals. However, there remains vigorous disagreement about what should be considered good for animals and about how we are morally obligated to treat them. Consensus about a definition of "animal welfare" is unlikely as long as such ethical disagreements continue. Because animal and veterinary ethics are in their infancy, it is advisable to let ethical debates about animal welfare continue for some time before attempts are made to define the term.

Finally, as we have also seen, definitions of "animal welfare" tend to remove competing ethical and scientific viewpoints from one's universe of discourse: alternative ethical and factual inquiries become literally unthinkable because they do not fit a preconceived definition of "welfare." Robust scientific and ethical inquiry about factors relevant to animal welfare is not facilitated by unexamined factual or moral propositions parading under the guise of purely "objective" definitions of central terminology.

There are many scientific questions about what animals experience and many ethical issues about what it is morally permissible to do to animals. Therefore it is simplistic and dangerous to suppose that, even in the absence of a good definition, all people will always agree that a given condition does or does not promote animal welfare. However, a great deal about animal welfare does seem clear and can serve as a basis for scientific and ethical inquiry.

ABSENCE OF PAIN, SUFFERING, STRESS, DISTRESS, AND OTHER SEVERE UNPLEASANT SENSATIONS. Although these unpleasant states are not always inimical to welfare,[48] we know that they often are. We also know that welfare can be more greatly affected the more intense or longer lasting the pain, suffering, stress, or distress. Among other kinds of negative sensations we know can negate welfare, or can lower the level of welfare, are severe or long-lasting feelings of hunger, thirst, heat, and cold.

ABSENCE OF DISCOMFORT AND OTHER LESS INTENSE NEGATIVE SENSATIONS. Although it may sometimes be argued that milder or transitory negative experiences are not sufficiently important to be regarded as inimical to welfare, we sometimes know that they ought to be so regarded. A short period of mild discomfort (or indeed a short period of intense pain) might not diminish an animal's overall welfare, but the same discomfort lasting for a significant time can negate or diminish welfare.

ABSENCE OF ANXIETY, BOREDOM, AND OTHER SOPHISTICATED UNPLEASANT PSYCHOLOGICAL EXPERIENCES. As argued in Chapter 23, one must be careful before ascribing to animals experiences, such as boredom, anguish, and anxiety, for these concepts presuppose sophisticated mental capacities that many kinds of animals probably do not possess. Nevertheless, we know that anxiety, for example, is extremely unpleasant. Therefore to the extent to which anxiety is experienced by animals, it would constitute a significant diminution of welfare.

PLEASURABLE EXPERIENCES. Pleasurable experiences or the satisfaction of preferences can be associated with behavior that is harmful to an animal. However, as Duncan argues, if experiencing negative sensations, such as pain and stress, are often part of welfare, there appears to be no reason why pleasurable experiences cannot *sometimes* be included in welfare to the extent that animals are capable of having such experiences.[49] We know that a dog that is allowed frequent enjoyment of toys, or a pig that devours its food with apparent pleasure, can thereby experience an elevated level of welfare. Moreover, to the extent that certain animals can experience very sophisticated pleasurable experiences (such as the exercise of curiosity or the enjoyment of company with other animals or people) we should want to include such experiences as components of animal welfare.

HEALTH, FITNESS, FULFILLMENT OF BASIC BIOLOGICAL DRIVES, ABSENCE OF ABNORMAL BEHAVIOR. Even those who deny that health and fitness are themselves components of welfare concede that "when an animal *is* ill, it will usually *feel* ill, so that health and welfare will be reduced together."[50] Absence of illness, disease, or injury are therefore often reliable signs of welfare, even if they should not be regarded as components of welfare itself. Likewise, we need not decide definitively whether patterns of stereotypical behavior, the inability to move about or behave normally, or the frustration of an animal's inborn nature or "*telos*" (see Chapter 11) are themselves diminutions of welfare or merely signs of something else—pain, stress, or distress—that are properly viewed as inconsistent with welfare. For we will often have good reason to know that abnormal or frustrated behavior are signs of negative experiences and for that reason if for no other diminish or negate welfare.

⟳ MAJOR ETHICAL ISSUES RELATING TO ANIMAL WELFARE

The number, range, and difficulty of ethical issues that confront the field of animal welfare are staggering. Table 13-1 lists some of these issues. The table does not purport to set forth all important ethical issues relating to animal welfare. Moreover, some of the questions listed are quite general and contain or imply further questions. (For example, there are many standard techniques in the handling of farm or laboratory animals that raise important welfare issues.) To a certain extent, the questions one lists as relevant to welfare will be a function of one's own value judgments. Thus those who oppose, say, the use of animals in research, would maintain that the appropriate ques-

TABLE 13-1

Major ethical issues relating to animal welfare

Farm Animal Welfare

- To what extent, if any, do standard agricultural practices (for example, indoor confinement rearing of pigs, intensive battery cages for laying hens, castration of cattle and pigs without anesthesia, debeaking of chicks, administration of subtherapeutic doses of antibiotics) make inappropriate compromises in welfare? Where an inappropriate compromise might be made, are there alternative methods that satisfactorily reconcile the interests of animals, farmers, and the public?
- How do various methods of stockmanship (including different kinds of contact between handlers and animals) affect welfare?
- Can modification in the design and construction of animal production equipment improve welfare consistent with legitimate economic needs of producers and the public?
- To what extent, if any, should farmers and veterinarians concentrate upon the welfare or productivity of herds rather than of individual animals?
- To what extent, if any, is it proper to tolerate disease in individual animals to promote overall productivity or profitability?
- Do conventional methods of handling and moving animals on farms comport with proper regard for welfare?
- Do present methods of transporting animals to feed-lots and slaughterhouses comport with proper regard for welfare?
- Should improvements be made in welfare aspects of slaughter and pre-slaughter procedures?
- To what extent, if any, should veterinarians argue for or insist upon procedures to further the patient's welfare when doing so is opposed by or runs counter to the client's economic interests?
- To what extent are emerging techniques in biotechnology designed to enhance production (for example, bovine growth hormone for dairy cows) conducive to welfare?

Laboratory Animal Welfare

- What are the welfare implications of variations in general housing and environmental conditions (for example, size and construction materials of cages, temperature, ventilation, quantity and quality of food, lighting, nature and quantity of bedding for nesting animals, ability to come in contact with other animals, opportunity for exercise)?
- To what extent should negative mental states, such as discomfort, stress, distress, pain, and suffering, be lessened or eliminated to comply with acceptable levels of welfare? Has there been sufficient attention to the development of anesthetics and analgesics for laboratory animals?
- Does laboratory animal welfare include positive mental states such as pleasure and psychological well-being, and to what extent, if any, should such experiences be provided to laboratory animals?
- To what extent, if any, should certain practices in cancer and immunology studies (for example, growth of large implanted tumors, use of Complete Freund's Adjuvant) be modified or abandoned to comport with appropriate levels of welfare?
- To what extent, if any, is it permissible to cause pain to or otherwise compromise the welfare of animals used in psychological experiments?
- What methods of euthanasia are appropriate in various circumstances and for various species? When do welfare considerations require euthanasia rather than continuing the experiment or allowing death as an experimental end-point?
- Is general animal welfare furthered or diminished by prohibiting the use of animals abandoned to pounds and shelters?
- In general, how should welfare considerations be weighed against economic costs of providing enhanced welfare or potential effects on research projects?
- Are certain species (for example, chimpanzees, certain monkey species) entitled to have various aspects of

Table 13-1 cont'd

Major ethical issues relating to animal welfare

Laboratory Animal Welfare (cont'd)

their welfare respected such that they should never be used in research or if used, may be used only in the most important and practically beneficial studies? To what extent, if any, is it appropriate to be more concerned about the welfare of certain "higher" species than about other "lower" ones?

- To what extent, if any, is it justifiable to compromise welfare in basic as distinguished from practically-oriented research?
- Are certain testing methods (for example, LD50, Draize Eye Irritant Test) sufficiently respectful of welfare?
- Does the moral appropriateness of such tests vary with the kind of substance or product (for example, medicine vs. cosmetics) being tested?
- To what extent is it possible or appropriate to reduce the use of animals in research or to replace animals with nonanimal modalities?

Companion Animal Welfare

- Are certain breed standards in dogs and cats so detrimental to health or comfort that they constitute an impermissible diminution in welfare? What should be the position of the veterinary profession regarding breed standards that have negative effects on welfare?
- Should veterinarians dock the tails or crop the ears of dogs?
- Under what conditions might welfare considerations argue against the declawing of cats and the de-barking of dogs?
- How should veterinarians respond when clients do not want to provide their animals medical care that would protect or promote these animals' welfare?
- How should veterinarians respond when clients cannot afford medical care that would protect or promote their animals' welfare?
- How should veterinarians approach clients who abuse or neglect their animals or whose ignorance about proper pet care leads them to harm their animals' welfare?
- When does due consideration for welfare argue in favor of euthanizing an ill or injured animal? How should veterinarians respond when clients elect to continue treatment when doing so causes the patient to suffer or to experience a greatly diminished quality of life? How should euthanasia be performed to protect welfare?
- Does the practice of euthanizing healthy, well-behaved animals "on demand" affect the ability of the veterinary profession to promote itself as a protector of animal welfare?
- To what extent are low-cost rabies and spay/neuter clinics consistent with due regard for patient welfare?
- Is there sufficient protection of the welfare of puppies bred in and transported from so-called "puppy mills"?

Sport and Entertainment Animal Welfare

- To what extent, if any, do certain pharmacological, medical, or surgical procedures (for example, pre-competition administration of drugs) pay due regard to performance animal welfare?
- Can the design (including track materials and geometry) and maintenance of tracks and racing surfaces be improved to promote welfare?
- To what extent are conditions under which racing animals are stabled or kenneled sufficiently conducive to welfare?
- Are conditions of training sufficiently respectful of welfare?
- To what extent do current practices, regarding the provision of emergency medical care and euthanasia of injured racing animals, pay due regard to welfare?
- Do current practices relating to veterinary pre-examination and track supervision sufficiently protect welfare?
- To what extent might animals be raced beyond the time when it is humane to do so? In general, is there sufficient respect for the welfare of animals that can no longer race or cannot meet the economic expectations of owners?

Continued.

TABLE 13-1 CONT'D

Major ethical issues relating to animal welfare

Sport and Entertainment Animal Welfare (cont'd)

- To what extent should veterinarians argue for or insist upon the provision of medical care to protect the patient's welfare when doing so is opposed for economic reasons by trainers or owners?
- Should surplus greyhound racing dogs be used in medical research?
- To what extent are conditions under which circus or amusement park animals housed and trained sufficiently respectful of welfare? Are some kinds of animal performance "acts" injurious to welfare?
- To what extent might certain current practices in the sport of rodeo be insufficiently respectful of welfare?
- Do current regulatory or voluntary procedures sufficiently protect the welfare of racing horses and dogs and show horses?

Wild and Exotic Animal Welfare

- Do welfare considerations argue against the keeping of certain species (for example, reptiles, amphibians, wolves) as pets?
- To what extent do various commercial and environmental practices (for example, discharge of treated or untreated sewage into the ocean, air pollution, deforestation, location of homes or farms in proximity to wildlife areas) affect the welfare of wild air, sea, and land animals?
- To what extent do various recreational practices (for example, motor-boating, whale-watching, human activities at national parks) affect the welfare of wildlife?
- Are current commercial or sport hunting and trapping practices sufficiently respectful of welfare?
- Is it preferable for government authorities to permit hunts of overpopulated groups of wild animals or to allow these animals to compete for limited resources on their own? How should authorities deal with wild animal populations that pose a threat to public health or safety?
- To what extent, if any, do welfare considerations argue against confining wild animals in zoos or aquaria? Is it ever inappropriate to confine certain species merely for human entertainment? What kinds of conditions or facilities are preferable from a welfare standpoint?
- To what extent should farmers, veterinarians, and the public be interested in or concerned about the welfare of fish in aquaculture facilities?
- Is sufficient attention paid to the welfare of surplus zoo animals that are auctioned or sold to private owners?
- When, if ever, should veterinarians treat wild animals that are not members of endangered or threatened species?
- To what extent are certain scientific practices to study wildlife behavior and habitat (for example, implantation of radio transmitters, various kinds of tagging) sufficiently respectful of welfare?
- Should scientists who come across injured or sick wild animals attempt to help them?
- Is it right to attempt to improve the welfare of animals in the wild by improving their environment, protecting them from predators, or treating them for illness or injury?
- In general, should veterinarians, scientists, and members of the public be concerned about the survival and welfare of individual wild animals as opposed to species or groups of animals or indeed of entire ecosystems?

tion should be not whether certain techniques or practices are conducive to welfare, but whether animals ought to be used in experimentation at all. I have attempted to include questions that would be regarded as important by some significant proportion of veterinarians, animal welfare investigators, animal users, and members of the public. I have tried to phrase the questions in a neutral manner, without indicating what answers to the questions might be proper.

～ WELFARE AND RIGHTS REVISITED: THE PRIMACY OF ANIMAL WELFARE

I began this chapter with definitions of animal welfare that contrast welfare with animal rights. We are now in a better position to return to the issue of what relationship there might be between animal welfare and animal rights.

Figure 13-1 illustrates several possible ways of viewing animal welfare and animal rights. Diagram A represents the view that animals have welfare, but no moral rights. Diagram B portrays the position of some animal activists that we should not speak of welfare but only of rights. Diagrams C and D portray both welfare and rights as applicable to animals. The circles are of equal size to indicate that animal welfare and animal rights are considered of equal importance. However, Diagram D represents the view that there is no overlap between animal welfare and rights; according to this position, welfare and rights can coexist but are still inconsistent concepts that cannot apply simultaneously to the same circumstances. In contrast, Diagram C represents the view that welfare and rights sometimes overlap—in the sense that animals can sometimes have a right to certain conditions conducive to their welfare. Diagrams E and F reflect the position that welfare and rights can overlap but are not of equal importance. Diagram E views animal welfare as much more important than rights. According to the position portrayed in Diagram E, animals have a moral few rights, and some of these rights are to conditions conducive to certain aspects of their welfare (such as freedom from pain or hunger). In contrast, Diagram F represents the view that rights are more important than welfare, but allows for the possibility that animals sometimes have rights to certain aspects of welfare.

Other diagrams reflective of other views are possible. One can draw circles representing welfare and moral rights in different relative sizes, and one can represent any overlap between welfare and rights as larger or smaller (to the point of inclusion). One can also draw different diagrams for different kinds of animals or for animals in different kinds of circumstances. For example, one can believe that higher nonhuman primates, such as chimpanzees and gorillas, have more extensive moral rights (and therefore merit a larger circle representing rights) than, say, laboratory mice.

I invite readers to select one of these diagrams, or to draw others that strike them as more representative of the relationship between animal welfare and animal rights. I shall indicate briefly why I think that, in general, the correct view is portrayed in Diagram E, or by another characterization in which welfare and rights intersect but in which welfare is viewed as much more important than moral rights.

As is discussed in Chapter 12, moral rights are very strong but also very limited in scope. Rights are such exceedingly powerful and central claims that they can be overridden infrequently, and then only for the gravest of reasons. To say, for example, that people have a moral and legal right to freedom of speech is to say that they almost always can say what they want, even if it bothers others to hear it. There are limited circumstances in which this right can be tempered or overridden. However, moral claims that are not important or that can be overridden frequently are too weak to be characterized as rights.

If rights are strong, they are also relatively few in number. Rights are a relatively small subset of morality, precisely because they reflect very important interests that are not easily compromised. People in the United States have a moral and legal right to

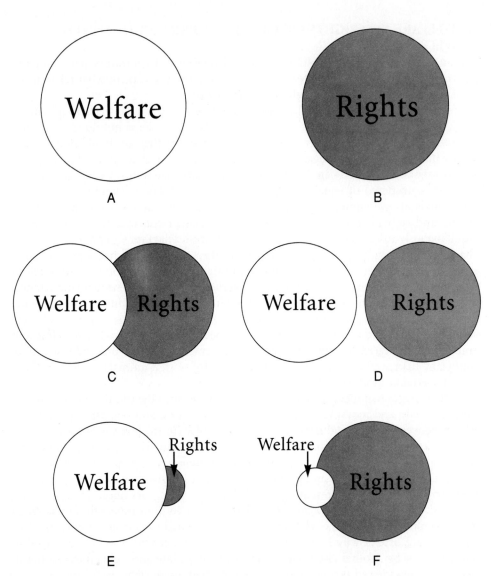

FIGURE 13-1. Some possible views regarding the relationship between animal welfare and animal rights.

own and use private property, to freedom of speech and religion, and to freedom from physical assault by others. We do not, however, have a moral or legal right to respectful and courteous behavior from passers-by, concern about our problems by strangers, or financial help from our neighbors. Such things may be morally admirable, and they may even on occasion be obligatory, but, in general, no one has a moral *right* to any of these and a myriad of other kinds of treatment.

In the animal area too, if moral rights exist, they are limited in scope—because of the nature of rights and because humans have a higher value than animals. If animals have moral rights, among these is the right not to be caused unnecessary or unjustifiable pain. Pain, we all would agree, is a *very serious* harm to animals, and animals are surely entitled not to be subjected to pain in the absence of a *very good* reason. At the same time, the claim of some animal activists that we should speak only of animal rights—that rights exhaust the field of our moral relations with animals—is counterintuitive. There are too many things that are good for animals but that just do not rise to the level of a right. It sounds highly overblown (and quite silly) to say that the family dog has a *right* to spend a few extra minutes on its morning walks to explore some extra territory, or to a certain number of bones or biscuits weekly, or to a game of fetch with its favorite ball each day. Yet, one can say without embarrassment that all these things are conducive to its overall welfare. One can also say that, because these things are conducive to its welfare, one ought to provide them from time to time.

In short, just as human rights have a limited area of application, if animals have rights, so must animal rights have limited scope. In contrast, animal welfare is almost everywhere. Almost anything one can do to animals can affect their welfare. A slightly changed diet, a different exercise regime, a bit more or less companionship, a somewhat larger or smaller enclosure, all such things, and a great many more, can be better or worse for certain animals. This does not mean that we must remain concerned each moment of the day with questions about whether we are providing our animals adequate welfare. Nor does it mean animals are always entitled to conditions that would benefit their welfare. The concept of welfare, unlike the concept of rights, allows for liberal balancing of human against animal interests and for deciding in many circumstances that human interests should prevail.

However, it is not enough just to argue that welfare is more important than rights, in the sense that we will find considerations of welfare in many more ethical situations involving animals than we will find questions of moral rights. As the policy of the World Veterinary Association on animal welfare quoted in Chapter 12 illustrates, welfare and rights sometimes intersect. Sometimes, a condition conducive to or constituent of animal welfare is so important to an animal that we can say the animal's claim to this condition rises to the level of a right. Adequate food and water are critically important to animal welfare. A hungry or thirsty animal can not only feel pain and distress (which are themselves inimical to welfare), but also can suffer physiological damage that might impair its ability to function or even survive. It is therefore not just wrong, but terribly wrong, to deprive an animal one keeps or uses of adequate food and water. One may subject animals to such treatment only for the most important of reasons. Here, those of us who believe that animals have some moral rights would say, is a right based on considerations of welfare.

REFERENCES

[1]Grady AW, Tambrallo L, and others: Animal rights jeopardize animal welfare, *Vet Econ* June 1989:122.

[2]Smith SJ, Hendee WR: Animals in research, *JAMA* 259:2007, 1988.

[3]American Veterinary Medical Association: Policy on Animal Welfare and Animal Rights, *1994 AVMA Directory*, Schaumburg, IL, The Association, p 56.

[4]*See*, for example, Dawkins MS: *Animal Suffering: The Science of Animal Welfare*, London, 1980, Chapman and Hall, pp 3-9; Duncan IJH: Animal rights—animal welfare: A scientist's assessment, *Poult Sci* 60:490, 1980; Fraser AF, Broom DM: *Farm Animal Behaviour and Welfare*, ed 3, London, 1990, Bailliere Tindall, p 4.

[5]*See*, for example, Curtis SE: Animal well-being and animal care, *Vet Clin N Am: Food Anim Pract* 3:373-374, 1987; Duncan IJH: An overall assessment of poultry welfare. In Sorensen LY, editor: *Proceedings of the First Dutch Seminar on Poultry Welfare in Egglaying Cages*, Copenhagen, 1978, National Committee for Poultry and Eggs.

[6]American Veterinary Medical Association: "Positions on Animal Welfare: Guiding Principles," *1994 AVMA Directory*, Schaumburg, IL, The Association, p 56.

[7]Fraser AF, Broom DM: *Farm Animal Behaviour and Welfare*, ed 3, London, 1990, Bailliere Tindall, p 4.

[8]Turner J: *Reckoning with the Beast*, Baltimore, 1980, Johns Hopkins University Press, pp 15-59.

[9]Rowan AN: *Of Mice, Models, and Men*, Albany,1984, State University of New York Press, pp 51-57.

[10]Curtis SE: Animal well-being and animal care, *Vet Clin N Am: Food Anim Pract* 3:377, 1987.

[11]Sainsbury D, Sainsbury P: *Livestock Health and Housing*, London, 1988, Bailliere Tindall, p 248.

[12]Fraser AF, Broom DM: *Farm Animal Behaviour and Welfare*, ed 3, London, 1990, Bailliere Tindall, p 366.

[13]*See*, for example, Wood-Gush DGM: *Elements of Ethology*, London, 1983, Chapman and Hall, p 196 ("All in all, the battery cage as built at present does not provide an environment conducive to the fulfillment of the hen's behavioural repertoire, but that does not mean that satisfactory cages cannot be designed."); Beilharz RG, Zeeb K: Applied ethology and animal welfare, *Appl Anim Ethol* 7:6, 1981 ("If we succeed in showing that animals are suffering under particular conditions of husbandry...there are two approaches. Either (1) we change the animals genetically and adapt them to the environment, or (2) we improve the environment."); Curtis SE: Animal well-being and animal care, *Vet Clin N Am: Food Anim Pract* 3:369, 1987 ("Still, even though well-being cannot be defined precisely, those of us who accept the responsibilities and obligations of caring for animals, particularly animals that are limited by us in their opportunities to care for themselves, must use any and all available knowledge, ways, and means to make our charges as comfortable, calm, and healthy as possible.") Curtis does not appear to be a proponent of the pure science model.

[14]Mill JS: *Utilitarianism*. In Cohen M, editor: *The Philosophy of John Stuart Mill*, New York, 1961, Modern Library, p 333.

[15]Fraser AF, Broom DM: *Farm Animal Behaviour and Welfare*, ed 3, London, 1990, Bailliere Tindall, p 257.

[16]Regan T: *The Case for Animal Rights*, Berkeley, 1983, University of California Press, pp 117-118.

[17]Hughes BO: Behavior as an index of welfare, *Vth Eur Poult Conf* 1976:1005-1014, cited with approval in Wood-Gush DGM: Housing systems and animal welfare research requirements—a review, *Anim Reg Stud* 2:275, 1979/1980.

[18]Lorz A: Tierschutzgesetz. Kommentar. Munich: Verlag C.H. Beck, quoted in Fox: *Farm Animals: Husbandry, Behavior, and Veterinary Practice*, Baltimore, 1984, University Park Press, p 178.

[19]Carpenter E: *Animals and Ethics*, London, 1980, Watkins, quoted in Duncan IJH: Animal rights—animal welfare: A scientist's assessment, *Poult Sci* 60:490, 1980.

[20]Banks EM: Behavioral research to answer questions about animal welfare, *J Anim Sci* 54:435, 1982.

[21]Beilharz RG, Zeeb K: Applied ethology and animal welfare, *Appl Anim Ethol* 7:3, 1981.

[22]Dawkins MS: *Animal Suffering: The Science of Animal Welfare*, London, 1980, Chapman and Hall, p 10.

[23]*Id*, p 25.

[24]Brambell FWR: *Report of the Technical Committee to Enquire into the Welfare of Animals Kept Under Intensive Livestock Husbandry Systems*, London, 1965, HM Stationery Office, Chap 4 par 2.5, cited with approval in Moss R, editor: *Livestock Health and Welfare*, Essex, UK, 1992, Longman Scientific & Technical, p 3.

[25]Simonsen HB: Role of applied ethology in international work on farm animal welfare, *Vet Rec* 111:341, 1982.

[26]Curtis SE: Animal well-being and animal care, *Vet Clin N Am: Food Anim Pract* 3:369-391, 1987.

[27]Fraser AF, Broom DM: *Farm Animal Behaviour and Welfare*, ed 3, London, 1980, Bailliere Tindall, p 256.

[28]*Id*, p 278.

[29]Duncan IJH: Welfare is to do with and what animals feel, *J Agri Environ Ethics* 6(special supplement 2):11, 1993, emphasis in original. Duncan also suggests that, at least in the future, we should attempt to "maximize...the positive feelings" of farm animals (*Id*, p 12), but he does not clearly include experiencing positive feelings in his definition of welfare.

[30]McGlone JJ: What is animal welfare? *J Agric Environ Ethics* 6(special supplement 2):28, 1993, emphasis in original. McGlone also states that "only when animals reach the prepathological state described by Moberg can we say that welfare is poor." *Id*. The prepathological states described by Moberg do not appear to require a *disturbance* of physiological function to the point that survival or reproduction are actually *impaired*. Moberg argues that alteration of biological function is inimical to welfare when "the stress is of such a magnitude that it results in a significant alteration of biological function..., placing the animal at *risk* for pathologies such as disease, abnormal growth, failure to reproduce or aberrant behavior. Moberg GP: Using risk assessment to define domestic animal welfare, *J Agric Environ Ethics* 6(special supplement 2):3, 1993, emphasis supplied.

[31]Moberg GP: Using risk assessment to define domestic animal welfare, *J Agric Environ Ethics* 6(special supplement 2):6, 1993.

[32]*Id*, p 3.

[33]Moberg GP: Using risk assessment to define domestic animal welfare, *J Agric Environ Ethics* 6(special supplement 2):1-2, 1993.

[34]Dawkins MS: Towards an objective method of assessing welfare in domestic fowl, *Appl Anim Ethol* 2:245-254, 1976; Dawkins MS: Do hens suffer in battery cages? *Anim Behav* 25:1034-1046, 1977.

[35]Hughes BO, Black AJ: The preference of domestic hens for different types of battery cage floor, *Br Poult Sci* 14:615-619, 1973.

[36]Baldwin BA, Meese GB: Sensory reinforcement and illumination preference in the domesticated pig, *Anim Behav* 25:497, 1977.

[37]Fraser AF, Broom DM: *Farm Animal Behaviour and Welfare*, ed 3, London, 1990, Bailliere Tindall, p 365.

[38]Dawkins MS: *Animal Suffering: The Science of Animal Welfare*, London, 1980, Chapman & Hall, pp 89-90.

[39]*Id*, p 10.

[40]*Id*, pp 94-95; *See also* Duncan IJH: The interpretation of preference tests in animal behavior, *Appl Anim Ethol* 4:197-200, 1978.

[41]Regan T: *The Case for Animal Rights*, Berkeley, 1983, University of California Press, p 357.

[42]Goodall J: *Through a Window: My Thirty Years with the Chimpanzees of Gombe*, Boston, 1990, Houghton Mifflin.

[43]Fox MW: Letter. A call for common understanding of animal welfare, animal rights, and animal well being, *J Am Vet Med Assoc* 196:832-833, 1990.

[44]Rollin BE: The concept of illness in veterinary medicine, *J Am Vet Med Assoc* 182:122-125, 1983. Indeed, as Rollin argues, one reason animal welfare is not value free is that typically welfare consists, at least in part, of the absence of disease or illness. Rollin BE: Animal welfare, science, and value, *J Agric Environ Ethics* 6 (special supplement 2):44-50, 1993.

[45]*See*, for example, Fox MW: *Farm Animals: Husbandry, Behavior, and Veterinary Practice*, Baltimore, 1984, University Park Press, 1984.

[46]Witttgenstein L: *Philosophical Investigations*, ed 3, New York, 1958, Macmillan, sections 66-85, pp 31-40.

[47]Duncan and Dawkins appear to speak for a majority of their colleagues when they claim that that "the *first* and biggest problem is one of definition" of welfare. Duncan IJH, Dawkins MS: The problem of assessing 'well-being' and 'suffering' in farm animals. In Smidt D, editor: *Indicators Relevant to Animal Welfare*, The Hague, 1983, Martinus Nijhoff, p 14. Duncan himself rejects health, lack of stress, or fitness as components of welfare on the grounds that "neither health nor lack of stress nor fitness is necessary and/or sufficient to conclude that an animal has good welfare." Duncan IJH: Welfare is to do with and what animals feel, *J Agric Environ Ethics* 6(special supplement 2):12, 1993. Duncan argues that feeling good is a necessary and sufficient condition for welfare. However, it seems incorrect to say that a racehorse with an underlying injury that is about to cause its leg to snap is in a satisfactory state of welfare seconds before disaster strikes because a pain-killing drug is making it *feel* good. The search for necessary or sufficient conditions for application of the term "welfare" seems doomed to failure.

[48]For example, as McGlone points out, the pain associated with parturition should not be considered a negation of welfare because it does not reflect an undesirable physiological state. McGlone JJ: What is animal welfare? *J Agric Environ Ethics* 6(special supplement 2):31, 1993. Likewise, pain, stress, distress, and a wide range of negative experiences can assist animals to survive and therefore in certain contexts should not be regarded as inimical to welfare.

[49]Duncan IJH: Welfare is to do with and what animals feel, *J Agric Environ Ethics* 6(special supplement 2):12, 1993.

[50]*Id*, p 11.

CHAPTER 14

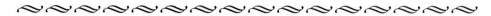

The Interests of Veterinary Clients

Clients also have interests that must be taken into account in determining how veterinarians ought to act. This chapter identifies some of these interests and demonstrates why they are entitled to great respect. The general principles developed here are applied in subsequent discussions of specific issues involving clients.

～ THE INTEREST OF ANIMAL OWNERS IN ACCESSIBLE, AFFORDABLE, AND COMPETENT VETERINARY SERVICES

Animal owners certainly have a legitimate interest in having available to them accessible, affordable, and competent veterinary services. Although obvious, these interests are far from trivial. As we shall see, they can play an enormous role in the determination of how veterinarians ought to act—sometimes by supporting, and sometimes by running contrary to, what veterinarians perceive to be in their best interests.

～ THE STATUS OF CLIENTS AS PURCHASERS OF VETERINARY SERVICES

Like other kinds of people, veterinary clients possess many legitimate interests. They may have an interest in furthering their careers, in earning a decent salary, in enjoying a happy life, and so on. Clients often seek veterinary services to promote some of these interests.

The most important reason clients are entitled to have certain of their interests respected by a veterinarian is not that clients have these interests, but that clients pay veterinarians for the specific purpose of furthering one or more of these interests. If one had to justify why a veterinarian ought, for example, to be honest with a farmer about the condition of his animals and ought to work diligently in the client's behalf, one would not begin by pointing out that farmers are entitled to make a living. Rather, we would say that the client deserves these things from his veterinarian because he is *paying* for them.

There are three major reasons paying for veterinary services entitles clients to have certain interests respected. First, the veterinarian who provides services to a client has made an agreement to serve the client. An agreement to provide veterinary services is a promise, and like other promises, it ought to be kept. Second, we believe that someone who pays for a service is entitled to his money's worth. Third, clients place reliance on their veterinarians and arrange their lives or business affairs accordingly. It is a fundamental principle of morality that if one person relies on another to do something, and the other agrees to let the first rely on him, the second person has an obligation not to let the first person down. If I have planned my day relying on your promise that you will pick me up in your car at a certain time, and you deliberately leave me in the lurch, you have done me a wrong in permitting me to act in reliance on your promise.

Likewise, the client who places his animal in the care of a veterinarian relies on her to do any of a number of things, and is likely to build part of his personal or economic affairs around this reliance.

From these three foundations of the obligations of veterinarians to paying clients, one can derive several general interests that are possessed by paying clients and that are entitled to great weight.

Honesty

Because a client pays for a veterinarian's services, a client has a strong interest in honesty from the doctor. Honesty from the doctor about what she will do is required for the client to be able to decide whether and under what conditions to retain the doctor's services. Honesty from the doctor about what she has done or failed to do is essential to enable the client to determine whether the doctor has fulfilled her agreements and kept her promises. As an employer of veterinary services, the client must also receive information that will enable him to determine how his animal is doing and whether he is spending his money wisely. Such information will be useless, and may even be harmful, to the client if it is not truthful.

Honesty is more than not telling a lie or telling the truth when a client specifically requests some information. Failing to inform a client about some condition or event about which he does not or could not know can also be dishonest. The following practices are all dishonest: charging a client for services not actually rendered, exaggerating the seriousness of an animal's condition to gain the client's business, recommending unnecessary procedures, and signing a health or inspection certificate without having examined the client's animal.

Loyalty and Protection of Confidences

Because a client hires a veterinarian to serve the client's interests, the client must be able to rely on the veterinarian's loyalty, his steadfast devotion to the client's interests and his unwillingness to compromise or undermine those interests. This does not mean a practitioner can never serve two competing clients. But it does mean that he cannot be a responsible party in determining which such client succeeds. He must, that is, either leave the competition to the clients or decline to serve one of them. For example, although an equine doctor may sometimes attend race horses of competing owners, he ought never to reveal anything about one owner's animal to another or do anything that would put one of them at a disadvantage.

A client has more than an interest in his veterinarian's loyalty to him as opposed to other clients or members of the public. Because a client engages a practitioner with the understanding that the doctor is serving his interests, the client has an interest in loyalty to him as opposed to the practitioner's own interests. This does not preclude the doctor from profiting from a professional relationship, but this profit must flow from the primary consideration of serving the client. A doctor who recommends an unnecessary procedure to increase his fee, or who refers a client to another doctor and accepts a rebate or commission from that practitioner, is committing an act of disloyalty to the client.

One way of assuring loyalty to clients is to keep confidential information received in one's professional attendance upon their animals. Such "information" includes not just statements made by a client or any of his employees or agents but also medical data gathered through diagnosis and therapy, as well as one's professional conclusions regarding such information.

Reasonable Fees and Payment Arrangements

The law gives veterinarians great leeway in determining what fees to charge and how to require payment of them. Indeed, provided a client agrees, and the fee is not so outrageous or overbearing as to be unconscionable, a veterinarian can obtain any fee arrangement from a client that she can get. However, as a purchaser of services entitled to his money's worth, a client has an interest in being charged a fee that is reasonable in the sense in which it truly reflects the amount of time, skill, materials, and training involved in the services actually provided. This does not mean that some products or services cannot be marked up so as to bear the necessary and reasonable costs of the entire practice—although there is, surely, a line between a legitimate mark-up and unconscionable gouging. Nevertheless, charges ought to bear some relationship to the services provided.

Clients also have a legitimate interest in obtaining payment arrangements that permit them to purchase services they can afford. Veterinarians are not charities. However, they are providers of services in an economy that is accustomed to permitting consumers to pay in installments, especially when large amounts are involved. Where a client's payment record is unreliable or incapable of verification, or where a practitioner's cash flow situation is precarious, a client's moral claim to flexibility regarding payments may rightly be overridden in favor of the doctor's legitimate needs. However, veterinarians should at least attempt to play by the rules that apply to the consumer economy generally and that make this economy possible. Just as a veterinarian would expect her car dealer or furniture store to structure their financial houses so as to permit flexible payment arrangements for her, so must she understand a client's interest in being able to make similar arrangements with a veterinarian.

∿ THE SIGNIFICANCE OF FREE OR REDUCED-COST SERVICES

A client's agreement to pay money to a veterinarian for professional services is an act of great ethical significance that invests the client with weighty interests and moral (as well as legal) rights. As a profession, veterinary medicine is not as heavily engaged in providing gratuitous services to the needy as is law or medicine. Nevertheless, as we shall see, a strong case can sometimes be made for such services, at least as a moral ideal if not an obligation. Moreover, some veterinarians do reduce fees for certain clients with financial problems. It is therefore important to understand that legitimate client interests do not derive solely from payment for veterinary services.

The law permits veterinarians to offer less extensive services for clients who do not pay or who pay reduced fees, if such clients understand that this is what they are receiving. However, once practitioners agree to provide any service, the law holds them to the same standards of competence regarding that service whether they charge their full customary fee, a reduced fee, or no fee at all. In general, someone who pays little or nothing has just as much right to sue a veterinarian for malpractice as a fully paying client.

Just as the law does not lower its standards for those who receive gratuitous or low-cost services, neither does morality, and for the same reasons. Such clients still rely upon an agreement by the doctor to provide veterinary services. They too require honest information to be able to make appropriate medical decisions for their animals. The doctor serves them and their interests no less than he serves the paying client, and they have no less need for his loyalty. Like other animal owners they too have an interest, as shall now be discussed, in trustworthiness and respectful treatment from the doctor because they too are animal owners and can have a great deal invested in the patient they bring to the veterinary office.

～ THE STATUS OF CLIENTS AS ANIMAL OWNERS

Clients' interests derive not just from the fact that they pay for or receive a veterinarian's services. Veterinary clients are not just consumers but are animal owners who entrust a particular *kind* of property to the care of their veterinarians. Typically, animals for whom veterinary services are sought are of significant emotional importance or economic value to clients. This fact affects profoundly the nature and weight of clients' interests.

The economic or emotional value of the animal strengthens and colors interests that can derive from the status of the client as a purchaser of the veterinarian's services. Although all consumers need honesty from merchants, for veterinary clients honesty can be especially important because an incorrect decision can result in economic or emotional disaster. Although all consumers have an interest in reasonable fees and payment arrangements, this interest can be enormously important when one is dealing with a living being in which the client can invest so much of himself. It is one thing to be denied the services of a television repairman because he insists on his entire fee up front, but quite another to lose forever a beloved companion because a veterinarian will not permit installment payments.

There are also several interests of veterinary clients that are better viewed as flowing not primarily from their status as purchasers of services but from their status as recipients of medical services for animals.

Trustworthiness

Although related to honesty, trustworthiness is a different concept. Trustworthiness goes beyond telling the truth. It includes carrying out a client's wishes and respecting her sensibilities. Today, when so many veterinary clients have treasured pets and economically valuable animals, trustworthiness is a central interest clients have in their veterinarians. Indeed, trustworthiness may well be more important in veterinary medicine than it is in human medicine or in any other profession. When people believe they have been wronged by a physician or lawyer they are usually able to complain about it and seek redress. Animals have no such ability. Barring some physical evidence of mistreatment, or statement by the veterinarian or a member of her staff admitting wrongdoing, a client must often rely solely on the veterinarian's trustworthiness to assure that competent and caring services are provided. The client may never know that his dog was hit to keep it quiet, that its water bowl was kept empty because of an employee's laziness, that a necropsy was performed on his animal without his permission, or that the body of another animal was substituted for that of his own for burial. Such things, however, are fundamental violations of the trust that clients place in their veterinarians.

Courtesy, Caring, and Respect

All consumers are entitled to be treated with at least a minimum amount of civility and courtesy; they deserve this much in return for their money. But because animals can be so important to veterinary clients, clients have interests in special kinds of courteous and decent treatment. These interests can, of course, vary greatly from one kind of client to another. A dairy farmer with a cow that must be killed, might not want from his veterinarian the kind of emotional solace that might be expected by a client who must contemplate the euthanasia of a beloved pet. The farmer, on the other hand, may expect sincere respect for his economic needs and an appreciation of the seriousness of a decision to put down one of his animals.

It would be impossible to list all the kinds of courteous, caring, and respectful treatment in which veterinary clients have an interest. Subsequent chapters discuss some of them in detail. I do, however, want to list some of the kinds of treatment veterinary clients and my veterinary students tell me they find most disrespectful in veterinarians. Some of these complaints may sometimes be unjustified when one takes into consideration not just the client's interest in decent treatment but also a veterinarian's interest in maintaining a competent and profitable practice. Nevertheless, these complaints are illustrative of what clients mean when they say—correctly—that they deserve to be treated with courtesy, care, and respect.

- Waiting two or three weeks for an appointment, and then having to sit for an hour before seeing the doctor, without receiving an apology or explanation for the delay
- Calling the doctor at lunch break or other times when the practice is in fact staffed and being greeted with a tape recording that makes it impossible to speak with someone
- Being urged to make important decisions quickly so that the doctor can proceed to the next appointment
- Seeing the doctor look repeatedly at her watch during an appointment
- Not having a private area away from the examining room to sit down with the doctor or family members so that important decisions can be made rationally and with dignity
- Not receiving a telephone call from the doctor reporting on the status of one's animal after a major procedure
- Not having one's telephone calls returned
- Being told that one's valued pet is only an animal, is getting old anyway, or is not worth the amount of money required to save it
- Being asked to state on an estimate or consent form the monetary value of one's animal
- Being repeatedly interrupted or ignored by the doctor during an examination of one's animal
- Receiving an impatient or rude response after expressing inability to understand the gravity or nature of the condition of one's animal
- Having the doctor dismiss as inappropriate, or leave the room at the first sign of, one's distress or grief
- Being served by a doctor or employee in dirty or disheveled attire

Treatment As an Intelligent and Autonomous Adult Entitled to Make One's Own Decisions

There is a specific kind of respect which clients have an interest in receiving from a veterinarian that derives from their status as owners of veterinary patients—respect in the sense of being treated as intelligent adults who are capable of making, and are entitled to make, their own decisions concerning veterinary care.

The animal as the client's property

Although some people object to this fact, it is nevertheless a fact of western legal systems and cultures that animals are considered property. One might attempt to argue for a client's interest in being able to make her own decisions about her animal by appealing to a general moral right of people to own animals. Such an argument is not necessary for our purposes here. A more immediate justification for permitting the client to make the decisions about her animal's veterinary care is that when client and veterinarian enter a professional relationship, they *accept* the fact that the animal is the client's property. Moreover, it is not part of the typical express or implied agreement between veterinarian and client that the veterinarian shall decide what is to be done with the client's property. Quite the contrary, both doctor and client usually understand (even if they do not state this understanding explicitly) that the doctor is working for the client, who retains the right to decide what services will be provided. Simply in virtue of having made such an agreement, the doctor is under an obligation to keep it.

"Informed consent"

Clearly, clients cannot make their own decisions about what will be done with their animals unless they are (1) permitted to do so without external pressure or influence and (2) given all the information they would reasonably need to make a decision. These requirements are stated simply but can place significant burdens on veterinarians. Pressure can be overt, but it can also be quite subtle. For example, the order in which a doctor states the alternatives to a client and the words she uses to state them can themselves push the client to make a decision that in fact is more the doctor's decision than the client's. Nor is it always easy to convey to clients the information they need. Some clients are less sophisticated than others and may require a lengthy or repeated explanation that can try the veterinarian's patience.

The law uses the term "informed consent" to describe the kind of decision a client must be permitted to make. It is a form of negligence for a veterinarian not to obtain from a client, before doing a procedure, the client's informed consent to that procedure. Unfortunately, the legal notion of informed consent does not afford complete guidance in characterizing the moral interests veterinary clients have in obtaining information and making their own decision.

First, although veterinarians clearly are legally obligated to obtain informed consents, it is not altogether clear what "informed consent" means in veterinary law. It is difficult to find court decisions that consider how much veterinary clients must be told and how much they must understand to exercise an informed consent. The legal concept of informed consent has been developed within the context of human medicine and dentistry and turns in large measure upon people's legal right to decide what shall be done with their bodies. Both in law and ethics, a person's own body is a sacrosanct matter, something not to be trifled with lightly by a physician or by anyone else. In contrast, the legal right of veterinary clients to exercise an informed consent derives not from their authority over their bodies, but from their authority over personal property. It may therefore be impossible to assume that everything courts or legislatures in a given jurisdiction require for informed consent in the medical context would be required in veterinary cases as well.

A second reason students of veterinary ethics may not find it very useful to speak about "informed consent" in the legal sense is that, even in the medical context, there are different definitions of the concept. One would think, as several courts did in the early 1970s,[1] that to make a truly informed consent, a medical patient must be given all the information a reasonable person in his circumstances would find necessary to make a decision. In recent years, however, the courts or legislatures of a number of states have decided that to make an informed consent, a patient must be given the information that an ordinarily competent and prudent physician would want to give the patient— even if a reasonable patient would want to know more. In these jurisdictions, it might follow that if most veterinarians believe that clients should be given information in a way that steers them toward a certain kind of decision, steering them toward that decision instead of letting them make up their own minds would meet the legal requirements for obtaining an informed consent.

"Informed consent" can be a useful term for normative veterinary ethics provided it is not restricted to its usual legal sense (or senses).

The owner's relations with the animal as a source of entitlement to the right to make an informed consent

The veterinarian's acceptance of a client's ownership of the patient is itself an important foundation of the client's interest in making his own informed decision about his animal. However, there is often another foundation—the fact that the animal is not just any kind of property but is something in which the owner has invested significant time, effort, money, or emotion. A farmer or horse breeder, for example, who has spent a good deal of money making an animal a part of his business operations has a very strong interest in seeing that his investment has its intended results. Such a client's commitment of time and money entitles him to decide how to handle his affairs with his animals, even if his veterinarian thinks she can help the client by pressuring him to make some other kind of decision. It is no less presumptuous, and wrong, for a veterinarian to push such a client's decisions in a certain direction than it would be for a banker to withdraw a depositor's money without authorization and use it in ways the banker thinks would benefit the depositor.

Regarding animals with whom clients have an emotional bond, there are different reasons arguing against intermeddling by a veterinarian.

First, veterinarians are not experts in human psychology. Nor would the few minutes they usually spend with clients enable even a psychologist to know very much about a client or his family and the precise nature of their relationship with their animal. The veterinarian may know more about the medical condition and prognosis of such an animal, and she may know a great deal about how she would feel if faced with the alternatives before the client. But although the doctor's technical knowledge should enable her to direct the client's attention to matters the client might not think of on his own, the doctor cannot presume to be able to judge for the client precisely what impact on a client's life these alternatives may have.

Second, even if veterinarians could ever know better than a client emotionally attached to an animal what is in the client's best interests, in the overwhelming majority of cases and therefore as a general rule, the client is still entitled to make his own decision. The client has undertaken the care of the animal, he has made the personal and financial sacrifices, he has arranged his life and that of his family around the life of his animal. Having made these commitments and decisions, he is entitled to decide, without subtle psychological pressure from a stranger who will not have to live with the decision, how his life and that of his family will proceed in the future.

An animal and human with a significant emotional attachment and reliance upon each other have a special relationship in which others, including a veterinarian, do not participate. My late Yorkie trusted me to throw him into the air in play but did not permit strangers do so. When he barked to me and not others for his dinner or walk, he understood we had a relationship he did not have with others. Perhaps it would be inappropriate to say that he "entrusted" me with his care (although I am not at all sure this is an inaccurate way of characterizing the matter) and that this gave me, and not our veterinarian, a special claim to make decisions concerning both of us. It is surely appropriate to say that my dog and I established a pattern of exclusive interaction that not only made it likely that I would want to do what was in his interests—but that *entitled* me to judge, for both of us, how matters of health or illness would affect the relationship.

This remarkable intermingling of the interests of animal and client brings us to the human-companion animal bond. The nature of this bond and its potential impact on normative veterinary ethics is the subject of Chapter 15.

REFERENCE

[1] *See*, for example, *Canterbury* v. *Spence*, 464 F.2d 772 (D.C. Cir. 1972).

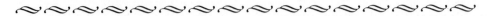

The Human-Companion Animal Bond

*T*he human-companion animal bond is gaining increasing prominence in the
veterinary world. "The bond" seems to be everywhere—in scholarly publications describing its value for promoting human health, in AVMA policy statements, in
practice management discussions touting its value for maximizing revenues, in advertisements appealing to the bond as an incentive for animal owners to buy pet products.

The concept of "the human-companion animal bond" can serve as an important
tool in ethical analysis. Unfortunately, it is showing signs of becoming little more than
a soothing, empty cliché.

∼ WHAT IS THE HUMAN-COMPANION ANIMAL BOND?

As I understand the phrase, the "human-companion animal bond" refers to a relationship between a human and an animal which has at least the following characteristics:

The relationship cannot be sporadic or accidental but must be continuous and
ongoing. We would hardly speak of a "bond," (as opposed, say, to an interaction)
between two beings unless they related to each other with some degree of frequency.

The relationship must also derive not just to a benefit, but to a significant benefit,
of both parties, and the relationship must benefit a central aspect of the lives of each. If
you and I alternate driving each other to work, our relationship is just too trivial to
describe as a "bond." If, however, we invest our life savings together in a business and
work long and hard at it, that begins to look very much like a bond.

To be a "bond," a relationship must also in some sense be voluntary. Prison cell-
mates who are thrown together for life do not thereby necessarily establish a bond.
Persons who choose to relate to each other can.

A bond must be bidirectional, with each party to the bond offering its attention to
the other. I can be extremely devoted to someone, showering that person with attention
and benefits. But if this attention is not returned, there is, as any unrequited lover
knows, no bond.

Insofar as is possible, each party to a true bond must treat the other not as a means
toward its own ends, but as something entitled to respect and benefit in its own right.
The antebellum slave owner certainly had a strong, continuous, significant relationship
with his slaves. However, this was not a bond, but bondage, because the relationship
was almost entirely one-sided and was severely detrimental to one of the parties.
Respect and benefit, however, are not sufficient. Churchill and Stalin had great respect
for each other. They also saw themselves and their nations as entitled in their own right

and for their own benefit to victory over the Nazis. But one would hardly describe their relationship as a "bond" because they distrusted and hated each other. A true bond requires at the very least something akin to admiration, trust and genuine good feeling of each party toward the other. Often, a bond involves love.

So, as I understand the phrase, a "human-companion animal bond" means at the very least a *continuous, bidirectional relationship between a human and an animal, which brings a significant benefit to a central aspect of the lives of each, which is in some sense voluntary, and in which each party treats the other not just as something entitled to respect and benefit in its own right but also as an object of admiration, trust, devotion, or love.*

Admittedly, one may be using some of these terms somewhat loosely in applying them to animals. For example, a family dog does not "voluntarily" enter the relationship in quite the same way as does its family. However, there is a sense in which we would say that a dog which must be tied down to prevent its running away, and which greets or interacts with its owner only when threatened with punishment or offered a treat, is not a member of a bond, precisely because it does not want to interact with its owner.

My definition reflects what we speakers of the English language generally mean when we talk about a "bond." It also leaves open, as I believe a useful definition of the human-companion animal bond must, questions regarding precisely what animals can be included. Some people seem inclined to restrict candidates for the animal side of the bond to dogs, cats, and caged birds. But it seems clear that other kinds of animals, such as some horses, ferrets, or rodents, can also qualify. The definition also allows for the possibility of stronger and weaker bonds between humans or animals. Nevertheless, as I have suggested, there will be a point at which a human-animal relationship simply becomes too trivial, or manipulative, to be called a "bond." It will also sometimes be appropriate to speak of human-animal "companionship" that is more significant than mere human-animal "interaction" but that still does not constitute a bond.

⁓ TRIVIALIZATION OF THE BOND

There are already signs that the concept of the human-companion animal bond will not become a useful tool in ethical discussion.

First, the phrase "human-companion animal bond" appears to be turning into a synonym for "owning or interacting in some way with any kind of pet." The phrase thus seems to denote the entire gamut of human-pet interactions. For example, small animal practitioner Dr. E. Garcia distinguishes several different attitudes towards pets, ranging from the most devoted to the almost entirely disinterested. He then proclaims that "regardless of the type of pet owner, there is some degree of bond between most owners and their pets that seems to transcend all others...[T]he bond between the pet and the owner, whatever it may be, has always been there, even as far back as our ancient ancestors."[1] The AVMA Committee on the Human/Animal Bond also equated "the bond" with pet ownership. It called for research about "the human/animal bond, especially patterns of pet ownership, motives for keeping pets, functions pets serve, and the nature of the physical interaction with pets." Having identified "the bond" with pet ownership, the Committee had no problem sweeping under this concept almost all human-pet interactions, including those involving "children of all ages" and apparently even owners who "view their pets as a nuisance and are unhappy with their pets' presence in the household."[2]

There are surely important ethical aspects and implications of many different kinds of human-animal interaction. The problem with equating the human-animal bond with pet ownership, however, is that it can draw one's attention away from human-animal interactions that are legitimately described as a bond and that have distinctive ethical features.

For example, if, as studies indicate,[3] people are soothed by touching a dog from time to time, or looking at fish in an aquarium or a bird in a cage, interesting ethical issues arise. A strong argument can be made that institutions which care for the ill or elderly ought to provide such animal contacts and should engage the services of a veterinarian to keep the animals healthy. However, there are important differences between these relatively casual human-animal interactions and those legitimately termed a bond. If someone is responding solely to the sight of a bird or dog, it would be difficult to argue that an institution entrusted with his care is obligated to spend a great deal of money on veterinary care for a very sick animal he happens to be looking at, if another animal could be substituted at much less cost. On the other hand, if the same person is permitted to keep for himself and comes to love a particular animal, it might be cruel and immoral to suggest to him that because veterinary care would entail some expense, his pet must be replaced with "another just like it." Likewise, it would be unfair to such a person and his devoted pet to take the animal away from him so that it can be passed around more casually to soothe the stresses of others. On the other hand, impressing an abandoned pound animal into this kind of service seems far less objectionable and indeed, could be a positive benefit to such an animal by assuring its continued life and some measure of human contact.

～ A ONE-SIDED "BOND?"

There is a second feature of much current thinking about the human-companion animal bond that may prevent it from achieving its rightful role in ethical deliberation. Most people who are studying the bond appear far more interested in its human side, and in promoting the interests of its human participants than in asking hard questions about what interests the bond might give to animals.

For example, Dr. Garcia remarks that appreciation of the bond "instilled in me the importance of my place in society—taking care of pets for people...[A]t no time in my practice life have I felt more an important element of society as far as contributing to people's happiness...If you look at yourself as a professional person who really does have a part in increasing the quality and happiness in people's lives, this should give you a warm feeling inside, and you have every reason to be proud."[1] An even more striking emphasis on people is found in the characterization of the bond offered by the 1988 Pew Report on *Future Directions for Veterinary Medicine*:

> The basis for the positive effect of health and well-being resulting from interactions with a pet has come to be known as the companion animal bond or the human/companion animal bond. It is based upon a biologically based set of actions called attachment behavior. As [a human] infant develops, it associates the nourishment, softness, and warmth provided by its mother with love and security. This contact releases endorphins which alleviate anxiety through their effect on the opiate receptors in the brain and forms the basis for social attachment, in this case between mother and infant. Attachment can occur between human beings, between humans and animals and even between a person and an inanimate object such as a security blanket. Endorphin-mod-

ulated good feelings are derived from interactions with an animal pet. The distinguished psychologist-psychoanalyst and pioneer researcher in animal/human relationships, Dr. Bernard Levinson, summed it up succinctly: "Love is the priceless ingredient with which our pets enrich our lives."[4]

This statement *defines* the human-companion animal bond as the basis for positive health and psychological effects on *people*. Its apparent interest in the bond solely as a tool to help people underscores the fact that the human animal bond—if it is a true *bond*—is a two-sided relationship. The bond is much more than a mechanism for releasing human endorphins or an animate alternative to a security blanket.

There is emerging a body of work studying the benefits animals can bring to the mentally ill, the retarded, the physically disabled, and the incarcerated.[5] However, it is difficult to find in such studies mention of what these contacts do to the animals.[6] It is difficult to find a concern about their needs or interests, and an appreciation that they are beings that count for something in their own right and are not just tools for making people healthy or happy.* The conclusion of one famous report on the use of dogs in a psychiatric hospital speaks volumes about the focus of most current research into the human-animal bond. Pet-facilitated therapy, this study determined, introduces "a non-threatening loving pet to serve as a catalytic vehicle for forming adaptive and satisfying [human] social interactions."[7] A discussion of the role of companion animals in childhood development speaks about pets as a "developmental asset" and the "pet-owner bond" as "optimally a flexible affiliation."[8] Another paper considers the "pet as an anxiolitic intervention," that is, as a means for reducing the anxiety of people.[9] A recent critique of the entire field of human-animal interaction studies proposes a new "unified theory base that allows evaluation of the impact and process of the human-animal interaction in a wide variety of samples."[10] This paper suggests that the concept of "quality of life" be utilized to measure "the potential benefit of the human-animal interaction."[11] However, the discussion makes no mention of how one might characterize and measure the effects of human-animal interaction on *animals*. The discussion restricts its conceptual analysis (supposedly of all scientific study of human-animal relations) to characterizing and measuring the effects of human-animal interaction on the quality of *peoples'* lives.

No one should dismiss the value of the human-animal bond in the promotion of human health and well-being. Nevertheless, it is inappropriate to speak of one member of a bond as "serving" as a "catalytic vehicle" or "developmental asset" for promoting the interests of the other. In a true human-animal bond, the animal must be seen in large measure as entitled to care and concern in its own right, not as a tool or vehicle.

Perhaps the concentration on the human side of the bond by researchers is a temporary, pragmatic approach aimed at obtaining the respect of scientists and veterinarians before greater attention is paid to the animals. However, as monkeys begin to serve as the arms and legs of quadriplegics, or cats and dogs are shuttled in and out of nursing homes to be petted by residents, or animals are placed in jails to relax or rehabili-

---

*This criticism cannot be made of the veterinarian founder of the human-animal bond movement, Dr. Leo Bustad. Bustad's interest in human-animal interaction began with a concern for animals. His devotion to both sides of the human-animal bond has gained him a place among the great figures in the history of veterinary medicine.

tate hardened felons, at some point, I suggest, one must ask whether all of this is fair to the animals.

It may not be clear how much we may morally do to animals in the service of human health and happiness. However, students of the human-companion animal bond must take this question seriously. They must take more seriously the task of understanding the effects of the bond on animals. Otherwise, "the human-companion animal bond" may become just another way of describing animals merely as objects for the use and enjoyment of people. This is a view of animals that many participants in true human-animal bonds find unacceptable.

～ SOME HARD QUESTIONS

Being a member of a human-animal bond, as this relationship is best understood, can create conflicts between animal owner and animal, as well as between both of these and others, including veterinarians and government. The following are among the hard questions raised by the bond that reflect some of these potential conflicts.

IS COMPANION ANIMAL OWNERSHIP SOMETIMES A MORAL RIGHT, WHICH CAN BE ABRIDGED, IF AT ALL, ONLY IN THE MOST EXTREME KINDS OF CIRCUMSTANCES? Thus far our society has treated ownership of companion animals not as a necessity of life but as a luxury. This is in part why the law believes it can require that pets be licensed, can place significant restrictions on their ownership, or under certain circumstances, can prohibit their ownership entirely. On the other hand, having children is not considered a luxury, but a fundamental right most adults are thought to have. To be sure, this right is sometimes overridden, as when the state takes a child away from its natural parents to protect it from abuse or neglect. But such intervention is, we believe, appropriate only in the most extreme kinds of circumstances, precisely because child-rearing is generally considered a fundamental aspect of life.

Now if for some people pets are every bit as important in the most central aspects of their lives as children, we must at least ask whether for such people having a companion animal is a moral, and should be a legal, right (at least in the sense that people should not be prohibited from having a pet if they want and can care responsibly for one). Should we make it difficult for such people to have pets, by charging them license fees they might be unable to afford, or by excluding pets from publicly supported or private housing? To what extent may we regulate how many, or what kinds, of pets can be possessed by participants in a human-companion animal bond? Are some common restrictions on pets and pet behavior unfair? For example, I must endure the racket caused by my neighbor's four children, because people have a right to have as many children as they want and because four children will in the nature of things make a lot of noise. Is it therefore not fair to expect my neighbor to accept without complaint the vociferous barking of my dog—because of his importance to me and the fact that such an animal will in the nature of things make some noise?

DO ANIMALS THAT CAN PARTICIPATE IN, OR HAVE PARTICIPATED IN, A HUMAN-ANIMAL BOND SOME-TIMES HAVE STRONG MORAL CLAIMS THAT CAN MAKE IT WRONG FOR THEIR OWNERS OR OTHER PEOPLE TO DO CERTAIN THINGS TO THEM, SUCH AS CONTINUING TO OWN OR MISTREAT THEM, EXPERIMENTING ON, OR EUTHANIZING THEM? Recently, several states abolished so-called "pound seizure" laws, which permit or require public pounds to release abandoned pets to research facilities (see Chapter 24). One of the arguments advanced by opponents of the use of pound animals in research is that because these animals once related to humans in a special way not experienced by purpose-bred animals, it is wrong to expose them to experimentation. According to this argument, once an animal is part of a human-companion animal bond, it is unfair to treat it as a research tool; it must live, if at all, the kind of role to which it has become accustomed and to which it is therefore entitled.

Whatever one thinks of this particular argument, it is difficult to dispute the general principle that animals which are members of a human-companion animal bond come to have certain moral claims in virtue of their having been in such a relationship. For example, it is wrong to neglect the adult dog that one showered with affection during its puppyhood, in part because the dog was permitted, indeed encouraged, to share in the joys of human companionship and affection. It is wrong to neglect the veterinary needs of one's loyal and faithful pet, in part because it has been loyal and faithful and thus deserves something in return.

The importance of the interests and moral claims of the animal party to the human-animal bond raises serious issues for veterinarians. To what extent should doctors act as advocates of the interests of patients, even if this means disagreeing with the wishes of clients? Should the profession rethink its attitude toward euthanasia—which is sometimes offered not just to clients whose animals are suffering painful terminal illness but also to people tired of their animals or inconvenienced by their behavioral problems? To ask such questions, one need not be a member of the animal rights movement or assert that humans and animals are of equal value. However, it seems to me that one cannot believe in the existence of a significant human-companion animal *bond* without believing that the animal members of such bonds have some significant moral rights (see Chapter 12).

TO WHAT EXTENT SHOULD THE LEGAL SYSTEM PROTECT THE INTERESTS OF ANIMAL MEMBERS OF HUMAN-COMPANION ANIMAL BONDS? Some have argued that the moral claims of companion animals cannot receive adequate protection unless such claims are given the force of law. Therefore, it is stated, we should test and license pet owners, prevent unworthy owners from keeping animals, and give animals legal "standing" so that their owners and veterinarians can be sued in their behalf.[12] A strong argument can be made that these measures would constitute too great an intrusion by government into peoples' private lives and would make pet ownership so expensive and aggravating to animal owners and veterinarians that they would deprive many people and animals of the advantages of the human-animal bond.[13] However, once one recognizes that at least some companion animals have strong interests that are not always respected, the question of whether and to what extent the law should be invoked to protect these interests is certainly a legitimate one, however we may ultimately come to answer it.

SHOULD VETERINARIANS PAY MORE SERIOUS ATTENTION TO BEHAVIORAL PROBLEMS OF COMPANION ANIMALS AND THEIR OWNERS? Human-companion animal bonds do not always go smoothly. Animals and their owners sometimes have behavioral problems, and not always, it seems clear, because the bond between them is too weak. Until recently, the veterinary profession seriously neglected the field of pet behavior. Perhaps the argument can be made (as it is still made by some physicians) that psychology is not a biological, and therefore not a medical matter. However, it is hard to see who would address the behavioral problems of pets and their owners if not veterinarians. To be sure, doing so will not be easy and will itself raise difficult issues. If the human-companion animal bond can give rise to or involve behavioral problems, the cause of these problems in either humans, animals, or both will sometimes come from the human side of the bond. Therefore veterinarians who want to address behavioral problems arising from the bond must become more knowledgeable about human as well as animal psychology. Much more effort will have to be expended by the profession and the veterinary schools to place into the hands of practitioners useful knowledge about behavioral implications of the human-companion animal bond.[14]

SHOULD VETERINARIANS OR SOCIETY PROVIDE FREE OR LOW COST VETERINARY SERVICES TO THE NEEDY, AND TO WHAT EXTENT SHOULD SOCIETY SUBSIDIZE THE HUMAN-COMPANION ANIMAL BOND IN GENERAL? Society has recognized some obligation to assist the needy in obtaining the services of physicians and hospitals. We sometimes provide public hospitals and publicly supported health insurance to the needy. We do this precisely because we believe that medical care, if not a right (and in many countries it is considered a moral and legal right), is so important and central a concern of life that society must help those with limited means to obtain it.

However, if, as research is now establishing, having a companion animal can be as important to one's physical and mental health as medical care itself, we must at least ask whether society has some obligation to help some people pay for or obtain veterinary services for their animals. Indeed, one might ask whether society sometimes ought to help those of limited means to purchase and keep companion animals in the first place.

The question of subsidized veterinary care is not one of which veterinarians need be afraid. First, it is by no means clear that government or the taxpayers can afford widespread subsidy of veterinary services. Second, just as subsidized medical care has been very good (some would say too good) to the medical profession, it might well offer veterinarians a means of substantially increasing their client base. Third, there are ways of helping the needy that do not involve taxpayer support. For example, veterinarians can volunteer some of their time, or offer financial support, to community animal clinics that serve the needy at reduced cost. If such services are limited to the truly needy, they need not cut into the regular practices of local doctors. At the very least, an appreciation of the importance of the human-companion animal bond and the concomitant need for affordable veterinary care provides an additional strong reason for veterinarians to support pet health insurance programs.

SHOULD THE VETERINARY PROFESSION RECONSIDER ITS OPPOSITION TO AWARDS IN MALPRACTICE SUITS FOR CLIENTS' EMOTIONAL DISTRESS? The organized veterinary profession enthusiastically supports "the human-companion animal bond." However, the profession continues to insist that courts in malpractice suits treat pets like other kinds of personal property, such as sofas and television sets, and deny awards for owners' pain and suffering resulting from animal loss or injury caused by veterinarian malpractice. But one cannot promote the human-companion animal bond as a vital part of clients' lives and at the same time tell pet owners that they cannot collect for their pain and suffering because animals are merely articles of personal property. Imposition of awards for client pain and suffering could make veterinary care more expensive and thus less frequent by dramatically increasing malpractice premiums. However, if veterinarians are serious about their advocacy of a significant human-companion animal bond, they must begin thinking more creatively about how this bond can be recognized by the law in ways which would not threaten the affordability of veterinary services.

To what extent should veterinarians and society treat members of true human-companion animal bonds differently from more causal or less devoted animal owners? Insofar as the human-companion animal bond may be good for revenues, the veterinary profession will have a motive to sweep within the bond as many clients and animals as possible. To be sure, an animal need not be a member of a true bond to need and deserve veterinary care. However, there are good reasons for veterinarians and others to try to understand and recognize when they are dealing with a bond properly speaking and when with mere pet ownership or human-animal interaction. For example, an argument can be made that the stronger the bond between client and patient, the more diligent a veterinarian should be in attempting to work out economic arrangements that will permit a client to pay for the best veterinary care available. In such a case the doctor can be dealing with a client and an animal for whom their continuing relationship is enormously important.

～ A CLICHÉ OR CHALLENGE?

The concept of a "human-companion animal bond" can describe a real and important relationship shared by some humans and some animals, a relationship that gives strong legitimate interests to both. The concept can stimulate one to raise important questions. It can suggest important considerations relevant to answering these questions. Normative veterinary ethics would therefore do well to resist those who would turn "the bond" into a soothing, hackneyed synonym for pet ownership or human-animal interaction. We must also challenge students of the bond to look carefully at both its sides.

REFERENCES

[1]Garcia E: Types of pet owners: Owner attitudes and the tie that binds, *Vet Forum*, July 1985:16.

[2]Committee identifies public health implications of human/animal bond, *J Am Vet Med Assoc* 189:18-19, 1986. Much of this language appears to have been adopted from McCulloch M: Companion animals, human health, and the veterinarian. In Ettinger SJ, editor: *Textbook of Veterinary Internal Medicine: Diseases of the Dog and Cat*, ed 2, Philadelphia, 1983, WB Saunders, p 228-229.

[3]Bird ownership is therapeutic, *J Am Vet Med Assoc* 189:1275, 1986; Katcher AH: Physiologic and behavioral responses to companion animals, *Vet Clin N Am Sm Anim Pract* 15:403-410, 1985.

[4]*Future Directions in Veterinary Medicine*, Durham, NC, 1988, Pew National Veterinary Education Program, p 32.

[5]*See*, for example, Katcher AH, Beck AM, editors: *New Perspectives On Our Lives with Companion Animals*, Philadelphia, 1983, University of Pennsylvania Press; Anderson RK, Hart BL, Hart LA, editors: *The Pet Connection: Its Influence on Our Health*, Minneapolis, 1984, University of Minnesota CENSHARE; Hines LM: Community people-pet programs that work, *Vet Clin N Am Sm Anim Pract* 15:319-332, 1985; Ryder EL: Pets and the elderly, *Vet Clin N Am Sm Anim Pract* 15:333-343, 1985; Beck AM: The therapeutic use of animals, *Vet Clin N Am Sm Anim Pract* 15:365-375, 1985; National Institutes of Health: *Summary of the Working Group on Health Benefits of Pets*, DHHS Pub No 216-107, Washington, DC, 1988, US Government Printing Office.

[6]For a response to this point, *see* Ianuzzi D, Rowan AN: Ethical issues in animal-therapy programs, *Anthrozoös* 4:154-163, 1991. The authors contend that "most animal-assisted therapy programs appear to have a relatively benign impact on the animals." However, this contention is based on a questionnaire distributed to registrants of the 1988 Delta Society Conference, only 5% of whom responded to it, and "phone calls to selected individuals who are very active in animal-assisted therapy to ask them about any concerns that may have come to their attention." Carefully conducted empirical studies of the effects of therapy programs on animals are required. Ideally, these studies should be included in investigations of the effects of animal-facilitated therapy on people. Moreover, evaluation of the animals should be made by veterinarians or animal behavior scientists who do not have a stake in the success of the programs being evaluated, and indeed, do not even know which animals are part of these programs.

[7]Corson SA, Corson EO, Gwynne PH: Pet-facilitated psychotherapy in a hospital setting, *Curr Psych Ther* 15:277-286, 1975, quoted in Schwabe CW: *Veterinary Medicine and Human Health*, ed 3, Baltimore, 1984, Williams & Wilkins, p 622.

[8]Davis JH, Juhasz AM: The preadolescent/pet bond and psychosocial development. In Sussman MB: *Pets and the Family*, New York, 1985, Haworth Press, pp 79-94.

[9]Wilson CC: The pet as an anxiolitic intervention, *J Nerv Ment Dis* 179:482-489, 1991.

[10]Wilson CC: A conceptual framework for human-animal interaction research: The challenge revisited, author's response, *Anthrozoös* 7:22, 1994.

[11]*Id*, p 4-5.

[12]Rollin BE: *Animal Rights and Human Morality*, Buffalo, 1981, Prometheus Books, p 168.

[13]Tannenbaum J: Ethics and human-companion interaction: A plea for a veterinary ethics of the human-companion animal bond, *Vet Clin N Am Sm Anim Pract* 15:438-439, 1985.

[14]McCulloch WF: The veterinarian's education about the human-animal bond and animal-facilitated therapy, *Vet Clin N Am Sm Anim Pract* 15:423-429, 1985.

CHAPTER 16

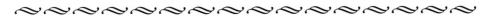

What Is a Veterinarian?
Who Will Decide?

This chapter considers some of the most important general interests of veterinarians. Veterinarians today face critical choices regarding how they wish to define themselves as professionals, and how they shall be viewed by the public. The chapter also asks a question as important as it is frightening: Will the increasing ownership of veterinary practices by nonveterinarians threaten the ability of the profession to shape its own moral character and destiny?

∼ SATISFACTION WITH ONE'S PROFESSIONAL STATUS

In considering their ethical obligations, veterinarians obviously must take into account the needs of patients and clients. However, the interests of veterinarians are also vitally important. It takes substantial time, effort, and expense to become a veterinarian. Veterinarians work hard to help clients and animals. In return, they deserve fair compensation, decent working conditions, respect from other veterinarians, and the esteem of the public. If veterinarians do not receive their due, the public and its animals will also suffer. Veterinarians who are not paid adequately or who cannot take pride in what they do will not approach their medical tasks with vigor and enthusiasm. The more difficult it will be for the profession to attract and retain bright and dedicated doctors. Anything that harms the profession is likely in the long run to harm its patients and clients as well.

∼ SELF-INTEREST: MONETARY GAIN

Veterinarians bring to their professional relationships with clients and animals an interest in earning an adequate living. This is, of course, only one kind of legitimate self-interest a veterinarian can have, but it is one shared to some extent at least by almost all practitioners.

It is sometimes difficult to assess how strongly a doctor's interest in financial success ought to count against the interests of patients, clients, employees, and others. Nevertheless, one should never underestimate the danger of undervaluing monetary reward. Veterinarians who are paid poorly do not receive what they rightly deserve. They may also suffer a lack of self-esteem that can lead to a more general denigration of their profession and of themselves. (I have seen this in students who are convinced that their skills, and indeed they themselves, are not of great value because they can earn more driving a bus or collecting garbage than practicing veterinary medicine.) Low salaries may result in a decline in the number and quality of veterinary school applicants. The ultimate outcome could be a lowering of the standards of veterinary practice, decreased public confidence in the profession, and lower earnings for all practitioners.

∾ PROTECTION OF THE PROFESSION

As members of a profession, veterinarians have a legitimate interest in strengthening their profession as an entity and in protecting it from conditions that could impair the ability of its members to function properly. Protection of the profession can include such activities as opposing the provision of veterinary services by unqualified persons, promoting a good image of the profession in the eyes of the public, and contesting legal actions by government or private citizens that threaten the interests of doctors.

Protecting the profession can assist in furthering veterinarians' legitimate interest in earning an adequate living. However, promoting a vigorous and respected profession brings other rewards. One of the benefits of being a veterinarian is enjoyment of interacting with colleagues.[1] Another is belonging to a profession that possesses talents not shared by members of the public generally and is respected for its values and good deeds. Just being a member of such a highly respected profession can provide rich personal satisfactions.

∾ INTERNAL CONSTRAINTS ON SELF-INTEREST

Veterinarians are not morally free to pursue their own self-interest. Some constraints on their pursuit of self-interest come, as we have seen, from the legitimate interests of patients or clients. For example, it is wrong for a veterinarian to recommend unnecessary services to earn more money, because doing this violates a client's right to obtain at a fair cost what she and her animal really require. Some moral constraints on a veterinarian's self-interest, however, come from within the profession itself—from the interests of its members or from its own central values.

One such limitation derives from the interest that other veterinarians and veterinary employees have in earning an adequate living. A veterinarian who hires employees has a moral obligation to respect this interest by paying them fairly for their services. It is not always easy to determine what constitutes just compensation for one's employees and fellow workers (see Chapter 25). However, if veterinarians ought to be fair in their economic dealings with clients, they must also be fair to their employees, including those who are veterinarians.

As the Veterinary Oath proclaims, the profession is committed to the general values of alleviating animal suffering, promoting animal health, and benefiting clients and members of the public. These are interests of the profession itself, and not just of its patients or clients. These interests can sometimes outweigh the interest of practitioners in monetary gain. This fact is recognized by the *Principles of Veterinary Medical Ethics*, which require, for example, that practitioners assure the availability of emergency services,[2] make a determination of therapy based primarily on the needs of the patient and client,[3] and provide high quality services, regardless of the fees charged, if any.[4]

∾ FOUR MODELS OF PROFESSIONALISM

A veterinarian's interest in monetary gain, economic justice, and benefiting animals and clients often must be considered in approaching particular moral issues.

Nevertheless, it is clear from current controversies among veterinarians about ethical issues that the problem is often not just determining the importance of certain specific interests in resolving particular issues. Rather, many veterinarians see normative veterinary ethics as a choice of competing *general pictures* or models of what a veterinarian ought to be. Included within each of these models is a weighting of such interests as monetary gain, animal welfare, and client satisfaction. For many practitioners, at stake is a definition of veterinary practice that contains an interrelated structure of valuations. From this definition, there then flow conclusions about appropriate behavior and attitudes in various kinds of circumstances.

There are many possible general models of private veterinary practice. However, at present there seem to be four major models that are vying for support in the profession. Each of these four models is very general and permits a range of values. Not all of the models are incompatible. Indeed, there are probably few practitioners who do not combine in their moral outlook elements from more than one of these pictures. Various kinds of practice may require certain combinations. Perhaps normative veterinary ethics will conclude that it is better for veterinarians to combine elements of the models, or to adopt a picture that should be characterized as an entirely new or different model, rather than to accept any of these four models in their pure form.

The Veterinarian as Healer

Many veterinarians see themselves as healers. According to this model, the veterinarian is to animals what many people want the physician to be to people—someone interested in a patient's welfare, who applies the healing arts with dignity and care, who works tirelessly for the patient's benefit, and who sees earning a living as the natural (and hopefully inevitable) outcome of serving the true needs of patients. This model of the veterinarian is expressed eloquently in Dr. Calvin Schwabe's description of veterinary medicine as:

> ...the gentle profession. Gentleness, compassion, and loving service to the especially dependent, helpless, and needy are qualities which most thinking individuals recognize as being basic to what we regard as humane behavior. The first veterinarians in ancient times were priests and a need for their secular ministry was never more evident than today.[5]

Dr. Schwabe's characterization of veterinary medicine as a "ministry" is especially apt. It reflects the contention of this model that healing is too important, too bound up with life and death, with pain and suffering, with human as well as animal welfare, to be cheapened by such things as discount coupons in newspaper advertisements, sale of water bowls and pet toys, and aggressive self-promotion. It is the model of the veterinarian as a healer that is at work when Dr. Robert Shomer complains that the practice of selling nonprofessional products (see Chapter 17) is replacing the question "Is there a doctor in the house?" with the question "Is there a salesperson in the store?"[6]

One must be careful not to make too much of an analogy between the veterinarian as healer and the physician steadfastly committed to saving the life or promoting the interests of human patients. Many people, and many veterinarians, subscribe to the anti-cruelty position (see Chapter 11) and do not see anything wrong with the painless killing of even healthy animals. Veterinarians participate in a good deal of killing of animals. They sometimes suggest or acquiesce in decisions that favor the interests of clients at the expense of patients. Whether such behavior is always morally correct is an issue for normative veterinary ethics. But an accurate descriptive model of veterinary practice must reflect what veterinarians actually think. And many veterinarians who see themselves as healers are not always committed to preserving animal life, or to promoting patients' interests when these conflict with the desires of clients.

This does not mean that the model of the veterinarian as healer excludes a doctor who refuses to kill healthy animals or takes an aggressive stand against clients who want to euthanize patients with curable conditions. It is altogether possible that such attitudes will gain enough support among veterinarians who describe themselves as healers that these attitudes will appropriately be seen as essential components of the model itself. If this occurs, we may want to split the current model of the doctor as healer into two different models, one which opposes painless killing of healthy or curable animals and one which does not. Today, however, the predominance of the anti-cruelty position in the profession and society does not appear to justify such a division of the model of the veterinarian as healer.

The Veterinarian as Friend and Counselor

In a landmark essay in legal ethics, philosopher Charles Fried observed that lawyers characteristically become so committed to serving the interests of their clients that it is appropriate to characterize them as their clients' friend.[7] Not all professional relationships involve what can accurately be termed a friendship. Sometimes, a service is provided with little emotional attachment on the part of either practitioner or client. However, like lawyers, veterinarians frequently care greatly about their clients and treat them as friends. One does not manipulate friends for one's own ends. Friends are people with whom one identifies so closely that many of their interests become one's own interests. Veterinarians who see themselves as friends and counselors listen to clients not just to earn a fee, or even to make a diagnosis or recommend an appropriate treatment—but also because they also genuinely care about helping clients to attain their own goals.

Many veterinarians tell me that serving as a friend and counselor to clients is a central part of their definition of themselves as professionals. Being a friend can involve touching an intimate part of a client's life, as when one discusses the options for a desperately ill pet. Being a friend can also involve sympathetic counseling about economic matters. A large animal practitioner who becomes involved in a personal and caring way in the efforts of a farmer to make a decent living is also a paradigm of the veterinarian as friend.

James Herriot, who is rightly regarded as the profession's most eloquent chronicler of the model of the veterinarian as healer, presents unequaled portraits of the veterinarian as friend. Herriot tells the story of a visit to an elderly client. One of her beloved dogs has just died. She senses that she will be next. She is troubled by the fact that some people say that animals have no souls, and asks Herriot whether she will see her pets again in heaven:

> ...I patted the hand which still grasped mine. 'If having a soul means being able to feel love and loyalty and gratitude, then animals are better off than a lot of humans. You've nothing to worry about there.'

'Oh, I hope you're right. Sometimes I lie at night thinking about it.'

'I know I'm right, Miss Stubbs, and don't you argue with me. They teach us vets all about animals' souls.'

The tension left her face and she laughed with a return of her old spirit. 'I'm sorry to bore you with this and I'm not going to talk about it again. But before you go, I want you to be absolutely honest with me. I don't want reassurance from you—just the truth. I know you are very young but please tell me—what are your beliefs? Will my animals go with me?'

She stared intently into my eyes. I shifted in my chair once or twice.

'Miss Stubbs, I'm afraid I'm a bit foggy about all this,' I said. 'But I'm absolutely certain of one thing. Wherever you are going, they are going too.' She still stared at me but her face was calm again. 'Thank you, Mr. Herriot, I know you are being honest with me. That is what you really believe, isn't it?'

'I do believe it,' I said. 'With all my heart I believe it.'[8]

The Veterinarian as Economic Manager and Herd Health Consultant

A new model of veterinary private practice is being advocated as a way of assuring the continued existence and profitability of farm and food animal practice. This model views the veterinarian as first and foremost a provider of herd management advice. Such advice typically is not in the form of answers to particular questions or medical problems. Rather, as Dr. David Galligan puts it, practitioners "offer a full-service program," the purpose of which is to "determine which combinations of services will offer the greatest return with the minimum risk on the dollar."[9]

Several things follow from the primary aim of providing a general profitable management system for animal herds. First, the veterinarian is no longer seen as someone whose primary function must be to examine animals, diagnose conditions, or dispense medications. Part of the veterinarian's "program" may involve hands-on veterinary care. However, she might leave most of this to clients, and may concentrate instead on providing advice about what animals to acquire, supervising the purchase of feed, designing methods of housing and husbandry, and counseling clients about when to sell and how much to charge for their products. As Dr. Galligan observes, one might "make more economic impact for the farmer pushing a pencil rather than pushing a syringe."[10]

Another aspect of the model of the veterinarian as economic manager is its disavowal of animal health as a necessary goal. As Drs. Barbara Straw and Robert Friendship note, "the concept of 'health' has traditionally conjured up images of a pathogen-free, or 'healthy' animal or herd; and customarily efforts have been directed toward control or elimination of the pathogenic agent to attain this state of 'health.' More recently, the veterinary professional has begun to appreciate that perfect health may not be synonymous with maximum productivity or maximum profitability."[10] "For years, " states Dr. Galligan, "we have recommended wiping out all disease in a herd, but now we're finding that this might not be cost effective. It might be more profitable for farmers and consumers to live with low levels of disease in herds."[9]

The model of the veterinarian as economic manager does not represent a complete break from the past. Veterinarians have long advised clients about herd management. They have provided guidance about matters not strictly speaking of a medical nature. They have recognized that economics sometimes dictates not treating certain animals or providing less extensive or expensive treatment than is available.

Nevertheless, the model of veterinarian as manager involves a momentous shift in attitude. Some farm animal practitioners tell me that when they have a situation in which it is cost-effective not to treat certain members of a herd, they inform the client that the *veterinary* approach would be to treat. They then either leave it to the client to decide whether he wants to go the veterinary route (or the best veterinary route), or they will advise the client to favor productivity with the understanding that this may not be the veterinary approach. Likewise, when these practitioners provide advice about feed, housing, or production that does not have medical consequences, they characterize what they are doing as providing a general program of management advice one of whose components is veterinary service.

In contrast, the model of the veterinarian as manager includes within the role of the practitioner *as a veterinarian* advising clients about purely economic, nonmedical matters and counseling toleration of certain kinds or levels of disease.

I suspect that veterinarians who are accustomed to the model of the veterinarian as herd health consultant may not appreciate how much the model is likely to surprise most laymen. Veterinarians, most people will say, are doctors, they are supposed to promote health and alleviate disease. It would be a mistake to dismiss this response on the grounds that it reflects ignorance about the economic needs of farmers or practitioners. Laymen can understand such things. They can also understand that because animals are not people we may often allow a farm animal practitioner to do in the name of economics certain things that would never be tolerated from a physician.

In their puzzlement about the model of veterinarian as manager, laymen might question the appropriateness of calling such a person a "doctor"—as opposed, say, to a "herd profitability manager" or "herd productivity and disease expert."[11] The dictionary defines the term "doctor" (in the medical and not just the degree-possessing sense) as someone "skilled or specializing in healing arts."[12] Puzzlement about the model is not necessarily a condemnation, but it is a reflection of how new and different a picture of the veterinarian this model presents.

The model of the veterinarian as an economic manager and herd health consultant faces a challenge that goes beyond the assumption by most people that veterinarians protect the health of their patients. This problem can be seen from a statement of the general objectives of herd health management offered in a leading textbook:

> The primary objective of a health and production management program for herds of food-producing animals is to maintain animal health and production at the most efficient level that provides maximum economic returns to the animal owner... .
> Some equally important secondary objectives include the provision of comfortable animal housing commensurate with reasonable animal welfare... .[13]

The discussion identifies as other "equally important secondary objectives" the minimization of pollution by animal wastes, prevention of zoonoses, and avoidance of contaminants and residues in animal products. However, it is stated again that the primary aim of herd health management is maximizing the economic return to animal owners:

> The objectives of herd health are achieved by the application of the concept of the target of performance. A target of performance is the level of animal health and production that is considered to be optimum and yields the best economic returns on investments.[13]

As argued in Chapter 23, it is doubtful whether the *best* economic return on investments is *always* consistent with acceptable levels of animal welfare. Moreover, the toleration of illness, which proponents of the model of the veterinarian sometimes recommend for economic reasons, will clearly sometimes cause a diminution of animal welfare. The authors quoted above appear to concede that animal welfare is a consideration independent of the "best economic returns on investments." This may be why they state that animal welfare is an "equally important" objective. But the statement is strained and problematic. One cannot at the same time say that animal welfare (and other societal goals) are *equally* important as maximization of returns on investment and are *secondary* objectives—unless one believes that animal welfare and these other goals always follow, inevitably and automatically, from maximization of returns. If animal welfare is equally important to producer profits, it must be regarded as a primary objective of the veterinarian's activities.

It is an ethical question whether animal welfare should be considered as important as producer revenues. Nevertheless, proponents of the model of the veterinarian as herd health consultant may have to convince the rest of the profession and the public that herd health management can give sufficient regard to the welfare of individual animals.

Veterinary Practice as a Business

The most controversial contemporary model vying for support from veterinarians (and, as we shall see, from nonveterinarians) is that of veterinary practice as a business.

It is probably incorrect to say that there is one picture of veterinary practice as a business. There may be several such pictures, which reflect varying views about the propriety of certain business techniques. For example, Dr. Robert Shomer includes "resorting to the tactics of merchandising and the sale of nonprofessional items"[6] within his conception of being a salesperson in a store rather than a doctor in the house. Some veterinarians tell me they are so opposed to self-promotion that they reject listing their practices in the Yellow Pages as "being a businessperson." In contrast, many veterinarians would probably object to any categorization that distinguishes being a healer or friend from being a businessperson. For them, management and promotion is no more than a means of achieving a veterinarian's traditional interests of helping animals and clients, and earning a living.

It is difficult at this stage in its development to offer a succinct characterization of the model of veterinary practice as a business. Nevertheless, it is an indisputable fact that some veterinarians (and some nonveterinarians) do define their practices as businesses and that this general perception colors their views about ethical behavior.

A 1987 *Veterinary Economics* editorial provides a good starting point for describing the model. The editorial opposed the provision of the *Principles of Veterinary Medical Ethics* permitting practitioners to sell nonprofessional items only if such products are generally unavailable or are difficult to obtain in the client's general vicinity.[14] The editorial discussed two successful doctors for whom merchandising of nonmedical products brought significant revenue. It characterized them as "young, talented, and innovative entrepreneurs." They "didn't feel obligated to carry on the customs of a dominant mentor like James Herriot. …[They] changed traditional customs and blueprints to fit their career goals, rather than altering the end to fit the means."[15]

It is entirely proper to speak of many kinds of practice management techniques as business techniques or business practices, because most if not all of these techniques are utilized in ordinary commercial businesses. However, the use of such techniques does not by itself turn a veterinary practice into a business, any more than a scientist who uses the tools of statistics in analyzing her data is transformed thereby into a mathematician. It is also entirely proper and—if the arguments of this chapter are correct—vitally important for veterinarians to believe that while certain business tools are essential in managing a veterinary practice, a veterinary practice is still something different from a business. Likewise, the goal of earning profits does not make a veterinary practice into a business. Even those who deny that veterinary medicine is just another kind of business can (and should) believe that a veterinary practice ought to be profitable and can (and should) engage in effective and ethical practice management.

The term "entrepreneur" best summarizes those who view their practices as businesses. By definition, entrepreneurs see themselves *as* businesspeople and not as people who must run a business to support their professional activities. They regard running a successful business and making money to be as important as the goods or services the business provides. They consider themselves entitled to engage in ordinary commercial practices that other entrepreneurs or tradespeople use, such as advertising and retailing. This does not mean that they recognize no ethical limits upon what they may do. But neither will they necessarily treat traditional values or approaches as boundaries within which their interest in monetary gain must operate.

Subsequent chapters of this book focus more directly on various approaches characteristic of the model of veterinary practice as a business. The following are among the kinds of behavior that are typical of the model. No one of these approaches is either necessary or sufficient for viewing veterinary medicine as a business. There may be practices conducted as businesses that do not exemplify some of these approaches, and practices not conducted as businesses that do. The following list sketches a general picture, which will be familiar to both supporters and opponents of viewing veterinary medicine as a kind of business.

- Referring to the practice as a "store" either in communications with the public or (perhaps more importantly) in one's own thinking
- Calling clients "customers" or "consumers"
- Referring to one's services and goods as one's "product," "products," or "product line"
- Referring to one's fees as "prices"
- Calling the practice a "business" or "just a business"
- Not including a traditional medical term (such as "clinic," "hospital," "veterinary," or "medical center" in the name of the practice)
- A physical layout or appearance that either makes the practice look like a typical retail business (for example, a heavy emphasis on nonmedical pet products), or places the practice within a facility (for example, a pet supply store or an all-purpose retail store) that is a business
- A heavy emphasis on selling nonveterinary items or services. Viewing the sale of such items as a critical source of profits
- A heavy emphasis on advertising; use of advertisements that look like those for typical retail businesses, that is, that announce "specials" or discounts in effect for

a limited time, contain dated coupons, or offer "free" goods or services
- Viewing one's practice as a "competitor" of other practices, in the sense in which being a competitor involves attempting to win over current clients of other veterinarians
- Referring to even medical services (such as in-house laboratory testing or dentistry) as "profit centers"
- Assessing the performance of employee veterinarians and staff based entirely or almost entirely upon "productivity," or "production," by which terms are meant the generation of revenues
- Viewing the primary purpose of the practice as the earning of profits
- Referring to the process of convincing clients to authorize services as "selling"
- Referring to the spending by clients for even medical services as "purchasing" or "buying"

Viewing veterinary medicine as a business involves not just perceiving profit as the primary aim of the enterprise but also engaging in sales techniques that are themselves characteristic of consumer businesses in our economy. In a discussion of merchandising to which we shall return in Chapter 17, Dr. Martin Becker offers an incisive description of some of these sales techniques.[16] Merely displaying products in the veterinary office, he observes, might have been adequate in the "old days" when people bought solely based on *need*:

> Today's consumers are drastically different, however. They have a lot of discretionary income and buy based on *desire*. Rather than just showing them what's for sale, we must tell a motivational story to encourage them to buy now.

Among the sales tools Dr. Becker recommends is to display:

> …the largest size of product on the right and graduate down to the left. This is called right-hand merchandising. Because more people are right handed it encourages consumers to reach for the largest size.

One can, of course, attempt to stimulate clients' desires to motivate them to buy what they and their animals really need. In another discussion, Dr. Becker advises taking advantage of the fact that "people buy almost everything based on emotion" to "improve the healthcare of your patients," and states that clients "want to be treated like a friend."[17] He warns that "failing to meet your clients' needs can have even more serious consequences than losing the sale" because it can cause "the premature or unnecessary death of the pet."[18]

The question, however, is not whether one *wants* to (or thinks one can) treat clients as friends and at the same time attempt to "encourage" them to "buy now." The question is whether conducting a veterinary practice as a business will, in fact, treat clients like friends and will, in fact, serve *only* the real and true needs of clients and patients.

To treat clients as friends one must (1) *avoid* attempting to take advantage of or to stimulate clients' desires, even as a purported tool to serve their needs; (2) *restrict* oneself to logical, rational, and truthful argument, devoid of subtle subliminal enticements, and directed at the needs of clients and their animals; (3) *not* view clients as sources of "discretionary income" a portion of which it is one's purpose to obtain for oneself; (4) *not* try to motivate clients to buy now (before they can change their minds) as distinguished from buying when it good for them; and (5) *refuse* to allow clients to purchase products or to authorize services they or their animals do *not* need. These requirements follow from what is meant by the terms "friend" and "friendship." Perhaps children must sometimes be motivated to do what is good for them by subtle (or not so subtle) appeals to their desires. However, true friends are treated differently. One recognizes their adulthood, maturity, and ability to decide for themselves. One does not think of controlling them for one's own ends or of serving anything other than *their* real *needs*. One would never think of encouraging them to do anything one knows is not in their interests.

In fact, selling by appealing to desires will sometimes result in selling things clients and their animals do not need. Satisfaction of immediate desires can be notoriously unreliable paths to the fulfillment of true needs, as many successful retailers know. Desires can focus on momentary pleasures as opposed to long-term goods. Desires can be based on considerations that the light of logic would not approve. "Right-hand merchandising" is a good example. If one displays the largest items on the right to "encourage consumers to reach for the largest size," one is encouraging *all* customers to reach for that largest size of shampoo, including owners not just of Newfoundlands but also of Chihuahuas. The client one wants to "encourage" automatically to reach for the right is not a person whose interests become so identified with one's own that one would never think of selling him the largest size simply because one wants to sell the largest size. A merchant who encourages people to reach for the largest size is doing this because *she* wants them to buy this size. The emphasis is on *oneself:* "How do *I* make the sale?" "How can I sell the item *I* want to sell?

A world in which people are encouraged subliminally if necessary to buy what a retailer wants to sell them—even if the retailer thinks the sale would be good for them too—does not evoke images of friendship. The model of veterinary practice as a business views both veterinarians and clients as what economists call "arms-length" participants in the marketplace: people with whom one has no intrinsic personal connection, but people with whom one deals on a self-interested footing. This approach, it is believed by classical economics, will benefit both buyers and sellers, not because benefiting buyers is the overriding goal of sellers but because the best way for sellers to benefit themselves is to try to satisfy potential buyers.

Indeed, for the model of veterinary practice as a business, the veterinarian-client relationship is itself a product for sale by the veterinarian. And if a doctor's affection for client and patient are part of the veterinarian-client relationship, this affection too is sold by the doctor and bought by the client. As Dr. Becker puts it:

> Our clients *want* to buy our positive emotion, care, and concern for them and their pets. It's only *after* they say 'yes' to our recommendations and buy into our care, concern, and enthusiasm that we have the opportunity to put our medical training to work.[18]

Speaking of "buying" or "buying into" care and concern may disturb even some veterinarians who believe their profession is a business. However, Dr. Becker's attempted use of this language is penetrating. For if the veterinarian-client relationship includes concern for clients and their animals, the model of veterinary medicine as a business must also try to view this concern as part of the veterinarian-client bargain. If the veterinarian-client relationship is a product for sale and purchase, it is entirely appropriate to try to describe this product in the terminology of the marketplace, with words like "buying," "selling," "prices," and "customer."

Whether veterinary practice ever really becomes a business will not be determined by veterinarians alone. Clients must be willing to accept the role of buyers. Although clients may someday consider themselves buyers of veterinary procedures, it will not be so easy for them to consider themselves buyers of veterinarians' care and concern. There is something odd in saying that one's care and concern can be offered for sale, in the same way that puppy shots or an ovariohysterectomy can be offered for sale. This is not just a psychological fact but a matter of what we *mean* by the concepts of "care" and "concern." To care about clients and their animals—to be a friend—means that one is really devoted to them because one believes that *they*, and not their payment of a fee, merits one's affections. One can act *as if* one cares in return for a fee, but one cannot *care* in return for a fee. True affection cannot be bought or sold. One either has it or one does not. If one begins with it, and then sells it for a price, it is gone. Again, this is not just a matter of the human psyche but also the way language uses terms that stand for genuine affection. To the extent that one believes care, concern, and positive emotion are tendered in return for one's fee, one thereby reduces the degree of care, concern, and positive emotion. To the extent that clients believe they are really purchasing care and concern do they reduce their own true, emotional bond with a veterinarian.

There can be no doubt that Dr. Becker and many other veterinarian advocates of the model of veterinary medicine as a business do care genuinely about clients and patients. However, care and concern for clients and patients derive from a more traditional ethic, which pre-dates the model of veterinary practice as a business. For most veterinarians, this ethic is firmly entrenched well before they graduate from veterinary school. The problem faced by advocates of the model of veterinary medicine as a business is fitting their sincere care and concern into a model that also wants to view professional life in terms of selling and buying. This task is like mixing oil and water. It just will not work, not because advocates of the model do not want it to work but because it cannot be done conceptually. The most strenuous efforts can never succeed in attaching the language of "buying" and "selling" to true care, concern, and positive emotion.

There are, I believe, three possibilities. To the extent that a completely consistent model of veterinary practice as a business becomes widely accepted, to that extent will true concern for clients and their animals diminish. To the extent that veterinarians preserve their traditional ethic of genuine concern, to that extent will the ability of the model to encompass the entire veterinarian-client-patient relationship be forestalled.

It is also possible that a variant of the model of veterinary practice as a business will be able to persist—inconsistently but tenaciously—attempting to intermix the opposed principles of buying-selling and caring. If this happens, we are likely to continue to see advocates of the model shifting paradoxically back and forth between statements about motivating consumers to buy now and affirmations of their true care for clients and patients.[17] My guess is that the model of the veterinary practice as a business will not be able to survive forever attempting to include both these opposing principles. Doctors will eventually have to choose between more traditional views of the veterinarian as healer and friend, and a consistently commercial model of veterinary practice as a business. As I suggest in the following, which of these choices prevails may depend upon whether veterinary practices that view themselves as businesses are owned by veterinarians.

Some veterinarians may find my characterization of the model of veterinary practice as a business cold and heartless. This is not a defect in the characterization. (Subsequent chapters will further demonstrate its accuracy.) Rather, unease with my description of the model reflects the fact that many veterinarians who *say* that their profession is just a business, really do not *believe* that veterinary medicine is just a business.

~ FROM A BUSINESS TO SOMEONE ELSE'S BUSINESS: THE OWNERSHIP AND CONTROL OF VETERINARY PRACTICES BY NONVETERINARIANS

There has recently been a significant development in the model of veterinary practice as a business. This development is disturbing even some of the most ardent defenders of the model. (Some of these doctors tell me they are now former advocates of the model.) An increasing number of veterinary practices are not only run as businesses. They are owned and controlled by businesspeople who are not veterinarians. This development could change forever the character of the profession as we have known it.

What Is Nonveterinarian Ownership?

There is a sense in which a nonveterinarian or nonveterinarian business can be said to "own the practice" if this layman or business owns the physical premises in which the practice is located and leases these premises to the practice. This is not what I mean by "nonveterinarian ownership." Rather, what I mean is ownership of the practice itself. Where one person owns a practice, nonveterinarian ownership would mean ownership of the entire practice, which might include the building, physical equipment, and medical records. Where a veterinary practice is a corporation or is owned by a corporation, nonveterinarian ownership means ownership by nonveterinarians of shares of the corporation. Where a practice is organized as a partnership or is owned by a partnership, nonveterinarian ownership means that at least one of the partners is a nonveterinarian.

There are varying possible degrees of nonveterinarian ownership. One or more laymen can, individually or collectively, own anything ranging from a small portion of a practice, to a majority interest in the practice, to the entire practice. Practices that are owned in part by nonveterinarians can also be owned in part by veterinarians.

Nonveterinarian ownership versus the "superstore" issue

Some veterinarians appear to identify the issue of whether nonveterinarians should own veterinary practices with the question of whether so-called pet supply retail "superstores" should contain veterinary practices. These two questions are different and should not be confused. It is possible for a practice to be owned by a nonveterinarian business that is not a superstore. Moreover, as is discussed in detail below, it is possible for a "superstore" to have within its premises a veterinary facility that is owned or controlled by veterinarians and that leases space from or shares space with the retail establishment. Such a facility need not adhere to the model of a veterinary practice as a business, even though the retail establishment in which the practice is located is a business. Therefore veterinarians who are concerned about the presence of veterinary facilities within retail businesses will not necessarily address this concern by objecting to nonveterinarian ownership of veterinary facilities.

Nonveterinarian ownership versus merchandising

Likewise, it is important to distinguish nonveterinarian ownership from merchandising, in the sense of the sale of nonveterinary goods and services by a veterinary practice (see Chapter 17). Some veterinary practices owned by nonveterinarians engage in such merchandising. However, a practice owned by nonveterinarians need not merchandise and may restrict itself to providing medical services.

Nonveterinarian ownership versus the model of the veterinary practice as a business

It is also possible for practices owned by nonveterinarians to conduct their affairs in ways that do not reflect the model of the veterinary practice as a business. This might occur, for example, where an owner-veterinarian has died and (if permitted by state law) his spouse assumes ownership of the practice. If the practice had been conducted by the doctor in accordance with more traditional approaches, the new owner may continue in this vein.

Although nonveterinarian owners need not view their practices as businesses, many do. Certainly, most nonveterinarians who purchase or invest in companies that own veterinary practices will regard their operations as businesses and themselves as entrepreneurs. This is not the only reason it is appropriate to include, as a general matter, nonveterinarian ownership within the model of the veterinary practice as a business. Acceptance of this model within the profession will lead inevitably to the ownership of practices by nonveterinarians whose primary interest is entrepreneurial. If *veterinarians* view themselves as businesspeople and their facilities as businesses, some businesspeople are bound to think they are just as qualified as veterinarians to own veterinary practices.

Indeed, if a veterinary practice is just a business like any other, there is no reason why a layman could *not* be as qualified as a veterinarian to own a veterinary practice. A veterinary practice would be like a jewelry store, which can be owned by someone who knows very little about gemstones, precious metals, or fixing watches. Such a business would not succeed without people knowledgeable in these areas, but these people can be hired and paid by an owner-entrepreneur whose sole interest is in earning revenues. Indeed, the owner of such a store need not even know how to manage the business, if he hires someone who does. He need never be present at his business. He need not care about, or even like, the kinds of goods and services his business provides.

What Is Nonveterinarian Control?

It is also important to distinguish nonveterinarian ownership of veterinary practices from nonveterinarian control. It is possible for laymen who own part or all of a veterinary practice to have nothing to do with its management. Such people could simply invest in the practice, allow it to be run by veterinarians, and collect their portion of the profits or assume their portion of the losses.

Although such arrangements are possible, they will surely be rare. Owners, and certainly majority owners, of businesses usually expect to have some say in the management of their business. In reality, nonveterinarian ownership is likely to mean a significant degree of nonveterinarian control. Thus, Dr. James Wilson believes that one potential benefit of such ownership—for veterinarians—is that doctors will not have to concern themselves with many of the details of management. "Think of the amount of time a big company…could allocate to practicing medicine, as opposed to managing practices, if it were to own 80 practices. The computing, payroll, and drug ordering are centralized, and the veterinarians devote all their time to practicing veterinary medicine."[19]

The Question Refined: Nonveterinarian Ownership and the Other Golden Rule

We can now better define the ethical question raised by nonveterinarian ownership. Taken in isolation, such ownership would present no ethical problems. A truly "silent partner" who never influences the running of the practice would have no effects on the services received by patients and clients, and no influence on doctors. Clearly, any important ethical issues raised by nonveterinarian ownership relate to whether nonveterinarian owners *control* or *affect* practices in ways that are not appropriate or acceptable.

One must separate the question of what effects nonveterinarian ownership might have from the issue of whether such effects would be ethically acceptable. The former is a factual question. Because at the time of this writing nonveterinarian ownership is only first emerging as a major trend, it is impossible to predict the effects of such ownership with great confidence. The influence nonveterinarian ownership may have on the interests of patients, clients, and doctors might differ in different kinds or sizes of practices, in different regions of the country, or in different states whose state licensing boards might approach potential problems or abuses with varying levels of vigor. For example, nonveterinarian ownership might have very different effects on how patients, clients, and employed doctors are treated depending upon whether a practice is owned by (1) a corporation which, though owned by nonveterinarians, is devoted only to the providing of veterinary service, or (2) a retail "superstore" in which the veterinary facility is only a part of the business and the veterinary staff is expected to generate revenues for the nonveterinary side of the operation. Likewise, the extent to which practices owned by nonveterinarians attempt to maintain an elevated image of veterinarians may vary depending upon the extent to which veterinarians are part owners.

Supporters of nonveterinarian ownership often paint a rosy picture of its benefits. It is therefore useful to consider the possibility of less salutary effects. More importantly, I assume the truth of a principle that is sometimes called the *other* Golden Rule: "He who has the gold, rules." Most nonveterinarian owners of veterinary facilities will view themselves as entrepreneurs and their facilities as businesses. They will invest in veterinary businesses primarily, and some may be in it entirely, for the money. There is nothing wrong with owning businesses and making money. However, people who own a business, people out of whose pockets the bills are paid and the salaries are tendered, people whose money is at risk, expect to have a significant influence on how the business is run. This fact alone may create serious problems for the profession.

The Legal Situation
The authority of the states to prohibit nonveterinarian ownership

Largely because of recent efforts by the Federal Trade Commission (FTC) to compel state veterinary licensing boards to allow nonveterinary ownership,[20] some veterinarians appear to be under the misapprehension that the ability of states to prohibit nonveterinarian ownership is an open legal issue. It is therefore important to explain briefly the law relating to nonveterinarian ownership.

The United States Supreme Court has held that the states, in the exercise of their governmental functions, are exempt from the federal antitrust laws.[21] Any state can restrict the ownership or operation of businesses or professional practices in ways that, if attempted by private parties, would restrain trade or competition—provided the state is not doing so to protect an enterprise it runs essentially as a business from competing private businesses.

The licensing and regulation of veterinarians are quintessentially government functions. Therefore it is clear that a state has the legal authority to pass a statute restricting the ownership of veterinary facilities to licensed veterinarians. Any state can decide, in its wisdom, that protection of the public and its animals requires that only licensed veterinarians may own all or any part of any veterinary practice or may employ veterinarians in a business that provides veterinary services. As of 1993, 21 states restricted ownership of veterinary facilities to licensed veterinarians.[22] Many more states (including many that allow nonveterinarian ownership) restrict ownership of practices organized as professional corporations to licensed veterinarians.

At the time of this writing, the only legal issue in some doubt concerns whether a state veterinary licensing board may, on its own without any explicit statutory directive, restrict ownership of veterinary facilities or the employment of veterinarians to its licensees. The Supreme Court has ruled that a state can adopt a policy, the effect of which is to restrain competition, but only if the policy is "clearly articulated and affirmatively expressed as state policy" and is "actively supervised by the State itself."[23] It can be argued that where a state veterinary board adopts a regulation restricting ownership of veterinary facilities to veterinarians, and where the practice act or some other statute does not explicitly require such a restriction or allow the board to impose the restriction, the *state* has not clearly enunciated an ownership restriction policy.[24]

In any event, the states can lawfully prohibit nonveterinarian ownership if they want to do so. The ethical and policy issue is whether the states should do so.

Ability to urge legal restrictions on ownership

Some veterinarians may also be under the misapprehension that they can subject themselves to legal action for restraint of trade if they voice support of state restriction of ownership to licensed veterinarians. As noted in Chapter 19, the antitrust laws do not preclude good faith attempts by individuals or organized groups to influence federal, state, or local government. Because it is lawful for state governments to restrict ownership of veterinary practices to veterinarians, it is lawful for veterinarians to ask state office holders to retain or institute this restriction on the grounds that prohibiting nonveterinarian ownership is good for the public, its animals, and the profession.

Prohibition against unlicensed practice of veterinary medicine

Even in states that allow nonveterinarian ownership, it is a criminal offense to practice veterinary medicine without a license. Supporters of nonveterinarian ownership appear to believe that this need not pose a problem for nonveterinarian owners. There is, these supporters assert, a difference between the management of a veterinary practice and the actual practice of veterinary medicine. As long as nonveterinarians restrict themselves to the former, it is claimed, they need not violate laws prohibiting unlicensed practice.

There are doubtlessly many situations in which everyone might agree that some action does not constitute the practice of veterinary medicine, but is merely part of "managing a practice." For example, a decision to charge a certain fee for a surgical procedure, or to stay open weeknights would be management decisions, which would not subject a nonveterinarian owner or manager to prosecution for the unlicensed practice of veterinary medicine. However, it might not always be clear where, in the eyes of the law, management ends and veterinary practice begins. The courts do not have a history of explaining the crime of unlicensed practice in the context of nonveterinarian ownership. Typically, prosecutions for unlicensed practice have been against people who engage in activities (such as spaying or neutering, or administering drugs) that involve direct hands-on provision of medical care to animals. It is not clear whether courts would interpret as the practice of veterinary medicine certain kinds of *influence* nonveterinarian owners might have on the medical care provided in their facilities. It could be argued, for example, that a decision by nonveterinarian ownership to use only certain kinds of suture material or to keep only certain kinds or brands of drugs in the practice are not purely matters of management, but cross over the line into behavior that substantially affects the medical care patients receive—and might therefore be classified as practicing or involving the practice of veterinary medicine. It remains to be seen whether a state licensing board, prosecutor's office, or court would view such kinds of influence as the practice of veterinary medicine.

If nonveterinarian ownership increases in states that permit it, veterinary licensing boards and courts in these states may be called upon to define more precisely what their laws regard as merely managerial as opposed to medical activities. This line may not always be easy to draw. It might not always be drawn by government bodies in predictable ways. Some nonveterinarian owners could find themselves caught on the wrong side of the distinction between management and practice.

⟿ THE CASE AGAINST NONVETERINARIAN OWNERSHIP
The Nonveterinarian Ownership Spectrum

I believe that nonveterinarian ownership will, in the long run, significantly harm the interests of veterinarians, clients, and patients. To make this case, I offer a spectrum of different possible arrangements in which the controlling interest in veterinary practices is held by nonveterinarians. The spectrum is not intended to portray all possible kinds of nonveterinarian ownership and control. The spectrum is not based on any actual veterinary practice or business, and any resemblance between anything in the spectrum (including the fictional "Petzilla's scenario") and any practice or business is purely coincidental.

Figure 16-1 summarizes this nonveterinarian ownership spectrum. Along the spectrum are various kinds of arrangements, more complete descriptions of which follow here:

1. A single facility practice owned by a nonveterinarian spouse of the deceased veterinarian former owner. The owner is consulted regularly and has the final say about basic economic and management decisions, but the veterinarians who work for her make most of the day-to-day decisions about how the practice is managed.

MORE TRADITIONAL ←→

LESS TRADITIONAL ←→

A single facility practice owned by a nonveterinarian spouse of a deceased doctor.	A business whose activity is restricted to the operation of veterinary hospitals; chief operating officer, top management staff are veterinarians.	A company which owns businesses other than veterinary hospitals; veterinary hospitals under a subsidiary company with substantial independence; chief executive officer and major management staff of the subsidiary are veterinarians; stand-alone veterinary operations.	A company which owns businesses other than veterinary hospitals; same central management for both veterinary and nonveterinary businesses; this management structure includes no veterinarians; stand-alone veterinary operations.	A company which owns businesses other than veterinary hospitals; same central management for both veterinary and non veterinary businesses; this management structure includes no veterinarians; veterinary facilities included in premises that offer nonveterinary goods and services.	The "Petzilla's scenario."

FIGURE 16-1. The Nonveterinarian Ownership Spectrum

2. A business owned by nonveterinarians whose activity is restricted to the operation of veterinary hospitals and whose chief operating officer and top management staff are veterinarians.

3. A company owned by nonveterinarians which owns businesses other than veterinary hospitals but which operates all its veterinary hospitals under a subsidiary company with substantial independence from parent ownership. The chief executive officer and major management staff of the subsidiary are all veterinarians. All the veterinary facilities operated by the company through its subsidiary are stand-alone veterinary operations, that is, they occupy premises that are veterinary hospitals only.

4. A company owned by nonveterinarians which owns businesses other than veterinary hospitals and which operates these hospitals via the same central management that operates all the company's business. This management structure includes no veterinarians. All the veterinary facilities operated by the company are stand-alone veterinary operations.

5. A company owned by nonveterinarians which owns businesses other than veterinary hospitals and which operates these hospitals via the same central management that operates all the company's business. This top management structure includes no veterinarians. All the veterinary facilities operated by the company are included in premises owned by the business that offer nonveterinary goods and services. The veterinary facilities are dignified in appearance and look much like traditional veterinary practices, except that they are located in the company's retail stores. Veterinarians working at these facilities are full- or part-time salaried employees. These veterinary facilities bear a strong resemblance to drug departments in stores that are still called "pharmacies," that is, retail operations that offer a wide range of goods and services one of which is filling prescriptions and selling pharmaceuticals.

6. The "Petzilla's scenario."

The Profession's Worst Nightmare?

Near, but perhaps not at the very end of the "Less Traditional" side of the nonveterinarian ownership spectrum is what I call "the Petzilla's scenario."

Imagine it is 5 years hence, and we are in the state of Nowhere. Several years ago a pet supply retail company owned and controlled by nonveterinarians decided to take advantage of the state's laws allowing laymen to own veterinary facilities. The company opened full-service veterinary hospitals in each of its stores. The stores are named "Petzilla's, The Monster Pet Supply Store." (Petzilla's is named after Godzilla, the famous Japanese movie dinosaur that came to the rescue of civilization when it was threatened by a series of evil dinosaurs.) There are now 10 Petzilla's in the state. Each store contains several departments, including "Groomzilla's, The Monster Pet Groomer," "Yummyzilla's, The Monster Pet Food Place," "Toyzilla's, the Monster Pet Toy Depot," and "Vetzilla's, The Monster Animal Hospital and Pet Repair Station." The symbol of Petzilla's is Bernice Brontosaurus, the huge but friendly dinosaur. Bernice appears in various guises in each Petzilla's store, in all its advertisements, and in letterheads of Petzilla's departments. For example, all stationery and invoices of "Vetzilla's, The Monster Animal Hospital and Pet Repair Station" feature a smiling Bernice in a white medical coat, a stethoscope hanging from her neck, and a white baseball-style cap on her head bearing the letters "DVM."

Each Petzilla's is laid out identically, to save costs and to assist customers to find what they want whichever store they visit. Each "Vetzilla's, The Monster Animal Hospital and Pet Repair Station" is at the back of the store. (Petzilla's wants consumers to see all the things for sale on their way to the clinic.) Next to each Vetzilla's is the Groomzilla's, with its 6-foot-high and 8-foot-long stuffed Bernice holding a pair of clippers and shampoo bottle.

Petzilla's offers somewhat lower fees for veterinary services than many other veterinarians in the state. Its costs are minimal for space allocated for the clinics. It purchases veterinary drugs and supplies in large quantities by buying for all its clinics in Nowhere and other states, and can offset "loss-leader" reductions in veterinary fees with profits from the sale of grooming services and pet supplies. There is an ample pool of veterinarians willing to work at Petzilla's clinics because Nowhere's veterinary school always graduates more doctors than the number of job openings in the state. Petzilla's can attract recent graduates by offering a salary well below the national mean for new graduates and by adding to this base a small percentage of the gross clinic revenues attributable to the doctor and a commission for sales of items (including grooming) purchased on the doctor's recommendations in the rest of the store. No doctor can own a portion of the business. There are only a few positions for the better paying job of veterinarian-manager in each clinic. However, Petzilla's easily replaces veterinarians who become dissatisfied with working conditions and salaries with other doctors, mainly recent graduates. Indeed, Petzilla's has begun lowering its clinic costs even further by utilizing a large proportion of part-time doctors, who can be paid even less in salary and benefits than full-time workers. Petzilla's is also able to keep expenses down by employing technicians who earn more than other technicians in the state but still considerably less than Vetzilla's veterinarians. Vetzilla's veterinarian managers try to assure that these technicians reduce to the absolute minimum allowable by law the time each doctor spends with patients or customers. To avoid making referrals to other hospitals, Vetzilla's clinics utilize the services of visiting specialists who can perform sophisticated diagnoses, treatments, and surgeries on Vetzilla's premises.

Petzilla's markets all departments of its stores aggressively. Full-page advertisements appear frequently in local newspapers. These advertisements always contain coupons (with expiration dates) that customers can redeem for discounts on veterinary services. Petzilla's customers receive two cards, one from the veterinary clinic and one from the rest of the store. Total purchases are punched out on each card. For each $100 spent on pet supplies, customers receive a $10 certificate for services at any Vetzilla's, and for each $200 spent at any Vetzilla's customers receive a $10 certificate for pet supplies at any Petzilla's. Present at all times in each Vetzilla's is someone dressed in a dinosaur costume to keep children brought by parents occupied, and to hand out Bernice-shaped lollipops and coloring books containing discount coupons for items offered throughout the store.

Among the veterinary services that Petzilla's advertises are "reasonably priced ear-cropping" of dogs and "the humane euthanasia of unwanted pets." To motivate customers to authorize medically advisable procedures, customers are given a 5% discount off a list of diagnostic, medical, or surgical services (such as all radiography, comprehensive blood work, spays and neuters, and teeth cleaning) if they agree to one of these procedures during the visit at which it is first recommended.

Petzilla's recently instituted a new promotional technique that has generated a great deal of excitement among its customers. At each Vetzilla's, for each office visit or inpatient diagnostic or treatment procedure, a card is filled out bearing the customer's and animal's name and the date and nature of the visit or procedure. The cards are placed in a huge glass bowl in the clinic's waiting room. The cards accumulate for a week, at the end of which Bernice Brontosaurus draws one card from the bowl. Each week the process is repeated with the cards for that week. Each week's winner receives a complete refund or fee waiver for the visit or procedure on the card and also gets a videotape of Bernice picking the lucky card. Several weeks ago, a customer of one Vetzilla's won a $750 surgical procedure. This new raffle is featured prominently in Petzilla's newspaper advertisements throughout the state, together with the names of the latest winners.

Petzilla's business is good. Several veterinarians in the state who have reached retirement age are having difficulty selling their practices to other veterinarians because of fears of potential purchasers that they cannot compete with Vetzilla's. Petzilla's expects soon to account for one-eighth of all annual client visits to veterinary offices in Nowhere. Petzilla's plans to open several more stores in Nowhere. But the story does not end here. Another national chain of pet supply superstores, convinced that it can do better than Petzilla's, is also planning to open stores in Nowhere containing veterinary clinics. A discount department store chain with over 1,000 stores across the country and over two dozen in Nowhere has announced that it will open veterinary clinics in its stores in the state. This is of great concern to Petzilla's management because this large chain has many stores in the state's most popular shopping areas. This chain can also offer consumers "one-stop shopping" that goes far beyond pet care to almost everything they might want to buy.

What Is Wrong With This Picture?
The interests of veterinarians, clients, and patients

Built deliberately into the conduct of Petzilla's business are features subsequent chapters of this book maintain are not in the interests of clients, patients, and the profession. For example, I argue that it is inappropriate to associate veterinary facilities with juvenile or demeaning depictions of animals or veterinarians, to advertise discounts, to motivate clients to make medical decisions quickly through offers of "savings," to pay employee veterinarians percentage commissions, to offer convenience euthanasia and nontherapeutic ear-cropping, and to keep veterinarian salaries as low as possible. If my arguments are correct, insofar as nonveterinarian ownership leads to these things, nonveterinarian ownership is not in the interests of clients, patients, and the profession.

Practices like Vetzilla's (if there are ever such) will harm veterinarians economically as well as professionally. Today, many practices begin with certain ideas about what they believe to be fair compensation for a veterinarian, and set their fees accordingly. This will not happen in operations like Vetzilla's, whose doctors are paid based not on what veterinarians believe to be fair to colleagues but on what nonveterinarian owners seek to earn for themselves. In a world filled with veterinary practices like Vetzilla's fewer bright and dedicated young people will endure the time, expense, and effort to become a veterinarian. For even if the money is acceptable, many will turn away from a profession whose members have little control over their professional lives and who exist as parts of a retail trade.

As a consequence of its subordination of veterinarians to nonveterinarian businesspeople, Vetzilla's and veterinary practices like it would harm clients and animals. The less veterinarians are paid or the less willing bright and dedicated people will become or remain veterinarians, the lower will be the quality of veterinary services. Clients will be harmed insofar as establishments like Vetzilla's manipulate them to purchase services or goods that they or their animals do not need. One potential consequence of practices like Vetzilla's would derive from a feature that I have not yet included in the scenario because I believe it is important to make the case against such practices with the assumption that they will not compromise the independent medical judgment of veterinarians. In fact, there is a strong possibility that in businesses driven by an overriding profit motive, economic decisions made by nonveterinarians will affect the nature and quality of medical care. Dr. Mary Beth Leininger put it well when she warned that:

> If the practice is a corporation [owned by nonveterinarians], somebody is making economic, bottom-line decisions that affect most aspects of medicine, such as the quality of vaccines and instruments. ...
>
> Most DVMs, whether economically right or wrong, are not necessarily bottom-line driven, but are driven by what is the best choice for both pet and client. ...I see corporate structure potentially eliminating that option with employed veterinarians since their paycheck depends on following a corporate management policy.[25]

The end of veterinary ethics?

Veterinarians too are capable of doing things that harm clients, patients, and their profession. Indeed, this is why official and normative veterinary ethics are so important: they can help us to discuss what is or is not morally appropriate so that the ethical as well as technical aspects of veterinary practice can be evaluated and improved. However, at least discussions of ethical issues among and with veterinarians are made within the context of shared values that derive from the professional status of veterinarians *as veterinarians*.

In contrast, the most important values that drive Petzilla's come from *outside* veterinary medicine. Two critically important provisions of the *Principles of Veterinary Medical Ethics* underscore obligations that can transcend, and may sometimes run counter to, maximizing profits:

> Veterinarians should consider first the welfare of the patient for the purpose of relieving suffering and disability while causing a minimum of pain or fright. Benefit to the patient should transcend personal advantage or monetary gain in decisions concerning therapy.[26]

> Determination of therapy must not be relegated to secondary consideration with remuneration to the veterinarian being the primary interest.[27]

The Petzilla's scenario should demonstrate even to veterinarians who say that their profession is "just a business" the extent to which values other than the profit motive are important to veterinary medicine. Veterinarians care about animals, not just so that they can earn money (which they rightly deserve!), but because they believe that animal health and welfare are important in their own right. Veterinarians care about clients because they believe that the psychological and economic relations people have with their animals are important in their own right. Veterinarians also care about their profession and its future. They want the profession to remain distinct and independent, and to prosper. They want future generations of veterinarians to enjoy and benefit from a profession so many doctors have labored for so long to establish and nurture.

In sum, beginning even before they enter veterinary school and continuing after retirement from active practice, veterinarians spend a lifetime immersed in a system of ethical values. Many of these values are distinctively *veterinary*. Many of these values accord independent importance to matters that are of no special interest to a purely profit-driven enterprise, unless its revenues are served thereby.

The fact that this is so can be seen by looking more closely at why Petzilla's behaves as it does. Petzilla's is motivated by monetary considerations only. It will adopt whatever approaches will generate a bottom line satisfaction to its owners. The decision whether to employ part-time instead of full-time veterinarians, to substitute technicians for veterinarians wherever possible, to offer convenience euthanasia or ear-cropping, or to offer discounted fees on certain services will be made on exactly the same basis as the decision whether to keep Bernice as the symbol for the business or even to retain the name "Petzilla's." If a certain approach generates satisfactory profits, it will be utilized. If not offering a certain service (such as nontherapeutic ear-cropping) would decrease profits, this will constitute a conclusive argument for offering that service. Thus Petzilla's has no special interest in attitudes about animal welfare that are evolving within the veterinary profession. Petzilla's would not consider attempting to guide public opinion on an issue such as ear-cropping or convenience euthanasia. Petzilla's is strictly market-driven. As long as enough people want and will pay for various services, this is fine with Petzilla's. If people no longer want such services, this is also fine, and Petzilla's will stop offering them, for business reasons.

Nor does Petzilla's have any special loyalty to or concern about the veterinary profession or its future. This business has no independent interest in maintaining high salaries for veterinarians or in preventing the veterinary profession from becoming one in which part-time rather than full-time doctors predominate. As long as it can find veterinarians to generate acceptable revenues, Petzilla's does not care about whether the prospect of joining a profession in which operations like its own deter the best and the brightest college students from choosing veterinary medicine as a career. Indeed, Petzilla's has no permanent commitment to providing veterinary services. If some day having veterinary clinics in the stores generates less than acceptable revenues, the clinics will be closed for the same reason they were opened—profitability. Indeed, if Petzilla's parent company decides that there are higher profits in fast food than pet supplies, it can close down the entire pet supply operation, without any compromise in its central aim of earning profits for its owners.

The Petzilla's scenario would pose at least three grave ethical problems for the profession.

First, many ethical values that have traditionally been embraced by the profession are irrelevant to the way this business offers veterinary services. Veterinary ethics has no independent significance for it. Official and normative veterinary ethics may have to be given some attention, not because ethics deserves attention in its own right, but if some attention to ethics turns out to be necessary to keep the business profitable.

Second, the larger the proportion of veterinary practices like these, the more restricted will be the ability of the organized profession to argue effectively that veterinary ethics should play a role in the providing of veterinary services. If 70% of practices are run by nonveterinarians simply as businesses, businesspeople may decide whether the veterinarians at 70% of practices will perform convenience euthanasia, offer volume discounts, and urge clients to purchase commercial pet foods their parent retailer can sell most profitably. To the extent that veterinary practices are run by businesses without ties to the profession and its ethics, the profession will have little if any ability to convince doctors to practice in accordance with ethical standards. I included at the end of the Petzilla's scenario the entrance of other nonveterinarian competitors into the veterinary services market. If this occurs, much of the nature of veterinary practice could be determined not by one business, but by competition among nonveterinarian-owned businesses. There is no telling how far a nonveterinarian-owned business will go, if its competitors are willing to engage in just a bit more commercialism or tacky behavior to attract customers.

Third, even if practices like Vetzilla's do not dominate the veterinary market, they can substantially harm the ability of all veterinarians to earn a decent living. For there still may be a sufficient number of places like Petzilla's—with their low-paid veterinarians, undignified advertisements, aggressive attempts to turn sales, and view of veterinary practices as retail shops—to establish an image of veterinary medicine as a second-rate, perhaps even disreputable, occupation. As I note in Chapter 17, very few lawyers advertise. Yet those lawyers who seem to fill the media or Yellow Pages with undignified and commercialistic advertisements have managed to convince the public that many lawyers are greedy, self-serving, and unethical. The same thing can happen to veterinarians, if there are enough facilities like Vetzilla's, and if enough animal owners turn away with revulsion from these practices and veterinarians who work in them.

Can It Happen?
The driving force of revenues

The Petzilla's scenario can indeed happen. Allowing veterinary practices to be run by laymen as businesses assures that there is only one consideration which will determine whether operations like Petzilla's exist—revenues. If establishments like Petzilla's make enough money for their owners, there might be such operations.

Because businesses run strictly as revenue-generators will not be motivated by an independently obligatory system of professional values that sometimes run counter to the maximization of profits, the only effective bar to the Petzilla's scenario must be the marketplace itself. Only resistance by enough clients can prevent operations like this from succeeding. Unfortunately, Petzilla's does not need acceptance of its approach by all veterinary clients, or indeed by most clients. Operations like this can profit with only a portion of the market. As we know, there are many people and many pet owners who do not have a high regard for animals. Moreover, there are already some veterinarian-owned practices that look like retail stores. Some of these facilities attract a sufficient clientele. One can find in the Yellow Pages in various parts of the country advertisements that feature foolish caricatures of animals, deceptive claims, unfair comparisons with other veterinarians, and characterizations of veterinary facilities as one-stop shopping centers only one of whose services is animal medical care (see Chapter 18). The fact that such behavior continues means that there are people who will accept it.

It is not paternalistic, antidemocratic, selfish, or anticompetitive for veterinarians to turn away from something even a significant portion of the public wants, or is at least willing to tolerate. As readers of this book will learn, I accord great weight to client interests. I argue that clients should control the medical decisions affecting their animals, even where veterinarians might sometimes make wiser choices. At the same time, part of what distinguishes a true *profession* from a trade, is that professionals have a high moral obligation to *educate* the public, to *lead*, to show people a *better* way. Veterinarians have an ethical obligation—not just to their profession but to their patients and clients—to convince the public of the great worth and value of animals. People must know that one ought not to purchase a pet as a temporary amusement, to ignore it when it becomes old or sick, or to neglect its medical needs. People must understand that taking their animals seriously means that veterinary care is, like medical care, a serious enterprise that sometimes requires economic sacrifice. The fact that a significant portion of the public will tolerate certain ways of dealing with animals or certain ways of offering veterinary care does not render these ways acceptable. As professionals, veterinarians should reject behavior that harms the interests of clients and their animals.

It is possible for veterinarians who own veterinary facilities to do the things envisioned in the Petzilla's scenario. However, if only veterinarians can own and control veterinary practices, facilities like Vetzilla's will be far less likely. Standing as a barrier to such operations should never be illegal attempts to restrain trade or competition, but the ethical values of a noble profession, internally absorbed and exemplified by individual doctors as a matter of individual decision. To be sure, these ethical values will be effective in preventing the Petzilla's scenario only to the extent that current and future veterinarians reject the scenario. But if it is individual *veterinarians* who will determine whether operations like Petzilla's exist, the profession will have at least a reasonable chance of convincing doctors that high ethical ideals are better in the long run for the profession and the animals and clients it serves.

Nonveterinarian ownership and the instability of veterinary values

Some proponents of nonveterinarian ownership may legitimately object that they have no intention of operating facilities like the fictional Petzilla's. Some will claim, correctly, that veterinary operations owned by laymen can be concerned about the interests of clients and patients and indeed, can sometimes sacrifice pecuniary interests as is required by the *Principles of Veterinary Medical Ethics*. It is possible that, at present, the great majority of nonveterinarian controlled practices occupy the "More Traditional" regions of my nonveterinarian ownership spectrum. Indeed, at the time of this writing, several of the profession's most talented and distinguished members were employed by hospitals with nonveterinarian owners.

The issue, however, is whether, in the *long* run, veterinary practices owned by nonveterinarians will remain as connected to the values of the profession as those owned by veterinarians, who, as veterinarians, are permanently connected to the profession. In fact, any tendency toward the maintenance of veterinary values by nonveterinarian owners must be unstable, precisely because the primary motivation of most such own-ers is earning profits. A widow who inherits her husband's practice might maintain its adherence to professional values. However, if she needs money, she can sell the practice to a company none of whose executives are veterinarians and none of whom care as much about the profession as she does. A company that owns only veterinary facilities and whose chief executive officer is a veterinarian may identify itself with the profes-sion and its values. However, the owners of this company may sell the business one day to another operator of veterinary hospitals none of whose top managers are veterinari-ans. And there is nothing to prevent the owners of *this* company, or the owners of any practice, from selling to a business whose major activities are not in veterinary medi-cine. Such a sale might be made to people who respect veterinarians. But the sale could also be made to a company most of whose revenues also derive from the sale of such things as toys, shoes, and fast food—and for whom veterinary services is just another potential profit center.

In sum, because the function of a business is to earn money, over time, many vet-erinary practices that are viewed by their nonveterinarian owners simply as businesses are likely to be owned by people who have no particular connection to the values of the veterinary profession. The less respect such owners have for the profession, the more the veterinary facilities they operate may come to resemble Petzilla's.

Potentially troublesome aspects of "more traditional" nonveterinarian-owned practices

Figure 16-1 recognizes that nonveterinarian-owned practices can respect the inter-ests of patients, clients, and veterinarians. However, the further one moves toward the "Less Traditional" end of the spectrum, the greater the danger that business motivation will predominate over the internal values of the veterinary profession. Businesses that are at least managed by veterinarians are more likely than those managed by laymen to reflect independent concerns for patients, clients, and the veterinary profession. Where veterinary hospitals are operated as stand-alone facilities, they are more likely to retain the appearance of a veterinary facility and its ambiance of medical care, and they are less likely to be used as a tool to sell other things.

An especially troublesome argument commonly raised in favor of nonveterinarian ownership is that it can lift the burdens of management from veterinarians, who are then "free" to do what they do best, practice veterinary medicine. Does this mean that veterinarians will no longer choose the equipment they use or the kinds or brands of drugs they dispense? If such decisions are made by nonveterinarians whose interest is solely in the bottom line, is there not a strong possibility that clients and patients will receive what is best for the practice's bottom line, instead of what is best for them? Does removing the "burdens of management" mean that doctors will not set fees, or will be unable to make particular fee or payment arrangements for certain clients? As I argue in Chapter 20, it is important that veterinarians maintain control over fees. Only then can they know that their fees are fair, and will they be able to explain fees confidently and without guilt or embarrassment. Does taking the "burdens of management" away from veterinarians mean having someone else decide what kinds of advertisements the prac-tice will run, whether to offer volume discounts, whether to sell nonveterinary products and services, or whether to perform such services as convenience euthanasia? If so, important ethical decisions involving not just the interests of patients and clients but also the future of the profession will also be taken away from veterinarians.

The lesson of pharmacists

One need not turn to fiction to see what entrepreneurial ownership can do to a profession. One need only look at many of today's so-called "pharmacies."

Not too long ago, pharmacies were owned and operated by pharmacists. Their dominant activity was compounding and dispensing pharmaceuticals. As a convenience, some sold small retail items such as candy and cosmetics. Some had soda counters and offered limited meals. But even these pharmacies had the look and feel of drug stores, because they were owned by local druggists who retained their primary professional function. Many of these pharmacists owned their stores for years and established strong personal and professional ties with their clientele and communities.

Today an increasing number of pharmacies are owned not by pharmacists but by large corporations. Many pharmacists are now salaried employees. These stores now sell a wide range of products, including things (such as cigarettes and sweets) which some people need pharmaceuticals to counteract. Add the cosmetics, magazines, books, auto and home supplies, film developing services, and groceries and the total impression is that of a large retail store only one of whose services is selling pharmaceuticals and health-related products. The next logical step has already been taken: the inclusion of pharmacy departments (and pharmacists) within large grocery stores, department stores, and discount shopping "clubs" that are not even called pharmacies because dispensing drugs constitutes but a small portion of their operation.

This will be the fate of many veterinarians if nonveterinarian ownership expands. Veterinary facilities owned by laymen will not be limited to stand-alone animal hospitals. As of this writing, some pet supply retailers are already opening their own in-store clinics. If this trend continues, like many pharmacists, veterinarians in many of these stores will occupy but one portion of the premises. Their veterinary departments will be immersed in a sea of retail items many of which have nothing to do with animal health (and in all-purpose retail stores, nothing to do with animals). Like many pharmacists, many of these veterinarians will be salaried employees with no opportunity to own the practice—or *any* practice if most veterinary facilities come to be owned by large corporations. I have already asked whether practitioners employed by nonveterinarians will forever exercise sound and independent medical judgment on behalf of patients and clients. Here, I simply wish to ask how many people will think it is worth the time, money, and effort required to become a veterinarian if the most one can hope for is a salaried position in a place that might not even *look* remotely like an animal hospital.

~ ARGUMENTS FOR NONVETERINARIAN OWNERSHIP

Dr. James Wilson believes there are several potential benefits of nonveterinarian ownership. Because these purported benefits appear to reflect an important assumption, it is useful to relate them together. As noted above, Wilson believes that a nonveterinarian-owned corporation which owns 80 practices might reduce costs substantially and free doctors from the tasks of management. He observes that starting a veterinary practice can be expensive and that a practice with today's sophisticated facilities can require more capital than is available to some veterinarians. He argues that in California, which has allowed nonveterinarian ownership for some time, there have not been special problems with nonveterinarian-owned practices, and such practices do not appear to have generated more complaints to the veterinary licensing board. To allay fears that veterinarians would lose control of medical decisions in nonveterinarian-owned practices, Dr. Wilson cites a provision of the *Principles of Veterinary Medical Ethics* which directs veterinarians to be "especially vigilant in ensuring that their professional judgments and responsibilities are neither influenced nor controlled by such nonveterinary individuals to the detriment of the animal patient."[28] He asks how many veterinarians:

> …might like to sell or give away an ownership interest in their practice to a superb technician, receptionist, or office manager as an incentive to stay with the practice long-term and to help it thrive?
>
> Likewise, how many young veterinarians might like to purchase a practice in partnership with a business colleague or friend who has tremendous skills, energy, and desire—and who has considerable cold cash instead of a veterinary educational debt load of $60,000 and an associate veterinarian salary of a mere $35,000. Last, how many [veterinarians] would like their spouses or other family members to have the option of carrying on the management of the practices they have built up over the past 10 to 30 years, instead of being forced to sell after an untimely and unexpected death.[29]

All these predicted benefits of nonveterinarian ownership envision veterinary practices in which veterinarians retain control over medical care or in which values basic to veterinarians appear to remain firmly in place. Indeed, in most of the situations Dr. Wilson imagines, veterinarians retain either majority ownership or substantial control over the entire operation. This would certainly be the case where a doctor transfers a piece of the practice to an employee, or where a young veterinarian is helped by a friend to purchase a practice. One would also expect most family members of a deceased veterinarian owner to have great regard for the profession and to continue the practice accordingly. Even in a large company that owns 80 practices Dr. Wilson pictures the veterinarians exercising independent medical judgment.[19] Wilson's appeal to the *Principles* also presupposes a situation in which veterinarians retain substantial control. It would make no sense to counsel doctors working in nonveterinarian-owned practices to be "especially vigilant" in assuring that professional judgments are not compromised unless they *could*, in fact, resist attempts by owners to make such compromises.

It is surely significant if the state with the largest number of veterinarians has not yet seen abuses attributable to nonveterinarian ownership. However, such evidence does not demonstrate the long-term harmlessness of nonveterinarian controlled corporate practices and clinics in retail stores. Even in California, the history of such practices is still relatively short, and they still constitute a small proportion of that state's veterinary practices.

Perhaps no argument in favor of permitting nonveterinarian ownership is more appealing than the image of the family of a deceased veterinarian that is prohibited from carrying on the practice the doctor labored so hard to establish. There are three problems with this argument. First, it begs the question of how the law *should* view a veterinary practice. States which require veterinarian ownership do not view a practice as an independent asset or piece of property like a house or automobile that can be passed to one's heirs or sold on the open market, but as something ancillary to the activity of practicing veterinary medicine. Second, in fact, few families of deceased veterinarians are as capable of carrying on a practice as was the doctor-owner, which is why such practices (or shares in them) are often sold, or closed. Finally, the law can adequately protect the interests of remaining family members. Thus in states in which only licensed veterinarians can own shares in practices organized as professional corporations, typically a deceased veterinarian's estate, or beneficiaries of the estate, are allowed to maintain ownership long enough for shares to be sold to another veterinarian.

⁓ WHAT SHOULD BE DONE ABOUT NONVETERINARIAN OWNERSHIP?

I believe that it follows from this discussion that nonveterinarians ought not to be allowed by state laws to own veterinary practices. There is no clear need for nonveterinarian ownership. Americans are apparently extremely satisfied with veterinary services,[30] and such satisfaction does not seem to diminish where only veterinarians own veterinary practices. Prohibiting lay ownership may make it more difficult for some doctors to open a practice. Not every practice may be able to afford the most expensive equipment or facilities. A few family members of deceased veterinarians who are not already inclined to do so may have to try to sell to other doctors. A relatively small number of nonveterinarian entrepreneurs may have to find another area in which to make money. These are minor problems compared to the risks of opening the floodgates of ownership to any nonveterinarian or nonveterinarian business. There is in my view no need to subject the profession and the public to these risks, and very strong reasons not to.

At the very least, those states that do not now allow nonveterinarian ownership ought to keep this restriction in place, pending evidence of what will happen in those jurisdictions which allow such ownership. Let us wait and see whether, *over time*, nonveterinarian ownership leads to better or worse veterinary services. With slightly more than half the states now allowing lay ownership we can determine the actual effects of such ownership. Let us see how many practices are opened in retail operations. Let us see if any such operations denigrate the image of veterinarians and their patients and try to manipulate clients. Let us see how the incomes of most veterinarians actually fare when they work for laymen—not in the short term, when corporate owners still need to compete with veterinarian-owned practices for doctors—but in the long run when they control a substantial proportion of available veterinary jobs. Let us see whether nonveterinarian owners step over the line between management and the practice of veterinary medicine. Let us allow nonveterinarian ownership sufficient time to develop into various different manifestations. Given the potential impact on veterinary medicine there is no need for states that prohibit nonveterinarian ownership to rush to change their laws.

⁓ VETERINARIAN-OWNED FACILITIES IN NONVETERINARIAN-OWNED BUSINESSES

At the time of this writing, new hybrid arrangements between veterinarians and retail businesses are beginning to make inroads into the veterinary services market. Large pet retail superstore chains are placing within some of their stores veterinary facilities owned not by the stores themselves, but by independent veterinarian-controlled practices or companies.[31] The brief history of such operations already indicates a wide range of possible arrangements and facilities. A veterinarian-owned practice may lease space in the retail store or may pay the store a percentage of its revenues. Such practices may provide limited vaccination and "wellness" care, or offer a full range of services typical of traditional stand-alone veterinary hospitals. The practices may be owned by veterinarians (or a veterinarian-owned company) dedicated to running many clinics in the stores of a pet supply retailer, by individual veterinarians who limit themselves to owning one practice within one store, or by veterinarians who also own other practices in the community. These veterinary facilities can be located within a store (with the entrance inside the body of the store), off a corridor shared by an entrance to the store, or adjacent to or near the store.

Potential Benefits

Veterinarian-owned facilities associated with retail stores are capable of avoiding the potential problems of nonveterinarian-owned practices pointed out in this chapter. Indeed, such veterinarian-owned facilities may not only be better for clients, patients, and the profession than some traditional-appearing stand-alone veterinary practices owned by laymen. Veterinarian-owned practices within retail stores may be better in certain respects than some practices that are owned by veterinarians.

First, the arguments raised in this chapter against nonveterinarian ownership apply only to nonveterinarian-owned or controlled practices. There is no reason in principle why veterinarian-owned practices in retail stores cannot adhere strongly to traditional veterinary ethical values. Such practices can assure that only doctors make medical decisions or decisions of a managerial nature affecting medical services; accord independent value to the interests of patients and clients; value and protect the status of their doctors; and, in general, identify with the role of the veterinarian as a leader and educator in animal care and welfare. To be sure, veterinarian-owned facilities in retail stores can adhere to the model of veterinary practice as a business, in which case they would be subject to any objections that can be raised to this model of practice. However, such objections can be made to veterinary facilities owned by veterinarians and do not relate specifically to the association of a veterinary hospital with a retail store.

Second, and ironically, veterinarian-controlled facilities in retail stores should find it easier than veterinarian-owned stand-alone practices to avoid the substantial ethical problems associated with the merchandising of nonprofessional goods and services (see Chapter 17). It would be foolish just from an economic standpoint for a veterinary hospital that is associated with, say, a pet supply "superstore" to sell nonprofessional items the retailer could sell more efficiently and cheaply. Indeed, it would be surprising if a store that agreed to associate itself with a veterinarian-owned facility would allow the facility to merchandise nonveterinary products and services the store also sells.

Thus both ethical and economic considerations argue strongly in favor of having veterinarians own and operate veterinary facilities within pet "superstores" and other retail businesses—*if* such retailers believe they must have veterinary facilities in their stores. From a business standpoint, retailers would be able to rely on people who know much better than they how to provide veterinary care; would therefore have a better chance of having satisfied customers for all of their store's operations; would not risk legal problems that could arise from the unlicensed practice of veterinary medicine by lay owners or managers; and would presumably be able to have in-store veterinary facilities in states that limit the ownership of veterinary practices to licensed veterinarians. From an ethical standpoint, leaving the veterinary operations to veterinarians would be better for all the reasons discussed in this chapter.

The best way for veterinarians to assure that the profession and its clients and patients are truly served by veterinary facilities associated with pet "superstores," may be for practitioners to convince such retailers to allow only veterinarians to own these facilities.

Important Issues
Maintaining independence

Although veterinarian-owned clinics associated with superstores can escape objections to nonveterinarian-owned practices, there are several important questions that must still be asked of them.

To avoid the dangers of nonveterinarian influence, doctors who operate clinics in retail businesses must maintain their independence from the stores with which they are associated. Decisions affecting medical care (including the setting of fees) must rest entirely with veterinarian management. There is nothing wrong with the veterinary practice taking advantage of the superior purchasing ability of the retailer to buy physical equipment and some kinds of medical supplies. It can be appropriate for the retailer to charge the veterinary practice a reasonable mark-up on such purchases. However, the retailer should not influence purchase decisions, for example, by offering a kickback to the practice if it agrees to buy items on which the retailer can obtain an especially good deal for itself or by retaining the right to decide what kinds or brands of equipment or supplies the practice shall use. Nor should veterinary facilities which pay the retailer a portion of their revenues permit themselves to be influenced by subtle or unsubtle pressures, for example, by a threat that the arrangement will be terminated unless the clinic expands its services to generate more money for the retailer. Veterinarians should also maintain control over the content and style of advertising for the practice.

No kickbacks for recommendations

Veterinarian-operated clinics in retail businesses should not receive kickbacks from the retailer for purchases (for example, of commercial pet food or grooming services) by clients in the rest of the store. Chapters 9 and 20 discuss why kickbacks are unethical. Soliciting or receiving a kickback in connection with a referral for nonveterinary products is specifically prohibited by the *Principles of Veterinary Medical Ethics*,[32] and by the regulations of several state licensing boards.

Dangers of veterinarian-retailer competition

In theory, independent veterinary facilities located in retail businesses will have a symbiotic relationship; each is supposed to benefit the other by the presence of animal owners. In fact, there is potential for significant competition between the veterinary and retail operations. Many people have limited funds to spend on their animals. Some who are influenced by the retailer's attempts to sell its goods may not have enough money left or may feel less motivated to pay for medical services recommended by the veterinarian.

Likewise, some people may be unable or unwilling to purchase retail goods after visiting the clinic. Sometimes, veterinarians may be medically and ethically obligated to advise clients not to purchase certain items (such as commercial food or pet treats) sold by the retailer, if such products are not in the patient's interests or the patient requires an incompatible medical product (such as a prescription diet). It will be interesting to see how, if such conflicts develop, veterinarians and retailers deal with them. Doctors should not resort to falsehoods or exaggeration to assure that clients leave their money at the clinic. Nor should retailers attempt to neutralize veterinarians' recommendations either by pressuring doctors not to make certain recommendations, or by stepping up promotional efforts to undermine or counteract doctors' recommendations.

Maintaining a dignified and professional atmosphere

Proper regard for the interests of clients, patients, and the profession requires veterinarians to approach all their professional activities in a dignified, tasteful, and elevated manner (see Chapters 17 and 18). Veterinary facilities should have an ambiance suitable for the important decisions of life and death that take place at a hospital. In all its encounters with individual clients and the public, each practice should proclaim respect for clients and animals. Conversely, juvenile, tasteless, degrading, and overly promotional behavior sends the message that animals and their owners are not important and do not deserve the kind of consideration people associate with medicine.

As I note in Chapter 17, pet retail stores can be places of great amusement and even greater promotion. There need be nothing wrong with this. However, even if a veterinary clinic is itself dignified in appearance and behavior, it can take on some of the ambiance of the store in or near which it is located. Protective measures may be required, such as completely separate entrances to store and hospital, or a "buffer zone" of somewhat less promotional activities around the hospital to enable it to maintain its own separate professional atmosphere. It is to be hoped that veterinarian-owned facilities associated with pet supply "superstores" or other kinds of retail businesses can maintain an ambiance which reflects both the independence of veterinarians and their sincere respect for patients and clients.

〜 THE SIGNIFICANCE OF "CHANGE"

Dr. Wilson argues that, whether nonveterinarian ownership is good or bad, the profession must adjust to it, because it is inevitable. He sees a general trend in the economy toward larger, corporate-owned businesses that can raise large amounts of capital. Among the industries which he views as examples of this inevitable change are "large-scale and convenience grocery stores…the optical world…the hotel industry…the automobile servicing industry, and the pharmacy world":

> Let's take off our blinders and open our eyes to the inevitable—that veterinary medicine is about to join the 21st century and that change requires access to far greater capital than currently exists among veterinarians. It also means that, whether we like it or not, and agree or disagree, things will be different than they have been in the past.
>
> What we need to do is adopt an attitude that change, no matter how threatening it may seem to some, will bring with it different risks and benefits for consumers and practice owners. With enough thoughtful, open minded questioning and planning, that difference can be the better for both groups.[29]

Unfortunately, we simply do *not* know whether, even with the most thoughtful questioning, nonveterinarian ownership can be *better* for clients or practice owners. (Nor should we forget the many veterinarians who may never get to be practice owners in a world dominated by large, nonveterinarian-owned corporate practices.) Moreover, the fact that something is a trend or a "change," is irrelevant to whether it is good or bad. Whether nonveterinarian ownership is good or bad is an issue that must be discussed in its own right. If it is good, and a change, it is a good change. If it is bad, and a change, it is a bad change and should be stopped or reversed.

Like claims about "change," assertions of inevitability tend to be a substitute for arguments. For centuries people have been claiming that various economic, social, or political developments were "inevitable." Rarely have these predictions been correct, often because most who made them viewed what *they* wanted as inevitable and hoped—mistakenly—that this piece of unfortunate news would soften the opposition. (Remember the Soviet Union?)

The growth and success of nonveterinarian-owned practices, large corporate non-veterinarian-owned practices or practices located in retail stores are not inevitable. Nonveterinarian ownership can be prohibited by states that choose to do so. In all states, veterinary licensing boards can assure that nonveterinarian owners do not engage in the practice of veterinary medicine. Where nonveterinarian ownership is allowed, veterinarians can battle the "change" in the open field of competition. They can offer alternatives to attempts (whether made by nonveterinarian or veterinarian-owned practices) to denigrate the image and earning power of the profession, to demean its patients, or to "motivate" clients to benefit a corporate bottom line. Veterinarians may be able to convince enough clients that there are good reasons to bring their animals to facilities that are owned, operated, and controlled by veterinary medical doctors. They may be able to convince clients that, wherever they might prefer to buy their groceries or home supplies, there are good reasons to bring their animals to a different kind of place. If enough veterinarians educate the public about the profession's traditional values, even nonveterinarian-owned practices may have to adhere to these values, as a matter of their economic survival.[*]

Veterinarians who defend traditional values and the independence of their profession may prove more than a match for those who see animal medical care as another investment opportunity. One thing is clear—nothing will accelerate any trend toward the model of veterinary practice as an ordinary business more effectively than acceptance by veterinarians of its inevitability.

---

[*]Forces internal to the development of large nonveterinarian-owned corporate practices or "superstore" veterinary facilities might also hinder their success. Some far-flung multi-practice companies could prove less profitable than profit-driven investors would like. Many clients might not find it all that convenient to take their animal to the doctor when shopping for pet supplies, or *vice versa*. Some pet supply retailers (and their in-store veterinarians) might not survive the increasing competition in this industry. Others might find it easier to do competitive battle without potential complications or competition from their own veterinary operations. It might take only a few instances of unprofitable or problem-ridden corporate or superstore practices to frighten investors away from the "business" of veterinary care. Nonveterinarian-owned large corporate practices are a relatively recent phenomenon. Pet "superstores" are even newer, and veterinary facilities within such stores still newer. Only time will tell whether such operations become a major or enduring force in the veterinary services market.

REFERENCES

[1]Herrick JB: The bond of being a veterinarian, *J Am Vet Med Assoc* 191:26-28, 1987.

[2]The American Veterinary Medical Association: *Principles of Veterinary Medical Ethics*, 1993 Revision, "Emergency Service," *1994 AVMA Directory*, Schaumburg, IL, The Association, p 44.

[3]American Veterinary Medical Association: *Principles of Veterinary Medical Ethics*, 1993 Revision, "Therapy, Determination of," *1994 AVMA Directory*, Schaumburg, IL, The Association, p 44.

[4]American Veterinary Medical Association: *Principles of Veterinary Medical Ethics*, 1993 Revision, "Fees for Service," *1994 AVMA Directory*, Schaumburg, IL, The Association, p 43.

[5]Schwabe CW: *Veterinary Medicine and Human Health*, ed 3, Baltimore, 1984, Williams & Wilkins, p 634.

[6]Shomer, RR: Letter, Is there a doctor in the house—or a salesperson in the store? *J Am Vet Med Assoc* 190:245, 1987.

[7]Fried C: Lawyer as friend: The moral foundations of the lawyer-client relation, *Yale Law J* 85:1060-1089, 1976; 86:573-587, 1987.

[8]*All Creatures Great and Small*, New York, 1973, Bantam Books, p 308. Copyright (c) by James Herriot. Quoted with permission from St. Martin's Press, Harold Ober Associates, David Higham Associates, and James Herriot.

[9]Quoted in Enrollment under the knife, *Vet Econ* March 1986:32.

[10]Straw B, Friendship R: Expanding the role of the veterinarian on swine farms, *Compend Contin Educ Pract Vet* 8:F69, 1986.

[11]Interestingly, the title of a regular series of articles in the Compendium of Continuing Education for Practicing Veterinarians was changed from "The Swine Health Advisor" to "Swine Production Management," *Compend Contin Educ Pract Vet* 9(2):101, 1987.

[12]Gove PB,editor: *Webster's Third New International Dictionary*, Springfield, MA, 1961, Merriam, p 666, emphasis supplied.

[13]Radostits OM, Leslie KE, Fetrow J: *Herd Health: Food Animal Production Medicine*, ed 2, Philadelphia, 1994, WB Saunders, p 2.

[14]As discussed in Chapter 9, this provision was removed from the *Principles* in 1989 because of objections by the Federal Trade Commission.

[15]Sollars M: Memo from the Editor, *Vet Econ* February 1987:1. James Herriot remains a favorite target of those who reject more traditional pictures of veterinary practice. Few defenses of the models of veterinary practice as a business or of the veterinarian as economic manager seem to be complete without an unkind reference to the "myth" or supposed "death" of James Herriot (Sollars M: Rest in peace famed James Herriot, *Vet Econ* March 1986:2), or to "the traditional approach…epitomized by the now renowned James Herriot." (Stein TE: Marketing health management to food animal enterprises, *Compend Contin Educ Pract Vet* 7:S330, 1986.) Opponents of more traditional models of practice rightly perceive Herriot's great popularity, among veterinarians as well as the public, as an obstacle to their views. If the arguments of this book are correct, Herriot, who died in 1995, will remain a great moral beacon for the profession for some time to come.

[16]"Storyselling" merchandising display encourages clients to buy products, *DVM* 20(3), March 1989:62.

[17]Becker M: What does it take to get clients to say "yes?" *Vet Econ* March 1994:52-55. Dr. Becker asserts that after people buy on emotion they "then back up their decisions with logic." (p 52) But his discussion does not convincingly demonstrate this contention. He compares buying in the veterinary office to car-shopping and observes that people often buy cars they do not need but emotion tells them to buy. "In the same way, logic tells you that you don't need that dress or that tie in the store window, but emotion tells you to 'go ahead and buy it.' To justify the purchase you say, 'I need a new dress for a special occasion,' 'The tie goes with my navy suit,' or the ever-popular, 'It's on sale.' Sound familiar? The buying-on-emotion phenomenon applies to veterinary practice as well" (p 52). Will clients who are encouraged to buy at the veterinary hospital, such as the people in Dr. Becker's example who buy at the clothing store, always buy what they or their animals really need? How many clothing store salespeople would insist that their customers buy only what they need? How many clothing store salespeople even care whether their customers buy only what they need? Dr. Becker's example illustrates further the impossibility of attaching standard sales practices to an ethic that regards clients as true *friends* and regards as paramount their needs and those of their animals.

[18]*Id*, p 54.

[19]Quoted in Zuziak P: Courtroom scene for debate over ownership of practice facilities, *J Am Vet Met Assoc* 202:1795, 1993.

[20]Verdon D: Ownership: US Circuit Court to decide fate of FTC actions, *DVM* 22(2):1, 1991.

[21]*Parker* v. *Brown*, 317 U.S. 341, 350-351 (1943). *See generally*, Areeda PE, Hovenkamp H: *Antitrust Law 1993 Supplement* Boston, 1993, Little, Brown, pp 128-221

[22]Courtroom scene set for debate over ownership of practice facilities, *J Am Vet Med Assoc* 202:1793-1796, 1993.

[23]*California Retail Liquor Dealers Association* v. *Midcal Aluminum*, 445 U.S. 97 (1980).

[24]This argument would probably lose in a court of law. In 1990 a very important federal appellate court overturned a proposed rule by the FTC to prevent state boards of optometry from restricting the ownership of optometry practices or the employment of optometrists to licensed optometrists. This Court held that such a

restriction was a legitimate exercise of these boards' governmental function of licensing optometrists, even in the absence of specific statutory authorization of the restriction. *California State Board of Optometry* v. *Federal Trade Commission* [1990-2 TRADE CASES ¶ 69,155], 910 F.2d 976 (D.C. Cir. 1990). The FTC decided not to seek appeal of the decision in the U.S. Supreme Court. It can be argued that because the highest court of the land did not endorse this opinion, it is not clearly the law. However, this appellate court has jurisdiction over FTC actions and is regarded as having special expertise in matters of administrative law. Thus even in the absence of a U.S. Supreme Court ruling on the matter, the opinion retains great authority.

[25]Quoted in FTC actions change DVM profession, rules, practice, *DVM* 22(10) October 1991:45.

[26]American Veterinary Medical Association: *Principles of Veterinary Medical Ethics*, 1993 Revision, "Guidelines for Professional Behavior," paragraph 2, *1994 AVMA Directory*, Schaumburg, IL, The Association, p 42.

[27]American Veterinary Medical Association: *Principles of Veterinary Medical Ethics*, 1993 Revision, "Therapy, Determination of," *1994 AVMA Directory*, Schaumburg, IL, The Association, p 44.

[28]American Veterinary Medical Association: *Principles of Veterinary Medical Ethics*, 1993 Revision, "Policy Pertaining to Corporate Ownership and Management of Veterinary Practices," *1994 AVMA Directory*, Schaumburg, IL, The Association, p 45. Dr. Wilson's suggestion that this provision protects patients and clients is unconvincing. The *Principles* do not govern the behavior of nonveterinarian practice owners. Moreover, as noted in Chapter 9, veterinarians facing any allegation of a violation of the code can simply resign their AVMA membership. A lay owner bent on affecting medical decisions need only find employee veterinarans to whom a paycheck is more important than adherence to the *Principles*.

[29]Wilson J: Letter. Nonveterinarian ownership of practice facilities, *J Am Vet Med Assoc* 203:608-609, 1993.

[30]The 1992 comprehensive study of the veterinary service market conducted by the AVMA indicated, for example, that approximately 90% of clients with companion animals are satisfied their current veterinarian. The American Veterinary Medical Association: *The Veterinary Service Market for Companion Animals*, Schaumburg, IL, 1992, The Association, pp 16-17.

[31]*See*, for example, Lofflin J: Who is Dr. Scott Campbell and why is he bringing full-service veterinary care to PETsMART? *Vet Econ* June 1994:26-43; Stultz TB: Petstuff to offer wellness care, *DVM* 25(8):22, 1994.

[32]American Veterinary Medical Association: *Principles of Veterinary Medical Ethics*, 1993 Revision, "Commissions, Rebates, and Influences on Judgment," *1994 AVMA Directory*, Schaumburg, IL, The Association, p 43.

PART THREE

Problems and Issues in Veterinary Ethics

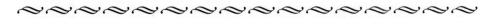

CHAPTER 17

The Sale of Nonprofessional Goods and Services

Toward the Choice of a Model of Veterinary Practice

*M*any ethical issues are forcing veterinarians to choose among different models of practice. None has created more controversy within the profession, or is more crucial to its self-definition, than the question of how far veterinarians may go in order to generate revenues. Different commercial activities raise different ethical concerns. This chapter focuses upon the selling of nonprofessional goods and services. Chapter 18 considers marketing techniques in veterinary practice. Chapter 19 discusses competition among veterinarians.

∼ THE MERCHANDISING OF PRODUCTS
What Is Merchandising?

Merchandising can be defined as the selling of a product or service not involved in or necessitated by the direct medical care of a patient.[1] Merchandising in this sense is different from "dispensing," which refers to the sale or supply of products (for example, drugs or pesticides) to clients for medical reasons by veterinarians, or by their facilities under their direct order.

Merchandising can include the sale of nonprofessional products such as ordinary commercial pet food, toys, bedding, and clothing. Merchandising can also encompass selling an ordinarily professional product for other than legitimate medical reasons. This can occur where a doctor has been given oral information by a client insufficient to justify dispensing a product for medical reasons, where a client insists on purchasing a product for his own reasons, or where a doctor simply wants to make some money. Merchandising also includes selling professional products to people who have no professional relationship with the practitioner.

As I use the term, "merchandising" is distinct from marketing, which can be defined as the promotion of one's services or goods to the public or to other veterinarians. It is possible to market without engaging in merchandising, by promoting purely professional services. One can merchandise professional or nonprofessional products without marketing, by selling them with a minimum of promotion and within the confines of one's office.

It is important to understand the distinction between merchandising and market-ing. Some veterinarians erroneously interpret arguments against the former as criti-cisms of the latter. I shall argue that although merchandising by veterinarians is usually objectionable, many forms of marketing can be ethical.

When Are Products "Medical" or "Professional?"

Virtually anything a veterinarian might sell could, under certain circumstances, have a direct and legitimate medical purpose and therefore not be a "merchandised" product. For example, a fabric halter might be indicated medically for a dog that has been injured by a metal collar. Nevertheless, few people would be inclined to say that halters, scratching posts, beds, sweaters, conditioning shampoos, or any of a myriad of other things that could under special circumstances be of medical importance, ordinarily are professional products.

It might not always be clear whether a product ought to be characterized as med-ical/professional. Moreover, insofar as merchandising is perceived to be profitable, there will be a tendency to categorize ambiguous products as generically medical/profession-al in nature—and thereby sweep them within the veterinarian's traditional role as a dis-penser rather than merchandiser. For example, one discussion recommends the sale of "fly repellents, pet colognes, spot removers, medicated shampoos, vitamins, coat condi-tioners, and chew bones" on the grounds that "most of these products are health-relat-ed and not only help improve our income but help provide a one-stop service for the client as well."[2] There has long been a strong push among proponents of merchandis-ing to classify ordinary, commercial pet food as a "nutritional," and therefore a medical or quasimedical, product. Thus one advocate of the sale of such foods recommends calling the waiting room display of these products the "nutrition center." Doctors are urged to include brochures about "feeding pets during the different stages of their lives; this will help educate clients as to what foods, vitamins, and minerals are necessary. …Then, when clients come into your exam room, you can ask what the dog or cat is being fed and remind clients about the nutrition information and foods."[3]

This example shows that although it generally may be useful to distinguish between the merchandising of medical/professional and nonmedical/nonprofessional products, in considering the appropriateness of merchandising, one should not become fixated on the question of how to define what is a medical/professional product. This is a difficult ques-tion that is not entirely ethical in nature: it relates to, among other things, the issue of whether the healing professions ought to be as concerned with preventing as curing disease and therefore ought to consider such things as nutritious food to be a medical product.

The major ethical question regarding merchandising is not whether veterinarians may morally *recommend* a number of things that are good for patient health or well-being. The issue is whether veterinarians may morally *sell* items that generally can be sold by nonveterinarians—because these items are not directed toward a specific med-ical condition, do not generally cause medical problems if misused, or do not require continuing medical supervision.* To facilitate discussion, I shall refer to all such items

---

*The "sale" and "selling" of nonmedical products are not restricted to instances in which a client takes possession of the products at the veterinarian's facility. A doctor who recommends nonprofessional items that are purchased elsewhere, in return for a commission or other kind of monetary benefit from the manufacturer or sales outlet, would be engaged in the sale, and merchandising, of these products. So would a veterinarian who receives payment from the manufacturer for taking orders for nonprofessional products that are delivered by the manufacturer directly to clients. Receiving a commission, rebate, or kickback, even for the sale of a nonprofessional product, is unethical (see Chapters 9, 14, and 20).

as "nonprofessional" or "nonmedical." There still might be some dispute about whether certain things should be categorized as nonprofessional items in this sense. However, ordinary commercial (that is, nonprescription) food, as well as such products as water bowls, clothing, grooming accessories (brushes, combs, perfumes, etc.), bedding, and toys clearly should be included in such a definition of "nonprofessional" products.

The Argument against the Merchandising of Professional Products

It is not difficult to appreciate why merchandising medical products is wrong. By definition, such products require dispensing by a veterinarian to protect the patient, and often the client and other persons. A veterinarian who merchandises medical products can cause patients to become ill and clients to suffer economic, physical, or psychological damage. He also endangers his own interests. Because it involves the sale of a medical product without a legitimate medical reason, merchandising medical products is negligent veterinary practice. It can subject a doctor to legal action by a client or one's state veterinary board.

The *Principles of Veterinary Medical Ethics* unequivocally condemn the merchandising of medical or professional products.[4] There appears to be little opposition in the profession to this prohibition, at least in principle. However, there are things veterinarians do that ordinarily are medically appropriate but can cross over the line between legitimate dispensing and merchandising. One such practice is diagnosing and prescribing over the telephone. If a doctor knows the animal and client, this can be perfectly appropriate medical practice but without adequate first-hand information, it can constitute merchandising of professional services or products. Among other practices that under certain circumstances (but not always) can constitute merchandising are selling clients professional items by mail order upon their written or telephone requests; dispensing enough medication to be used over an extended period of time on the patient; supplying additional amounts of a medication without examining the animal to determine whether the drug is still indicated; and permitting one's receptionist to sell professional items (such as prescription diets) originally dispensed for medical reasons without having current knowledge about the animal's condition.

The merchandising of professional products need not be motivated by greed, although it can be. A doctor who merchandises a medical product might believe sincerely that she is acting in the interests of patients and clients. What characterizes the merchandising of professional items is inadequate familiarity with the patient. Therefore it will sometimes be more appropriate to describe the merchandiser of a medical item as negligent rather than unscrupulous. But whether negligent or mercenary, the merchandising of professional products is ethically objectionable.

The Argument against the Merchandising of Nonprofessional Products

There are few controversies in the profession more intensely fought than that involving the propriety of merchandising nonprofessional products. The literature is fairly bursting with defenses and denunciations of the practice.[5]

I have suggested that problems in normative veterinary ethics should be approached, at least initially, by considering how various alternative solutions would affect the legitimate interests of all concerned (see Chapter 10). Such an analysis, I submit, argues *very strongly* against the merchandising of nonprofessional products, at least by the great majority of veterinarians.

The interests of veterinarians: Is it profitable?

The argument raised most often in favor of merchandising nonprofessional products is increased profits. There is no shortage of reports about practitioners who have made a great deal of money engaging in such merchandising.[6]

However, the question for the profession is not whether some veterinarians have increased their revenues through merchandising, but rather whether, for the profession *as a whole and in the long run*, merchandising will prove profitable.

As the late Dr. Robert Knowles observed,[1] it is far from clear that merchandising will increase the incomes of most practitioners. Merchandising nonprofessional products has a relatively small profit margin. Ordering, storing, displaying, and selling such products requires time and space that might be devoted to professional services. Moreover, most businesses that move large quantities of pet products (such as supermarkets, animal feed and supply stores, grooming establishments, and the new pet supply "superstores") are far better merchandisers than veterinarians. Once such establishments perceive that veterinarians are making inroads into their profits, they can quickly undercut veterinarians' prices. They can use their advertising and marketing expertise to make even the most ambitious veterinary "nutrition center" or pet product display an unprofitable nightmare.

Since the publication of the first edition of this text, quite a few doctors have reported to me that they no longer sell commercial pet food because they found it unprofitable, or just not worth the time and effort. Interestingly, many also concede that after they began to doubt whether selling these products was in *their* interest, they questioned whether the practice is good for clients and patients. Dr. Ronald Whitford, a successful practice owner and respected management consultant, writes that he has discontinued selling nonprescription food because (1) today, unlike in the past, the food he can sell is no better than that available commercially; (2) he cannot compete with retailers in his area and maintain a satisfactory markup; and (3) the business of selling nonprescription foods requires marketing, storage space, allocation of staff, and paperwork that detract from his ability to practice veterinary medicine. Dr. Whitford was led to these conclusions by ethical as well as management considerations:

> We need to fully weigh the marketing potential of pet food and look carefully at all the possible side effects. It's all not positive. For example, do clients really view us as salesmen when we're selling them a product? We'd be better off developing a working relationship with pet industry professionals in our communities. By increasing their volume, we in fact help our clients by making these products much more available and affordable.
>
> Ten years ago, providing food to our clients was important. In my opinion, we're doing both our client and the pet a disservice when we go into the exam room today and spend one-third of the 15 minute office visit trying to sell a bag of dog food.[7]

The most dangerous potential result of the merchandising of nonprofessional products is the erosion of the model of the veterinarian as healer and of the image of veterinary patients as beings entitled to first-class medical care. These views of veterinarians and their patients did not spring into existence overnight. It has taken the profession generations to improve its scientific base and the techniques, drugs, and services it can offer to animal owners. The profession has also labored hard to inculcate in the public an appreciation of the value and importance of pets as well as other animals. It did so long before the popularity of the concept of the "human-companion animal bond" or even before the advent of modern veterinary drugs and techniques. It did so by discouraging crass commercialism and insisting that veterinarians strive as far as possible to approach their animal patients with much the same dignity and professionalism people expect from physicians.

Veterinarians can now take advantage of this fortunate confluence of advancing veterinary science, traditional professionalism, and an enhanced appreciation of animals to improve revenues. People who care greatly about their animals and who consider veterinary medicine a calling as worthy and scientifically advanced as medicine will pay for competent and caring veterinary services.

However, it would be a grave mistake for veterinarians to take high regard for their profession for granted. Many people still do not look upon veterinarians as "real" doctors. As all veterinarians know, for every animal owner who seeks high-quality veterinary services, there are many who do not. There is still much more work to be done to convince animal owners and society at large of the value of veterinarians and their animal patients.

The routine merchandising of nonprofessional products threatens to reverse this continuing elevation of the veterinarian and the potential for profitability this elevation promises. What would we think of a pediatrician who might sell bassinets, baby bottles, and tricycles, or of an internist who peddled exercise equipment or granola? Aside from immediate revulsion, we would suspect that they do not consider themselves, or their medical areas of expertise, to be good or valuable enough to enable them to earn a decent living. We would also think that they are more interested in their own monetary gain than in helping their patients. We would say that they are showing their patients great disrespect.

Such reactions are not attributable just to the historical fact that physicians happen to have been able to survive without merchandising nonmedical products. These reactions stem from our fundamental belief that the physician's power over matters of life and death, and health and illness is so important that medical care must be approached in a dignified manner and with as few trappings of commercialism as possible. We afford physicians an elevated status because of the importance we attribute to ourselves, their patients, and the momentous reasons for which we seek their assistance.

Veterinarians who merchandise nonprofessional products tell their clients and the public not to be offended by commercialism in the veterinary context. They send the message that animal health and disease, pain and suffering, and life and death are not important enough to be separated from ordinary commercial activities. In fact, they promote precisely the view that has prevented veterinarians from achieving the respect long afforded physicians and dentists—the view that a veterinarian's patients are "only animals." As Dr. Robert M. Miller warns:

> …excessive concentration on selling products instead of rendering professional services is incompatible with the image that guarantees success for the practitioner. Unfortunately, we are so influenced by some colleagues and other professionals in the business world or in industry that we're progressively losing our identity as a learned, scientific profession, dedicated to the

control of disease in animals. If we lose that identity by causing the public to see us as salespersons, merchants, pet-shop proprietors, or anything else but doctors of veterinary medicine, it will cause us irreparable harm.[8]

Ironically, the veterinarian-merchandiser is also mounting a direct assault against the profession's most powerful marketing tool, the human-companion animal bond itself. For if the bond means anything at all, it implies that many animals ought to be given love, respect, and dignified medical care, in virtue of their great worth and importance. There is hard evidence that dignified veterinary practice can be profitable.[9] Practitioners who treat animals that are increasingly coming to be seen as beings of great worth and value are doing better. People, especially those with small animals and horses, are willing to pay for first-rate veterinary care.

The interests of veterinarians: Beyond profits

The potential for increased revenues, however, does not constitute the only, or indeed the most important, reason for concluding that the merchandising of nonprofessional products is not in the interests of the profession as a whole. As Dr. Robert Shomer has observed,[10] veterinarians receive many nonmonetary benefits from placing greater emphasis on professional services than on material award. They can rest assured that they are indeed serving the interests of their patients, clients, and society. They also benefit from perceiving themselves, and from being perceived, as true professionals who by virtue of special training, skill, and service deserve a special kind of respect and admiration afforded only to the few. If veterinarians sometimes must choose between their heritage of professionalism and acting like ordinary storekeepers to make some extra dollars, it still remains very much in their interests to choose professionalism.

The interests of clients and patients: From service to manipulation?

There are also many reasons why the merchandising of nonprofessional products is not in the interests of most clients and their animals.

First, such products will usually cost clients more at veterinary facilities than at retail stores, especially large chain operations that buy in great bulk and pass their savings along to consumers. On items purchased infrequently, the difference might be trivial. But on pet food, a client could pay substantially more over an animal's life by buying from a veterinarian. This money could be used for other worthy purposes, including veterinary care. Supporters of merchandising frequently claim that clients are getting their extra money's worth in the expertise of the veterinarian and in the convenience of being able to buy pet items when they are at their veterinarian. These are spurious arguments. Many nonprofessional items require no veterinarian recommendation or advice. Regarding others (such as pet foods), veterinarians can still recommend without actually selling; this approach would enable clients to benefit both from lower prices and professional recommendations. In fact, convenience argues for the selling of nonprofessional items in supermarkets or department stores, which most people frequent far more often than their veterinarian.

Aside from increased costs to clients, there are potentially darker sides of veterinary merchandising that can make it quite manipulative. Some clients will undoubtedly buy such things as toys or snacks because they feel guilty they have made their animal endure an examination or treatment. Veterinarians should not take advantage of such fictional anthropomorphizing by clients. Some merchandisers will surely fall prey to the temptation of appealing to the model of the veterinarian as healer—a model that rejects commercialism—to sell nonmedical items. This may be accomplished by playing upon the belief of most clients that veterinarians do not recommend things for their own monetary gain but to benefit patients and clients. Even if a veterinarian does not consciously appeal to the image of a healer for monetary gain, the client may still be influenced into buying something because the doctor recommends it. (Of course, merchandising will eventually kill the goose that can lay these golden eggs. For once clients come to see veterinarians as shopkeepers rather than doctors, they will not be so impressed by product recommendations.) Finally, because the primary motive for merchandising nonmedical items is profit, there is a distinct danger that merchandisers will push a particular product or brand not because it is the best one for their patients but because it yields a higher profit for themselves.

Some veterinarians will insist that they can merchandise without manipulating clients. However, once one begins to accept maximization of profit as a legitimate aim of one's practice, one is subjected to enormous pressure to push clients to do things they would not otherwise consider. This is sometimes the only way to persuade customers to part with as much money as they can be motivated to spend. For example, among the techniques recommended by one discussion are the following:

> Use wood shelving wherever possible to promote a look of warmth and permanency.
> Line up at least two consecutive rows of each item if possible; grocery stores use this technique to attract the eye of hurried customers.[11]

Another proponent of waiting room displays reports that in:

> …a recent survey conducted by the Point of Purchase Institute regarding the purchase of pet accessories, nearly 80% of those questioned stated that they did not plan on making that purchase…five minutes before they did. What does this tell you? Pet accessories are primarily an impulse sale. Did you ever wonder why your local supermarket crams all those candy bars, safety razors, nylons, and magazines at the checkout stand? You guessed it. Idle minds make for impulse spending.[12]

Dr. Martin Becker has offered an incisive characterization of the goals and methods of successful merchandising.[13] Merely displaying products, he points out, might have been:

> …adequate in the "old days" when people bought solely based on *need*.
> Today's consumers are drastically different, however. They have a lot of discretionary income and buy based on *desire*. Rather than just showing them what's for sale, we must tell a motivational story to encourage them to buy now. Please reread that last sentence, because it's vitally important that you understand it if you ever hope to grasp the real importance of merchandising.

One who wishes to motivate a purchase does not, as Dr. Becker observes, rest content with selling what consumers might *already* want. Selling involves *stimulating desires*—bringing already existing (but perhaps not clearly articulated) desires to the fore, or creating new desires. This is done partly by sending explicit, implied, or sometimes even subliminal messages that, in their totality, say to a customer "Buy *this*! Buy this *now!*" Thus Dr. Becker recommends employing the smallest possible peg hooks and shelves:

> This makes the display look full...Consumers like to buy from well stocked displays. The merchandise appears to be popular and bought in large enough quantities to get good prices. Empty displays signify defective merchandise, close-outs, or poor buying power.

Perhaps the most interesting of Dr. Becker's recommendations is the use of human physiology:

> Display the largest size of product on the right and graduate down to the left. This is called right-hand merchandising. Because more people are right handed it encourages consumers to reach for the largest size.

Dr. Becker is entirely correct that the most successful retailers do not restrict their efforts to logical argument directed at the needs of potential customers. These retailers know that, unlike the reasoned recognition of a need, desires can be impulsive, irrational, and unreasonable. To stimulate desires, therefore, a successful retailer may be able to use subtle suggestion and innuendo. If a retailer actually told customers they are getting a good price on an item, he might or might not be telling the truth, and he might have to demonstrate to particular customers why, for them, an item represents good value. A retailer can avoid these problems by merely leading customers to *think* they are getting a good price because the merchandise *appears* to be bought by the store in large quantities. Instead of having to demonstrate the merits of a particular product, a retailer can make it *appear* that a product is popular, and hope that customers associate popularity with quality and satisfaction. Instead of having to demonstrate the merits of a particular size of a product, a retailer can try to take advantage of a tendency to reach for the right, so that the largest size will be chosen, whether or not this is what any particular customer actually needs.

Veterinarians might ask themselves a few questions. Is this how clients should be approached? What will happen if clients ever *learn* that this is how veterinarians attempt to "encourage them to buy now?" Will they come to think of the veterinary office as just one more place where someone is trying to separate them from their money? Will such a perception make it easier or more difficult to persuade clients of the necessity of medical services for their animals? Will the veterinarian-retailers of the future long for the "old days," when people were called (and thought of themselves as) clients and not customers, when clients brought their animals to a veterinary hospital and not a store, and when clients assumed that if their veterinarian recommends something, they and their animal must really need it? Will veterinarian-retailers of the future long for the "old days" when clients came to the hospital with the question "Doctor, what would you do if this were your animal?" instead of the phrase "*Caveat emptor*" (Let the buyer beware)?

Arguments of Merchandisers

Because there is significant support among veterinarians for merchandising nonmedical products, it is useful to consider briefly some of arguments commonly offered in its favor.

"Merchandising does not compromise my skills."

One argument is that it is possible to sell nonmedical items and still provide highly skilled veterinary services.[14] As I have argued, this is a dubious proposition regarding some doctors, who will have to expend time and money that could otherwise be spent practicing or improving technical skills. However, even if merchandising did not affect technical ability, this would not defeat the argument I have made against it. The most important issue raised by merchandising is not one of skill, but whether veterinarians want to be perceived as doctors or storekeepers. Auto mechanics and plumbers can be extremely skilled and still merchandise. However, these tradespeople do not occupy the same position of admiration and respect accorded to medical professionals. Perhaps some technically skilled veterinarian-merchandisers will be able to make a good living. But ultimately they will not occupy the elevated status of healers and will not benefit from the many advantages that this status can bring.

"I can't be a physician and should not feel guilty or inferior about it."

Some supporters of merchandising accept the fact that their position is incompatible with the high level of professionalism we expect of physicians, but maintain that it is foolish for veterinarians to think they can ever be like physicians. Veterinarians, it is said, should accept the fact that they are veterinarians. They should realize that their rung on the professional ladder is not incompatible with merchandising. Those practitioners who resist merchandising are diagnosed as frustrated physicians who are attempting to hide their feelings of inferiority by espousing unattainable professional ideals. As one supporter of merchandising puts it, "if these insecure, ultraprofessional veterinarians want to look, act, feel, and smell like a physician, why didn't they go to medical school?"[15]

The notion that veterinarians cannot be perceived as occupying as elevated a status as physicians is just inaccurate. Many people already regard veterinarians at least as highly as physicians.[16] To be sure, veterinary patients are animals, and animals will never be regarded as the equals of human beings. Therefore veterinarians can never expect to be viewed exactly as are physicians. But it hardly follows that veterinarians should not behave in many important respects as do physicians.

The detractors of "ultraprofessionalism" are themselves making a fundamental conceptual mistake. They are the ones who begin with a picture of the physician as the purest and most exalted practitioner of the healing arts. They then measure veterinarians against this model. They believe that other veterinarians who want to behave in certain ways as do physicians must also be measuring themselves against physicians. And because the merchandisers understand that there cannot be a complete fit between this pure physician model and veterinary practice, they attribute some misunderstanding or psychological infirmity to veterinarians who strive to apply some of the ideals of human medicine to veterinary medicine.

In fact, there is no need to measure veterinarians against some idealized picture of physicians. What is obligatory or ideal in veterinary practice will flow from features of veterinary practice itself. Sometimes, these features will demand of veterinarians kinds of behavior one would expect of physicians; sometimes they will not. If veterinarians should behave similarly to physicians in certain respects and under certain circumstances, it does not follow that they are to this extent approaching closer to being physicians. It means that veterinarians share certain moral obligations and ideals with another healing profession. The fact that veterinarians might want to appeal to medicine, dentistry, law, or other learned professions to illuminate issues in veterinary ethics does not mean that they are striving to be members of any of these other professions.

"My clients don't mind my selling nonprofessional products."

Another argument made by supporters of merchandising is that their clients do not find the practice offensive and do not have a lowered image of them as professionals because they merchandise. Studies have not yet been done regarding how the merchandising of nonprofessional products affects the public's image of veterinarians. There are, surely, many clients who will stay away from practices that merchandise. Other clients might dislike merchandising but might remain with a practice out of convenience or because they like a particular doctor. The fact that merchandisers can maintain or even increase their client base does not prove that clients in general accept merchandising, but only that there are some clients who do not mind it and some who do not mind it enough to go elsewhere.

Let us grant for the purposes of argument that some veterinary clients do not find the merchandising of nonprofessional products offensive or unprofessional. If this is so, it would only show that in the minds of these people, veterinary medicine is still not regarded as belonging on the same level of professionalism as medicine or dentistry. This should surprise no one. Every practitioner has seen clients who do not regard their animals, or veterinarians, with great admiration or respect. Other clients might be accustomed to a view of veterinarians that distinguishes them from "real" doctors, and therefore might forgive them a kind of commercialism they would not tolerate in physicians or dentists.

The issue for the profession is whether it wants to foster an image of veterinary practice that so elevates the practitioner, the patient, and the client, that selling nonprofessional products will be considered offensive by clients and the public.

"Merchandising nonmedical pet products is necessary in today's market."

The argument raised most frequently in support of merchandising is that it is forced upon practitioners by current market conditions, especially the influx of new graduates into the profession. Indeed, it is common to hear that unless they sell nonprofessional products, practitioners will be committing economic suicide.[15]

If the profession as a whole really had to choose between merchandising and extinction, one would have to tolerate merchandising, however offensive it might be. It would be wrong to insist on a prohibition that would force the profession to close down. That would cause great harm not just to doctors but also to clients and animals.

There might be some doctors who must choose between merchandising and economic suicide, but I have yet to find a small animal practitioner who can make the case convincingly. A practitioner's economic "suicide" would mean more than that one's present practice cannot survive but that one cannot practice veterinary medicine anywhere. Moreover, to show that a particular practice faces the choice between merchandising and suicide, not only must it be shown that the practice will literally fold without the sale of nonmedical products. It must also be the case that nothing else can be done to cut costs or increase revenues to keep the practice afloat. If a practice requires the sale of commercial pet food or leashes to survive, it is surely already in very bad shape.

In fact, almost all veterinarians who claim that they "must" merchandise nonprofessional products mean either that they cannot maintain present income levels without merchandising, or that they cannot make as much money as they would like without merchandising. There are two appropriate responses to these claims.

First, as discussed in Chapter 18 most veterinarians have at their disposal an enormous range of potential professional services that can be used to maintain or increase revenues. Moreover, these professional options can be promoted by a wide range of professionally dignified marketing techniques.

Second, it might just be the case that the ethical standards of the profession place limitations on what some practitioners can earn. In this regard, veterinary medicine is no different from any of the other professions, each of which prohibits certain activities that could arguably earn its members more money. (Lawyers, for example, are not permitted to encourage their clients to commit crimes so that they can earn a fee defending these clients.) Some veterinarians appear to believe that their profession is treated especially badly by the marketplace and for that reason, is entitled to engage in merchandising to bring incomes to higher levels. But in fact there are many valuable and hard-working professionals (including public school teachers, college professors, nurses, social workers, government attorneys, and public hospital physicians) who probably will never earn what most veterinarians can. The U.S. economic system does give veterinarians who want significant economic reward the opportunity to try to attain it. However, there is no guarantee that veterinarians' income will reflect their moral worth or value to society.

A Possible Exception: Merchandising of Nonprofessional Products by Farm and Food Animal Practitioners

The argument against merchandising nonmedical products turns in large measure on the worth and importance of the veterinary patient. Among those kinds of animals that most people would regard as sufficiently important to merit dignified care are dogs, cats, caged birds, and other family pets, as well as many pleasure, show, and race horses. However, some veterinary patients are not regarded, and are never likely to be regarded, with great love, admiration, or respect. A draft horse or dairy cow might be an object of affection for some owners, but it is more often viewed as an economic asset. Cattle, chickens, pigs, sheep, and goats produce—or indeed can themselves become—products in the marketplace.

A veterinarian who treats such animals need be no less skilled or dignified than a small animal practitioner. But the patients of these doctors are themselves components of commerce. It seems paradoxical to ask veterinarians whose very professional activity is aimed at putting products into the stream of commerce to refrain from "engaging in commercialism" connected with the merchandising of nonmedical products.

Additional arguments can be made in favor of merchandising of nonprofessional items by farm animal practitioners. Much of large animal practice, like the industry it serves, is economically depressed, and additional sources of revenue might well be imperative. Moreover, although some farm animal practitioners decry this fact, many farmers do not want their veterinarian to be the sole dispenser of medical goods or services. Some clients purchase medical items from nonveterinarians and medicate their animals themselves; others want to be able to administer medications left by the doctor. Farm animal practitioners may rightly wonder whether it makes sense for them to restrict themselves to dispensing medical products if their clients do not even regard them as the sole source of medical items.

These arguments do, I believe, provide some support for the view that farm and food animal veterinarians may merchandise nonmedical products. However, there are also counterarguments.

First, even if it does not appear inherently offensive for farm animal practitioners to merchandise, the profession as a whole might still have a strong interest in arguing against such merchandising. For merchandising by farm animal doctors could make it difficult for other veterinarians, who today make up the great majority of the profession, to convince the public that merchandising in their kinds of practices is inappropriate.

Second, to be successful, merchandising in farm animal practice might have to involve the kinds of activities recommended by the model of the veterinarian as economic manager (see Chapter 16). There probably is not a great deal of money to be made selling occasional farm implements or food supplements; successful merchandising to farm clients might require large-scale sales of feed and equipment necessary for sizable herd management programs. However, such activities might in the long run injure the interests of many veterinarians, clients, and farm animals. Veterinarian merchandising of nonmedical items might make it even more difficult for doctors to convince clients that veterinarians should administer medicines—and thus could reduce revenues that practitioners would otherwise gain from providing professional services. Additionally, many food and farm animal practitioners are just not trained to provide the kinds of services required of a large-scale economic manager.[17] Other doctors might find the model of the veterinarian as economic manager esthetically displeasing or morally unsatisfactory. Widespread adoption of the model could drive into extinction many of these traditional, hands-on, medicine-oriented practitioners. This could harm not only these doctors but also clients who want or can afford the kinds of services they have been providing.

As the 1987 *AVMA Report on the United States Market for Food Animal Veterinary Medical Services* acknowledged, much investigation is required before the profession can determine "what services are needed by producers and how veterinarians can economically deliver those services."[17] Time will tell whether the economic survival of food and farm animal practice requires significant merchandising of nonmedical goods and services, and whether practitioners who engage in such merchandising can do so with a level of professionalism that is consistent with the interests of the profession as a whole.

ᔒ THE FOUR PHASES OF VETERINARY MERCHANDISING

Veterinarians who take up merchandising should understand that they do not just participate in behavior that threatens the interests of clients, patients, and the profession. Every small animal doctor who retails nonprofessional products could be contributing to a much larger historical process. This process might result in consequences far beyond what doctors who merchandise intend or would find acceptable. The ultimate outcome of this process could be the end of veterinary practice as we have known it.

There will, I believe, be four phases of development that flow from the merchandising of nonprofessional products and services. Each phase follows logically from the phase preceding it. All follow logically from the single principle that veterinary practice may include the retailing of nonprofessional goods and services.

Phase One: The Sale of Patient-Related Nonprofessional Products and Services by Veterinarians

We have already considered the first phase of merchandising: the sale of nonveterinary products that are related to animal health, welfare, or happiness, or to the enjoyment members of the public derive directly from their animals. Although such items as ordinary nonprescription diets, water bowls, and pet toys are not medical in nature at least they pertain to the animals clients bring to the veterinary facility. It is this fact, indeed, which has allowed merchandising to gain acceptance among many veterinarians. For these doctors can say, truthfully, that merchandising is still part of their overriding purpose to help their patients.

Nevertheless, veterinarians who participate in this first phase of merchandising have taken the critical psychological and ethical steps that will lead to Phase Four. As Dr. Robert M. Miller puts it so well, these veterinarians themselves have "blurred the line" between their status as a medical professional and ordinary commercial retailing.[8] They have accustomed themselves to working in an environment that is not dedicated solely to animal health. They also send a signal to the public, and to nonveterinary commercial retailers, that there is nothing special—nothing sacrosanct and inviolable—about the practice of veterinary medicine that would prevent its intermixture with ordinary retailing.

Once these steps are taken by the profession as a whole the rest, as the saying goes, is history.

Phase Two: The Sale of Non-Patient-Related Nonprofessional Products and Services by Veterinarians

If veterinarians accept retailing of nonprofessional items as part of a process of serving client convenience, there is no reason in principle why all the nonprofessional items they sell should relate directly to clients' animals. In the second phase of merchandising, veterinarians will supplement their stock of patient-related items with goods that are not related to their clients' animals or may not be related to animals at all. This phase may begin with the retailing of products that have an animal theme, such as greeting cards with animals or stuffed animal dolls. But again, there is no reason in principle why retailing must restrict itself to animal-related matters, so long as one can offer something people who come in with their animals are willing to buy.

One practitioner reports success supplementing animal-related nonprofessional products (such as toys, pet treats, food dishes, shampoos, and kitty litter) with what he calls "human interest" items:

> Stuffed animals, key chains, items that will interest a client, such as sweat shirts with an animal on it. We even offer a photo studio at our center. …
>
> To display your products, I do not recommend the pegboard. Remember, you are not a pet shop. I use slapboard which gives a professional appearance. The products I offer are higher-priced items. Homemade collector's items are a big seller, like some stuffed bears which cost $300

and give me the feel of class. They all sold. I just purchased a life-sized dog from Europe. They are absolutely gorgeous and sell for $695. I had several sell for Christmas.[18]

Phase Three: The Sale of Veterinary Professional Products and Services by Animal-Oriented Commercial Retailers

In 1991 a large national grocery chain announced that its pharmacies in Maryland would begin selling pet vaccination kits to the general public. These kits, containing a hypodermic syringe with distemper, hepatitis, leptospirosis, parainfluenza, and parvovirus vaccine, were priced at $4.99. Each kit came with a set of instructions, and pharmacists were available to answer questions of pet owners about how to administer the vaccines. The Maryland Veterinary Medical Association objected to the planned sale of vaccines, which, according to an article in the *Baltimore Sun*, were available in 61 pharmacies owned by the grocery chain in the middle Atlantic states as well as its stores in the Phoenix area. Maryland veterinarians called on the chain to stop selling the vaccines because of risks to pets as well as to people who could use the cheap syringes for their own drug habits. The vaccination kits did not, however, violate Maryland law, which required only that consumers who purchase syringes show identification and sign a register book.[19]

In 1993 the New Jersey VMA succeeded in temporarily suspending a mobile vaccination clinic to be held at a pet supply "superstore" in Paramus. The city health officer canceled the clinic because the Pennsylvania-based vaccination service did not hold a required New Jersey medical waste generator's license. The superstore promptly applied for the license and moved to make arrangements to comply with the state veterinary practice act requirements relating to emergency coverage, record-keeping, and veterinarian-client relationships. At this point, there was nothing the state veterinarians could do to stop the clinic.[20]

Many veterinarians are outraged by such incursions by commercial retailers into the area of animal health. However, all veterinarians should understand that this is but the next phase in the development of merchandising: the retailing of veterinary medical services—and the employment of veterinarians—by nonveterinarian retailers whose businesses are animal-related. Veterinarians who merchandise pet clothing, toys, food, and assorted nonmedical paraphernalia have themselves blurred the line between veterinary practice and ordinary commercial retailing. They then step over the line into the new territory to compete with pet shops, pet "superstores," department stores, and supermarkets by retailing items traditionally sold by such businesses. These veterinarians should not be surprised when retailers take advantage of the same blurred line to compete with veterinarians by providing services traditionally offered by veterinarians. Veterinarians cannot have it both ways. They cannot seek to compete with retailers by claiming that veterinary medicine is "just another business" and then appeal to their special status as *doctors,* as protectors of animal and public *health,* when commercial retailers accept the challenge.

If retail stores sell pet vaccines or offer vaccination clinics, and if they compete with veterinarians in the sale of nonmedical products like commercial pet foods and toys, many of these stores will conclude that it is economically inefficient for them to force consumers to choose between their store and a neighboring veterinarian for *anything* either could provide. For once a consumer enters a veterinary facility, there is the possibility of a lost sale for the retail establishment. Therefore some of these retailers will try to compete with veterinarians by hiring their own veterinarians and placing them inside their stores. This will decrease the probability that consumers will go elsewhere for veterinary services as well as nonveterinary items. And if veterinarians object that retail stores ought not to be providing medical services for animals, these stores will surely respond that they are offering the public *exactly* what veterinarian advocates of merchandising themselves promote—truly "one-stop shopping."

In principle there is nothing to prevent nonveterinarian retailers from maintaining their facilities as veterinary operations, that is, as distinctive and recognizable animal hospitals whose major function is providing veterinary care (see Chapter 16). However, acceptance of merchandising by veterinarians, together with nonveterinarian ownership and employment of veterinarians, will result in many "veterinary" facilities that are owned by nonveterinarians losing their distinctive veterinary character. This will happen not because the retail operation will be part of the veterinary operation but because the veterinary operation will be part of the retail operation.

A *New York Times* article on the recent success of pet "superstores" indicates how the atmosphere of a retail facility can differ from that of a traditional veterinary hospital. At one superstore, according to this report:

> There are basic groceries and gourmet goodies like pricey peanut butter cookies and soda water in offbeat flavors. The freezer case holds all manner of frozen entrees and desserts. Down one aisle are health and grooming products like toothpaste, deodorant and apricot-scented shampoo. In the clothing aisle, you find a trendy new outfit in a neon Navajo pattern, a matching backpack, sunglasses—and look, Halloween costumes already.
>
> Of course the whining starts in the toy department, and by the time you get to the snacks displayed by the checkout, you're not surprised to catch one of your young charges engaged in some playful shoplifting. "Muffy," you say, "drop that dried pig's ear—now!"
>
> That's right, a purloined pig's ear.[21]

Such stores may well be pleasing to the eye and great fun, for both animal owners and pets. But is this the sort of atmosphere with which veterinarians wish themselves and their profession to be associated? Is this sort of atmosphere conducive to the making of serious medical decisions about animals? Will it enhance the image of veterinarians and their patients?

Phase Four: The Sale of Veterinary Professional Services by General Commercial Retailers

The third phase of merchandising will not be the end result of the mixture of merchandising and veterinary services. Although their focus is on supplying pets and their owners with animal-related items, pet "superstores" do not differ in any significant respect from other kinds of retail operations. They are another kind of consumer retail business. If pet "superstores" make money employing veterinarians and selling pet products, it will only be a matter of time before full service department stores, discount department store chains, large grocery stores, so-called "pharmacies," and members-only wholesale discount "clubs" do the same. Many of these stores—which tend to dwarf even the largest pet "superstores"—already proclaim themselves as "one-stop shopping" centers. Many already have on their premises full-service pharmacies and opticians. If they perceive the pet market, including the market for veterinary care, to be profitable, they will not leave the field to the pet superstores, just as the pet superstores will not leave the field to veterinarians. Some of these retailing giants could find it profitable, and quite easy, to add a veterinary department where allowed by law to do so. These retailers would have absolutely no interest in having animal care as the dominant theme of their operations. Nor would they need or want ownership or management of their stores by veterinarians. Veterinarians would occupy a very small portion of the physical space, and ambiance, of these stores.

Can anything be done?

Unfortunately, practitioners who reject both the sale of nonveterinary products by veterinarians and the sale of veterinary products by retailers may suffer because of doctors who merchandise. As discussed in Chapter 16, veterinarians in states that allow nonveterinarians to own veterinary facilities can urge their state legislatures to change the law to prohibit lay ownership. Veterinarians who practice in states that allow members of the public to purchase syringes and associated vaccines without a prescription from a licensed health professional should work to change these laws.

Where one cannot rely on the law to prohibit laymen from owning veterinary practices or selling medical products, veterinarians will have to convince the public that they offer something ordinary retailers do not. The coming years will see increased discussion of purchasing, management, and marketing techniques that can effectively attract potential "customers" of superstores and nonveterinarian-owned corporate mega-practices.[22]

It is clear, however, that the road to certain failure lies in attempting to beat retailers at their own game. *For their own survival, veterinarians must distinguish themselves as quickly and decisively as possible from retail stores.* They must stop selling nonmedical items. They must offer high quality, compassionate, and personalized medical services, in an atmosphere that is a world away from commercialism or manipulation. Most importantly, veterinarians must promote and proclaim the importance of dignified veterinary services for animals and clients so that it becomes *unthinkable* for the great majority of people to associate veterinary care with ordinary retailing.

～ GROOMING

The term "merchandising" is generally understood to refer to the sale of merchandise, that is, products. Veterinarians can also offer services that are not medical/professional in nature. One nonprofessional service frequently urged as a source of increased revenues is grooming.

Ancillary and Cosmetic Grooming

Two very different kinds of grooming can be offered by veterinarians. The first, which I call "ancillary grooming," is not performed because the client has the independent purpose of grooming his animal but because the animal is already at the facility for a medical reason and ought to be groomed during this time. Typically, ancillary grooming is done because it is necessary for the health or comfort of the animal, as when an inpatient is bathed after it has come in contact with its own excrement, or a horse receives a routine brushing and a cleaning of its hooves. Ancillary grooming also includes the situation in which an animal (such as a show dog) normally receives non-medical, purely cosmetic grooming at regular intervals and is groomed in a veterinary facility because it is there, for medical reasons, at one or more of these times. Ancillary grooming can also include grooming a patient prior to discharge from the hospital so that the client can have the animal in the same condition in which it was admitted.

Ancillary grooming is quite different from the services provided by a professional grooming establishment, to which owners bring their animals specifically for the purpose of having them groomed. I shall call such a service provided in the veterinary office or hospital "cosmetic grooming." Clients might bring their animals to a veterinarian solely for cosmetic grooming, or it can be provided to them in addition to some medical service such as a general physical exam. The latter would be an instance of cosmetic and not ancillary grooming because the animal could be groomed even if it were not present at the facility for some medical purpose.

Those who recommend grooming as a source of practice revenues typically have cosmetic grooming in mind. Moreover, they do not envision the groomer as someone who happens to be physically present at the veterinary office as a convenience to clients. Rather, the veterinary facility is supposed to offer the service and to collect the fees for it. The groomer is to be retained as a regular employee or an independent contractor with the doctor taking a percentage of the grooming receipts.[23]

The Argument against Cosmetic Grooming

There need be nothing wrong with ancillary grooming. It can be no different from giving a human hospital patient a shave or bath during his stay, for his health or comfort. Moreover, it seems perfectly appropriate for veterinarians to charge for ancillary grooming and to take a reasonable markup for supplies and labor, just as one would for supplies and labor expended in providing professional services.

The typical arguments in favor of cosmetic grooming are the same ones that are raised for merchandising nonprofessional products: revenues, client convenience, patient welfare, and still more revenues. According to one proponent:

> ...(t)he groomer can detect skin, ear, dental, and other problems that can be referred to a staff veterinarian. Vaccination programs that have been lagging can be brought up-to-date. Sales of home grooming supplies and equipment can be stimulated. Proper nutrition can be counseled. Sales of...coat conditioners...can be stimulated.[24]

These words undoubtedly are motivated by a sincere desire to help patients and clients. Yet the picture that emerges unavoidably from such a passage—and, I submit, will ultimately be perceived by the public—is different. The veterinary office will no longer be seen as a place where sincere, dedicated people seek to serve the patient and client. It will rather be like a pack of vultures, who swoop about patients, twice a month if possible, picking over their skin, teeth, and whatever, seeking relentlessly to find another way to take another bite out of clients' wallets.

Can anyone seriously doubt that using grooming to get clients and their dollars into the office will lead to the purchase of unnecessary nonprofessional and professional items? Can anyone think that clients for whom the veterinary office becomes a place of successive requests for money will be more eager to visit veterinarians, or will be more trusting of their recommendations?

However, even if we suppose that some doctors who offer in-office cosmetic grooming will never manipulate clients for their own monetary gain, these practitioners, also, will be assisting in the demise of the image of the veterinarian as a dignified provider of medical care. Poodle cuts, shampooing, colognes, and fancy ribbons do not belong in the same place in which momentous issues of life and death are confronted by a healer. These things, together with the sale of nonmedical products, will inevitably transform the veterinary hospital into a one-stop animal supply store and service station.

None of this means that grooming is unimportant or that professional groomers should not play a role in promoting animal health. A professional groomer who discovers or suspects a medical condition can suggest that the owner see his veterinarian, and can recommend a doctor if asked to do so. Likewise, if an animal needs grooming for its health or comfort, the doctor can suggest that it be taken to a groomer. However, a beauty parlor does not belong in a medical office.

Separate Grooming Facilities

Some veterinarians do not have a groomer within their veterinary office but nevertheless profit directly from a grooming business. The doctor might own all or part of a grooming establishment, which might be adjacent to the veterinary office. Or one might lease space located in another place to a groomer in return for some percentage of the groomer's gross revenues. A veterinarian can also lease space to a groomer for a fixed rent.

The unprofessional appearance of a beauty parlor in the veterinary office can sometimes be avoided by separate veterinary and grooming establishments. (However, there are adjacent veterinary and grooming facilities with identical storefront designs that make their connection obvious.) Nevertheless, separate facilities can still pose some of the same problems as in-office cosmetic grooming. Indeed, these problems can be even more insidious. For when clients visit a veterinarian with an in-office groomer, they will at least suspect that there is a financial connection between the two. Even where facilities are separate, the trip to the groomer can be used as a pretext for urging appointments with the veterinarian. And the doctor or staff can still make it a practice to comment on the appearance of patients and thereby use the sanctity and authority of the medical office to get the client's animal into the beauty parlor.

It is perfectly appropriate for doctors to recommend grooming for legitimate health reasons. But it is no more professional for a veterinarian to recommend grooming for purely cosmetic reasons than it would be for a physician to comment on a patient's hairdo and urge a trip to a human beautician or barber. If a veterinarian's separate grooming and medical facilities conduct themselves separately and professionally, it might be possible for a doctor to avoid manipulating clients by trying to sell them one kind of service each time they are utilizing the other.

~ BOARDING

In-facility boarding offers far less potential for manipulation of clients, and can constitute far less a departure from the image of the veterinarian as a medical person, than does cosmetic grooming or the sale of nonprofessional products. The decision to board an animal is not as likely to be made on impulse or to be influenced by subtle commercialistic appeals. Moreover, although some boarding establishments do have a veterinarian on call, for many clients, leaving their animal at a veterinary facility has special advantages. It can assure prompt medical attention if something goes wrong. Special diets or prescribed medications can be administered. Some clients feel more comfortable leaving an animal in a facility whose essential professional service includes the prevention of illness. If an animal is boarded with its regular veterinarian, its records will be available should medical care be required. Unlike veterinarians who operate a grooming parlor, doctors who board animals can give clients not just a service they may want, but also one that is directly related to a veterinarian's special professional training and expertise.

Some people might be inclined to think that it is as offensive for a veterinary hospital to board healthy animals as it would be for a human hospital to set aside several floors as a hotel for tourists. Yet, there are important differences between hotel guests and boarded animals. The latter need assistance and supervision to remain healthy and indeed to survive. Many are, in a real sense, bereft of their families and companions, and in such unaccustomed surroundings, they can be in special need of kind and considerate caretakers. It is more accurate to compare the boarding of a pet in a veterinary facility to the temporary stay of a person who is not ill but nevertheless in need of supervision in a custodial care facility. We do not consider it offensive or unprofessional for such facilities to be owned and operated by physicians precisely because good medical care should be available to people who must stay in them.

～ ETHICS AND MERCHANDISING

In 1986 the AVMA House of Delegates voted to eliminate a 32-year-old provision of the *Principles of Veterinary Medical Ethics* which considered it "unprofessional for veterinarians to display leashes, collars, meats, foods, and other nonprofessional products in their offices, hospitals and waiting rooms."[25] The vote was close and followed heated debate. AVMA President Dr. A. F. Hopkins (who stated he himself had "no intentions of displaying leashes, collars, dog food dishes, and the like") predicted that the prohibition could well be reinstated in the future.[26]

Indeed, there was so much dissatisfaction with the new permission of merchandising that the next year, a serious attempt was made to reinstate the old prohibition. The House of Delegates settled on a compromise, which was intended to allow merchandising only when it clearly served the interests of clients. The 1987 Revision of the *Principles* stated that "display of nonprofessional products is undesirable, but is permissible if such nonprofessional products are generally unavailable or are difficult to obtain in the general vicinity of the client being served."[27]

The prompt reinstatement of a partial prohibition against merchandising illustrated that a substantial proportion of the profession finds merchandising unacceptable. Unfortunately, even the 1987 modified restriction of merchandising violated federal antitrust laws and was removed following the FTC inquiry into the code (see Chapter 9). The *Principles* no longer attempt to restrict the lawful display and sale of nonveterinary products. The AVMA is now powerless to prevent what I have argued will be the terrible consequences of merchandising. Now, each individual practice must decide for itself, whether it shall maintain its distinctive status as a medical facility or carry on as a retail store.

This situation is both good and bad. It is good because ethics now takes on increased importance. Practitioners can no longer be *compelled* to behave in ways that preserve their status as medical professionals. They must decide for themselves that this is what they want. This decision must be based on inner ethical beliefs about the value of their clients, their patients, and themselves.

At the same time, the inability of the profession to compel practitioners to act like veterinarians instead of retailers means that the image of the entire profession may suffer, even if only a minority of practitioners merchandises. Many people have a negative view of the legal profession. They associate lawyers with tacky and misleading advertising, unconscionably high fees, and a self-serving attitude. In fact, only a tiny proportion of the legal profession advertises at all, and the great majority work very hard to protect their clients' interests. A relatively few bad apples have tarnished an entire profession's image. The same thing can happen to veterinary medicine. Even if veterinarians who retail or retailers who employ veterinarians remain in the minority, if enough people come to view veterinary facilities not as places of healing but places of selling, this may be the image most people will have of the profession.

REFERENCES

[1] Knowles RP: Merchandising in veterinary medicine, *Trends* 2(3):49-50, 1986.

[2] Clark R: *The Best of Ross Clark on Practice Management*, Lenexa, KS, 1985, Veterinary Medicine Publishing, p 75.

[3] Lofflin J: Use marketing leverage to lift your bottom line, *Vet Econ* October 1986:89-94.

[4] American Veterinary Medical Association: *Principles of Veterinary Medical Ethics*, 1993 Revision, "Dispensing, Marketing, and Merchandising," *1994 AVMA Directory*, Schaumburg, IL, The Association, p 46.

[5] Lofflin J: Merchandising: It works for him. Does it work for you? *Vet Econ* May 1992:37-51.

[6] For example, Walterscheid E: Retail displays pump new life into practice income, *Vet Econ* February 1987:36-48; Shouse D: Making the move to merchandise, *Vet Econ* July 1988:46-56; Lofflin J: Merchandising: It works for him. Does it work for you? *Vet Econ* May 1992:37-51.

[7] In Peterson C: What role will nutrition play in your practice? *Vet Econ* May 1989:62.

[8] Miller RM: Is service subjective? *Vet Econ* May 1992:43.

[9] Between 1989 and 1991 alone, mean professional incomes for all veterinarians in private clinical practices increased 21.9%, from $51,745 in 1989 to $63,069 in 1991. Percentage increases during this period were greatest for equine and small animal practitioners. Mean income jumped 27.1% for equine doctors, 26.9% for small animal predominant practitioners, and 25.9% for small animal exclusive practitioners. In contrast, increases were 10.5% for large animal exclusive, 9.3% for large animal predominant, and 7.8% for mixed animal practitioners. Wise JK: *Economic Report on Veterinarians and Veterinary Practices*, Schaumburg, IL, American Veterinary Medical Association, p 11.

[10] Shomer RR: Letter, Is there a doctor in the house—or a salesperson in the store? *J Am Vet Med Assoc* 190:245, 1987.

[11] Walterscheid E: Retail displays pump new life into practice income, *Vet Econ* February 1987:46.

[12] Levy JC: Merchandising in veterinary medicine: Another view, *Trends* 2(5):52, 1986.

[13] Becker M: "Storyselling" merchandising display encourages clients to buy products, *DVM* 20(3), March 1989:62.

[14] Dunn TJ: Alternatives to economic suicide. *Vet Econ* March1987:124; Gragg C: Those who merchandise will survive, *Vet Econ* February 1987:43; Becker M: Letter, Dr. Becker's bandanna article draws fire, *Vet Econ* March 1994:17.

[15] Dunn TJ: Alternatives to economic suicide, *Vet Econ* March 1987:124.

[16] Miller RM: Don't tarnish the image, *Vet Econ* March 1986:88.

[17] Wise JK: US market for food animal veterinary medical services, *J Am Vet Med Assoc* 190:1532-1533, 1987.

[18] Allesio ET: What products sell best, *Vet Forum* February 1990:35.

[19] Rivera J: Veterinarians fear misuse of over-the-counter vaccines, syringes, *Baltimore Sun*, September 11, 1991, p 1D.

[20] New Jersey DVMs help stall Petco vaccination clinic, *DVM* 24(12), December 1993:4.

[21] Eaton L: Hey, big spenders: three rival chains are bringing the 'category killer' concept to the $15 billion market for pet supplies, *New York Times*, September 11, 1994: Section 3, p 1.

[22] *See*, Gavzer KM: How to avoid getting steamrolled by pet superstores, *J Am Vet Med Assoc* 205:554-556, 1994, which offers several suggestions, including cooperative purchasing of materials, promoting client word-of-mouth referrals, finding a distinctive niche for one's practice, and computerized inventory control and financial records.

[23] Clark R: Practice management Q&A, *Vet Econ* September 1986:42.

[24]Clark R: *The Best of Ross Clark on Practice Management*, Lenexa, KS, 1985, Veterinary Medicine Publishing, pp 85-86.

[25]American Veterinary Medical Association: *Principles of Veterinary Medical Ethics*, 1985 Revision, "Displays in Waiting Rooms," *1986 AVMA Directory*, Schaumburg, IL, The Association, p 454.

[26]AVMA Says OK to product displays and merchandising, *Vet Econ* September 1986:11.

[27]Displays and reciprocity emerge as key House issues, *J Am Vet Med Assoc* 191:625, 1987; American Veterinary Medical Association: *Principles of Veterinary Medical Ethics*, 1987 Revision, "Displays in Waiting Rooms," *1988 AVMA Directory*, Schaumburg, IL, The Association, p 476.

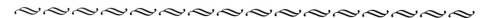

CHAPTER 18

Promotion and Marketing

∾ WHAT IS PROMOTION AND MARKETING?

In this book I use the terms "promotion" and "marketing" interchangeably, to refer to the activity of urging others to avail themselves of one's services or products. Some people might object to this definition. They might, for example, want to reserve the word "marketing" for selling techniques, such as advertising, directed at large numbers of people (that is, at "the market"). Others might be offended by any application of the word "marketing" to veterinarians, on the grounds that the term has connotations of commercialism and manipulation. I am as opposed to unprofessional commercialism in veterinary practice as anyone. However, it is more important to determine what kinds of promotional techniques are morally acceptable than to spend a great deal of time passing judgment on terminology—especially because the word "marketing" has already gained acceptance in the profession.

Two different kinds of marketing can be employed by veterinarians. "Internal" marketing is directed at present clients. "External" marketing is directed at the general public and is intended primarily to attract people who are not current clients. Some techniques can constitute both internal and external marketing. For example, a program in which one offers discounts off one's customary fees if clients bring in more than one pet at a time may be directed at both existing and potential clients. However, one could further promote such a program by using internal marketing (for example, by sending a mailing announcing the discounts to present clients) or external marketing (for example, by advertising the discounts in a local newspaper).

Marketing by veterinarians can be aimed at a wide range of audiences, including potential new clients, current clients, former clients, the public at large, and other veterinarians. The goals of marketing can be specific (for example, to remind clients to bring their dogs in for a heartworm test) or extremely general (for example, to educate the public about the benefits of good veterinary care). Marketing can be undertaken by individual doctors for their own practices and can be done by veterinary associations for their members or for veterinarians in general. Veterinarians can also participate in promotional campaigns of nonveterinarians, such as pet food companies.

There are many different ways of promoting one's practice, ranging from overt appeals for business in advertisements, to more subtle statements in one's letterhead, newsletter, or announcements of new staff. Virtually any contact between a practice and the public (including the manner in which the receptionist handles clients and how employees speak about the practice to others) can afford opportunities for promotion. As the profession becomes more interested in marketing, creative and hitherto undreamed-of promotional techniques can be expected to surface. Some of these might prove morally objectionable. This discussion does not attempt to address the ethical implications of all current and potential marketing techniques, but focuses on several that have recently aroused interest or controversy in the profession.

Can marketing be ethical?

One of the general themes of this book is that veterinarians will benefit themselves, their clients, and their patients by not viewing monetary gain as the overriding aim of their professional lives. Monetary reward is important. But a veterinarian should, I have urged, try to earn a decent living through practicing in a dignified and professional manner, and should not view practice as primarily the road toward an income.

Almost any marketing technique can be used for commercialistic and unprofessional ends. Some techniques are so undignified, dishonest, or predatory that they must be considered inherently unethical. It is also clearly the case that many veterinarians are becoming increasingly interested in marketing because they want to maintain or increase practice income. However, it does not follow from any of these things that all marketing is necessarily unethical. Certain promotional techniques can be used out of a sincere desire to convince clients to take advantage of veterinary services because these services are beneficial.

⮑ THREE GUIDEPOSTS FOR ETHICAL MARKETING

Each proposed marketing technique must be considered in its own right with due attention to how it might affect the legitimate interests of patients, clients, practitioners, and others. Nevertheless, I want to suggest three general requirements any marketing technique must meet if it is to be ethical.

Dignity and Tastefulness

First, a marketing technique must exhibit the dignity and tastefulness that is expected of a member of a medical profession. Such things as singing radio commercials, flashing or neon practice signs, and raffles for free puppies do not accord with the conservative behavior people expect of a professional who deals with matters of health and illness. It might not always be easy to decide whether a certain kind of marketing approach meets the requirement of dignity and tastefulness. Indeed, attempting to make such decisions might sometimes involve defining the boundaries of what we mean by the terms "dignity" and "taste." However, few veterinarians would dispute that marketing must be dignified and tasteful, even if they might sometimes disagree about what this means in practice.

Honesty and Respect for Clients

As the discussion of the merchandising of nonprofessional products in Chapter 17 emphasizes, one objectionable feature of the commercialization of veterinary practice is its tendency to manipulate clients. Treating clients as autonomous decision-makers requires honesty toward them and respect for their ability to decide for themselves (see Chapter 14). Many clients have a soft spot in their hearts for their animals and understand that veterinarians know a great deal more about animal health than they do. They are therefore likely to believe whatever a veterinarian says. An advertisement claiming that Dr. X is a specialist when in fact she is not board-certified can prevent clients from making a choice they would want to make. A newsletter that ominously threatens the demise of clients' cats if they are not brought in immediately for leukemia vaccinations puts undue (and dishonest) pressure on clients. Our society is accustomed to marketing techniques that shade the truth and exaggerate the importance of goods and services. If veterinary marketing is to remain professional, it must avoid such tendencies.

Fairness to Other Practitioners

Promotion can affect not only clients but other veterinarians. An advertisement or telephone directory announcement stating that Dr. Y has "the most modern facilities anywhere" is doubtlessly directed at potential clients. But it appeals to clients by making an explicit or implicit claim about other doctors. If such a statement is false or misleading, it can treat the public unfairly by depriving it of important correct information. A false statement can also be unfair to other veterinarians by making claims about them that they are unable to contest.

Marketing can place pressure on doctors even when it is not intended consciously to draw clients away from other veterinarians. For example, some practices distribute their own client leaflets on medical topics. With the advent of computerized "desk-top publishing," such offerings can look professionally printed. A doctor who produces such brochures might have no intention of belittling other veterinarians. Nevertheless, clients who visit neighboring facilities might wonder whether these doctors are as up-to-date as the veterinarian with the fancy leaflets.

No veterinarian can claim a lucrative client base as a moral or legal right. However, if veterinary marketing turns doctors against each other, forces them to expend resources that would otherwise be devoted to the improvement of skills and facilities, and makes flashy promotion more appealing to the public than excellent medicine, many good veterinarians, clients, and animals will suffer. Determining the proper balance between the right to promote oneself and the importance of keeping promotion secondary to practicing medicine is one of the most challenging tasks faced by normative veterinary ethics.

~ INTERNAL PROMOTIONAL TECHNIQUES
Good Medicine

Good, thorough medicine may well be the most profitable—and is certainly the most dignified—marketing tool available to veterinarians. There is an enormous range of professional services that veterinarians can recommend because they constitute good medicine. The late Dr. Robert Knowles offered the following examples of procedures that can be suggested to caring pet owners: laboratory examination before each surgery; electrocardiography on all aged surgical patients; pre- and postoperative radiographs on all orthopedic patients; chest radiographs on all aged surgical patients; tracheal wash and cytology on all chronic coughers; rabies vaccinations and feline leukemia (FeLV) tests and vaccine for cats; vigorous promotion of heartworm prevention; and annual physical examinations.[1] Dentistry is another important medical service that is a significant potential source of practice revenue.[2]

The following thoughts of Dr. Knowles are more valuable than any extended dissertation on good medicine as a marketing tool:

Be pleasant, friendly, genuinely interested in your client, your patient, and their problems. Offer high-quality veterinary medicine, encourage your clients to accept the care that their pets should have. Don't do so timidly, but boldly and with confidence that this is what is needed and confidence that your client WILL accept that care you offer. You will far outstrip the merchandiser and have a meaningful measure of pride in the doing.[1]

Displaying Professional Products

Many veterinarians display professional products such as flea preparations and prescription diets. Displaying professional products (including some veterinary drugs) need not be undignified or unprofessional. A tasteful display can inform clients about items the doctor can recommend should the need arise. It can also educate clients about the fact that today's veterinarians have at their disposal a scientifically sophisticated armamentarium of drugs and medical products.

It is negligent and unethical for a doctor to relinquish to a client the decision of whether a medical product will be recommended. Doctors must suggest medical goods and services, and they must do so only when they are indicated medically. Therefore a display of professional items should never be used to encourage or induce clients to purchase specific displayed products. Clients certainly may be permitted to ask whether a displayed item would help their animal, and they may ask general questions about a displayed item. However, if one is going to recommend a displayed item, one must do so only for medical reasons, irrespective of whether it is displayed and whether the display has caught the client's attention.

Informational Brochures and Leaflets

Some veterinarians provide clients brochures containing information about certain diseases, conditions, and treatments. These publications range from professionally printed booklets with color illustrations to one-page photocopied handouts. They are sometimes devoted solely to medical matters, but might also contain information about the practice and its services. They can be produced by or for individual doctors, or by veterinary associations. There are also booklets printed by nonveterinary enterprises (such as pet food companies) that contain advertisements for these companies' products, and sometimes, discount coupons.

Informational brochures, like displays of professional items, can enhance clients' image of the doctor and of the profession as a whole. This, in turn, can assist doctors in convincing clients to accept their recommendations for medically indicated services or products. Brochures can also help clients in making their own informed and voluntary decisions by providing them with explanations of medical problems and suggested treatments. Thus client brochures have an enormous potential in benefiting the interests of patients, clients, and veterinarians.

There are, however, potential dangers. As is the case with the display of professional items, brochures should never be used to urge clients to ask for something only a veterinarian should recommend. Dr. Mary Beth Leininger has observed that many clients are especially impressed by printed documents; they tend to believe that if something is in writing, it must be so.[3] Doctors must therefore be careful not to use written material that is untruthful or that tries to influence clients other than by an appeal to rational argument. Entitling a client handout "Do You Want Your Dog to Survive this Year's

Heartworm Epidemic?" would be an example of an unacceptable appeal to client fear and insecurity.

A potential ethical problem is raised by materials produced by companies (typically, pet food manufacturers) whose products can be purchased directly by clients from retailers. Such publications can enable doctors who do not have a large promotional budget to provide informational pamphlets to clients. The practice of displaying posters and booklets furnished by commercial pet product companies has become so widespread that most veterinarians probably think there is nothing remarkable or problematic about it. Indeed, I have found that some doctors are surprised anyone could object to using such material, especially because much of it contains useful information.

The problems, of course, come from the impression that such publications will undoubtedly give some clients. Some may think that the doctor endorses this particular brand when in fact one might not. Moreover, whether or not a doctor endorses the brand that supplies one's booklets, one becomes part of a third party's promotional campaign for a commercial product. As I argue below, it is inappropriate for veterinarians to allow their waiting or examination rooms to serve as billboards for any company's products. Doctors who want to distribute informational material should find that the client brochures prepared by the AVMA, or their own photocopied handouts, do the job quite well and are appreciated by clients.

Newsletters

One recent development in veterinary marketing is the advent of practice newsletters. Newsletters afford doctors the opportunity to reach clients in a dignified manner with information that will assist them in making informed decisions about veterinary care. Newsletters can avoid the appearance of commercialism so often associated with advertisements in the print or broadcast media, for, unlike the latter, newsletters need not be presented alongside usual commercial appeals for consumer products. Moreover, newsletters targeted at current clients are less likely to be seen by other doctors as an attempt to steal away their clients.

Because the distribution of newsletters is still an emerging area of veterinary marketing, it is premature to attempt to set forth specific ethical guidelines concerning them. However, one might keep in mind the three general requirements of all marketing: dignity and tastefulness; honesty and respect for clients; and fairness to other doctors. Dignity includes treating medical matters with seriousness (though not necessarily without some humor); informing clients about available services, office hours, and clinicians without making blatant appeals for business; and not bombarding clients with so many newsletters that they will believe they are being hustled rather than informed. Honesty and respect for clients includes not attempting to influence them with sensationalistic language that frightens them or with scientific prose they cannot understand. Fairness to other doctors means, in part, that a newsletter should attempt to inform clients about medical issues and the opportunities their doctor provides for addressing them—and should not be a disguised attempt to compare one's own virtues with alleged shortcomings of other practitioners.

As is the case with brochures, newsletters should avoid giving the impression that the doctor is endorsing commercial products. Likewise, newsletters should not be produced by commercial firms in return for inclusion of advertisements for their products, nor should commercial advertising be accepted in order to defray publication costs. (Including an announcement of a nonprofit organization, such as a humane society animal adoption service, need not be undignified or improper.) Because much of a newsletter's impact depends on its appearance, design components such as titles and artwork should be dignified and tasteful. The entire production should reflect the doctor's sincere desire to provide truthful and useful information.

Reminders and Sympathy Cards

If newsletters are an appropriate means of informing and reminding clients of a doctor's services, so are direct mailings to clients reminding them that their animals are due for tests, vaccinations, scheduled visits, and routine physical exams. Nor does it seem particularly undignified to send a reasonable number of additional reminders to follow up an initial mailing.

Some doctors send sympathy cards to clients after the death of their animals. Although such mailings might in fact improve clients' image of their veterinarian, sympathy cards should *not* be considered a marketing tool and should never be sent with the intention of promoting the practice. The death of a beloved animal is too sensitive a matter to be used as an opportunity for promotion. Indeed, to avoid the possibility of misinterpretation, it is important that sympathy cards not even give the appearance of having a promotional aim. Thus while the signature or the name of the doctor would be appropriate for such a message, such things as the hospital's office hours or a list of its services are not.

"Fun" Facilities

Another proposed internal marketing technique is turning the veterinary hospital into a place where all members of the family have an enjoyable, fun-filled time. According to one discussion, doctors must make sure that:

> ...clients say "yes" if they were asked: "Did you have a good time at the veterinarian?" Whoever said visiting the veterinarian *shouldn't* be fun? In all seriousness, this question is being asked about physicians—who are frightened by the answer and its implications. Medicine doesn't have to be cold, sterile, or impersonal. Pet owners have a choice. And as most are incapable of discerning medical competence, they can only assume their pets are treated as they are.[4]

Dr. Becker offers several suggestions for making a practice "seem 'user friendly' and warm-n-fuzzy,"[5] including a refreshment center with complimentary beverages for clients.[6] He also recommends several ways of entertaining and occupying the attention of children, such as "balloons, a coupon for free yogurt, or coloring sheets. ...You'll make the kids smile, please their parents, and be seen as 'user friendly.'"[6]

It is, surely, good for both clients and veterinarians for a practice to be comfortable and uplifting. If clients associate animal hospitals with cheap furniture, drab walls, dark and dingy lighting, and bad smells, many might be less motivated to seek medical care for their animals. Pleasant surroundings show that a doctor cares about clients. A positive environment makes it easier for clients to understand and make important medical decisions affecting their animals. It is therefore appropriate that architects and interior decorators are helping veterinarians to transform the image of the veterinary hospital from the somewhat homey places of old to more modern and pleasant medical facilities. Nor is there anything wrong with making available certain creature comforts such as up-to-date magazines or a beverage. As all veterinarians know, children do sometimes arrive with parents and patients. Occupying them with harmless pleasures can be conducive to the atmosphere all clients and patients in the hospital require.

Creature comforts for clients and their children should be unobtrusive and serve as a tool for assisting clients (and patients) through what can be an unnerving or difficult experience. Such comforts should not constitute a major portion of the ambiance of the practice. Nor, in my view, should veterinarians do what the first authors quoted above recommend—attempt to assure that clients always "have a good time" and "fun" at the veterinarian. The phrase "warm-n-fuzzy" may also be an unfortunate way of characterizing methods of making people comfortable that might otherwise be appropriate.

Veterinary hospitals must not be cold or imposing, but neither should they be, in their general behavior or ambiance, "fun." It is not fun to decide to euthanize a desperately ill animal. It is not "warm" or "fuzzy" to authorize a surgical procedure, even if it is routine or has a good prospect of success. It is not always fun to pay for veterinary care. Medical decisions must be approached by clients with a sense of seriousness because of their potential consequences. These decisions can be serious and important because veterinary patients are important. These decisions can be serious and important because veterinary clients are important.

It is but a short step from viewing a veterinary facility as a "store" to demanding that it provide a fun-filled experience for the entire family. Stores and shopping malls are, after all, places of entertainment, diversion, and instant gratification for "kids from 8 to 80." Aside from what it might do to the image of veterinarians and veterinary medicine, making animal hospitals "fun" could in the long run make it more difficult for doctors to convince clients to do the best for their animals. If clients expect that visiting a veterinarian must be fun, they will not come back when a visit is no longer fun. They will feel deprived or swindled when there is bad news, when a difficult decision must be made, or when a bill must be paid.

Clearly, no one who seeks to make the veterinary office a place of fun *wants* to lessen the seriousness with which people approach the responsibility of animal ownership. We must, however, sometimes attend to possible effects rather than intentions. Veterinarians should discourage the notion that human-animal interaction in all its manifestations, including taking an animal to the veterinarian, should always be fun. The attitude that animal ownership should be all pleasure is partly responsible for the terrible pet overpopulation problem, and for the appalling lack of concern some owners exhibit regarding appropriate medical care for their animals. When the new kitten or puppy is cute and "fun," there is no problem. But when it needs to be house-trained, when it grows older or more demanding, when it gets sick—when the fun is gone—then it is taken to a veterinarian for euthanasia, tossed out on to the street to fend for itself, or left in a shelter to join millions of other pet corpses.

As I argue in Chapter 21, a critical ethical task faced by the profession relates to what must happen before an animal is brought to the office, indeed before an animal is obtained by its owner. Clients must begin the relationship with their animals with the understanding that ownership is a serious responsibility that can bring sacrifice as well as pleasure. It is also important that responsible attitudes begin in childhood. For adults and children, visiting a veterinarian must be placed in the context of one's entire relationship with an animal throughout its life. This relationship will likely include times of seriousness, difficulty, and responsibility, as well as times of pleasure and enjoyment. Unfortunately, illness and even the prevention of illness belong on the more serious side of our relationships with our animals. Veterinarians must never allow or encourage clients—or their children—to forget this fact.*

ᴥ EXTERNAL MARKETING TECHNIQUES
Practice Names

The first contact many potential clients have with a practice is seeing or hearing its name. The AVMA has attempted to avoid confusion and prevent deception in the use of practice designations in its "Guidelines for Naming of Veterinary Facilities."[7] The Guidelines define the terms "animal medical center," "hospital," "clinic," "office," "mobile facility," "emergency facility," and "on-call emergency service." For example, an animal medical center is "a facility in which consultative, clinical, and hospital services are rendered and in which a large staff of basic and applied veterinary scientists perform significant research and conduct advanced professional educational programs." A hospital is "a facility in which the practice conducted includes the confinement as well as the treatment of patients." In a "clinic," "the practice conducted is essentially an outpatient type of practice."

The AVMA definitions seem useful in preventing misleading practice names. However, there are probably so many possible ways of abusing practice names that a complete set of guidelines would be unfeasible. Among the kinds of designations not mentioned by the AVMA that might sometimes mislead the public are the following: those that couple the name of the region of the country or state with a term like "animal medical center;" using the name of a neighboring college or university in the practice designation when it has no connection with the educational institution; and practice designations that imply the facility provides better care than others.

Signs and Logos

The 1940 AVMA *Code of Ethics* stated that "display signs of reasonable size and dimensions on veterinary hospitals are not regarded as objectionable, provided that they do not announce special services, such as bathing, plucking, clipping, x-ray work, etc., which characterize the ways of the charlatan."[8] The current code does not include a section on signs, but the matter of signs is worthy of consideration. Many practices are located in commercial districts in which businesses vie for attention by confronting the public with large, and sometimes extremely ugly and distracting signs. A veterinary practice might feel compelled to erect a conspicuous sign or billboard so that it does not get lost in the morass.

Even when it is located in a commercial district, a veterinary hospital, clinic, or office is still a medical facility. Practice signs must therefore be a reasonable size. They should avoid style or content that is demeaning to medical professionals, such as garish colors, flashing or neon lights, juvenile animal caricatures, commercialistic slogans, and

---

*In his novel *Brave New World*, Aldous Huxley predicted the ultimate transformation of medical facilities into places of fun and frolic. Young children are taken regularly to hospitals in which people are dying, where they play among these patients' beds. The aim is to assure that dying too is associated with pleasure and that no one will feel grief, sorrow, or unpleasantness because of another's passing.

insipid spelling or diction (for example, "We care 4 pets."). Signs should also avoid making statements that are themselves unethical, for example, that the hospital provides better veterinary care than others in the area.

Many practices have adopted logos, or graphic designs, that are used internally or externally for identification and promotion. Some of these logos are designed by professional artists. A logo might be included in external practice signs as well as on stationery, invoices, business cards, and newsletters. Logos can say much about the attitude and professionalism of a practice. They can promote a practice by indicating the kinds of animals it treats as well as the doctors' caring and compassionate attitudes toward patients and clients. Some logos are extremely beautiful and elegant. Others demean patients, clients, and doctors with juvenile or tasteless animal caricatures.

Discounts and Giveaways

Some veterinarians offer discounts on services to attract new clients and to motivate current clients to bring in their animals. Clients can be given a volume discount, that is, they can be charged a certain percent less than the ordinary fee for each animal if they bring in more than one during a visit to the facility. Or a doctor can offer a discount off the regular fee; this can be done for new clients only, or for all clients who bring in a specified species of animal or who bring in their animals during a specified time period. A variant of discounting is offering a "free" service or product with the payment of the usual fee for some service. Offering discounts or giveaways is usually a means of getting someone into one's practice. Discounts are therefore typically found in public advertisements, although they can be presented in client newsletters or redemption coupons distributed in such places as pet stores and grooming parlors.

In 1987 a provision was added to the *Principles of Veterinary Medical Ethics* prohibiting the advertising of discounts and discounted fees.[9] This provision was removed as a result of the 1988 Federal Trade Commission inquiry (see Chapter 9). However, that veterinarians can no longer be compelled to avoid discounts does not render discounts or the advertising of discounts appropriate.

It is in the interest of veterinarians, clients, and their animals that veterinary patients be viewed as important beings entitled to first-class, dignified medical care. Such a perception is undercut by discounts. We would be revolted by a pediatrician who offered a discount for each additional child brought to the office. ("One baby, $30, two for $55, three for $80.") We would say that such a marketing technique cheapens the patient. Discounts analogize veterinary patients not to human medical or dental patients but to such commodities as tires, cans of motor oil, and lawnmowers, for which volume or seasonal discounts are commonplace. By cheapening the patient, discounts also cheapen the image of the veterinarian.

It is difficult to believe that there are many clients who would pay, say, $20 for an examination for one cat but would bring in a second only if its exam cost $2 or $3 less. Moreover, there are more dignified ways of allowing clients to pay less than one's usual fee and thereby to encourage them to obtain care for their animals. One can reduce one's fee, not as a discount, but as a special accommodation to a client in need. Certain basic services such as heartworm tests or vaccinations may be offered for a lower fee than is charged for complete examinations. Like medical health maintenance organizations, one can offer prepayment plans encompassing a range of services that, if paid for individually, would cost clients more. Some doctors, for example, offer prepaid puppy and kitten packages that include several examinations and vaccinations. Participation in pet health insurance programs can also translate into reduced cost per visit for clients.

Veterinarians should not assume that the public will accept discounts and give-aways. One doctor mailed coupons offering a free flea collar or canister of flea powder to clients who would bring in their cats for routine vaccinations and a fecal test. The coupons were sent to 10,000 households. There was one response. Interestingly, the doctor interpreted the results as an indication of "the reluctant feline client."[10]

Nor do veterinarians help their image or earning power by attempting to entice clients with so-called "free" services. Only the most naive clients could think that any-thing is really free and that they are not paying somewhere. As Dr. Ronald Whitford observes, "everyone knows nothing of *real* value in this world is ever "free."[11] Nor, sure-ly, should veterinarians utilize a promotional gimmick that denigrates the value of their services and the importance of their expertise. It is a mystery why any veterinarian would promote a free *professional* service and thereby analogize one's expertise to the extra few ounces of diet soda or toilet bowl cleaner a manufacturer can add with little skill to a container and offer as "free." To be sure, if veterinarians start competing with each other in offering "free" professional services the costs of which are *not* passed along to clients, the people who will pay are these doctors themselves.

Client Bonuses and Incentives

A marketing tool that has recently gained some adherents is offering present clients bonuses or incentives to motivate them to refer new clients. As one proponent explains, this technique saves time and money because clients are doing work doctors would otherwise have to do themselves. Clients become "practice promoters" and participants in what the marketing trade calls "multilevel marketing" or "MLM":

> First, MLM shifts the cost and reward for promotions from the conventional channels of adver-tising and distribution to a network of distributors. Next, MLM uses word of mouth advertising. Finally, MLM leverages your time. Translation: instead of spending hard cash on printing (pro-motion) and mailing (distribution) newsletters, for example, you can enlist your clients to talk to their friends about your quality services (saving you this marketing time).[12]

Dr. Becker has advocated client bonuses which increase with the number of clients referred. For the first three referrals, clients receive a thank-you card, a handwritten note from the doctor, and a certificate for a free video rental at a local video shop. The fourth referral earns a scented candle and another handwritten note. However, because one's "ultimate goal is multiple referrals, ...we market our 'frequent-referral program' with the lure of a 10% preferred customer discount after five referrals." A flyer distrib-uted to clients begins with the following words, in capitalized large boldface type: "EARN A LIFETIME 10% DISCOUNT...STOREWIDE."[13]

Several objections can be made to such bonuses or incentives. As Dr. Whitford observes, such discounts can lead to anger and resentment by clients who do not receive them, perhaps because all of their friends are already clients.[11] As is always the case with "discounts," clients may wonder whether the doctor's fees are too high to begin with, if substantial savings, indeed, substantial lifetime savings, can be offered to some people.

However, the most fundamental ethical problem with paying clients for referrals is that it turns clients from ends into means. Clients (and their animals) are no longer one's sole objects of attention. They are also marketing tools which function to serve the doctor. There is a world of difference between earning a fee because one has served a client loyally, and turning clients into paid promoters for one's practice. The former situation involves benefits that flow deservedly from the professional relationship. The latter appeals to interests that can have nothing to do with helping others.

It seems appropriate to cite the Golden Rule, which the *Principles of Veterinary Medical Ethics* rightly proclaim as a pillar of professional morality. The Golden Rule counsels us to treat others as we would want to be treated by them. If one were a client—not a current client seeking to earn a referral bonus, but a prospective client being solicited for a veterinary practice by a current client—would one be comfortable knowing that the reason for the solicitation might be a potential bonus for the solicitor? Would one trust a veterinarian more or less, who pays current clients to bring in new clients? I suggest that the answers to these questions are obvious.

∿ ADVERTISING

The most conspicuous form of external marketing is advertising. The *Principles of Veterinary Medical Ethics* define "advertising" as "newspaper and periodical announcements and listings; professional cards; office and other signs; letterheads; telephone and other directory listings; and any other form of communication designed to inform the general public about the availability, nature, or prices of products or services, or to attract clients."[14] This definition is extremely broad and includes several marketing tools (such as simple telephone listings, letterheads, and business cards) most people would usually not include within that term. There is, however, an important point to such a definition. It draws attention to the fact that veterinarians who market their practices to the public can be doing much the same thing whether or not we would, strictly speaking, call their promotions "advertisements." The broad definition also enables the *Principles* to set forth guidelines applicable to a wide range of marketing techniques.

The Legal Situation

It was not so long ago that advertising by veterinarians was prohibited, both by state practice acts and the AVMA. The 1940 AVMA *Code of Ethics*, the predecessor of the current *Principles of Veterinary Medical Ethics*,[15] reflected the view of advertising that lasted into the 1970s. According to the *Code*:

> Advertising as a means of obtaining patronage is objectionable in the practice of any branch of medicine. It is denounced as unethical and unprofessional. Veterinary medicine is not an exception. *Per contra*, on account of its widely misunderstood objectives, it is the branch of medical practice that is most vulnerable to fair and unfair criticism from other scientific pursuits.

Among the practices categorized as "unprofessional advertising" and singled out for specific condemnation were advertising in a "city, commercial, telephone or any widely circulated directory;" allowing one's "name to be printed in public directories as a specialist in the treatment of any disease or in the performance of any service," and the "distribution of cards or circulars by mail or otherwise reminding clients that the time is at hand for rendering certain services (vaccinations, worm-parasite treatment, *et al.*)." Veterinarians were permitted by the *Code* to include in their local telephone directory a simple listing of their name, address, and telephone number, but all such listings had to have "identical visual prominence." No veterinarian could use boldface type, or state "his name or hospital or institution in any way differing from the standard style, type, or size used in the directory for the listing of professional groups (physicians, dentists, lawyers, nurses)."

In 1977 the U.S. Supreme Court wiped away such prohibitions when it struck down as violative of the First Amendment to the Constitution, a total ban on advertising of fees imposed upon attorneys by a state bar association that all lawyers in the state were required to join.[16] This decision is frequently misinterpreted as standing for the proposition that veterinarians and other professionals have a legal right to use "established marketing and advertising techniques."[17]

In fact, although the Court did hold that restrictions on certain kinds of professional advertising violate the constitutional protection of freedom of speech, it did not give professionals a blank check to use any advertising technique acceptable in the commercial world. The Court held that false and misleading advertising by professionals could be banned either by state boards of registration or professional associations. It left open the possibility of restricting in-person solicitation and advertising claims about the quality of services. The Court speculated that it might be proper for government and professional associations to regulate the time, place, and manner of professional advertising. The Court also warned that "the special problems of advertising on the electric broadcast media will warrant special consideration." The Court made it clear that government and professional associations have a legitimate, though limited, role in the articulation and enforcement of ethical standards regarding advertising by professionals.

In recent years, the Court has increasingly emphasized false, deceptive, and misleading advertising as legitimate targets of state and professional association regulation. In one decision, the Court stated that commercial speech that "is not false or deceptive and does not concern unlawful activities...may be restricted only in the service of a *substantial* governmental interest, and only through means that directly advance that interest."[18] One example of potentially truthful advertising the Court still considers open to regulation is in-person solicitation by lawyers.[19] However, the Court has cast doubt on whether it would allow government authorities or professional associations to regulate advertising by professionals that is undignified or tasteless if such advertising is truthful.[20]

The AVMA Response and the Post-1989 *Principles*

The AVMA response to the 1977 U.S. Supreme Court decision was to place in the *Principles of Veterinary Medical Ethics* a section entitled "Advertising Regulations." This section began with the general rule that advertising "is permissible when it includes no false, deceptive, or misleading statement or claim." The section then listed 14 general categories and specific examples of false, deceptive, or misleading representations.

The treatment of advertising in the old code was lengthy and specific. The list of false, deceptive, and misleading claims was not intended to be exhaustive but rather illustrative of kinds of prohibited representations. Among explicitly prohibited kinds of advertising were those (1) predicting "future success or guarantees that satisfaction or a cure will result from the performance of professional services;" (2) containing "a combination of a veterinarian's name or photograph and identifying a veterinarian as part of a testimonial, endorsement, or sales promotion of a nonveterinarian service or product, to the extent that the testimonial or endorsement represents implicitly or explicitly that the endorser's knowledge as a veterinarian gives him or her expertise with respect to any feature or characteristic of the nonveterinary product or service;" (3) containing "statistical data or other information based on past performance or case reports;" (4) including a "statement of opinion as to the quality of professional services or representation regarding the quality of professional services which is not susceptible of verification by the public;" and (5) containing statements of fees for a range of services that do not also include "reasonable disclosure of all relevant variables and causes affecting the fees so that the statement will not be misunderstood or be deceptive."[21]

The FTC inquiry into the *Principles* wrought major changes in the code section on advertising. The section is no longer called "Advertising Regulations," but "Advertising," perhaps to weaken the implication of the old title that the rules will be strenuously enforced. The post-FTC section is shorter, less specific, and considerably watered-down. All the provisions quoted in the previous paragraph were removed. The code still prohibits "false, deceptive, or misleading claims." Moreover, several of the kinds of such claims still included in the *Principles* can be interpreted (though, perhaps, with some stretching) to include some of the kinds of statements omitted after 1989. For example, the code still lists as an example of a prohibited representation one that "contains a representation or implication that is likely to cause an ordinary prudent lay person to misunderstand or be deceived, or fails to contain reasonable warnings of disclaimers necessary to make a representation or implication not deceptive."[22] This statement could, perhaps, be interpreted to include guarantees of cures, on the grounds that laymen might misunderstand that a veterinarian can never guarantee a cure because of the variability of individual patients and the inability to predict what will happen in every case to each patient. On the other hand, a member of the AVMA who might be charged with guaranteeing a cure in violation of the *Principles* could well argue that because the specific prohibition against such guarantees was removed from the code, the code can no longer be interpreted to prohibit guarantees.

In my view, none of the omissions or modifications made in the advertising section of the *Principles* were necessary to assure conformity to the antitrust laws administered by the FTC. (This is not to criticize the AVMA for making these changes, faced as it was with potentially disastrous litigation from a powerful government agency.) More importantly, all the kinds of statements specified by the pre-1989 *Principles* as false, deceptive, or misleading but eliminated or modified in the new code are useful examples of false, deceptive, and misleading representations—and can expected to be viewed as such by any state licensing board.

For example, it is inherently false, deceptive, and misleading for a veterinarian to guarantee a cure or results. Laymen are also likely to be misled by, or to misunderstand, claims purportedly backed by past performance or case reports because they cannot see, understand, and evaluate all relevant scientific evidence. Statements about fees that merely indicate a range without warning about specific variables are likely to mislead the public, and indeed have been specifically prohibited by at least one veterinary licensing board.[23] The omission from the post-1989 *Principles* of the prohibition against claims of quality of services flies in the face of the explicit statement by the Supreme Court that such representations may be banned by private associations and licensing boards because they are not susceptible to verification by the public.[16]

Advertising in the Print and Broadcast Media

I have found that some practitioners and clients feel comfortable about modest advertisements in newspapers or magazines but object to veterinary advertising on radio or television. Perhaps because broadcast advertising is usually expensive, it has not yet become a major issue among veterinarians. There has, however, been no shortage of undignified newspaper advertisements. A typical tasteless veterinary advertisement might include multiple coupons for various services. The coupons might offer discounts (for example, $1 off a cat spay) that an unsuspecting client might not know are minuscule. The coupons might also contain tiny expiration dates so that the public knows they must be redeemed before it is too late, just like supermarket coupons for laundry detergent. There might be an offer of a package deal for a series of related services—with a large "X" drawn through the usual price total, and a new, much lower amount emblazoned in enormous type. The advertisement might be further decorated with an insipid cartoon animal reminding readers about the great savings to be had.

The advertising section of the *Principles* does address some of the offensive features of such advertisements. However, the *Principles* are restricted to prohibiting false, deceptive, and misleading substantive claims and do not address what is often the most important problem with advertisements: their disregard for style and taste. Fortunately, professionals can still try to be dignified in their communications with the public, even if the courts decide they can no longer be compelled to be so.

Yellow Pages Advertisements

Advertisements in Yellow Pages telephone directories can present many of the same kinds of ethical problems as other promotional techniques. There are Yellow Pages advertisements that, for example, claim that doctors specialize in areas in which they are in fact not board-certified; use impressive but undefined terms ("A Full-Service Veterinary Hospital"); falsely imply a facility is the only one of its kind in the area ("Capital City's Full-Service Animal Hospital"); falsely imply a hospital has features not possessed by others in the area ("A Hospital with Surgical Facilities on the Premises"); and that make or imply a claim of higher quality service not susceptible to verification by the public ("High Quality Facilities to Serve You Better"). Some advertisements also appear in red, an adaptation of the flashing or neon sign to the print medium.

Yellow Pages advertisements can be truthful and dignified. They can provide potential clients useful and essential information. However, there appears to be an inherent tendency within the medium toward exaggeration and tastelessness. Unlike other forms of advertising, the Yellow Pages impose severe pressures upon doctors to advertise. Doctors know that the Yellow Pages are usually consulted by people who are looking for a veterinarian. Doctors who are not listed might have no chance of obtaining the patronage of such people. Many doctors rightly wonder whether a basic listing of name, location, and telephone number is sufficient, for to most people, one veterinarian's name will mean no more than another. Many people probably are attracted to a listing that contains more information. Many undoubtedly will be attracted to the largest advertisement for a practice in their locality.

Thus a distinct burden is placed on veterinarians to place a full-blown advertisement (as opposed to a simple listing of name, address, and telephone number) in the Yellow Pages. And the larger or flashier the advertisements of competing doctors, the more pressure there will be to place an advertisement at least as conspicuous as those of one's competitors. To distinguish oneself, a doctor may feel compelled to do what ordinary commercial advertisers do to attract attention to their messages—puff and puff again until the truth is stretched beyond recognition.

To their credit, many veterinarians have managed to resist the tide of exaggerated and undignified listings. But for some, the Yellow Pages war is like a mini-nuclear arms race. Once they have begun placing large and flashy advertisements, it can become impossible to stop, as they feel compelled to outdo each other for their own survival. (I invite readers skeptical about this characterization to compare the last several years of veterinarian Yellow Pages listings for their area. One will probably find a steady increase in the number of full-blown advertisements, their size, use of color, and the number of exaggerated and misleading claims.) Who loses as a result? The public, which is subjected to misleading claims. And honest doctors, who might lose clients and suffer the consequences of a diminished image of the profession.

Ironically, it is not even clear that Yellow Pages advertisements are effective, which makes the risks they can pose to clients and the profession's good name even less defensible. Several experienced practice management consultants question whether much revenue is attracted in the first place by Yellow Pages listings.[24] Additionally, as consultant Donald Dooley observes, the advertisements represent an inefficient allocation of limited resources:

> Yellow Page advertising is used to steer clients from one hospital to another. It does nothing to try to reach those who aren't already using veterinary services. We spend millions as a profession to steal a client from one hospital to the next and nothing to try to get new clients into the profession.
>
> Veterinarians spend millions of dollars across the nation in the Yellow Pages, while state and national veterinary organizations have a tough time raising even $100,000 for a budget to do a smattering of advertising for the profession as a whole—advertising that would encourage more people to utilize veterinary medical services.[25]

The 1992 AVMA report on the veterinary service market for companion animals also appears to confirm that Yellow Pages advertising is not enormously effective. The report documents that for dog, cat, and bird owners, convenient location and hours, reasonable fees, and recommendations of others were the reasons cited most often by clients for the first visit to their veterinarian. Yellow Pages advertising and other kinds of advertising were at or near the bottom of the list. For example, among dog owners 67.8% cited convenient location as a reason for first choosing their veterinarian, 47.3% reasonable fees, 38.8% convenient hours, 36.4% recommendation, 5.1% Yellow Pages listing, 4.8% the outdoor sign, 2.0% advertising, and 9.8% other.[26]

It is not clear precisely how far state boards and professional associations may lawfully go in compelling adherence to standards governing Yellow Pages advertisements. Certainly, the courts would not uphold the requirement of the 1940 AVMA *Code of*

Ethics that all veterinarian telephone directory listings have "identical visual prominence."[27] However, there is no legal impediment to the enforcement of current administrative and official prohibitions against false or misleading advertisements. Thus, in
1988 the California Board of Examiners in Veterinary Medicine decided to give its
licensees two years to correct "illegal advertising in the Yellow Pages or any other advertising medium," including fraudulent or misleading price advertising or the use of
"misleading phrases such as 'as low as,' 'and up,' 'lowest prices,' or any other inexact
comparative expressions."[23]

Application of constitutionally permissible prohibitions against false, deceptive, or
misleading claims to Yellow Pages advertisements might bring the added bonus of
eliminating much of the tastelessness. Deception and tastelessness often seem to be
found together.

To assist practitioners who want to clean up their advertisements on their own, or
state boards that might want to provide some encouragement, Table 18-1 lists kinds of
false, deceptive, or misleading statements made by veterinarians that appear most commonly in advertisements, and especially Yellow Pages advertisements. Practitioners
must understand that whether a statement is deemed by the law to be false, deceptive,
or misleading does not turn on whether *they* understand—or think they understand—
the meaning of the statement. Nor is the test whether doctors intend to deceive the
public. The test is whether an ordinarily reasonable member of the public, a prospective client, who sees an advertisement is likely to be given a false impression or to be
misled. For example, some doctors may think that they know what "complete" facilities
are. Some may honestly believe that their practice is "complete" in some sense. The
word "complete," however, may mean something quite different to a layman. It must
also be emphasized that whether a statement is false, deceptive, and misleading
depends on all the relevant circumstances, including what else might be stated in an
advertisement and all relevant facts about a practice. Thus the claim that a practice
provides "complete" care or services is often false and misleading. This representation
probably implies, to members of the public, that *this* practice can do *everything* available in veterinary medicine for *all* patients. This, in turn, appears to imply, among
other things, that there are on the premises members of all the recognized specialties,
and that the practice offers the latest and most effective diagnostic, medical, and surgical procedures. On the other hand, some veterinary hospitals, including veterinary
school facilities and several very large private practices, can truthfully claim they provide "complete" services.

The extent to which the statements listed in the table are commonplace provides
strong evidence of the need for remedial action by many individual doctors and some
state licensing boards.

Solicitation

Solicitation is advertising directed toward specific persons. Solicitation can be done
through the mail. It can also be accomplished through oral or in-person communication with prospective clients by a veterinarian or someone hired to promote the doctor's practice.

Solicitation, especially in-person solicitation, can be extremely coercive.
Accordingly, the American Bar Association (ABA) *Model Rules of Professional Conduct*

TABLE 18-1
∼

False, deceptive, or misleading claims
commonly found in Yellow Pages and other advertisements

CLAIM OR REPRESENTATION	COMMENT
"Complete" care, services, medical or surgical facilities "Full service" facility or hospital "All" medical or surgical facilities	Unclear representations that can imply to laymen the availability, on the premises, of all available procedures and services for all species. These claims can be made truthfully only by a few facilities, or where a state licensing board provides definitions of such terms that are then applied properly.
"All your pet's needs"	Implies the availability, on the premises, of all necessary services, including those of a specialist if required. Such a claim is often false.
"High quality" care or services "Quality" care or services "Modern" facilities	Can imply that other practices do not offer "high quality" or "quality" care, or have out-of-date equipment. All veterinarians are required by state practice acts to offer quality care and modern facilities. Any representation relating to quality or level of quality is incapable of verification by the public, and when reasonably interpreted as a claim of higher quality than that provided by other facilities is also usually false.
"Superior" care or services	States that a practice provides better care or services than others. This claim is incapable of verification by the public and is usually false.
"Trustworthy" "Dependable"	Can imply that other veterinarians are not trustworthy or dependable. All veterinarians are required by state practice acts and principles of malpractice liability to be both trustworthy and dependable.
"State of the art" facilities, care, or services "The standard of excellence" The "best" facilities, care, or services "Highest standards"	Represent that a practice offers facilities and services that are as advanced in nature and as excellent in quality as those offered by any practice anywhere. These claims are false when made by most practices. They are also usually incapable of verification by members of the public, who are unlikely to be able to determine whether a facility can truthfully be characterized in any of these ways.
"Safe" surgery "Effective" vaccines "Accurate" diagnoses	Imply that other practices offer surgery or vaccines that are different, and less safe or effective, and diagnosis that is not correct. May imply a guarantee of cure or result.
"Low cost"	Can imply that the fees of this practice are generally lower than fees of other practices. This claim is often false, and incapable of verification by members of the public, who are unlikely to be able to determine whether a given fee is "low" compared to the fee of another practice for the same animal with the same condition and under the same circumstances.
"Reasonable fees"	Can imply that the fees of other doctors are not reasonable or are too high.
"Affordable fees"	Can imply that the fees of other doctors are not affordable or too high.

Continued.

TABLE 18-1 CONT'D
~

False, deceptive, or misleading claims
commonly found in Yellow Pages and other advertisements

CLAIM OR REPRESENTATION	COMMENT
"Specializing in…" "Jane Doe, DVM, Dermatology, (Cardiology, Internal Medicine, etc.)" "Cardiology," (Ophthalmology, Internal Medicine, etc.)"	False and deceptive when applied to doctors who are not diplomates of the indicated specialty or of a specialty recognized by the AVMA.
"We take the time to examine your pet." "A veterinarian who is compassionate." "You and your pet receive personalized care here." "You can trust us to care for your pet." "A hospital where the doctors have time for you and your pet." "A hospital where the doctors take the time to talk to you."	Such claims need not always be false, deceptive, or misleading, but they are when they make unfair, and false, comparisons with other practices. At the very least such statements can be ethically objectionable because they may give an unfair and inaccurate picture not just of one's colleagues but the profession in general.

state that "a lawyer shall not by in-person or live telephone contact solicit professional employment from a prospective client with whom the lawyer has no family or prior professional relationship when a significant motive for the lawyer's doing so is the lawyer's pecuniary gain." Written or recorded solicitations are not prohibited, but like oral or in-person solicitation cannot occur either if the prospective client has made known his desire not to be solicited or the solicitation "involves, coercion, duress, or harassment."[28]

As the ABA *Model Rules* explain, a person solicited in person or by telephone:

…who may already feel overwhelmed by the circumstances giving rise to the need for legal services, may find it difficult to evaluate all available alternatives with reasoned judgment and appropriate self-interest in the face of the lawyer's presence and insistence upon being retained immediately. The situation is fraught with the possibility of undue influence, intimidation, and over-reaching.[29]

These arguments seem no less relevant to solicitation by veterinarians, especially when the practitioner making a solicitation knows that the potential client has an animal in need of treatment. Moreover, either in-person or written solicitation will sometimes involve trying to win over people who are satisfied with their current veterinarian. It is unclear how the peace of mind of such people and the good names of other doctors will survive a solicitor's claim that clients will be happy with the solicitor's services.

Even before the Federal Trade Commission inquiry, the *Principles of Veterinary Medical Ethics* took a relatively permissive attitude toward solicitation. According to the pre-1989 code:

Written solicitation is permissible provided it does not exert undue influence, pressure for immediate response, intimidation, or overreaching. Oral or in-person solicitation, although permissible with the following caveats, is nevertheless undesirable because its very nature provides no evidence that can be examined by a regulatory body.[30]

Although the code failed to prohibit oral or in-person solicitation, at least it condemned solicitation that exerts undue influence, pressure, or overreaching. In the post-1989 code, this is gone. Now:

Written solicitation is permissible. Oral or in-person solicitation is undesirable because it provides no evidence that can be examined by a regulatory body.[22]

If the ABA *Model Code* can prohibit all solicitation that exerts undue influence or harassment, and can prohibit oral or in-person solicitation intended primarily for the solicitor's pecuniary gain, so can the AVMA *Principles*. The antitrust laws prohibit the restraint of fair and lawful competition, not the restraint of coercion or harassment.

The solicitation of a client by a veterinarian can be morally permissible when the practitioner happens unintentionally upon an animal requiring immediate medical care. Here, the animal's need for treatment would appear to outweigh the potential dangers of manipulation inherent in solicitation. However, even in such a situation, the interests of the animal owner would argue strongly in favor of the doctor encouraging the owner to seek continuing or follow-up care from his own regular veterinarian if medically possible.

～ THE VETERINARIAN AS A PROMOTER FOR OTHERS
Free Supplies and Waiting Room Advertisements

It is not uncommon for veterinarians to permit for-profit businesses to use the veterinary office to market their products or services, even if doing so provides no direct economic benefit to the practice. This can be done by displaying free supplies (such as puppy food or skin care preparations), or by permitting businesses to place advertisements or brochures in the waiting room.

A doctor who permits such third-party marketing might be motivated by a sincere desire to assist clients. However, turning one's office into a billboard for businesses raises the same ethical problems as distributing brochures containing advertisements for non-medical products. It gives the impression that the doctor is endorsing products generally and without the need to tailor a recommendation to the particular patient. It also makes the veterinary office an arm of the promotional activities of a nonveterinary business.

Nothing prevents a doctor from recommending a puppy food, pet photographer, grooming parlor, or pet-sitting service to clients who ask one's advice about such matters. Moreover, if a doctor believes that a certain product can be recommended on legitimate medical grounds for a particular patient, there seems nothing wrong in giving the client a free sample of that product provided by the manufacturer. But imagine what one's reaction would be if one encountered in a pediatrician's office a display of free baby foods or brochures for a baby photographer. Veterinarians who permit similar third-party marketing in their practices need not, surely, be committing a heinous moral offense. However, they are undermining the image of the veterinary office as a medical facility as opposed to a general all-purpose animal advice and service center. As I have argued, this latter image is not in the long-term interests of patients, clients, or veterinarians.

Third-party Coupon Redemption Programs

A perennial issue relating to the ethics of marketing concerns third-party promotional campaigns, in which veterinarians participate not only with the purpose of marketing their own practices, but with the effect of promoting the business of someone else.

In a typical third-party promotion, a nonveterinary business supplies to animal owners a coupon or certificate entitling them to free or discounted services from a participating doctor. To obtain these coupons, owners must, of course, purchase the company's products. Redemption schemes need not entail that the participating veterinarian be reimbursed by the company; the expected benefit to the doctor can be solely the entrance of a client and patient into the veterinary practice. Prior to 1989, the *Principles of Veterinary Medical Ethics* prohibited such redemption programs on the grounds that they implied an endorsement or testimonial by the doctor of the commercial product associated with the coupon.[31]

Although the FTC inquiry resulted in the elimination of the prohibition from the code, the prohibition never had much effect. Veterinarians then, and now, continue to become mired in such campaigns. The result is often aggravation and discord.

Veterinarian participation in coupon redemption programs is unprofessional when it implies doctors' endorsement of commercial products, and when it turns veterinarians into an arm of a commercial enterprise interested in selling its own, nonmedical products for profit.

However, these are not the only evils of coupon redemption schemes. They can lead the public to make unnecessary and invidious comparisons among doctors. Those who choose not to participate must explain to clients why and risk being perceived as greedy or unhelpful. Sometimes, certain doctors may not be permitted to participate. This occurred when the American Animal Hospital Association and 9 Lives® Cat Food announced a program entitling consumers to services at AAHA hospitals. The promotion led many non-AAHA doctors to complain that the public would think they were not as competent as AAHA members.[32]

Coupon redemption schemes can also give the impression that the entire profession endorses a company's products. This happened in 1987, when the Friskies Pet Care Division of the Carnation Company announced a program in which purchase of its Friskies® brand foods would entitle consumers to a "free checkup" from a member of the AVMA. Many veterinarians interpreted the campaign to imply endorsement of this brand of food by the AVMA. The AVMA and Carnation explained that there was no such endorsement, and Carnation agreed to send all AVMA members a letter stating that the AVMA was not a cosponsor of the program.[33]

The AVMA can also become associated with the marketing campaigns of manufacturers of commercial products, and thereby give the impression (intended or not) of its endorsement of these products. A 1990 issue of the *Reader's Digest* included an eight page section containing brief "articles" about various aspects of pet care together with advertisements for various products.[34] According to a notice attached to copies of the magazine mailed to AVMA members, the section was "done by the AVMA" with "support" from three manufacturers. At my talks to several regional and local VMAs, a substantial number of doctors expressed anger at the advertising section. They objected to the fact that each of the three "articles" on specific health problems contained on the same page on which it was printed an advertisement for an associated product and also faced a full-page advertisement for the same product. For example, the piece on fleas, ticks, and Lyme disease had advertisements for a pet insecticide spray; the "article" on dental care had advertisements for dog biscuits and rawhide strips claiming to prevent tooth and gum disease. I was told by some doctors who recommended the products featured in the advertisements that they did not like the apparent implication that the AVMA, and *all* veterinarians, endorsed these products. Especially unhappy were doctors who did not recommend one or more of these products. One doctor related that a client who had seen the advertising section could not understand why he refused to recommend a product endorsed by the AVMA itself. Clearly, the AVMA had no intention of endorsing any of these products or implying that all veterinarians recommend them. But this was not how some people read the advertising section, and their interpretation was entirely predictable.

It is unrealistic for the profession to blame pet product manufacturers who want to use the good name of veterinarians to promote their own products. These businesses undoubtedly wish to promote good pet care. But they are not charitable institutions. They cannot be expected to market veterinary practices without some return for themselves. If anyone is to blame for misunderstandings or misinterpretations, it is the profession itself for allowing its image to be associated (even unintentionally) with third-party promotional programs. There is only one appropriate response when companies attempt to garner explicit or implicit support for their promotions from individual doctors or veterinary associations: a clear and resounding *no!*

Testimonials and Endorsements

Veterinarians can also participate in promotional campaigns of businesses by giving testimonials for or endorsements of their products or services. There are three potential problems with such endorsements. First, they render veterinarians part of the promotional activities of commercial enterprises. This process can sometimes involve undignified, commercialistic behavior by someone who ought to be viewed as a healer and a friend (see Chapter 16). Such behavior can make it difficult for the profession to present itself as interested first and foremost in helping patients and clients. Second, some people might tend automatically to believe an endorsement by a veterinarian, especially if the doctor is well-known. Third, when a doctor is compensated for an endorsement or has some personal connection with the company using it, her words can be motivated more by self-interest than a desire to state the truth; the public will therefore want to know of the connection in order to evaluate the endorsement's credibility.

Two sections of the *Principles of Veterinary Medical Ethics* discuss testimonials and endorsements. Endorsements for nonveterinary, that is, nonprofessional or nonmedical, goods or services are treated in the code's advertising section. This provision prohibits any statement or claim that "contains, in a manner which is false or misleading: a testimonial about or endorsement of a veterinarian, or a combination of a veterinarian's name or photograph and identification as part of a testimonial, endorsement, or sales promotion of a nonveterinary product or service."[35] This general language replaces the stricter provision of the pre-1989 code that prohibited all veterinarian endorsements of nonveterinary products manufactured by commercial, for-profit companies.[36] The older provision astutely placed all such endorsements in the category of "false, deceptive, or misleading," on the grounds that there is nothing in a veterinarian's training or abilities that could give one special expertise regarding a nonveterinary product or service. For it would be a rare advertisement indeed that would not utilize a veterinarian's endorsement of a nonveterinary product without attempting to state or imply that a veterinarian must have special expertise regarding the product.

A separate section of the *Principles* is devoted to testimonials for and endorsements of veterinary products, services, and equipment.[37] Where an endorsement represents that the endorser uses the product, the endorser must be a *bona fide* user of the product. There must be adequate substantiation that the endorser's experience with the product is representative of what consumers will experience. Adequate substantiation implies "publication of a report in a journal wherein articles are subjected to peer review or in a publication recognized by reputation as a source of reliable scientific information." An endorser's qualifications must give him or her the expertise to evaluate the product, and an endorsement must be supported by the actual exercise of this expertise. Finally, "where there exists a connection between the endorser and the seller of the advertised product which might materially affect the weight or credibility of the endorsement, such connection must be fully disclosed." Among such material information would be whether the endorser was solicited to give the endorsement, and whether "the veterinarian is being compensated in the form of product or monetary benefit."

These guidelines regarding the endorsement of professional products derive largely from the 1988 proposed revision of the code undertaken prior to the FTC inquiry. If enforced, they will protect the public from false, deceptive, and misleading endorsements of and testimonials for veterinary products. Regrettably, the code does not apply the same strict specific standards to endorsements for nonveterinary products.

∾ CORPORATE SPONSORSHIP OF PROFESSIONAL ACTIVITIES

Any discussion of promotion and marketing must mention the activity of veterinary and animal supply businesses in sponsoring professional functions and events. From continuing education seminars offered by state and local VMAs, to annual conventions of VMAs and various specialty and practice groups, scarcely a professional gathering does not receive some monetary support from companies from which veterinarians purchase goods or services. Sometimes one company underwrites an entire event. At some of the larger meetings several pet supply or pharmaceutical companies subsidize the costs of lectures, including speaker honoraria. Exhibitors pay fees that help defray an organizing body's expenses. There is also substantial corporate support in the form of advertising in professional journals and newsletters of state and local VMAs.

A 1993 survey conducted by the AVMA Center for Information Management found that although 97% of veterinarians support commercial exhibits at meetings, there was some opposition to other corporate activities. Approximately 12% opposed advertising in AVMA journals, 15% corporate sponsorship of collaborative market research, and 13% corporate contributions to conventions and speakers.[38] These figures, I would argue, reflect the ethical situation relating to corporate sponsorship of professional activities. In the main, such support appears to be useful and appropriate. There are, however, relevant questions. There are also problem areas.

There are two major arguments in favor of corporate sponsorship of professional activities. The first relates to the clear benefits such support bestows on the profession, its patients, and clients. Some veterinarians may not realize how fortunate they are regarding the availability of first-class opportunities for continuing education. For a small, relatively poor profession, the possibilities are staggering. Not only are there several annual gatherings of national scope, many smaller local, state, and regional VMAs invite speakers with international reputations. These meetings enable doctors to keep current about the latest information, learn about the availability of specialty care, and maintain their licenses in states in which continuing education is a requirement of registration. Much of this would not be possible without corporate support. Corporate exhibits also provide opportunities for doctors to learn about available equipment, services, and textbooks, and to look for the best values for themselves and their clients and patients.

Corporate sponsorship of professional activities is also appropriate because, in our economic system, companies have a legal and moral right to engage in it. If veterinarians can lawfully and ethically promote their services to the public, so may companies market themselves to veterinarians.

Relevant Questions
Does corporate support compromise doctors' independent exercise of professional judgment?

There are, however, ethical questions that can appropriately be asked about corporate support in general or any given instance of such support. As the *Principles of Veterinary Medical Ethics* recognize, "veterinarians should not employ professional knowledge and attainments and nor render services under terms and conditions which tend to interfere with the free exercise of judgment and skill or tend to cause a deterioration of the quality of veterinary service."[39] Thus corporate support would be wrong if it compromised doctors' independent exercise of their professional judgment.

Companies would not sponsor professional activities if they did not hope they would benefit thereby. It hardly follows, however, that doctors are influenced in their decisions by corporate sponsorship, and for at least three reasons. First, veterinarians are sufficiently clever to know when a company supporting some event or activity is attempting to sell its products. If, as is surely the case, doctors must ordinarily be trusted to decide among competing products or services, there is no reason to think their judgment will somehow be clouded by an event sponsored by a company whose salespeople they may already encounter on a regular basis. Second, corporate sponsorship is often discreet and understated. Sometimes, all doctors will know of the sponsorship is a statement in program brochures or proceedings. Third, there is so much corporate sponsorship that is difficult to conclude that any companies really gain an advantage over their competitors. If today's meeting is sponsored by ABC pet food company, tomorrow's will likely be supported by the XYX pet food company. Indeed, a large meeting might be sponsored by both, and by several pharmaceutical companies. Corporate sponsors may not like to hear this, but the matter of corporate sponsorship is very much a "buyer's market." Veterinarians seem to *expect* the opportunity to listen to several competitors making the strongest case for the quality and value of their products.

This is not to say that in particular instances corporate representatives cannot attempt to undermine a doctor's exercise of independent judgment, say by offering a kickback or rebate. But such dangers are not inherent in corporate sponsorship itself, and can in any event be resisted by doctors and prohibited by state licensing boards.

Does corporate support affect the content of professional activities?

Veterinarians must also demand that corporate support never compromise the independent exercise of judgment of conference organizers and speakers, and of journal editors and authors. Organizers and editors must never be influenced in their choice of contributors by corporate sponsorship, nor should speakers or writers be asked or required to include in their contributions stated or implied endorsements of the product, or the kind of product, offered by the sponsor.

I have attended meetings where a speaker is a veiled (and sometimes not-so-veiled) advertisement for a company sponsor. In each such instance, the attempted sales pitch was apparent, and the negative reaction of the audience unmistakable. In general, there does not appear to be a problem, faced even by smaller organizing bodies, with interference from sponsors. Indeed, speakers typically do not know beforehand that their talk is supported by any company or a particular company; usually all they know of any such support is what any attendee may read in a program proceedings or poster. I myself have been invited several times to make the arguments against the sale of nonprofessional products at meetings sponsored by companies which urge veterinarians to sell such products. Sometimes, these very talks have been supported by such companies. The response of company representatives has always been polite and professional.

Promotional overkill

Although corporate support does not seem to improperly influence the judgment of many veterinarians, promotion can be so blatant that it becomes offensive. There is nothing wrong with brief remarks by a company's representative before a program or a sponsored dinner. However, compelling attendees to sit through a 15-minute demonstration before the speaker is introduced is another matter. A poster or two indicating a company's support can be informative, but signs plastered on every wall or photocopied advertisements for each attendee can exceed the bounds of good taste. At one large convention a colleague of mine found two screens in the room in which he was to speak: one for his slides and the other immediately adjacent, projecting the logo of the company supporting his lecture. He demanded that the promotional slide projector be turned off so that he and the audience could concentrate on the presentation.

Such promotional overkill may be like the glut of billboards on a highway. These advertisements become so omnipresent that people cease even to notice their messages. But they can still lend an atmosphere of ugliness to the whole experience. Even if company sponsorship does not affect anyone's behavior, organizing bodies and sponsors themselves should assure that a professional gathering avoids the *appearance* of being little more than a promotion.

REFERENCES

[1]Knowles RP: Merchandising in veterinary medicine, *Trends* 2(3):49-50, 1986.
[2]Gants R: A no-more-excuses look at veterinary dentistry, *Vet Econ* June 1990:44-51.
[3]Quoted in: Newsletters — Keep you in touch with your clients, *J Am Vet Med Assoc* 190:957, 1987.
[4]Wood F, Watson W, Putman K: Outsiders spot problems, opportunities in practice, *Vet Econ* November 1993:88.
[5]Becker M: 60 hot practice tips that will make you money, *Proceedings of the North American Veterinary Conference* 7:876, 1993.
[6]Becker M: 38 resolutions for a *great* year, *Vet Econ* January 1994:43-44.

[7]American Veterinary Medical Association: *Principles of Veterinary Medical Ethics*, 1993 Revision, "Guidelines for Naming of Veterinary Facilities," *1994 AVMA Directory*, Schaumburg, IL, The Association, p 89.

[8]*Code of Ethics of the American Veterinary Medical Association*, "Advertising by Display Signs," *J Am Vet Med Assoc* 96:93, 1940.

[9]American Veterinary Medical Association: *Principles of Veterinary Medical Ethics*, 1987 Revision, "Advertising Regulations," *1988 AVMA Directory*, Schaumburg, IL, The Association, p 476.

[10]Lofflin J: Practice growth comes from feline favor, *Vet Econ* March 1986:68.

[11]Whitford R: Letter, Rewards undermine professional credibility, *Vet Econ* November 1992:17.

[12]Calhoun B: Give word of mouth promotion new meaning, turn TLC into MLM, *Vet Forum*, March 1992:36.

[13]Becker M: Three steps to *dramatically* increase your referrals, *Vet Econ* September 1992:73.

[14]American Veterinary Medical Association: *Principles of Veterinary Medical Ethics*, 1993 Revision, "Advertising," *1994 AVMA Directory*, Schaumburg, IL, The Association, p 42.

[15]*Code of Ethics of the American Veterinary Medical Association*, *J Am Vet Med Assoc* 96:93-94, 1940.

[16]*Bates v. State Bar of Arizona*, 433 U.S. 350 (1977).

[17]McCurnin DM, Thompson A: Professional advertising, *J Am Vet Med Assoc* 188:1387, 1986.

[18]*Zauderer v. Office of Disciplinary Counsel of the Supreme Court of Ohio*, 105 S.Ct. 2265, 2275 (1985), emphasis supplied.

[19]*Id*, at 2277.

[20]*Id*, at 2280 (asserting that "although the State undoubtedly has a substantial interest in ensuring that its attorneys behave with dignity and decorum in the courtroom, we are unsure that the State's desire that attorneys maintain their dignity in their communications with the public is an interest substantial enough to justify the abridgment of the First Amendment rights").

[21]American Veterinary Medical Association: *Principles of Veterinary Medical Ethics*, 1987 Revision, "Advertising Regulations," *1988 AVMA Directory*, Schaumburg, IL, The Association, p 476.

[22]American Veterinary Medical Association: *Principles of Veterinary Medical Ethics*, 1993 Revision, "Advertising," *1994 AVMA Directory*, Schaumburg, IL, The Association, p 43.

[23]Legal advertising as perceived by the BEVM, *Calif Board Exam Vet Med News* Spring 1988:1.

[24]Lofflin J: Is your Yellow Pages ad working? *Vet Econ* May 1989:35-41.

[25]Quoted in, *Id*, p 41.

[26]American Veterinary Medical Association: *The Veterinary Service Market for Companion Animals*, Schaumburg, IL, 1992, The Association, p 39.

[27]*Code of Ethics of the American Veterinary Medical Association*, "Directory Advertisements," *J Am Vet Med Assoc* 96:93, 1940.

[28]*ABA Model Rules of Professional Conduct*, Ethical Rule 7.3, "Direct Contact with Prospective Clients." In Gorlin RA, editor: *Codes of Professional Responsibility*, ed 2, Washington, DC, 1990, Bureau of National Affairs, p 380.

[29]*Id*, p 381.

[30]American Veterinary Medical Association: *Principles of Veterinary Medical Ethics*, 1987 Revision, "Advertising Regulations," *1988 AVMA Directory*, Schaumburg, IL, The Association, p 476.

[31]American Veterinary Medical Association: *Principles of Veterinary Medical Ethics*, 1987 Revision, "Redemption Coupons," *1988 AVMA Directory*, Schaumburg, IL, The Association, p 477.

[32]*See*, for example, Shomer R: Letter, Objects to examination coupon program, *J Am Vet Med Assoc* 182:852, 1983; Friedman J and others: Letter, Alleged discriminatory advertising, *J Am Vet Med Assoc* 182:1300, 1983.

[33]No AVMA sponsorship of Carnation's free checkup program for pets, *J Am Vet Med Assoc* 190:1087, 1987.

[34]*Reader's Digest*, March 1990: 187-196.

[35]American Veterinary Medical Association: *Principles of Veterinary Medical Ethics*, 1993 Revision, "Advertising," *1994 AVMA Directory*, Schaumburg, IL, The Association, p 42.

[36]American Veterinary Medical Association: *Principles of Veterinary Medical Ethics*, 1987 Revision, "Testimonials and Endorsements," *1988 AVMA Directory*, Schaumburg, IL, 1988, The Association, p 475.

[37]American Veterinary Medical Association: *Principles of Veterinary Medical Ethics*, 1993 Revision, "Testimonials and Endorsements Relating to Veterinary Products, Services, and Equipment," *1994 AVMA Directory*, Schaumburg, IL, The Association, p 43.

[38]Wise JK, Yang JJ: Veterinary issues survey—Part I: Professional association activities, *J Am Vet Med Assoc* 204: 726-727, 1994.

[39]American Veterinary Medical Association: *Principles of Veterinary Medical Ethics*, 1993 Revision, "Guidelines for Professional Behavior," paragraph 3, *1994 AVMA Directory*, Schaumburg, IL, The Association, p 42.

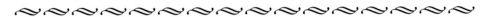

CHAPTER 19

Are Veterinarians Colleagues or Competitors?

*M*any veterinarians are uneasy about their economic future. In general, veterinarians are not nearly as well-compensated as members of other professions with comparable educational backgrounds and importance. The 1993 median professional pre-tax income of U.S. veterinarians in private clinical practice was $47,316, and the mean was $59,188.[1] The substantial difference between these figures indicates that many veterinarians earn well below what, compared with some other professions,[2] is a modest income. Perhaps even more significantly, although private practitioners in most practice categories saw increases in mean incomes between 1983 and 1991, mean incomes declined in all these categories between 1991 and 1993. The declines ranged from a low of 0.7% for large animal exclusive doctors to a high of 7.7% for small animal practitioners.[1]

Veterinarians' concerns about their ability to earn adequate income have contributed not just to a general interest in finding ways of generating revenue, such as merchandising and marketing, but also to questions about how practitioners can coexist in the marketplace with colleagues. Issues regarding competition and relations among doctors can be expected to grow in number and intensity as perceived economic pressures increase.

∾ THE MAJOR CONCERN

Statistics are not kept about which ethical issues are of greatest interest to veterinarians. I have spent many years speaking at VMA meetings, continuing education seminars, and classes at veterinary schools. The topic people want to discuss most often is not euthanasia, fee setting and collection, animal rights, or even animal welfare. I believe I can state with confidence that the ethical area most troublesome to veterinarians relates to competition. Is it ethical to try to win clients over from other veterinarians, and if so are there limitations on how this may be done? Is it proper to tell a client that another doctor made a mistake? Is it ever ethical to criticize another veterinarian? Can veterinarians associate with each other, and engage in cooperative efforts to advance veterinary care, when they are being told even by some veterinarians that they ought to be competing aggressively with other doctors? In short, should veterinarians consider themselves as colleagues or competitors?

The proposed 1988 Revision of the *Principles of Veterinary Medical Ethics* (see Chapter 9) had an answer to this last question. Veterinarians, it declared, "should consider themselves as colleagues rather than competitors."[3] Predictably, this provision did not survive the Federal Trade Commission (FTC) inquiry into the code, nor will this statement ever be in the *Principles*. The statement seemed intended to discourage competition, and any attempt by a professional association to discourage its members from competing against each other violates federal antitrust laws. However, whether individual veterinarians should—as a matter of *ethics*—consider themselves as colleagues rather than competitors remains very much a legitimate question.

~ WHAT IS COMPETITION?

Before one can discuss legal and ethical aspects of competition it is essential to understand what is meant by the term. There is a sense in which each veterinary practice that functions in an area having at least one other veterinary practice is, by definition, in "competition." In this sense, to say that there is "competition" is to say that there is more than one provider of veterinary services to which clients can take their animals. In this sense, a client can state that if she is not pleased with her current veterinarian, she can always go to "the competition"—even if "the competition" never engages in any activity designed to attract new clients or to win over other doctors' current clients. In this sense, merely by practicing and accepting cases a veterinarian is "competing" with other practices.

It is important to identify this definition of "competition" because it is misused by some proponents of aggressive marketing and promotion in support of the claim that because "competition is inevitable," veterinarians might as well accept the fact and act accordingly, that is, engage in aggressive rivalry.

This first sense of "competition" is not the one employed in this book, nor is it what most veterinarians have in mind when they think about competition. "Competition" as I understand it involves, necessarily, the attempt by two or more doctors or practices to obtain the patronage of the same person or persons. The following definitions offered by *Webster's Third International Dictionary* make clear that as the word is used in ordinary, commercial, and legal parlance, competition involves a contest in which each participant attempts to win out over, or best, the others[4]:

- "the act or action of seeking to gain what another is seeking to gain at the same time and usually under or as if under fair or equitable rules and circumstances: a common struggle for the same object..."
- "a contest between rivals: a match between contestants"
- "the effort of two or more parties to secure the custom of a third party by the offer of the most favorable terms"
- "a market condition in which a large number of independent buyers and sellers compete for identical commodities, deal freely with each other, and retain the right of entry and exit from the market"

"Competition" in this sense does not follow merely from the presence of more than one practice to which clients can take their animals. Competition involves *active attempts* by two or more veterinarians or veterinary practices, each to gain what only one can have: the same client and animal in the practice at a given time. These targets of competition can be members of the public who are not currently clients of any veterinarian. They can also be current clients of other doctors.

"Competition" also requires more than merely telling the public of one's services or fees, in advertisements or brochures, for example. Competition requires more than a willingness to accept new clients, including clients of other doctors. These things can be done without an active attempt to gain clients at the expense of any other doctor. Competition requires, by definition, an additional element: an attempt to gain *for one-self* a piece of business that one thereby *prevents* another competitor from having. Competition is more than a struggle *for* clients and patients. It is a struggle *against* one's competitors. As the dictionary indicates, competition involves rivalry, and head-to-head contest among combatants. Competition can create more than one "winner," if the market is large enough (or through the efforts of competitors becomes large enough), and more than one competitor does well. However, with regard to the patronage of any one customer at any one time, there can be only one winner. This is the essence of competition.

～ LEGAL ASPECTS OF COMPETITION

The general issue of competition among veterinarians is fraught with legal dangers. U.S. federal and state laws protect certain competitive practices and prohibit or restrict others. Some veterinarians have not been beyond suggesting solutions to ethical issues that could expose them to very serious legal troubles.

The Sherman Antitrust and Federal Trade Commission Acts

The most important laws affecting competition among veterinarians are the federal Sherman Antitrust Act and the Federal Trade Commission Act.

Passed over 100 years ago, the Sherman Antitrust Act was intended to curb the power of giant monopolistic collections of businesses, or "trusts," which dictated prices and prevented small or new firms from competing in the marketplace. The Act prohibits "(e)very contract, combination in the form of trust or otherwise, or conspiracy, in restraint of trade or commerce among the several States, or with foreign nations."[5] The Act also states that "(e)very person who shall monopolize, or attempt to monopolize or combine or conspire with any other person or persons, to monopolize any part of the trade or commerce among the several states, or with foreign nations shall be deemed guilty of a felony."[6] In addition to providing criminal penalties for violators, the statute permits private persons (such as veterinarians or veterinary clients) who are damaged by anticompetitive practices to sue violators (such as other veterinarians or veterinary associations), and to recover triple damages, court costs, and attorneys' fees. Consumers can also institute class action suits against violators. The Sherman Antitrust Act and additional statutes that extend its scope to other kinds of restraints of trade are enforced by the U. S. Department of Justice and the FTC.

The Federal Trade Commission Act provides that "(u)nfair methods of competition in or affecting commerce, and unfair or deceptive acts or practices in or affecting commerce, are declared unlawful."[7] This statute is enforced by the FTC. Although the FTC Act is technically not part of the antitrust laws, conduct violating these laws will also constitute a violation of the FTC Act because anticompetitive practices are deemed by the FTC Act to be unfair. However, the FTC Act's prohibition against "unfair" trade practices also includes such tactics as false and deceptive advertising and "bait and switch" inducements. The FTC Act's prohibition against unfair trade practices functions as a counterweight to the Sherman Antitrust Act's policy of promoting competition. By prohibiting deceptive, unfair, and underhanded trade practices, the FTC Act limits the most egregious forms of competition.

State Antitrust and Unfair Trade Practices Acts

Many states have statutes that are modeled on federal antitrust and fair trade practices laws. These state laws also prohibit businesses and professional people from engaging in anticompetitive or unfair trade practices, such as price-fixing. Such statutes usually are enforced by the state attorney general. Some states also specifically prohibit anticompetitive behavior by veterinarians in their veterinary practice acts or state licensing board regulations (see Chapter 7).

The Underlying Policy of Federal Antitrust Law and Its Application to the Professions

As the U. S. Supreme Court has explained, the purpose of the federal antitrust laws is to protect freedom of competition, in the second sense of "competition" defined above. Underlying this purpose was a determination by Congress that "the unrestrained interaction of competitive forces will yield the best allocation of our economic resources, the lowest prices, the highest quality and the greatest material progress."[8]

It is essential that veterinarians understand what the antitrust laws do and do not say. These laws reflect a philosophic judgment by the legislative branch that competition is good. The antitrust laws also require the courts to utilize the underlying goal of promoting competition in determining whether any given trade practice violates the law. However, the antitrust laws do not themselves require any individual person, business, or professional practice to engage in any form of competition. The antitrust laws prohibit two or more persons, businesses, or professional practices from unfairly *restraining* or *attempting to restrain* lawful competition. People are free to compete if they so desire, but they are also free not to engage in full-blown competition if this is their choice.

The U.S. Supreme Court made this point clearly in a case involving the National Society of Professional Engineers (NSPE), a private professional association similar to the AVMA. The NSPE's code of ethics prohibited competitive bidding by its members. Builders were required to determine which engineer or engineering firm to employ on their projects without any consideration of an engineer's fees. After a builder decided which engineer to use, based solely on engineering considerations, the builder would then learn the engineer's fee. If the builder decided this fee was not satisfactory, it could reopen the process and seek another engineer. The NSPE's stated rationale for its prohibition against competitive bidding was that the quality of buildings and engineering projects would be assured if builders did not base their choice of an engineer, at least initially, on the amount of an engineer's fee.

The Court held that the NSPE's prohibition against competitive bidding violated the antitrust laws because it restrained free competition by preventing builders from fully considering price. However, the Court stated that the "Sherman Act does not require competitive bidding; it prohibits unreasonable restraints on competition."[9] In other words, any individual engineer and builder could decide not to raise the issue of the engineer's fee during initial consideration of the engineer's proposal. It is unlawful, however, for a group of engineers to try to impose such a practice on any engineer or builder.

Antitrust law is complex and technical, and it is impossible to summarize it here. Although its purpose is to prevent unreasonable restraints upon competition, the law does not provide an exhaustive list of illegal activities. The courts have identified certain practices they consider automatically anticompetitive; among these are organized boycotts against a selected enterprise to drive it out of business, price-fixing by groups of businesses or professional associations, and bans on competitive price-bidding. Regarding behavior not deemed inherently anticompetitive, courts will determine whether, given the facts peculiar to the kind of business involved, the history of the alleged restraint, and the reasons it was imposed, the behavior at issue has an *unreasonable* negative effect on competition.

Although it may not always be clear whether a given activity violates antitrust law, certain features of the law are beyond dispute.

1. Antitrust law prohibits restraint of trade by more than one person or business acting in concert. This is why the Sherman Antitrust Act speaks of a "contract," "combination," or "conspiracy" to restrain trade.

2. Because professional associations such as the AVMA, or regional, state, or local VMAs, consist of two or more persons, they are subject to the antitrust laws. So are any two or more veterinarians who might attempt on their own to discourage, inhibit, or restrict competition. However, the U.S. Supreme Court has also indicated that professions, such as veterinary medicine, have distinctive aims and activities and might not always be treated by antitrust law identically to ordinary commercial businesses. The Court has said that:

It would be unrealistic to view the practice of professions as interchangeable with other business activities, and automatically to apply to the professions antitrust concepts which originated in other areas. The public service aspect, and other features of the professions may require that a particular practice, which could properly viewed as a violation of the Sherman Act in another context, be treated differently.[10]

Thus the Court has indicated that claims of superior service and in-person solicitation by professionals raise special dangers and may therefore be prohibited by state licensing boards.[11] However, the Court has also made clear that "textbook" examples of anticompetitive behavior by professionals, such as attempts to fix minimum fees for services or to restrict the range of services provided by members, are illegal.

3. The antitrust laws do not prevent joint attempts to influence federal, state, or local government even when the basic objective of such attempts is to achieve government action that has anticompetitive effects, provided these attempts are not a "cover" or "sham" to gain protection from the antitrust laws.[12] Thus although concerted attempts to run mobile vans out of town to reduce competition would be unlawful, practitioners clearly may express to their state veterinary licensing board sincere and good-faith reservations about the ability of particular facilities to provide adequate care to certain kinds of patients.

4. Finally, although unreasonable attempts by veterinarians to restrict free and lawful competition are unlawful, neither the antitrust laws nor any governmental agency enforcing these laws can compel any individual practitioner who has not otherwise violated the law to engage in advertising, marketing, any form of self-promotion, or the sale of nonprofessional products. The law does, however, prohibit two or more veterinarians from agreeing or attempting to restrict, discourage, encumber, or burden any lawful competition or lawful sale of goods and services by themselves or by any other veterinarians.

Thus veterinarians remain free, individually, to decide whether or to what extent they want to battle against their colleagues for the same clients. Provided they do not attempt to impose their views on others, or violate other laws relating to practice, they may seek their own individual counsel and do what they think is right. The antitrust laws do restrict substantially the power and authority of official veterinary ethics—the process by which the organized profession imposes moral values on its members (see Chapters 8 and 9). However, the antitrust laws, like the constitutional protection of the freedom to advertise, elevate the importance of normative ethics—the activity in which each person must decide ethical questions for himself or herself (see Chapters 5 and 10).

The Role of the FTC and Potential Antitrust Violations by Veterinarians

Although both the U. S. Justice Department and the FTC enforce the antitrust laws, the latter has been more active in regulating the veterinary profession. For example, in 1986 the FTC applauded the Virginia state veterinary board's withdrawal of certain restrictions on truthful advertising, but criticized proposed regulations prohibiting claims of superiority and the use of solicitors to attract business.[13] As discussed in Chapter 9, a 1988 FTC inquiry about 52 possible antitrust violations in the *Principles of Veterinary Medical Ethics* led to substantial changes in the code. The FTC also takes an interest in the activities of local veterinary associations. It accused the Madison County, Alabama VMA (MCVMA) and four Alabama veterinarians of illegally agreeing not to participate in a program offering discounted spays and neuters and of illegally agreeing to restrict their advertising in the Yellow Pages. The FTC proposed a consent decree in settlement of the charges, which according to one report included the requirement that "for 10 years, the MCVMA would be prohibited from continuing a meeting in which any member states his or her intention not to participate in a program promoting discounted veterinary services, unless the member is ejected from the meeting. If more than one member makes such statements, the meeting must end immediately."[14] The FTC can also take legal action against veterinary state licensing boards. In 1989 it demanded that the Oklahoma State Veterinary Board remove from its regulations a prohibition against the ownership of veterinary practices by nonveterinarians, on the grounds that the prohibition restrained competition. After 2 years of litigation, the Board agreed to the demand because it could no longer afford to battle the FTC.[15]

What happened in these cases illustrates why veterinarians must exercise extreme caution in approaching issues relating to competition.

1. In its determination to protect freedom of competition, sometimes the FTC reaches interpretations of the law that are at least open to debate. The FTC's criticisms of the Virginia licensing board's proposed regulations prohibiting claims of superior quality and solicitation contradict the statement of the U. S. Supreme Court that claims of superiority and in-person solicitation by members of professions pose special dangers and may therefore be prohibited by state licensing boards.[16] Although, as noted in Chapter 9, several provisions of the pre-1989 *Principles of Veterinary Medical Ethics* did violate the antitrust laws, several provisions that were removed did not. As discussed in Chapter 16, a 1992 federal appellate court decision appears to reject the FTC's contention that state professional licensing boards cannot issue regulations restricting the ownership of practices to their licensees.

2. As what happened to the *Principles* and in Oklahoma also show, even when it might not be correct in its interpretation of the law, the FTC may still be able to impose its interpretation on people who lack the money, time, or will to contest their case. Veterinary associations are not wealthy and eager for litigation, and in most states, veterinary licensing boards are not among the most powerful or well-financed agencies of government.

3. Finally, because the FTC may interpret ambiguous behavior (activities that might but also might not be intended to restrain trade) as attempted restraints of trade, veterinarians must do more than avoid clear violations of the antitrust laws. They must be careful to avoid actions that present even the *appearance* of illegality. The FTC is likely to look askance at any discussions during any veterinary meeting or among any group of veterinarians in which activities that could restrain trade are even raised, however casually. Thus it would be dangerous to have a discussion at a meeting of a VMA in which members talked about what they charge for various services. Indeed, it would be unwise for any two veterinarians from different practices serving the same geographical area ever to discuss their fees, even in private. Although such a discussion might in fact not be intended to gain agreement about prices, it could give the appearance of such an intention, and could result in FTC action.

State Civil Causes of Action

Veterinarians should also be aware of state laws that permit them to be sued (or to sue) for actions relating to competition. In many states, business and professional people may be sued for wrongful interference with a competitor's right to seek and retain customers. Among such civil causes of action are the following:

- *Injurious falsehood*: "the publication of matter derogatory to the plaintiff's title to his property, or its quality, or to his business in general, or even to some element of his personal affairs, of a kind calculated to prevent others from dealing with him, or otherwise to interfere with his relations with others to his disadvantage."[17]
- *Interference with contractual relations*: the intentional and improper interference with the performance of a commercial contract between another and a third person by the intentional inducement or causing of the third person not to perform the contract.[18]
- *Intentional interference with prospective advantage*: the deliberate attempt by wrongful means to prevent the plaintiff from carrying on his trade, including such tactics as harassment of the plaintiff's customers or employees; obstruction of the means of access to his place of business; threats of groundless suits; and inducing employees to commit sabotage or to undermine the plaintiff's business.[19]

Veterinarians who make false statements so harming the reputation of a competitor as to deter clients or colleagues from associating or dealing with him might also be sued for defamation of character.[20]

⌇ IS COMPETITION AMONG VETERINARIANS BENEFICIAL?

Whatever may be the benefits of full-blown, head-to-head competition in other areas of the economy, it is doubtful whether "competition" in the classic sense serves the interests of clients, animals, and veterinarians. Restrictions of space allow me only to offer several observations that should stimulate individual practitioners to make their own judgments. I wish to make clear at the outset that my doubts about competition among veterinarians are not intended to question the potential benefits of competition generally. Competition often brings improvements in the quality, price, and availability of consumer goods. Rather, I believe there are distinctive facts about medical care for animals, and about the market for veterinary services, which raise questions about the wisdom of aggressive, full-blown, head-to-head competition among veterinarians.

Invidious and False Comparisons

There are in my view two major reasons why it is not in the interests of clients, patients, and veterinarians for practitioners to actively battle each other for clients. First, if a veterinarian competes with colleagues for clients, he must convince prospective clients that there is some reason it is advantageous for them to come to *him*. Competition often leads competitors to make unflattering representations about other competitors. As the 1992 comprehensive study of the veterinary service market conducted by the AVMA indicates, the overwhelming majority—approximately 90%—of clients with companion animals are satisfied with their current veterinarian.[21] This means that full-blown competition for clients will usually require attempting to win away another practice's current clients. It will often be difficult to do this without telling these people that their present veterinarian does not merit their patronage.

One danger of criticizing one's colleagues is that it can lead to a diminished view not just of them but of the profession in general. But criticizing one's fellow veterinarians will also often involve something at least as bad: making false, deceptive, and misleading claims. This will often be the case because (as the AVMA survey of client satisfaction indicates) the great majority of veterinarians do provide excellent services. To be sure, some practices have equipment or kinds of practitioners that others do not, some may be more convenient in terms of location or hours of operation, some may have lower fees, and some will have doctors that just happen to "hit it off" better with particular clients and animals. However, in general, clients in most areas of the country can obtain highly competent services from more than one veterinary practice.

Therefore to convince people to leave their current veterinarian, or to come to *their* practice, some practitioners will have to deceive or mislead to give people the impression that they are preferable. The Yellow Pages of various localities provide evidence of this. As related in Table 18-1, claims of superiority, higher quality, state-of-the art services, complete services, low cost, and safety often are simply false. These claims are often made by practices that offer no better, more advanced, more affordable, safer, or complete services than others in their community. Veterinary practice acts do prohibit false, deceptive, and misleading advertisements. The extent to which such advertisements persist shows that some doctors either do not know about these laws, do not care about them, or are willing to push their competitive efforts as far as regulatory authorities will allow. The end result is the same: falsehoods motivated by the perceived need to best one's colleagues. These falsehoods help neither the public nor the profession.

The Nature of the Veterinary Services Market

However, the major reason full-blown competitiveness among veterinarians will not benefit clients, patients, or the profession is that competition among veterinarians misreads the nature of the market for veterinary services. Head-to-head competition addresses a problem that does not exist in this market, and fails to address the serious problem that does.

As the 1992 AVMA report on the veterinary service market for companion animals shows, the major problem faced by the profession—and by animal owners and their animals—is that not enough owners seek veterinary services. The report relates that in 1991 approximately 34.6 million households in the United States owned a total of approximately 52.5 million dogs; 29.2 million households owned a total of 57 million cats; 5.4 million households owned a total of 11.7 million birds; and 1.9 million households owned a total of 4.9 million horses.[22] Yet, despite these impressive numbers, a substantial proportion of owners did not seek veterinary care for any of their animals. Although 82% of dog-owning households obtained veterinary care in 1991, the figures were only 62% for cat-owning households, 54% for horse-owning households, and 11% for bird-owning households. Moreover:

> ...mean veterinary visits per households for dogs was 2.64 visits per year in 1991, up from 2.37 visits per year in 1987. For cats, mean veterinary visits was 1.78 visits per year in 1991, up from 1.62 visits per year in 1987. Mean visits per household for birds was 0.22 visits per year in 1991, up from 0.15 in 1987. For horses, mean visits per household was 2.40 visits per year in 1991, up from 1.85 in 1987.[23]

These statistics demonstrate that not enough people are taking their animals to a veterinarian. Many *millions* of animals do not receive *any* veterinary care, and many millions that are sometimes taken to a veterinarian probably ought to be taken more often. The figures for cats and birds are especially significant, because cats now outnumber dogs and because the percentage of bird owners seeking veterinary services is so small.

Full-blown, head-to-head competition among veterinarians will not be of significant value to clients, animals, and practitioners because such competition will not substantially increase the number of owners who bring in their animals, nor will it persuade people to take their animals to their current doctor more often. Rather, competition—the struggle among practitioners for the same business—will at best tend to shift members of the profession's existing client base from practice to practice. The Yellow Pages provide evidence of this. In Chapter 18, I quoted remarks by practice management consultant Donald Dooley about the cost and effectiveness of Yellow Pages advertisements. His comments merit quotation again here. Dooley observes that:

> Yellow Page advertising is used to steer clients from one hospital to another. It does nothing to try to reach those who aren't already using veterinary services. We spend millions as a profession to steal a client from one hospital to the next and nothing to try to get new clients into the profession.
> Veterinarians spend millions of dollars across the nation in the Yellow Pages, while state and national veterinary organizations have a tough time raising even $100,000 for a budget to do a smattering of advertising for the profession as a whole—advertising that would encourage more people to utilize veterinary medical services.[24]

The Yellow Pages are the quintessential paradigm of head-to-head competition. Here, in one place, are advertisements that are clearly intended to attract clients who could go to other practices. Here can sometimes be found, in one place, advertisements that make invidious comparisons with other practices. If such competition is not terribly effective and at best shifts current clients from one practice to another, there is no reason to think that other forms of competition against other doctors will work differently.

The capture of another veterinarian's clients by the capturer may be good for him, but it is not likely to benefit the losing veterinarian. More importantly, because the great majority of veterinarians provide competent services at fees that are usually comparable to those of other practices in their area, most clients and patients are not benefited either. The tragedy, as Dooley states, is that most people who need to be convinced to seek veterinary services remain untouched. Moreover, some of these people may be less and not more motivated to take their animals to a veterinarian by competition and advertisements that do not give the profession a good image.

Veterinarians, therefore, would do better for themselves and those they serve by promoting the value of veterinary services to people who do not yet have a veterinarian, rather than competing for current clients of other doctors. They would then face the critical task (one largely of internal rather than external marketing) of convincing current clients to provide their animals the best services they can provide.

It might be argued that full-blown competition will help everyone at some point, when the market for veterinary services becomes both large and permanent. Competition among manufacturers of automobiles and television sets, for example, benefits consumers because there is virtually universal demand for these products. Competition therefore functions to keep quality high and prices low for those who want these products. The situation of universal demand which allows competition to work for the benefit of purchasers of consumer goods will probably never be characteristic of the veterinary services market. Veterinarians will *always* have a problem convincing all owners who should bring their animals for medical care to do so. This is so because veterinary patients are *animals*. Although many people have high regard for animals, others do not. Moreover, animal medical care surely will never have the same priority for many households as human medical care, or indeed a wide range of non-medical human expenses. Money spent on an animal will usually come out of a family's discretionary income, and there will often be matters that appear to some more urgent or worthy than veterinary care.

Thus it will likely always be a struggle for veterinarians to convince enough people to employ their services, and to convince people to employ their services as often as they should. It is precisely because this struggle is important, for animals as well as veterinarians, that the scarce resources of an undercompensated profession should not be frittered away on competitive head-to-head battles for the same clients, when these battles do not substantially increase the overall client base and tend to give the profession a bad image to boot.

Aggressive Competition versus Availability, Service, and Information

To doubt whether full-blown, head-to-head competition for clients is beneficial is not to question other approaches that are clearly ethical and beneficial. Each practice should, wherever its caseload allows, accept new clients and patients. This affords the public a choice. Each practice should provide the very best services it can offer and should try to meet or exceed the level of care provided by other facilities in the community. This also affords the public a choice and assures that clients can obtain competent services. Each practice may, through internal and external promotion, inform the public about its facilities, services, doctors, and fees. This can assure that members of the public know what is available and will help potential clients to choose a practice that is best for them and their animals. No practice should—as a matter of ethics as well as law—ever agree or attempt with other practices to restrict the full availability of veterinary services to the public.

However, availability, service, and information, even when expressed in advertisements, need not be aimed at winning current or prospective clients away from other doctors. Availability, excellent service, and providing information to the public about one's practice can be motivated by the desire—inherent in the values of true professionals—always to do one's best for all one can help. This is a positive attitude of aiming for excellence, rather than a negative attitude of attempting to tear down someone else to benefit oneself.

As I have already observed, but cannot emphasize enough, the legal profession provides important lessons to veterinarians about commercialism and competition. Many people associate lawyers with aggressive, sleazy, and deceptive competition because of certain advertisements in the Yellow Pages and in the print and broadcast media. In fact, very few attorneys ever advertise. Indeed, as odd as this may sound to some people, most lawyers do not actively compete against other lawyers for clients. Most rely mainly on word-of-mouth referrals. The fact that a small number of so-called "ambulance chasers" and aggressive competitors have managed to tarnish the image of the entire legal profession should serve as a warning to veterinarians that the same thing can happen to them.

Individual Choice

Finally, in light of the antitrust laws it must be emphasized again that no veterinarian or veterinary association should ever attempt to inhibit lawful full-blown competition or do anything that even presents the appearance of attempting any restraint of competition. All the arguments of this book are directed at individual doctors, who retain the legal right and moral duty to decide for themselves how they shall approach issues relating to competition. What veterinarians do in the marketplace must be chosen doctor by doctor and practice by practice without outside compulsion, restraint, or influence.

~ SOME CURRENT CONTROVERSIES REGARDING COMPETITION
Competition from Humane Societies

One of the most bitter controversies regarding competition for veterinary clients concerns the operation of veterinary facilities by nonprofit humane societies. Because such organizations are tax-exempt, some are able to charge clients much less than private practitioners for the same services. Some veterinarians have reacted by asking the courts to close down humane society veterinary hospitals, and at least one such suit has been successful.[25] In 1983 the AVMA, the American Animal Hospital Association, the American Humane Association, and the Humane Society of the United States proposed model legislation "limiting the full-service humane hospital or government veterinary hospital to service only those who cannot afford private veterinary care."[26] The AVMA has adopted two policy statements relating to veterinary services provided by humane organizations, the 1982 Memorandum of Understanding for Humane Organizations and Veterinarians[27] and the 1983 Guidelines for Veterinary Associations and Veterinarians Working with Humane Organizations.[28] The former encourages private doctors and veterinary associations to "provide veterinary service to animal shelters at a mutually agreeable fee."

The argument usually raised in favor of full-service, low-cost humane society hospitals is that they benefit both clients and animals by making veterinary care less expensive. In the short range, this could be so. But over time, there is a danger that some private practices that cannot compete with humane societies will disappear. This will harm the interests of clients and animals. A reduction in the number of doctors would not only make it more difficult for clients to obtain veterinary services; it would reduce the diversity of practices and approaches that a thriving community of veterinarians can offer the public.

Full-service, low-cost humane society hospitals can also be profoundly unfair to private doctors with whom they compete, even if these doctors can maintain satisfactory revenues. The government, by exempting such facilities from taxation, subsidizes their operation in a manner in which it does not subsidize the ordinary practitioner. This arguably might be acceptable if only the needy were being served by humane society hospitals; helping the needy is a traditional governmental function. However, by permitting tax-exempt organizations to offer the same services to the same clients at a lower cost, the government steps into the market and gives selected participants an advantage in the absence of any compelling need to do so.

The debate about humane society veterinary facilities is likely to continue for some time. The following suggestions are offered for consideration by the profession and government:

1. Humane societies should be permitted to operate full-service hospitals without imposition of taxes if they do not use their tax-exempt status to undercut fees charged by private practitioners, and if they charge fees that are within the normal range of those generally charged in their communities. Although humane societies ought not to be given a competitive advantage because of their tax-exempt status, neither would it be fair to make it more difficult for them to compete with private doctors just because they are operated by nonprofit organizations.

2. An argument (though not, in my view, a very strong one) can be made for permitting tax-exempt humane society facilities to provide at reduced cost to all members of the public a limited number of veterinary services essentially related to the mission of these societies. Because these organizations are viewed as serving a public function in protecting people from animal disease and predation, it can be maintained that they ought to be permitted to offer low-cost rabies vaccinations. Because they are involved in efforts to control animal populations and place unwanted animals, it can be argued that they may offer the public low-cost sterilizations, certainly of animals that they themselves place for adoption, as well as euthanasia of unwanted animals that would otherwise become a public nuisance. An argument can also be made that, given their traditional concerns with animal suffering and their function of ministering to injured animals on public ways, humane organizations should be allowed to maintain emergency facilities that can serve all emergency injury cases.

3. Because assisting the needy is widely recognized as a legitimate function of government, a strong case can be made for permitting humane societies to offer government subsidized services at reduced cost only to such persons. However, the problem of defining "need" in the veterinary area requires considerable thought before one can be comfortable about government subsidy of humane society veterinary services. When people require medical care costing many times their annual income, it is not difficult to conclude that they might need financial assistance or a publicly subsidized facility. In the veterinary area, however, where fees are usually much lower, it is often the case that clients can literally afford a procedure—but come to the conclusion that they do not want to pay for it, or that paying for it would be an undue burden. Such clients might well say that they "need" help, and their pleas can seem especially poignant if they foist upon us the choice of subsidizing them or having their animals killed. It seems grotesquely unfair to clients whose love for their animals enables them to dig deep into their resources, to subsidize other people who might place a relatively low value on their animals. Those who urge that humane society facilities should serve the needy must be prepared to engage in the difficult and unpleasant task of determining whether some clients believe they are in "need," not because of financial hardship but because they do not have as much regard for their animals as they ought to have.

4. Ideally, humane societies providing lower-cost services should use local practitioners to staff their veterinary facilities. Local practitioners might be more likely than salaried humane society staff to care about whether the facility is indeed providing an essential public service or assistance to the needy, rather than unfair competition against established private practices.

5. Under no circumstances may veterinarians serving in humane facilities provide inferior medical care or deviate from their usual ethical obligations to patients and clients.

6. In a provocative discussion, Dr. Gordon Robinson suggests that veterinarians might be able to prevent unfair competition from humane society hospitals by doing spays and neuters at sharply reduced fees. As he explains, humane societies detest the fact that they are in the "killing business." To avoid killing so many animals, many open spay and neuter facilities. Once constructed, such facilities can be used in other kinds of cases, and it is difficult for doctors working in them to turn away animals and clients that need or want their services. Dr. Robinson argues that low-cost humane society facilities that take clients from struggling practitioners might not open in the first place if these doctors could make sterilization more affordable.[29]

Vaccination and Testing Clinics

Whenever there is a legitimate medical objection to some activity, it is proper for the profession to raise it, even if it might appear to some that the objection is being made for economic reasons. Approaches that are bad medically cannot be good ethically. This can be a problem with vaccination clinics in which doctors immunize or test large numbers of pets without being able to conduct a physical examination, take a history, or advise clients regarding follow-up care. The *Principles of Veterinary Medical Ethics* distinguish between mass clinics designed to protect the public, such as rabies vaccination programs, and those designed to protect animal health. The code recognizes that the former function can usually be accomplished without the opportunity for examining the animal. However, "when the primary objective is to protect the animal's health, clinical examination of the patient including proper history-taking, is an essential and necessary part of a professionally acceptable immunization procedure."[30]

Supporters of animal health-oriented mass clinics might respond that it is better that animals be vaccinated or tested, even if this means that some will suffer because they cannot be examined properly. But veterinarians, who are committed to animal health and competent care, should not settle for such a choice. When brought an animal for the purpose of protecting its health, they should impress upon the client what must be done to fulfill this purpose. Veterinarian participation in clinics without adequate medical attention can only perpetuate acceptance by some of the legitimacy of a choice between poor care and no care.

Spay and Neuter Clinics

Some veterinarians offer clients greatly reduced fees in spay and neuter clinics in which large numbers of animals are processed through a limited surgical service. (Often these clinics are operated by humane societies, whose tax-exempt status contributes to the lower fees.) Some practitioners believe that these clinics, like mass vaccination programs, can lead to medical problems because of their limited focus. Dr. Richard Fink, for example, has seen patients that must undergo subsequent surgeries because procedures (such as removal of papillomas) were not conducted during treatment at limited sterilization clinics.[31]

The approach of the *Principles of Veterinary Medical Ethics* to spay and neuter clinics is obscure. The relevant section states that doctors should always "exercise individual judgment in deciding whether to undertake the care of any particular patient, regardless of whether the patient is referred by a humane organization, a spay and neuter clinic, or others."[32] This section does not appear to deal with the propriety of participating in a spay and neuter clinic itself (as opposed to taking a referral from such a clinic), a matter that ought to be addressed if such programs are harming some patients. Because veterinarians are always supposed to exercise "individual judgment," it is unclear what the section is supposed to mean. Presumably, it is not meant to condone turning away an animal in need of follow-up or referral care to voice one's opposition to a low-cost sterilization clinic or humane society hospital.

Mobile Veterinary Facilities

The AVMA "Guidelines for Naming of Veterinary Facilities" define a "mobile facility" as a "practice conducted from a vehicle with special medical or surgical facilities or from a vehicle suitable only for making house or farm calls."[33] A mobile facility is thus to be distinguished from the situation in which a veterinarian who maintains a fixed-premise facility visits a home or farm in a motor vehicle containing a limited supply of medicines or implements to be used in or on the client's premises.

Today's mobile veterinary facility is usually a motor trailer or large van. Some provide only vaccinations and testing. In others, animals are also examined and treated. Some doctors with mobile facilities practice only in such facilities. Some mobile facilities are part of practices that include a fixed-premise office, clinic, or hospital in which animals are regularly seen or to which they are referred when they cannot be adequately diagnosed or treated in the mobile unit.

In certain locations and under certain kinds of conditions, mobile facilities can play an enormously beneficial role in providing veterinary care. To those in the inner city without means of transporting their animals to the doctor, to many elderly, to residents of nursing homes and public housing projects, and to people in rural areas that cannot support a fixed-premise veterinary office, a mobile van might be the only source of veterinary services. Some of these people might also have difficulty affording standard veterinary fees and would not frequent a standard fixed-premise facility with higher fees even if it were available to them.

There has been considerable opposition in the profession to mobile facilities because some of them seek clients who can come to, and can afford the fees of, fixed-premise practices. Such mobile facilities are perceived by some as just another variant of the street peddler, whose low overhead enables him to undercut the prices ordinary establishments must charge, who might not contribute his fair share of taxes, and who cannot offer the variety or quality available in more standard kinds of businesses.

"Unfair" competition

To some doctors, the mere fact that mobile facilities do not have the same overhead costs of fixed-premise hospitals gives the former an unfair competitive advantage. Some practitioners also believe it is unfair that a mobile facility can simply show up at a shopping center or parking lot and lure away from them clients whom they have served for years.

The quickest answer to such complaints is that they contradict certain basic features of our economic system. Our system does not regard as unfair—indeed, it rewards—those who can find less expensive ways of serving the public's needs. The fact that a mobile facility is cheaper to operate than a fixed facility does not itself make the former unfair, any more than a fixed-premise hospital that can cut costs by hiring fewer but more productive employees is being unfair to other fixed-premise practices.

Compliance with zoning ordinances, payment of taxes and fees

A much stronger charge of unfairness can be brought against any mobile facility that violates local zoning ordinances. Zoning rules represent a community's collective judgment concerning esthetic values and the proper manner of reconciling the interests of various segments of the population. Some communities ban street vendors altogether. Some permit them only in certain locations and at certain times and only after receiving a permit. Still other communities require that all street operations be conducted by businesses with a permanent location in the area.

A mobile practice that knowingly violates zoning rules is showing contempt for a community by attempting to profit from it while rejecting rules it has set down for all enterprises. There is little doubt that if a fixed-premise veterinary facility attempted to violate zoning rules either by placing a building in an inappropriate area or by operating its own mobile facility in violation of zoning standards, city officials would be able to find and stop it. If fixed practices must abide by zoning rules, so must mobile ones. If mobile practitioners find a community's zoning rules overly restrictive, they can, like anyone else, ask for a variance or challenge the rules. A mobile facility would also be unfair to fixed practices and to the community if it failed to pay all required taxes and permit fees.

Quality of service

The argument against certain mobile facilities most likely to impress the public and government is that they provide inadequate veterinary care. This charge can certainly be made against patient health-oriented mass veterinary clinics offered through mobile facilities. As noted above, such operations are deemed medically inappropriate by the AVMA. All practitioners, as well as the state veterinary boards, have an interest in preventing mobile facilities from accepting patients they are not equipped or qualified to handle.

Nevertheless, doctors who object to mobile facilities that do provide high quality care and obey the law might find that the public will interpret their criticism to be motivated by naked self-interest. Fixed practices can explain to clients why their fees sometimes must be higher than those of mobile vans; they can include examinations within vaccination fees; they can conduct their own lower-cost vaccination clinics (with the possibility of appropriate examinations); they can sponsor or participate in community clinics for the needy; and they can explain to clients the advantages of bringing animals on a regular basis to a full-service fixed facility.

Ethical obligations of mobile facilities

Mobile facilities have important moral obligations that flow from their nature as limited and movable operations.

First, these facilities must never attempt to undertake diagnoses or perform procedures that can only be accomplished, or can be accomplished better, in a larger fixed-premise hospital. All veterinarians are morally obligated to make treatment choices based primarily on the needs of patient and client and not their own pecuniary interests.[34] It would be profoundly immoral for a mobile facility to fail to inform clients of alternative approaches because these options cannot be done at such a facility.

Second, any veterinary facility must be able to be found on a continuing basis by clients and regulatory authorities. Otherwise, patients in need of follow-up care will be left in the lurch, and it will be impossible for state licensing boards to determine whether good quality care is being provided.

～ RESTRICTIVE COVENANTS OF NONCOMPETITION

So-called "restrictive covenants of noncompetition" involve an agreement between a veterinarian and the practice in which he or she works that he or she will not, after leaving employment, practice veterinary medicine (or practice in specified fields of veterinary medicine) for a specified period of time within a specified geographical area of the former practice. The U. S. Supreme Court has ruled that such covenants need not violate federal antitrust laws, even though they clearly restrict competition, because it is reasonable to encourage the growth of businesses by protecting them temporarily from competition by former employees.[35] Individual states have the authority to determine whether and under what conditions they shall recognize such agreements.

Restrictive covenants of noncompetition involving veterinarians are allowed in most states. Even where such agreements are enforceable, they will not be upheld unless the restrictions they impose are reasonable. Each requirement of the agreement must be reasonable, including the length of time of the restriction, its geographical scope, and the nature of the restriction given the interests of the parties to the agreement and the public. (In some states, agreements deemed unreasonable will be voided altogether, and in others, courts will substitute reasonable restrictions for those upon which the parties agreed.) Whether a restriction is found reasonable will also depend on all the relevant facts, which can vary from case to case. For example, a covenant prohibiting a former employee from practicing within a 10-mile radius might be reasonable in a rural area, but unreasonable in an urban area in which a 10-mile radius could include millions of potential clients. Likewise, a court might not uphold a covenant prohibiting a former employee from "the practice of veterinary medicine," where the former employer is a large animal exclusive practice and the employee seeks to work in a small animal exclusive practice. In such a case, the former employer's interests would not be harmed by the employee's new job, and the harm to the employee and the public would clearly outweigh any benefit to the former employer.

In the first edition of this book,[36] I asserted that restrictive covenants are ethically acceptable. I noted that in bringing a doctor into a practice, owners provide immediate access to their most valuable "asset," their clients and patients. Practice owners are entitled to some protection against associates who might want to use this asset for their own benefit. I also suggested that because the law will only enforce reasonable restrictions, associates usually need not worry about signing away more than what is morally fair. If they do so, the law will not hold them to the promise.

Since the publication of that edition, I have been compelled by mounting evidence to conclude that restrictive covenants are doing employee veterinarians much more harm than they are bringing demonstrable benefits to employers and the public. I now believe that all states should prohibit restrictive covenants involving veterinarians, at least those involving nonowner doctor employees. Although the requirement that restrictions must be reasonable might in *theory* protect legitimate interests of employers and employees, in *fact*, too many employees are being forced to sign unfair agreements. Some employers are using these agreements more to manipulate or punish employees than to protect themselves against unfair competition.

I have heard from many veterinarians, many of them recent graduates, who have been harmed unfairly and unreasonably by restrictive covenants. They point out that new doctors often do not have a wide choice of employment opportunities. Given the large number of new doctors seeking work, one can be fortunate to obtain a single offer. There may be student loans to repay, which can make it difficult to turn down a position with the hope that another will come along without a restrictive covenant attached to it. One may need to locate in a certain area because one's family resides there. These doctors also point out that even if the provisions of a contract are unenforceable because they are unreasonable, it may be impossible for a young veterinarian to afford the legal fees or take the time to defend against an injunction or suit for damages by a former employer.

By themselves, such facts would not make restrictive contracts unethical. The fact that a recent graduate needs employment does not render any less legitimate a prospective employer's interest in protecting his client base. However, I have become convinced that too many veterinarians are taking unfair advantage of restrictive covenants and their superior bargaining power to unfairly burden employed veterinarians.

The following story illustrates how these covenants can actually function:[*]

Dr. Smith, who graduated from veterinary school 6 months ago, signed a restrictive covenant with a small animal practice prohibiting him from "engaging in the practice of veterinary medicine, surgery, or dentistry for 2 years within a 10-mile radius" of the practice. Smith was required to sign the covenant as a condition of his employment. When he voiced concerns about it, he was told the covenant could not be deleted from the employment agreement.

After a few months at the practice, Smith, who grew up on a farm, decided that he would be happier in equine and farm animal practice and so informed his employer. The employer was outraged that Smith wanted to leave so soon, and reminded Smith about the restrictive covenant. Smith responded that he was willing to stay on until the employer could find a replacement. Smith also tried to convince the employer that because he wanted to enter equine and farm animal practice, he would not be a threat to the employer even if he remained in the area. The employer, angered more by Smith's intention to leave than by the possibility of damaging competition, told Smith that he would sue to enforce the agreement.

Smith now faced the dilemma of staying with an employer who was already mad at him, or seeking a large animal position in the area and being sued. He felt that given the employer's reaction to what he thought was a fair and reasonable proposal, he had no future at the practice even if he abandoned his plans to become a large animal doctor.

Although he could have argued in court that he should be allowed to practice large animal medicine, an attorney Smith consulted could not guarantee he would prevail. Nor did Smith have the money, time, or psychological stamina for a legal battle.

Although there was a large animal practice within the geographical area encompassed by the restrictive covenant that was interested in hiring Dr. Smith, he decided that it would be safer to look elsewhere. He located a position many miles away, in another state. His wife remained in their old home with their children until they finished the school year and she could locate a job in the area to which Smith moved.

The following examples represent the kinds of abuses reported to me most often by recent graduates:

- Requiring an employee to sign a restrictive covenant prohibiting "the practice of veterinary medicine" within what would otherwise be a reasonable geographical area for what would otherwise be a reasonable amount of time—and then threatening to sue an employee who seeks to work for another facility that cannot possibly compete with the employer's hospital because it is engaged in a different kind of practice
- Offering a doctor a limited term of employment (for example, as an intern or resident) without the possibility of an extension and requiring the employee to sign a restrictive covenant prohibiting practice in the area for several years—even though the employee doctor will be at the practice for a short time, and it is the employer who does not want to keep him on any longer

---

[*]This story, like all the cases in this book, is realistic in the sense that it is derived from actual events, but is not based on any individual case or situation. Any similarity between actual situations and this and other examples in this text is not intended and is purely coincidental.

- Requiring an employee doctor to sign a restrictive covenant prohibiting the practice of veterinary medicine for a specified time in a specified geographical area of any facility owned by the employer, where the employer owns several clinics located throughout a large geographical area, the resulting geographical restriction encompasses a very large portion of the state, the employee would not see cases in all the satellite facilities, and the employee has neither the intention nor ability ever to practice in all the territory encompassed by the restrictive covenant
- Threatening to take a former employee doctor to court for violation of a restrictive covenant where the doctor wants to do part-time relief work for several facilities nights and on weekends and will not be in a position to take clients away from the employer with whom she signed the contract
- Threatening to take a doctor to court for violation of a restrictive covenant, where the doctor's working for another practice is unlikely to harm the former employer, but the employer is angry that the employee has left and wants to punish her
- Utilizing a restrictive covenant as a tool to make it more difficult for presently employed doctors who are unhappy with salaries or working conditions to complain—by threatening them that if they quit the covenant will prevent them from finding a better position in the area
- Requiring an employee to sign a restrictive covenant that one knows is probably unenforceable because it specifies too long a time or too extensive a geographical area, believing that the employee cannot afford legal counsel to challenge the contract or defend against a lawsuit
- Refusing even to talk with an employed doctor about overlooking a violation of the covenant where adhering to the agreement would cause the employee severe economic hardship, or where the employee is prepared to demonstrate that going elsewhere will not harm the practice

I do not mean to suggest that all, or even most, restrictive covenants are abused in such ways. However, the law must ask whether, in general, restrictive covenants really protect practice owners more than they harm employee doctors, and whether these covenants benefit or harm the public. I have met very few owners who can demonstrate that they have been threatened by a former employee stealing away clients or that they *ought* to be protected from having to convince clients to stay with them. In contrast, I am now convinced that the overwhelming majority of recent graduates and employee veterinarians who wish to practice in a way that could violate the terms of a restrictive covenant do not seek to leave an employer with the intention of *competing* with that employer. The great majority are seeking better employment conditions: more favorable hours, a better salary, or colleagues whose company they think would be more enjoyable. Many seek work in a practice that, in fact, offers little opportunity for direct competition. Many doctors who are subject to restrictive covenants are young, relatively inexperienced, and financially incapable of owning their own practice and taking away a former employer's clientele.[37]

Prohibiting restrictive covenants would not cause disaster. In Massachusetts, the medical practice act bans restrictive covenants involving physicians, without apparent effect on the ability of physicians to maintain their practices. California, which has the largest number of veterinarians of any state,[38] prohibits their signing restrictive covenants. The time may be at hand for legislatures in all states to consider prohibiting restrictive covenants among veterinarians. At the very least, data should be gathered to determine whether restrictive agreements benefit the profession, and its clients and patients.

In states where restrictive covenants of noncompetition are enforceable, employers should exercise sensitivity in the presentation of them to employee doctors. No jurisdiction requires such agreements. Practices that do not really need them should not ask doctors to sign them. Where a practice reasonably believes it does need some protection, and insists on having employees sign a restrictive covenant, the agreement should be written as narrowly as possible so as to address the kind of competition the practice reasonably fears. (Thus a small animal exclusive practice should not attempt to prevent an employee doctor from "the practice of veterinary medicine or surgery.") It is wrong to try to induce an associate to accept restrictions that are not enforceable, hoping that their invalidity will not be discovered or challenged. One should also consider not enforcing a covenant against an employee who can demonstrate a hardship or the improbability of actual competition. A prospective associate should always be given the opportunity to consider any written employment agreement, and to consult an attorney, before signing it. Perhaps most importantly, employee doctors, and especially recent graduates, should assume that the worst *can* happen and that an employer *will* attempt to enforce a restrictive covenant. No such agreement should be signed unless one is convinced one will be able to live with it.

⚬ CRITICIZING COLLEAGUES

If the ethical topic of greatest interest to veterinarians concerns their general relations with colleagues, the specific ethical problem that appears to trouble practitioners most relates to criticism of one's performance by another veterinarian. In many years of addressing meetings and classes both large and small, I have found that always—not often, but *always*—a discussion of relations with other doctors turns to complaints about how some veterinarians are unfairly criticizing others.

The Arguments Against Criticizing a Colleague

Some examples

The following cases illustrate why criticism by a colleague or someone who works for a colleague can be damaging and unfair.

Case 19-1 Mr. and Mrs. Client's cat begins vomiting at 8 p.m. and is in great distress. They call their veterinarian's office and hear a taped message stating that the practice is closed until 9 a.m. the next morning. They look in the Yellow Pages and find a listing for the ABC Animal Clinic, which is open evenings. They bring the cat to ABC. It is examined by Dr. Z, who asks Mr. and Mrs. Client when the cat was last seen by a veterinarian. They respond that they had taken the cat to their doctor 2 weeks ago for a flea problem. Dr. Z spots several fleas. He screws up his face and says, "Jeez, I don't know what kind of vet you are going to. This is unbelievable." Dr. Z then rattles off a number of approaches he would have taken to the flea problem. Mr. and Mrs. Client look at each other and think to themselves that this is a really good veterinarian.

In fact, the Clients' old (and now former) veterinarian gave them appropriate instructions about how to deal with their cat's fleas, but they were not scrupulous in following these directions.

Case 19-2 Ms. Client uses Dr. X for veterinary care for her dog, but takes the animal regularly to Dr. Y's facility for grooming. Dr. Y has an in-practice groomer.

As she is leaving the dog with Y's groomer, the groomer tells her, "You should have Dr. Y take care of your dog. There have been a lot of problems with Dr. X, and his fees are very high."

Ms. Client tells her friends what the groomer said and decides to switch to Dr. Y.

In fact, Dr. X is quite competent and does not charge fees that are higher than those of other practices for comparable services. Dr. Y's groomer receives a bonus for each client who sees Dr. Y on her recommendation.

Case 19-3 Dr. Q is presented with a 5-year-old intact female Golden Retriever. She has never been pregnant, despite efforts to breed her. Dr. Q strongly urges an ovariohysterectomy. The clients want very much to have her puppies and ask whether there isn't anything else that can be done. Dr. Q, who is aware of prostaglandin hormonal therapy being conducted at a veterinary school in a neighboring state tells the clients that he can refer them to a doctor there. Dr. Q does so even though he thinks it would be inhumane to put the dog through the therapy because it does not always work, can be distressful to the animal, and will not guarantee permanent relief from pyometra. He telephones Dr. R, a theriogenologist at the veterinary school and makes an appointment for the clients.

Upon examination of the dog, Dr. R recommends prostaglandin treatment. When told by the clients that Dr. Q thought surgery was the best option, Dr. R, shaking her head benignly, remarks with a smile "Well, these GPs aren't up on the latest advances. We're specialists here. Did you know that veterinary medicine has specialists just like human medicine?"

The clients opt for prostaglandin and vow to use only specialists in the future. In fact, it is at least arguable that the hormonal therapy is not humane (see Chapter 22). Dr. Q did nothing wrong or incompetent, and he went out of his way to assure that the clients were informed of all available options.

Case 19-4 Mr. Client has an 8-year-old Tabby cat he takes to Dr. C, who owns a feline-exclusive practice. His 10-year-old Pomeranian is the patient of Dr. D, who has a small animal hospital in the area. On a visit with the cat to Dr. C's hospital, Mr. Client looked through an open door into Dr. C's surgical suite and noticed some impressive looking machinery. While Dr. C was examining the cat, Mr. Client asked her about it. C told him this was the latest inhalation anesthesia equipment. Dr. C took him to see it and explained how it worked.

Mr. Client remarked to Dr. C that when his Pomeranian needed surgery, he recalled Dr. D saying that he was going to use an injection to anesthetize the dog.

Dr. C responded that she had some bad experiences with injectable anesthetics and that not every veterinarian could afford this kind of equipment. Mr. Client left very upset about Dr. D.

In fact, Dr. D, who is a board-certified veterinary surgeon, has advanced inhalation anesthesia equipment, but sometimes uses an injectable anesthetic on older dogs because in his experience, they do well on it and it is quickly reversible.

Case 19-5 Mrs. Client's 6-year-old Collie returned home limping on its left hind leg after a vigorous jog with Mr. Client. Mrs. Client is very fond of the dog but has been unable to find a veterinary hospital that, in her opinion, "does a good job at a decent price." She was unhappy with the MNO Animal Hospital, because they once charged her $45 for an x-ray, so she decided to take the Collie this time to the TUV Veterinary Hospital.

Dr. T, owner of the hospital, examined the dog and suspected a cruciate ligament injury. He advised Mrs. Client that the Collie would have to be examined under anesthesia. He also suggested that radiographs be taken.

Dr. T performed his examination and determined that the dog indeed had a ruptured cranial cruciate ligament. When Mrs. Client arrived to pick up the Collie, he told her that there was some good and some bad news. The good news was that he had ruled out the possibility of cancer, infection, and a broken bone. The bad news was that the dog had a rupture of a ligament and needed surgery immediately.

Mrs. Client asked "what all this will cost" and was told several hundred dollars, in addition to the fee for the anesthesia and diagnostic work. She thought to herself that here was another veterinarian who was trying to pressure her into paying a lot of money. She told Dr. T she wanted a day or two to make up her mind. Dr. T told her it would be a mistake not to operate on the dog immediately, but that if she absolutely needed some time to think about it, she should restrict the dog's movement and activity until the operation, which, he stressed again, should be done as soon as possible.

Angry about being "rooked by another one of those horse doctors," Mrs. Client waited several days to see if the dog would get better on its own. After it appeared to be getting much worse, she took it to the FGH Animal Hospital, the last veterinary facility in her town which she had not yet tried.

Dr. F, the owner of the hospital, examined the dog and took a history from Mrs. Client. She told him that she had taken the dog to another veterinarian. She did not name this doctor but complained that she didn't think he did a good job. When she told Dr. F this veterinarian said he thought it could be cancer, Dr. F said "No, I don't think so." Dr. F also said that if this was what he thought it was (namely, a ruptured cruciate ligament), there was no way he could, in good conscience allow this dog to go home without having surgery. Mrs. Client authorized Dr. F to examine the dog and to do the surgery if necessary.

As she left for home, Mrs. Client was pleased that Dr. F's fee for the examination and surgery was 5% lower than Dr. T's. "Just let that thief Dr. T try to collect from me for that x-ray and exam!" she said to herself. "The guy is obviously incompetent, Dr. F said so himself. And Dr. F had better do a great job for all the money he's asking!"

The interests of practitioners

It is certainly not in the interests of most veterinarians to be criticized by another doctor or another doctor's employees. At the very least, clients to whom such a criticism is made can suffer doubt or anxiety about the care their animal may have received from its first doctor. A criticism by a second doctor, if strong enough, could lead the client not to pay the first doctor's fee. The client may decide to choose another veterinarian. The client may spread bad words about the first doctor to other current or potential clients. The client may decide to sue the first doctor for malpractice or even to file a complaint with the state licensing board.

All these things can occur whether a criticism is true or false. These consequences can be especially unfair when a criticism is unjustified. And one of the major problems with criticism of a colleague is that it most likely will be unjustified.

Unfair criticism: Recurring situations

As the above cases illustrate, there are several reasons criticism of a colleague to a client can be inaccurate, unfair, or both.

NOT THE SAME CASE. First, and perhaps most importantly, a second doctor examining an animal will often not see exactly the same case as was seen by the first. The patient's condition may have developed further and not as a result of any improper action by the first doctor. Something entirely new may have occurred, either unexpectedly or as a result of an injury to the animal or lack of compliance by the client with the first doctor's instructions. In Case 19-5, for example, although the first doctor advised immediate surgery, it may still have been possible to postpone the operation for a short time. However, when the second doctor saw the dog, the condition might have been considerably worse (because of the client's inaction), and the second doctor, unaware of how long the client delayed, may have drawn an incorrect conclusion about what the first doctor saw from his own examination of the patient.

LACK OF KNOWLEDGE ABOUT WHAT TRANSPIRED DURING THE FIRST DOCTOR'S CARE. As cases 19-1, 19-4, and 19-5 illustrate, a fertile source of inaccurate and unfair criticism is a second doctor's ignorance about what actually happened when the first doctor attended the patient. What did he find? What did he tell the client? What did he recommend, and why? How did the client respond to his recommendations? In all these examples, the first doctor acted correctly. But the client may not have appreciated the appropriateness of that doctor's actions because veterinarians do not, nor need they, always tell clients precisely why they make a certain diagnosis or recommend a particular approach. A client's lack of knowledge about what happened during a previous doctor's care can become a second doctor's lack of knowledge—if the latter accepts as true or complete what the client says transpired when the first doctor saw the animal.

IGNORANT OR CONFUSED CLIENTS. A client's lack of understanding about what really happened when the first doctor saw the animal can result from the client's ignorance or confusion. The client may not have understood precisely what the first doctor said, and this might not be the first doctor's fault. Some clients are unsophisticated and have difficulty understanding complex or subtle medical information. Some clients are so upset that they may be unable to understand completely. This need not be a problem, if the client remains with the first doctor, who has the opportunity to make sure the client understands what is happening before treatment is authorized. But lack of clear understanding can cause problems, if the client transmits faulty information to a second doctor. The client's ignorance or confusion can cause problems if, as in Case 19-4, it leads him to question the first doctor's judgment or competence.

IMPRESSIONABLE, NONCOMPLIANT, AND CONTENTIOUS CLIENTS. As cases 19-1 through 19-4 illustrate, some clients are extremely impressionable. Some may have a great deal of respect for veterinary medicine, and as in Case 19-3, may believe whatever is said by a practitioner who appears authoritative. Because some clients believe whatever a veterinarian says—even when what is said is based on faulty information provided by the client—criticizing a colleague can harm that colleague.

To be sure, some clients are far from impressionable. Especially dangerous are those who forget or ignore a first doctor's instructions. They can transform their animal's condition into something quite different from what the first doctor saw, and can place that doctor in an especially bad light if they fail to mention their noncompliance to the second doctor.

Most, dangerous, however, is the kind of client in Case 19-5. Such people are looking for a reason to think ill of a previous doctor. They can interpret what is ordinarily a harmless statement or question as a criticism. Some may want a reason for not paying a fee. Some, like the client in Case 19-5, may lie about what a previous doctor said or did. Clients like these can be like roving time bombs that are destined to explode in the direction of *any* veterinarian they visit. People who are looking for bad opinions about veterinarians who served them well are likely to find objections to anything done by any doctor—including the latest.

Outright criticism aimed at harming a colleague. Some veterinarians take advantage of client receptivity, or predictable reactions, to criticize a colleague in order to deliberately harm that veterinarian. Because its aim is usually winning over the client to whom it is made, such criticism is properly viewed as a form of competition. When made, as in Case 19-1, without sufficient factual basis, it is patently false. When made, as in Case 19-3, by a veterinarian who seeks to discredit a doctor who has clearly done nothing wrong and indeed is responsible for the client's consulting him in the first place, the criticism is mean-spirited as well as inaccurate.

Careless or misinformed statements that can be interpreted as criticisms. Unfortunately, a statement that might not be intended as a criticism can sometimes be interpreted as one. It is sometimes impossible to know that an ordinarily harmless statement will be taken by a client as a criticism because one cannot always know a client's motivation or her experiences with another doctor. On the other hand, there are some kinds of statements which, though perhaps not intended to criticize, ought to be seen by any doctor to amount to a criticism under the circumstances. Thus Dr. F, in Case 19-5 might not have intended to call Dr. T's performance into question. Yet given the complaining attitude and statements of the client, he should have been aware that his remarks about the dog not having cancer or needing immediate surgery could have been interpreted as criticisms.

Careless remarks made to praise oneself that can be interpreted as criticisms. Sometimes, statements made to clients might be intended merely to praise one's own actions or to promote one's practice but can be interpreted as a criticism of another doctor. It is quite possible that when she talked about her experiences with injectable anesthetics and showed Mr. Client her surgery suite, Dr. C, in Case 19-4, never meant to suggest that such anesthesia was inappropriate for his dog or that the veterinarian who treated it did not have inhalation equipment. Yet, Mr. Client reached this conclusion. Veterinarians cannot anticipate everything a client might think, but in the context of the conversation, Dr. C probably should have understood that her remarks could be interpreted as a criticism.

Arguments in Favor of Criticizing a Colleague
The Golden Rule

The most frequent response practitioners and veterinary students appear to have to cases such as those presented above is to cite the Golden Rule. It is important, most will say, not to criticize a colleague because one could be criticized by another veterinarian. How, it is asked, would *I* feel if another veterinarian said that I made an improper diagnosis, had faulty or out-of-date equipment, or mishandled a case?

This was precisely the approach to the criticism of colleagues taken by the pre-1989 *Principles of Veterinary Ethics*. One was told to:

> Handle new clients, their sick animals, and the veterinarians they have consulted previously in a manner consistent with the Golden Rule. *To criticize or disparage another veterinarian's service to a client is unethical.* If your colleague's actions reflect professional incompetence or neglect or abuse of the patient, call it to your colleague's attention and, if appropriate, to the attention of officers or practice committees of the local or state veterinary associations or the proper regulatory agency.[39]

As discussed in Chapter 9, the Federal Trade Commission (FTC) objected to the absolute condemnation of criticizing or disparaging another veterinarian's service to a client as an unlawful restraint of trade: the prohibition would deprive clients of information that could be truthful and important in their determination of which veterinarian to employ. Indeed, the FTC suggested that the Golden Rule itself could be seen as intended to restrain competition. The italicized sentence was removed from the code. The Golden Rule remains, but in another section of the *Principles* that does specifically relate to competition.

The FTC was correct in viewing the absolute prohibition of criticism of colleagues as a violation of the antitrust laws, and in objecting to the apparent intention of the code to associate the Golden Rule with a prohibition of criticism. Indeed, the Golden Rule sometimes argues in favor of criticizing a colleague. Consider the following case.

> *Case 19-6 Mrs. Miller comes to your hospital for the first time with her male cat, Tiger. Growing out of Tiger's front left paw are three misshapen claws. The area is oozing pus. She tells you that she had the cat declawed at Dr. X's hospital. She asks you to examine the animal and advise her what to do. You determine that whoever did the procedure did not remove the whole claws, leaving the pieces of bone that caused the regrowth and infection. Tiger needs another procedure to correct the problem.*
>
> *What do you tell her?*

FIRST REACTIONS. I use this case frequently with doctors and veterinary students. Typically, there are two different kinds of reactions. Some people will respond that one really does not know what Dr. X confronted and what he did. Perhaps, they say, Dr. X did nothing wrong and there was some reason, unbeknownst to us, why the whole claws were not removed. Others who consider this case will react by suggesting that before one does anything else, one should contact Dr. X to see what actually happened.

For reasons I will discuss shortly, these are both excellent responses. They are motivated by a desire to be fair to Dr. X and indicate a reluctance to assume he must have done something wrong. Nevertheless, the story must be continued.

> *Case 19-6 (cont'd) You are quite certain that Dr. X failed to properly remove all of the claws and that this is the cause of Tiger's present condition. You telephone Dr. X and tell him about your examination of the cat. He says "Oh boy! I guess I goofed on another one."*
>
> *What do you tell Mrs. Miller now? Do you tell her that Dr. X was responsible for Tiger's problem? In considering your response, do you think it is relevant that the law does not permit veterinarians to collect a fee for incompetent services, and would also entitle Mrs. Miller to receive reimbursement from Dr. X for the cost of correcting his errors? Would your response to these questions and this case be different if only one of Tiger's claws had been involved? If this were the first time Dr. X ever had a problem with this procedure?*

SECOND REACTIONS. At this point, there tend to be three responses. Some doctors and students, usually a very small number, will say that one should tell Mrs. Miller that Dr. X performed the procedure on Tiger improperly. A somewhat larger number will respond that one should not state outright that Dr. X erred, but say *something* (for example, "The procedure on these claws didn't quite work out.") that might lead a client of normal intelligence and sophistication to conclude—by herself—either that Dr. X erred or to ask Dr. X whether he made a mistake. The majority of practitioners and students, when confronted with the supplemented case, respond that it would be wrong to say *anything* negative about Dr. X's performance. Some will suggest that one might say something to the effect that, "This sort of thing sometimes happens from time to time with declawing." Perhaps, some will suggest, one should speak to Dr. X in a way that might lead to his not making the same mistake again. But the great majority of doctors and students believe that one should not dwell on what Dr. X did or did not do, but should focus on what needs to be done now to remedy the situation. Doctors and students who give this response will point to the dangers of criticizing other doctors and to the Golden Rule. "How," they ask, "would I feel if *I* were Dr. X?"

Now we are ready for the following case, which is addressed to those who would give this last response.

Case 19-7 Several months ago, you had surgery on your foot after a bad fall. You are still limping and experiencing pain. You decide to see a second surgeon to determine if anything is wrong. After a complete examination, she discovers that the first surgery was performed incompetently. She contacts the first physician, who admits his error. She has not yet told you of her discovery or the first surgeon's admission.

Imagine, just for the purposes of this case, that you are not a sophisticated veterinarian or veterinary student with extensive knowledge of medicine and anatomy. You are a person of ordinary intelligence and knowledge and would not know that the first surgeon erred unless you were told by the second surgeon.

What would you want the second surgeon to tell you?

I have found that veterinarians have a hard time considering how they would want to be treated in Case 19-6 if they were Mrs. Miller and she were the veterinarian. Practitioners are so sensitive to the dangers of criticism by colleagues that many are unable to accept that any ethical principle—much less the Golden Rule—could require speaking ill of a colleague. Case 19-7 can lift what might otherwise be an impenetrable barrier by abandoning the veterinary context altogether. Many practitioners and students respond to it before they realize the implications of their response. For the overwhelming reaction to Case 19-7 is that the second physician should, *of course*, tell me what the first doctor did. It is *my* body. Even if I decide not to seek legal remedy against the first surgeon, most will say, I am entitled to know what happened to me. For the second physician not to tell me is to treat me like a child, many will say. After all, they will say, the second physician owes me this information because she works for *me* and not for the first doctor.

The relevance of such responses in the veterinary context is clear, and disturbing. The Golden Rule must be applied first and foremost by a physician or veterinarian to the person with whom there is a professional, and personal relationship. It is not another veterinarian who is paying one's fee or who is being entrusted with a patient's health and safety. Unless one is willing to say that a physician's first loyalty is to her colleagues and not her patients, one must concede that veterinary clients too sometimes are entitled to know that a previous veterinarian caused their animal harm. A client's animal, like a client's own body, is his property. He may sometimes be entitled to learn from a second doctor if the previous veterinarian harmed his animal.

The interests of clients and patients

Unfortunately (for veterinarians), it is sometimes in the interests of a patient, client, or the public for a veterinarian to tell a client about a colleague's misdeeds. The following kinds of situations can and do occur.

Situation 1: The first doctor (Dr. 1) has committed an act of negligence that the second doctor (Dr. 2) has every reason to believe will not be repeated. However, the law holds that a veterinarian is not entitled to a fee for negligent services. If Dr. 2 does not tell the client what happened, the client will never know that he paid Dr. 1's fee unnecessarily and is legally entitled to its return.

Situation 2: Dr. 2, a specialist to whom the patient was referred by Dr. 1, knows that Dr. 1's approach to the patient was improper. She has also seen and heard of other examples of Dr. 1's incompetence and believes it is pointless to confront Dr. 1. Dr. 2 knows that if she does not say something to the client, the client will return to Dr. 1, thereby risking further injury to the patient.

Situation 3: Dr. 2 concludes that Dr. 1 intentionally abused the animal and mistreated the client. When Dr. 2 confronts Dr. 1, Dr. 1 refuses to acknowledge his error and continues to heap abuse on the innocent client.

Situation 4: Dr. 2 believes that Dr. 1 is frequently incompetent but will never be able to bring herself to lodge a complaint with the state VMA or board of registration. If Dr. 2 does not tell the client about Dr. 1's incompetence, there might never be any investigation of Dr. 1, and Dr. 1 will continue to harm animals and clients.

Situation 5: The client comes to Dr. 2 suspecting that Dr. 1 injured her animal and asks Dr. 2 whether Dr. 1 was negligent. After reviewing the case and speaking with Dr. 1, Dr. 2 concludes that Dr. 1 was indeed negligent.

These situations are undoubtedly atypical. They also state as fact certain things (for example, that Dr. 1 was negligent) that may often be far from clear. Yet, the cases illustrate circumstances in which a doctor's failing to tell the client that a colleague erred, can harm the client, the patient, or both.

Situation 1 refutes a claim I sometimes hear from veterinarians: that when a second doctor can confront a previous doctor privately and can see to it that the former's mistake will not recur, no one is really harmed. However, even under these circumstances, the client can be harmed because she might be deprived of money that should have remained in her pocket. The animal might also have experienced unnecessary pain or illness.

In all the situations, a decision by the second doctor not to criticize the first can deprive the client of her legal and moral right to complain to somebody about the first doctor's behavior, for the client might not otherwise know that anything was amiss. In *Situations 2* and *4*, the second doctor's silence can threaten the health of the patient and other animals. And in *Situation 5*, the second doctor's silence might entail his lying to the client and failing to give the client a piece of information the client wants and for which she is paying.

Those who would insist that even in these five kinds of situations, a second doctor must never say anything bad about the first to the client are exhibiting an attitude that many clients would surely find disturbing—the view that a veterinarian does not work for the client who is paying the fee but rather for another veterinarian, whom the doctor might not even know. Clients might well wonder whether such an attitude reflects the kind of loyalty to them and their animals they assume is part of the veterinarian-client and veterinarian-patient relationship.

The Approach of the Post-1989 *Principles of Veterinary Medical Ethics*

The *Principles* is a document of official and not normative ethics. Therefore one would expect it to lean toward the interests of veterinarians rather than clients, and it does. Accordingly, the *Principles* do not provide completely satisfactory advice regarding criticism of colleagues. However, as a result of the FTC inquiry the code's treatment of the issue is greatly improved, from an ethical as well as legal standpoint.

The *Principles* now take two approaches toward the issue of criticism. First, following holdings of the U. S. Supreme Court allowing professional associations to prohibit representations that are false, deceptive, and misleading, the code now states that:

> Veterinarians should respect the rights of clients, colleagues, and other health professionals. No member shall belittle or injure the professional standing of another member of the profession or unnecessarily condemn the character of that person's professional acts *in such a manner as to be false or misleading.*[40]

Another section requires a doctor who is called into consultation "to avoid criticism of the [referring] veterinarian by the consultant or the client, if that criticism is false or misleading."[41]

The requirement that any criticism of a colleague at least be truthful is extremely important. If followed, this requirement would prevent the great majority of critical statements, because the great majority of criticisms of one doctor by another are factually incorrect or are based on insufficient information. Perhaps even more importantly, prohibiting false or misleading criticisms places a heavy procedural burden on practitioners. Because it is usually impossible to determine whether a previous doctor acted appropriately without obtaining from that doctor her side of the story (including relevant facts about the patient and client), it follows from the prohibition that a practitioner should *always* attempt to contact the previous doctor before making any statement, even one that might be truthful.

The code's second approach to the issue of criticism is less satisfactory. A section devoted to referrals, consultations, and attendance on patients by a second doctor advises one to attempt to learn whether a previous veterinarian has attended the case and to contact that doctor to ascertain his diagnosis and treatment. This is fine and clearly serves the interests of obtaining facts and being fair to one's colleague. However, this section of the code then repeats a key sentence that was contained in the pre-1989 *Principles,* and justifies this statement with what appears to be a derogatory assertion about clients:

> If your colleague's actions reflect professional incompetence or neglect or abuse of the patient, call it to your colleague's attention and, if appropriate, to the attention of officers or practice committees of the local or state veterinary associations or the proper regulatory agency. Remember that a client who is abruptly changing veterinarians is often under severe stress and is likely to overstate or mis-state the causes for differences with the other practitioner.[41]

There are many things wrong with this paragraph.

1. Although the paragraph does not repeat the absolute prohibition of the pre-1989 code of criticism of a colleague to a client, this appears to be its intent. For the paragraph lists appropriate approaches to a colleague's misdeeds, and telling the client what happened is not on the list.

2. The paragraph appears to counsel silence to the client even when a previous doctor has engaged in the most egregious acts—not just incompetent behavior

but also outright abuse. All professionals make mistakes in a lifetime of practice. A case might sometimes be made for not revealing a previous doctor's mistake to a client when it was an honest error that is unlikely to be repeated. But abusing an animal is absolutely unacceptable behavior for any veterinarian. Surely, if one *knows* that, say, a colleague has beaten the patient this might be something the client is also entitled to know.

3. The paragraph does not appear to include among the reasons for contacting a previous doctor before saying anything to a client the need to assure that any statement about that doctor would be correct and truthful. For if one should not tell a client about a previous doctor's error when one already knows the doctor erred, the point of contacting that doctor can never be to enable one to make a truthful statement about that doctor's performance to a client.

4. The actions recommended by the paragraph other than contacting the colleague are ones very few veterinarians will take. Most doctors are wary of making a complaint about a colleague's performance to a state or local VMA because they would not want to air such a matter in public. (Some are afraid of being sued for defamation of character by the criticized veterinarian.) In years of discussing this issue with many hundreds of veterinarians, I have never met one who has initiated a complaint about a colleague's performance with the state licensing board. Doctors prefer that complaints be filed by clients because they do not want to be perceived as attempting to cost a colleague his or her license.

5. Finally, it is not fair to include in the code's only discussion of how to handle a previous doctor's incompetence, neglect, or abuse a statement about clients who have "differences" with another doctor, who are "abruptly changing" veterinarians, or who are under "severe stress." Clients who do have differences with a previous doctor or who are abruptly changing doctors *are* notoriously inaccurate and dangerous. However, there is absolutely no reason to associate such clients generally with veterinarians whose actions "reflect professional incompetence or neglect or abuse." Nor is there evidence that most people to whom one could ever say something negative about a previous doctor are such clients. It is also highly doubtful that most clients who change doctors either do so "abruptly" or are under such "severe stress" that they cannot understand what a previous doctor did or what might be told to them by a second doctor. The last sentence of the paragraph quoted above conveys a very unfortunate tone. It appears to respond to the issue of when, if ever, another veterinarian may be criticized with a criticism of *clients*.

Reconciling the Interests of Veterinarians and Clients
Basic principles

It may not be possible to find an approach to the issue of criticism of colleagues that always pays sufficient regard to the legitimate interests of both veterinarians and clients, but one must try. The task should be begun, I would suggest, by setting forth several basic ethical principles. One can then determine what follows from these principles and from indisputable facts about situations in which veterinarians can criticize the actions of colleagues. I want to offer the following principles, and several corollaries of these principles, which I believe follow from the discussion in this and other chapters.

PRINCIPLE 1: BECAUSE A VETERINARIAN WORKS FOR THE CLIENT, ONE HAS FIRST AND FOREMOST THE DUTY OF LOYALTY TO *THIS* CLIENT AND THIS CLIENT'S ANIMAL. A veterinarian is therefore morally obligated to truthfully answer a client's questions to the best of his or her ability. One is also morally obligated to tell a client what any ordinarily reasonable client would regard as essential information about her animal or medical treatment of her animal, past or present. However, it does not serve the interests of clients to give them false information or to make statements one does not have sufficient evidence to support. One must also be careful not to allow one's self-interest (for example, any desire to win over the client for oneself) to color one's perception of whether there is sufficient evidence to make a negative statement about a colleague.

PRINCIPLE 2: VETERINARIANS ARE ENTITLED TO BE TREATED FAIRLY BY FELLOW VETERINARIANS. Part of what constitutes fair treatment is not making false, deceptive, or misleading statements about a colleague's performance. Therefore veterinarians are morally obligated not to make statements about colleagues that they know, or should know, are false, deceptive or misleading. Veterinarians are also morally obligated not to make statements about colleagues that put them in a bad light unless they have good evidence that such statements are true.

PRINCIPLE 3: IT IS IMPOSSIBLE TO GIVE CLIENTS RELIABLE INFORMATION ABOUT WHAT ACTUALLY TRANSPIRED DURING A PREVIOUS DOCTOR'S ATTENDANCE OF THE CASE WITHOUT ATTEMPTING TO LEARN FROM THAT DOCTOR, OR HER RECORDS, ABOUT HER DIAGNOSIS AND TREATMENT. This would be the case even where a client is a dependable source of information about what happened during the first doctor's care of the animal.

PRINCIPLE 4: IT IS IMPOSSIBLE TO BE COMPLETELY FAIR TO A COLLEAGUE WHO ATTENDED A CASE WITHOUT GIVING HER THE OPPORTUNITY TO RESPOND TO WHATEVER QUESTIONS OR CONCERNS ONE MIGHT HAVE ABOUT HER CARE OF THE ANIMAL. This follows as a matter of common courtesy, from the fact that clients can be unreliable sources of information, and from the fact that there is often more than one side to any story.

Recommended approaches

From these basic principles, and related facts, one can derive a number of more specific approaches to the issue of criticism of colleagues. Table 19-1 presents a list of such approaches. The table is not intended to be complete. Even more specific recommendations can be generated from some of the approaches in the table, and the table does not purport to contain all approaches that would follow from the basic principles. The table contains recommendations that relate not just to the general issue of criticizing colleagues, but also to a more specific kind of criticism that will be discussed below: statements made by specialists about general practitioners. Also included in the table are some general recommendations for veterinary associations.

Most of the approaches recommended in the table are identical to or build upon statements made in the *Principles of Veterinary Medical Ethics* about criticizing colleagues. However, the approach of the code loses some of its persuasiveness because, as I have discussed, it seems intended primarily to protect veterinarians. Therefore wherever possible, I attempt to ground approaches recommended in the *Principles* on the interests of clients as well as doctors. This is done to assure that the recommendations are not offered to protect only veterinarians, and to recognize that veterinarians *should* serve first and foremost their clients and patients.

Table 19-1

Approaches to the issue of criticism of colleagues

1. OUT OF FAIRNESS TO THE CLIENT, RESIST ANY INITIAL TEMPTATION TO CRITICIZE A COLLEAGUE'S HANDLING OF A CASE.
- Diagnosing a colleague's performance without having all relevant facts is no better from a purely technical (much less ethical) standpoint than reaching a diagnosis of a patient's medical condition without examining the animal.
- There is often more than one way to approach a case medically. That you might have approached a situation differently does not mean that the previous doctor erred.

2. IF YOU SUSPECT OR ARE TOLD THAT THE PATIENT WAS SEEN BY ANOTHER DOCTOR REGARDING THE MATTER AT HAND, TRY TO DETERMINE HIS OR HER NAME, DIAGNOSIS, AND TREATMENT. ASK FOR PERMISSION TO CONTACT THE DOCTOR AND TO OBTAIN THE PATIENT'S MEDICAL RECORDS.
- Out of fairness to the client as well as a previous doctor, do not say anything about a previous doctor's performance if the client will not reveal his or her identity, for it will then be impossible to obtain all relevant information.
- It is appropriate, when seeking to speak with the previous doctor to obtain records, to tell the client that this is necessary for appropriate care of the patient. Malpractice on your part can result from initiating a course of treatment without sufficient history and background information.

3. BE ESPECIALLY CAREFUL, AND CLEAR TO THE CLIENT ABOUT YOUR DIAGNOSIS AND INTENDED TREATMENT WHEN YOU SUSPECT OR ARE TOLD ANOTHER DOCTOR HAS BEEN INVOLVED. THE CLIENT MAY RETURN TO THE FIRST DOCTOR, OR GO TO A THIRD DOCTOR, AND COMPLAIN ABOUT YOU.

4. NEVER MAKE UNJUSTIFIED OR FALSE STATEMENTS ABOUT A COLLEAGUE.

5. IF YOU DO NOT KNOW A COLLEAGUE, OR HAVE NO SPECIFIC REASON TO DOUBT HIS OR HER COMPETENCE, ASSUME THAT HE OR SHE IS AS COMPETENT AS YOU.

6. MAKE SURE THAT YOUR EMPLOYEES DO NOT MAKE UNNECESSARY OR FALSE CRITICISMS OF OTHER DOCTORS OR HOSPITALS TO CLIENTS.

7. IN CONSULTING WITH A PREVIOUS DOCTOR—OR IF YOU ARE THE PREVIOUS DOCTOR BEING CONSULTED BY ANOTHER VETERINARIAN WHO HAS SEEN THE PATIENT—TRY TO BE NON-COMBATIVE AND COOPERATIVE.
- Remember that clients have a legal right to employ the veterinarian of their choice, and that you have a legal obligation to provide medical records to another doctor at the client's request.
- A hostile atmosphere, or a desire by the second doctor to undermine the first, is not in the interests of the client or patient because these things hinder the cooperative sharing of information.

8. EVEN AFTER CONSULTING WITH YOUR COLLEAGUE, EXERCISE EXTREME CAUTION BEFORE COMING TO THE CONCLUSION THAT HE OR SHE ACTED IMPROPERLY. THIS FOLLOWS FROM THE FACT THAT THE CASE MAY BE DIFFERENT FROM THE SITUATION CONFRONTED BY YOUR COLLEAGUE. IT ALSO FOLLOWS FROM THE FACT THAT NEGLIGENCE CANNOT BE CONCLUDED FROM AN UNFORTUNATE RESULT ALONE.

9. IT IS IMPORTANT TO BE TRUTHFUL TO CLIENTS. THEY DESERVE HONESTY, AND THEY MAY BE PAYING YOU A FEE FOR COMPETENT AND HONEST ANSWERS TO THEIR QUESTIONS. THE FOLLOWING STATEMENTS CAN BE TRUTHFUL DEPENDING ON THE CIRCUMSTANCES:
- "I honestly cannot say that Dr. X made a mistake because I cannot tell you what your animal's condition was when he saw it."
- "Your animal's condition could be caused by something entirely unrelated to Dr. X's diagnosis or treatment."
- "I really can't say that I would have done anything differently."

10. IF, AFTER CONSULTING WITH A PREVIOUS DOCTOR AND REVIEWING ALL APPROPRIATE RECORDS, YOU COME TO THE CONCLUSION THAT THIS DOCTOR DID DO SOMETHING WRONG, AND IF THE CLIENT ASKS WHETHER SHE DID SOMETHING WRONG, OR YOU BELIEVE THAT YOU MUST IN GOOD CONSCIENCE SAY SOMETHING, ATTEMPT TO CONVEY INFORMATION IN THE LEAST INFLAMMATORY AND DEROGATORY MANNER POSSIBLE. THIS PRINCIPLE FOLLOWS FROM THE FACT THAT, AS A DOCTOR, YOU ARE NOT AN EXPERT IN POLEMIC, OR PUNISHMENT, BUT IN VETERINARY MEDICINE.
- Describe the situation or respond to a question as objectively as possible, describing facts. For example, if, as in Case 19-6 you conclude that the previous doctor did not perform the declaws properly, you might tell the client the facts: "The claws were not completely removed. They grew back from remaining bone, with associated infection."

TABLE 19-1 CONT'D

Approaches to the issue of criticism of colleagues

- Do not advise the client to see a lawyer or respond to a question whether she should sue a previous doctor. As a veterinarian, one can honestly say that it is not part of one's role to give such advice.

11. *IF YOU ARE A SPECIALIST, BE PARTICULARLY CAREFUL TO KEEP IN MIND THAT GENERAL PRACTITION-ERS ARE NOT HELD TO THE SAME STANDARDS AS SPECIALISTS. IT DOES NOT FOLLOW FROM THE FACT THAT YOU MIGHT HAVE DIAGNOSED OR TREATED A CASE DIFFERENTLY, THAT A GENERALIST WHO SAW THE PATIENT FIRST ACTED INCOMPETENTLY OR IMPROPERLY.*

12. *VETERINARY MEDICAL ASSOCIATIONS SHOULD EXERCISE CAUTION IN RESPONDING TO VETERINARI-ANS WHO MAY BE MAKING UNFAIR CRITICISMS OF COLLEAGUES.*

- A VMA, or any group of two or more doctors, must be careful not to violate antitrust laws or the FTC's interpretations of these laws. Never attempt to censure or put pressure on a doctor who criticizes other doctors because this could be viewed as a conspiracy to restrain competition.
- VMAs can encourage members to think about the general issue of professional relations and organize lectures and seminars on the issue.

~ ETHICAL ISSUES IN REFERRALS AND CONSULTATIONS

Competent veterinary practice sometimes requires referral to a specialist, a practitioner with equipment or facilities not available to the referring doctor, or to a facility that operates during times the referring practice is closed.

In some cases, a receiving doctor might be tempted to use the referral as an opportunity to win the client away from the referring doctor. Clearly, if this became a general practice, the legitimate interests of many clients and patients would be harmed. Doctors would stop making referrals out of fear of losing clients. Referring doctors would be harmed because of their inability to keep some of their clients satisfied, and receiving doctors would be harmed by not obtaining referrals.

In considering how receiving doctors ought to handle referrals, it seems appropriate to distinguish two general kinds of cases: (1) the routine situation in which the receiving doctor has every reason to believe that the patient will obtain appropriate care upon return to the referring doctor, and (2) the unusual situation in which the receiving doctor concludes that returning to the referring doctor is not in the best interests of the patient or client.

In the first kind of case, it seems clear that the receiving doctor should encourage the client to return to the referring doctor for continuing care. Neither the interests of the patient or client require a change in doctors, and the receiving doctor has benefited from the referral. Difficulties arise, however, if the client insists upon using the receiving doctor in the future for care not related to the purposes of the referral. When the receiving doctor is a specialist in a limited area (such as ophthalmology or cardiology) and does not practice with other doctors who can provide general continuing care, the answer might be easy: the receiving doctor cannot accept the patient because he is not equipped to provide the kind of care the patient will need. However, what ought to be done might not be so clear when a receiving doctor or other doctors in his practice can provide continuing care and the client wants him or his practice to take over care of the patient. If the receiving doctor agrees to do so, he probably will be violating the implicit understanding he had with the referring doctor that the case would be returned, and he might lose future referrals from that doctor. On the other hand, it is far from clear that the receiving doctor should automatically reject the wishes of a client who now insists on using his services. For clients do have the moral and legal right to decide how their animals should be treated, and what veterinarians they shall employ.

The situation becomes murkier and potentially even less pleasant when the receiving doctor believes that it is not in the best interests of the patient to return to the referring doctor. There are different possibilities here, ranging from the case in which the receiving doctor believes that the referring or original doctor will provide grossly inadequate care, to the case in which it might be just somewhat better for the patient to remain with the receiving doctor or to be seen by a third doctor.

Where the interests of a patient clearly would be harmed by its returning to the referring doctor, it seems to me that a strong argument can be made for the receiving doctor doing something to urge against such a return, provided that the receiving doctor has taken steps (by speaking with the referring doctor, for example) to assure himself that the patient would not be well-served by returning. Moreover, the desire of clients to choose their own veterinarian must always carry some weight on the scales of moral deliberation. Therefore it can be argued that where the client comes to the receiving doctor already unhappy with the first doctor or simply wants to change doctors, the receiving doctor need find less deficiency in the referring doctor's performance to be absolved of one's ordinary obligation to encourage the client to return to the referring doctor.

∾ WHEN A CLIENT CHOOSES ANOTHER VETERINARIAN

However much one might object to a client's choice of another doctor, and however much one might hold the second veterinarian responsible for this choice, it is essential that a referring or original doctor not do anything to frustrate the wishes of the client or jeopardize the health of the animal. One must not refuse reasonable requests to provide copies of the patient's records to the client or a second doctor, nor may one withhold essential information to make it more difficult for a second doctor to do her job or to motivate the client to return. Such actions could have serious legal consequences. The veterinary practice acts and regulations of many states require practitioners to furnish medical records when these are requested by the client or another veterinarian. Moreover, it is wrong to hold the patient, who might need treatment and probably had nothing to do with the change in doctors, hostage to a doctor's dissatisfaction with a colleague's acquisition of the case.

The *Principles of Veterinary Medical Ethics* agree with these recommendations but with an interesting twist. The code states that doctors should be willing to honor a client's request that the case be referred to another practitioner. The first doctor is said to have "an obligation to other veterinarians that the client may choose" to withdraw from the case and to forward the patient's medical records to another doctor who might request them.[41] In truth, the first doctor's moral obligation regarding forwarding of records is to the client and to the animal. If a subsequent doctor can be said to have a "right" to these records, it is only indirectly—because the client's wishes must be respected and because the animal can suffer if appropriate records are not made available to its new veterinarian.

～ SPECIALIZATION AS A COMPETITIVE WEAPON

Specialists can be an enormous assistance to front-line general practitioners. However, some general practitioners are concerned about the potential use by specialists of their board certification as an unfair competitive weapon, that is, as a means of attempting to convince the public that they will provide better care for an animal even when a general practitioner would be perfectly capable of handling the case. Additionally, animosity has arisen between general practitioners and some specialists brought into communities by breed associations to conduct diagnostic clinics of purebred animals.[42]

The best known controversy regarding specialization as a possible competitive advantage involved a decision by the Canine Eye Registration Foundation to certify purebred dogs as free from hereditary eye disease only upon examination by a board-certified ophthalmologist. In 1979, four general practitioners sued the foundation, the American College of Veterinary Ophthalmology (ACVO), the AVMA, and several board-certified ophthalmologists, charging them with violating the Sherman Antitrust Act. The defendants countersued. The plaintiffs' claims against the ACVO, the AVMA, and several of the veterinarian defendants were dismissed. A federal magistrate found in favor of the remaining defendants on the complaint, which judgment was then upheld on appeal. The court then issued summary judgment in favor of the defendants on their counterclaim. The plaintiffs were required to pay $416,893.99, and the amount was then tripled in accordance with the Sherman Antitrust Act. In 1986 the U. S. Supreme Court refused to review the lower court judgment, thus letting the award stand.[43]

Any attempt by specialists to convey the impression that they are *ipso facto* better qualified to care for clients' animals is unethical, and is already prohibited by official and administrative rules against false and misleading claims.

Such prohibitions have not had much effect on Yellow Pages advertisements. The typical Yellow Pages contain advertisements in which specialists proclaim their board certification, not to local practitioners, who already know of the specialists in the area, but to members of the public. It seems clear that some specialists place such advertisements with the precise intention of using their certification as a means of attracting clients, knowing full well that many potential clients will conclude incorrectly that a specialist must be better for their animals than a general practitioner. However, because board certification is a fact about specialists, it might be extremely difficult to prove that specialists are publicizing their board certification with the intent to mislead or deceive. Moreover, the suggestion that specialists should not mention their board certification in advertisements is likely to strike many specialists as an unfair attempt to restrict their ability to compete, and as an infringement of their moral and constitutional right to inform the public about their services.

REFERENCES

[1]Wise JK, Gehrke BC: Professional incomes of US veterinarians, 1993, *J Am Vet Med Assoc* 205:1405-1408, 1994. Although the mean incomes for all categories of private practice declined between 1991 and 1993, median incomes remained constant for small animal practitioners and increased for large animal-exclusive and large animal-predominant doctors.

[2]Smith MT: The wild new word of health care for your pet, *Money* April, 1994:149 (stating that "the average doctor of veterinary medicine earns $63,466 a year, compared with $177,400 for an M.D.").

[3]American Veterinary Medical Association: *Principles of Veterinary Medical Ethics*, Proposed 1988 Revision, "Guidelines for Professional Behavior," paragraph 1, *AVMA 1988 Annual Convention Delegates' Agenda*, Schaumburg, IL, The Association, Appendix A, p 17f.

[4]Gove PB, editor: *Webster's Third New International Dictionary,* Springfield, MA, 1961, Merriam, p 464.

[5]15 U.S.C. § 1.

[6]15 U.S.C. § 2.

[7]15 U.S.C. § 45(a)(1).

[8]*Northern Pacific Railway Co.* v. *United States,* 356 U.S. 1, 4 (1958).

[9]*National Society of Professional Engineers* v. *United States,* 435 U.S. 679, 694 (1978).

[10]*Goldfarb* v. *Virginia State Bar,* 421 U.S. 733 at 778-789, n. 17 (1975).

[11]*Bates* v. *State Bar of Arizona,* 433 U.S. 350, 383-384 (1977).

[12]Vakerics TV: *Antitrust Basics,* New York, 1994, Law Journal Seminars-Press, pp 6-27, 6-28; *Eastern Railroad Presidents Conference* v. *Noerr Motor Freight, Inc.,* 365 U.S. 127 (1961); *United Mine Workers of America* v. *Pennington,* 381 U.S. 657 (1965).

[13]FTC staff lauds veterinary board's ad proposals, *BNA Antitrust Trade Reg Rep* 50:694, 1986.

[14]Lofflin J: Government takes potential violations seriously, *Vet Econ* August 1991:32.

[15]Zuziak P: Courtroom scene set for debate over ownership of practice facilities, *J Am Vet Med Assoc* 202: 1793-1796, 1993.

[16]*Bates* v. *State Bar of Arizona,* 433 U.S. 350, 383-384 (1977).

[17]Prosser WL, Keeton WP: *The Law of Torts,* ed 5, St. Paul, MN, 1984, West Publishing, p 967.

[18]RESTATEMENT (SECOND) OF TORTS § 766 (1979).

[19]*See,* Prosser WL, Keeton WP: *The Law of Torts,* ed 5, St. Paul, MN, 1984, West Publishing, pp 1005-1015.

[20]RESTATEMENT (SECOND) OF TORTS § 559 (1979).

[21]American Veterinary Medical Association: *The Veterinary Service Market for Companion Animals,* Schaumburg, IL, 1992, The Association, pp 16-17.

[22]*Id,* pp 6-7.

[23]*Id,* p 18.

[24]Quoted in Lofflin J: Is your Yellow Pages ad working? *Vet Econ* May 1989:41.

[25]*Virginia Beach Society for the Prevention of Cruelty to Animals* v. *South Hampton Roads Veterinary Association,* 329 S.E.2d 10 (Va. 1985); *see also,* Dildine D: Silent settlement resolves clinic suit, *DVM* 13(1):1, 1982 (relating events regarding the Michigan VMA suit against the Macomb County Humane Society).

[26]Animal health care symposium cosponsored by veterinary profession and humane groups, *J Am Vet Med Assoc* 183:393, 1983.

[27]American Veterinary Medical Association: "A Memorandum of Understanding for Humane Organizations and Veterinarians," *1994 AVMA Directory,* Schaumburg, IL, The Association, p 70.

[28]American Veterinary Medical Association: "Guidelines for Veterinary Associations and Veterinarians Working with Humane Organizations," *1994 AVMA Directory,* Schaumburg, IL, The Association, p 69-70.

[29]Robinson GW: How to keep a humane society hospital out of your community, *Vet Econ* June 1990:32-41.

[30]American Veterinary Medical Association: *Principles of Veterinary Medical Ethics,* 1993 Revision, "Vaccination Clinics," *1994 AVMA Directory,* Schaumburg, IL, The Association, p 45.

[31]Quoted in Clark R: *The Best of Ross Clark on Practice Management,* Lenexa, KS, 1985, Veterinary Medicine Publishing, p 102.

[32]American Veterinary Medical Association: *Principles of Veterinary Medical Ethics,* 1993 Revision, "Humane Organizations and Spay and Neuter Clinics: Examination and Surgical Sterilization of Pets," *1994 AVMA Directory,* Schaumburg, IL, The Association, p 45.

[33]American Veterinary Medical Association: *Principles of Veterinary Medical Ethics,* 1993 Revision, "Guidelines for Naming of Veterinary Facilities," *1994 AVMA Directory,* Schaumburg, IL, The Association, p 90.

[34]American Veterinary Medical Association: *Principles of Veterinary Medical Ethics,* 1993 Revision, "Guidelines for Professional Behavior," paragraph 2, *1994 AVMA Directory,* Schaumburg, IL, The Association, p 42.

[35]*National Society of Professional Engineers* v. *United States,* 435 U.S. 679, 694 (1978), citing *Mitchel* v. *Reynolds,* 1 P. Wms. 181, 191, 24 Eng. Rep. 347, 350 (1711).

[36]Tannenbaum J: *Veterinary Ethics,* ed 1, Baltimore, 1989, Williams & Wilkins, pp 295-296.

[37]Dr. James Wilson reports similar experiences to those described here. Wilson J: Is your noncompete clause too restrictive? *Vet Econ* March 1994:60-64. He finds among veterinarians "excessive paranoia over future competition from employed veterinarians," states that some veterinarians ask employee doctors to sign "demeaning, oppressive, and often unenforceable non-compete clauses," and believes that "excessively harsh covenants not to compete are more likely to add—justifiably and unnecessarily so—to the vast number of unhappy associate veterinarians." (p 64) Wilson, however, does not call for elimination of restrictive covenants but urges that veterinarians use them fairly and draft them carefully. I would prefer to be able to endorse Dr. Wilson's approach. However, I have seen too many ethically and legally bad restrictive covenants and too many cases in which practitioners have attempted to use these agreements to make life difficult for present or former employees. I doubt whether even carefully drafted agreements will stop all the abuses (assuming doctors who want to abuse restrictive covenants seek to have them drafted carefully).

[38]American Veterinary Medical Association: "AVMA Membership by Member Status by State (as of September 30, 1993)," *1994 AVMA Directory*, Schaumburg, IL, The Association, p 23 (reporting 4,502 active AVMA California members, the next closest states being Texas with 3,510 Florida with 2,518, and New York with 2,365).

[39]American Veterinary Medical Association: *Principles of Veterinary Medical Ethics*, 1987 Revision, "Professional Relations with New Clients," *1988 AVMA Directory*, Schaumburg, IL, The Association, p 477, emphases supplied.

[40]American Veterinary Medical Association: *Principles of Veterinary Medical Ethics*, 1993 Revision, "Guidelines for Professional Behavior," paragraph 5, *1994 AVMA Directory*, Schaumburg, IL, The Association, p 42, emphases supplied.

[41]American Veterinary Medical Association: *Principles of Veterinary Medical Ethics*, 1993 Revision, "Referrals, Consultations, and Relationships with Clients," *1994 AVMA Directory*, Schaumburg, IL, The Association, pp 43-44.

[42]American Veterinary Medical Association: *Principles of Veterinary Medical Ethics*, 1987 Revision, "Diagnostic Clinics, Guidelines for Conducting," *1988 AVMA Directory*, Schaumburg, IL, The Association, p 478.

[43]*Rickards* v. *Canine Eye Registration Foundation, Inc.*, 704 F.2d 1449 (9th Cir.), *cert. denied*, 104 S.Ct. 488 (1983); 783 F.2d 1328 (9th Cir.), *cert. denied*, 107 S.Ct. 180 (1986).

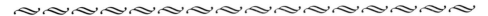
Treating Clients Fairly

Clients cause as many ethical problems for veterinarians as animals. It is clients with whom practitioners communicate, from whom they receive payment, and by whom any complaints are likely to be made. Moreover, because a client's interests sometimes conflict with the patient's, a veterinarian can be torn between serving the two.

There may be as many different possible ethical issues involving client relations as there are clients and veterinarians. This chapter discusses some of the more common of these problems that can often be considered apart from potential conflicts in interest between clients and patients. Chapters 21 and 22 consider ethical issues that routinely involve such conflicts.

∼ ACCEPTING NEW CLIENTS

A veterinarian may lawfully refuse to serve a client willing to pay for services,[1] provided the reason for doing so is not specifically prohibited by law, such as racial or religious discrimination, and provided one has not held oneself out (for example, as an emergency facility) to the public as available for certain kinds of cases (see Chapter 4). The law often requires far less of people than does morality. Our legal system generally holds that people often ought to have the freedom to act ethically or unethically if that is their choice.

The *Principles of Veterinary Medical Ethics*, which is a document not of law but of morality, appears to accept the minimal legal standard regarding freedom to choose clients as an *ethical* rule. "Veterinarians," the code states, "may choose whom they will serve."[2]

It is not difficult to appreciate why this is an unacceptable general ethical standard. Imagine a client who appears for the first time at a veterinarian's office when the doctor is free. The animal desperately needs treatment the doctor can provide with minimal effort, and the client is willing to pay whatever the veterinarian wants. However, the doctor turns the client away after flipping a coin to decide whether she will take the case, or because the client is wearing a polyester leisure suit, or because the client is overweight. Surely such a decision would be morally wrong. A veterinarian's job is to help clients and their animals, and these just are not morally valid reasons for refusing to do this job. One cannot approach the issue of when one may accept or refuse clients with the *legal* rule that "one may choose whom one will serve." Good reasons for turning away clients must be distinguished from bad.

The following discussion assumes that a doctor and facility are qualified to handle a particular patient and are able to do so. Obviously, if either of these things is not the case, and the client can safely take the animal to a facility that is able to treat it, declining to accept the case is both a medical and ethical imperative.

Questionable Payers

One legitimate reason for refusing to serve a new client can be a justified concern that the client is unable or unwilling to pay one's fee. The problem, of course, is that it can be extremely difficult to determine whether such a concern is justified regarding a client one has never served. Appearances can be deceiving. Moreover, many people who do not have a great deal of money have enormous regard for their animals and will make sacrifices elsewhere.

Veterinarians whose case load can accommodate new clients ought to presume that they will accept someone as a new client, and should accept new clients, unless there is some good reason not to. This conclusion follows from the fundamental principle that it is the function of a veterinarian to help people and their animals. There are ways of seeking to assure payment from new clients. One can accept credit cards, require a deposit before undertaking a procedure, or ask clients to specify their occupation and place of work or that of their spouse, which information can then be verified. One can have a frank talk with potential clients. Veterinarians, who are accustomed to counseling people concerning momentous decisions of life and death, can be very good at sensing the extent to which potential clients are committed to their animals and are prepared to be responsible for their medical care.

Disgruntled Clients of Other Doctors

Another kind of client one can sometimes be justified in turning away is the sort that comes to the office complaining about another doctor, or worse, about several veterinarians. Such people can be cantankerous and can make it impossible to treat the patient competently; they can attempt to embroil one in a dispute with another doctor; and they might be inclined to turn their complaints against you. A veterinarian's commitment to animals and clients does not imply that one must accept torture from clients or that one must constantly fear a lawsuit.

To be sure, one must be sensitive and cautious before turning away a disgruntled client of another doctor. Dissatisfaction is sometimes justified. There might have been a personality conflict between the client and the former doctor for which the doctor was partly responsible.

Strange or Potentially Troublesome Clients

Sometimes, even a brief encounter can indicate likely trouble from a potential new client. Some people are so obviously obnoxious and demanding or have such strange ideas about what should be done with their animals, that one can predict a professional relationship would be stormy. Some potential clients bring the possibility of entanglement in activities not befitting a veterinarian. For example, several practitioners have told me that they turn away people who appear to be using or breeding their animals for illegal dog fighting. Some veterinarians have had so much trouble catering to the medical opinions and demands of particular breeders, that they will not accept breeders as clients.

The Relevance of the Patient's Condition

The condition of the patient is a relevant factor in determining how strongly other reasons (for example, a potential client's obnoxiousness or financial condition) should count in the decision whether to accept a case. Where the animal is not ill or does not need immediate care, that one knows one will not get along with the client or may have problems obtaining one's fee may sometimes justify declining the case.

On the other hand, where a critical need of a potential patient must be served immediately, lest it suffer or die, a veterinarian's commitment to animal welfare will exert great moral force in favor of accepting the case. Sometimes, this force will be sufficient to outweigh one's legitimate qualms about the client. The fact that a client is obnoxious does not seem a sufficiently weighty reason for turning away an animal requiring immediate treatment to save its life. Sometimes, the force exerted by the animal's interests will not count in favor of taking the case. For example, where the animal requires an expensive procedure that the owner admits is beyond his means, one might be compelled to decline the case, or recommend euthanasia.

There are many possible different combinations of factors relevant to deciding whether one is morally obligated to treat an animal. There are different maladies with different prognoses, perceived potential problems with clients, and conditions relating to the availability of care elsewhere. Sometimes there are alternative approaches one can take to reconcile one's own interests with those of the client and animal. It might be possible to accept a patient on a temporary basis until it recovers from a particular malady. Sometimes, it might be morally preferable to stabilize the patient so that it can be transferred to another doctor who is able to accommodate the client's requirements.

The Problem of the Clientless Animal

Many small animal practitioners have faced situations in which a stray animal or one the owner of which is not yet known or present is brought into the facility requiring emergency care. In the case of a stray, even if a government body will compensate the doctor, such payments could represent a small fraction of one's fee. When the animal's owner is absent at the time of admission, there can be uncertainty about what the owner would authorize. One could face the prospect of suing for the fee.

Alternative approaches are sometimes available. The laws of some jurisdictions permit a veterinarian to stabilize owner-absent animals and to recover the fee from owners when they are located. Some doctors budget a certain amount for the treatment of stray and owner-absent animals over given periods of time. A most admirable approach was developed by Dr. Rodney Poling, a Massachusetts practitioner. He has established a stray animal fund to which civic organizations and clients contribute. When a stray or owner-absent animal is brought in for emergency care, the animal is treated. If it is not possible to find the owner, the fund pays the practice for the animal's care. The animal is helped, and the practice does not suffer. The Massachusetts Veterinary Medical Association has created such a state-wide fund, to which any member practice can belong and which will disburse contributions for appropriate cases. Such an approach, if adopted throughout the country, could end forever the terrible problem of whether to treat the stray or owner-absent animal.

⌣ WITHDRAWING FROM THE VETERINARIAN-CLIENT-PATIENT RELATIONSHIP

Clients can become financially unreliable, strange, or threatening after a professional relationship has begun. Under such circumstances, one sometimes will be morally justified in asking the client to find another veterinarian for the same reasons that would justify not accepting such a client in the first place. However, withdrawing from the professional relationship can present special legal and moral problems.

Once one has accepted an animal as a patient, one is legally obligated not to withdraw from the case as long as the patient cannot be transferred without harm to another doctor or until the client is given adequate notice of one's intention to withdraw and adequate opportunity to obtain the services of another doctor. A veterinarian who fails in this obligation and terminates the veterinarian-client-patient relationship prematurely can be held liable to the client for abandonment, which is a form of negligence. Abandonment is a concept that is based on the needs of the patient and not on the shortcomings of the client. Thus even if a client is falling behind in payments, or is making the doctor's life miserable, one cannot unilaterally terminate treatment if the patient is in immediate need of it or if the client has not been given a reasonable opportunity to obtain care elsewhere. The legal obligation not to abandon a patient reflects the ethical principle that it is wrong to take out one's frustrations with a client upon a patient requiring immediate care.[3]

A doctor who wishes to terminate the professional relationship with a client also has the moral obligation (which all professionals have in their dealings with clients and the public) to use courtesy and tact. There is no need to inflict unnecessary guilt or bad feelings on a client, or to risk becoming the target of an administrative complaint or lawsuit. It is important, however, not to tell falsehoods concerning the condition of the patient to make the parting easier. This could lead the client not to seek needed care for the animal or could cause him unnecessary distress or expense. Thus it is wrong to try to get rid of a client whose animal requires continuing visits to a veterinarian by telling him that his animal is just fine and does not need further care. Nor is it fair to terminate the professional relationship by claiming that the animal really requires more extensive and expensive specialty care than one is able to provide, when in fact the animal does not require such care.

∽ FEES AND COLLECTIONS
The Ethical Dimensions of a Fair Fee

The contemporary veterinary practice management literature devotes a substantial amount of attention to the setting of fees. However, there is relatively little consideration of how to assure that one's fees are ethically appropriate—that is, *fair*.

One approach to fairness: What the market will bear

There are two predominant approaches to fairness in fees in practice management articles and texts. One approach is to concede that fees should indeed be fair and then to assert as fair whatever a practitioner can obtain from clients. For example, one author advocates calculating surgery fees based on the number of minutes usually spent on each kind of procedure. To determine the amount to charge per minute, a mathematical formula is used that adds to the weekly salary a doctor wants the gross profit margin one desires, and divides this total by the number of minutes actually spent providing services per week. Although this author thinks that a 50% profit margin would be desirable, he settles in his formula on a profit of 30%, because this is what he believes most practitioners can realistically obtain. To obtain the total fee for a service, he adds to the time-based fee a charge for items and products consumed during the surgery, such as gloves and gowns. These are marked-up three times the cost. This author declares such a fee structure "equitable" but provides no argument to support the assertion. There is no consideration of how large a profit margin or mark-up it is *fair* for a doctor to *want*. (In some fields, such as grocery retailing, a 300% mark-up on items essential to consumers would probably be considered price gouging.) Such a consideration would be irrelevant, given this author's view that the only measure of fairness is to "allow clients to make the decision"[4] whether they want to pay one's fee. If they want to pay, the fee is fair, and an appropriate measure of one's value.

A recent management text offers a concise statement of this "what the market will accept" philosophy of fairness in fees:

> Concentrate on value, not price. Never apologize for your fee structure (and make sure your staff don't either). Teach staff that the approach always should be 'we can provide this service for as little as…' The level of fees is irrelevant—£50, $100, or ECU200 if the value of the service you offer is perceived by your clients as—£55, $120, or ECU250!!!
> …Don't ever get trapped by charging fees which are 'affordable.' Only your clients can decide what they can or choose to afford. It is all a question of priorities. Just offer the best, quote the price, and let the client decide.[5]

The denial of fairness

A second approach to the setting of fees dispenses altogether with any attempt to characterize whatever veterinarians can get as "fair." Advocates of this approach tend not to tackle the issue of making fees fair. Indeed, they tend not to talk about or mention "fairness" at all as they go about discussing how to set one's fees. One discussion in a leading practice management text at least presents its reasons for not considering fairness:

> The concept of what is "fair" will be different for any two persons and is certain to vary among clients as a group, veterinarians as a group, and between individuals. Practical is a better key word. Practical is what clients as [a] group can afford. Practical is what must be charged to be competitive with other veterinarians in one general location (as each practice will define the boundaries of such location.) Finally, but not the least important, practical is what each practitioner wises to have and can reasonably expect from a 'practice.'[6]

It is not clear whether the assertion here is that there is no such thing as fairness, or that fairness just cannot be a workable consideration in setting a veterinarian's fees. In any event, according to this discussion it is unnecessary to worry about whether one's fees are fair. What really counts is feeling comfortable about what one wants to charge, and then getting it if one can.

The unavoidability of fairness

The assertion that no two persons will ever agree on what is fair is incorrect, and obviously so. There may well be some disagreements among veterinarians and clients about whether fees are fair. But, as argued throughout this book, disagreements in veterinary medicine about what is fair, just, or right do not arise because there is no such thing as fairness, justice, or rightness. Rather, veterinarians, clients, and patients can have conflicting interests that are sometimes difficult to reconcile. One cannot turn away from ethics because ethical questions can sometimes be difficult to answer or might be answered differently by people in different positions.

The assertion that a fair or ethical price is one that the market will bear is also incorrect, and obviously so. Just as a house or car, it is said, has no intrinsic "worth" or "value" apart from what people are willing to buy and sell it for, so, it is claimed, a "fair" fee or price is simply what a particular doctor can charge and receive. If someone is willing to pay $1,000 for a routine spay, who are we to say that the fee is unfair?

Certainly, a client's willingness to pay a proposed fee is an important factor in determining whether it is fair to him. Often, people will not be heard to complain that they have been treated unfairly if they have knowingly and deliberately decided to pay what a doctor requests. Nevertheless, "fairness" is *not* just another way of talking about what the market will bear. Most people, surely, believe that it is sometimes fair for a specialist who has invested years of time and money developing her skills to charge more than a general practitioner for her services, not because (or just because) clients might be willing to pay more, but because her sacrifices and special skills entitle her to a higher fee. People believe that a doctor who travels to a farm in the middle of the night to attend a difficult case can fairly ask more than his usual fee for this service, not because the client will pay but because the hardship and inconvenience entitle him to a higher fee. Likewise, we would say that a doctor who demands triple his usual fee from a client who rushes through the door with a dog just hit by an automobile is acting unfairly by taking advantage of a desperate situation.

It is understandable that the practice management literature tends to avoid real discussion of fairness in setting fees. Most veterinarians need a simple and workable way of determining fees. They have an interest in avoiding procedures that allow revenue to drip through the cracks or that force them into complex (and potentially costly) ethical deliberation about a fair fee each time they are confronted with a case that raises special ethical problems. Unfortunately, fairness does not always lend itself to mathematical computation or unvarying formulae. Fairness sometimes raises issues that have no clear answers.

Some Considerations Regarding Fairness of Fees

The following thoughts are offered to stimulate further consideration of the issue of fairness in fees. As is the case with many suggestions offered in this book, their primary purpose is to probe and question rather than to pass final judgment. One general statement can be asserted as a matter beyond argument: because of antitrust laws, any consideration of fairness in fees must presuppose that a decision about what fees to charge will rest with individual practitioners deciding how ethical principles should affect their own independently-reached decisions (see Chapter 19).

Fairness to the practitioner

As discussed in Chapter 16, veterinarians are entitled to attend to the interests not just of patients and clients, but also of themselves and their families. It is therefore not only appropriate, but necessary, for practitioners to take their own legitimate needs into account when setting fees. Fees should be fair to doctors as well as to clients.

A veterinarian's role

Unfortunately, much of the practice management literature concerning fees appears to be concerned *only* with the veterinarian's interests. In recommending that fees be as high as clients will pay, some of these discussions seem to be saying that the veterinarian is the only one who matters. At the very least, such discussions place the burden of determining at what point a fee ceases to be fair solely on clients. The only task assigned to practitioners is to set fees as high as possible; the termination of this process is determined by *clients*, at the point where they will pay no more.

A client's willingness to pay a fee is often one factor in determining whether that fee is fair. However, it is ethically wrong to place on clients the entire burden of determining where fee levels should rest. Most clients have no way of knowing or understanding a veterinarian's expenses. They do not know the cost of medications, surgical equipment, insurance, associates' salaries, obtaining and keeping nonveterinarian support staff, and so forth. They do not know the general or particular economic pressures facing their veterinarian. They do not know what fee structure is necessary just to keep the operation afloat, much less at a level that compensates everyone working for the practice fairly. They do not know, and cannot adequately understand, the education and expertise required for procedures performed on their animals.

Declaring "fair" anything clients will pay is wrong because clients and practitioners are not on a level playing field in the matter of assessing the appropriateness of fees. This uneven field is not unethical. It is just a fact that distinguishes clients from doctors. But to know that there is an impenetrable curtain between clients and practitioners and then to exalt clients as the all-knowing, all-powerful arbiters of fairness is itself unfair. As is the case so often in considering relations with clients, here also the Golden Rule is an excellent guide. A veterinarian who is considering marking up a pill from $.25 to $2.50 because she can get away with it might ask how *she* would feel if this was done to her if she were a client or were done to her by her pharmacist when she needs a medication for herself or a family member. "But you will pay it!" is not likely to seem a conclusive argument for the fairness of the price under such circumstances—even if an appreciation of all the facts would indicate that such a mark-up *is* appropriate and fair. More needs to be said than that people will pay.

Because only veterinarians know the costs and needs of their practices, *they* must bear the major burden of determining whether their fees are fair. Clients will consider their ability to pay. This can be a difficult enough task without their having to worry about whether requested fees represent a reasonable and fair profit for the practitioner. If clients reach the point of routinely doubting whether veterinary fees are fair, persuading a client that one's fees are reasonable will become difficult indeed.

Fairness and general approach to fees

The question of whether a fee is fair always must be capable of being asked, whatever might be one's general approach to setting fees. There are currently two leading systematic methods for setting fees advocated in the practice management literature: the time-based method and the cost-plus method. In the former, the fee for a service or kind of service is calculated by estimating the amount of time spent on that service, and multiplying it by a charge for each unit of time (for example, 1 minute, a tenth of an hour, or 1 hour). The unit charge is usually calculated by dividing the total amount a doctor expects to gross (including salary) by the total amount of time that will be expended in providing services. In the cost-plus method, fees are calculated by taking the cost of a service (including salary and consumables) and adding to it a mark-up to reach a desired profit level.

Neither of these approaches lends itself to a completely satisfactory consideration of whether any given fee is fair.

First, both methods calculate fees utilizing pre-determined amounts for salaries or profits. When proponents of either method concede the relevance of "fairness" they usually urge adding a fair markup to *assumed* salaries and other expenses. Rarely is it asked whether the desired salary or profit is itself fair. Moreover, this is an extremely difficult question to answer. How does one determine when an annual salary is fair or equitable? Is a salary of $50,000 fair? $75,000? $100,000?

Second, both methods apply a criterion to setting the fee for a particular service that is *independent of the nature of this service and its value.* In the time-based method, a general per-time unit fee is applied *all* services or to all instances of a kind of service. In the cost-plus method, a general percentage of mark-up usually is applied to *all* services. Because the calculation of a fee is not related intrinsically to the service being performed, odd—and potentially unfair—fees are inevitable. For example, a doctor's training and level of expertise is a relevant factor in assessing the fairness of a fee. A veterinarian who has expended years of education, study, and practice learning how to diagnose and treat certain conditions, and who as a result becomes more efficient and better at it than most other doctors, can be entitled to higher fees that reflect this training and expertise. In both the time-based and cost-plus approaches, a doctor with such expertise will not always charge what a service is fairly worth. Both time-based and cost-plus approaches run the risk of asking too little for some services (for example, diagnosing unusual heart sounds) that might be done quickly or inexpensively by a skilled doctor but can also be of critical importance and require significant expertise, and too much for other services (for example, ear cleaning) that can be time intensive and require relatively little expertise. Ironically, the time-based method can charge clients more for the services of doctors whose lack of training or background requires them to spend more time on a case than would an experienced doctor.

Third, both time-based and cost-plus methods, by separating the percentage of mark-up from any particular service, make it difficult to address the issue of the fairness of any fees, much less the fee for a particular service. Just as it is difficult to assess the fairness of the salaries to be utilized in either method, so is it virtually impossible to evaluate the fairness of a *general* rate of profit. Is it fair for a veterinarian to earn 10%, 25%, 35%, 50%, or even 100% over total costs? How does one even begin to approach such a question? One could try to compare veterinarians with other professionals or businesspeople, but using them as standards would just presuppose the fairness of *their* fee structure and beg the question of the fairness of veterinarians' fees. For example, many retail stores double the wholesale price of items. Is this fair for veterinarians?

Given the difficulty of evaluating the fairness of a general profit level, it is not surprising that advocates of both time-based and cost-plus methods who concede the relevance of fairness resort to quick assertions about fair profit margins. The advocate of the time-based approach quoted above settles on a 30% level of gross profit because this strikes him as representative of what veterinarians are in fact now earning. But *why* is this fair? A discussion that recommends the cost-plus method suggests that the profit level over and above the practice owner's salary "should at least reflect the rate of return if a similar investment of capital were put into a relatively secure investment such as treasury bills."[7] This is a puzzling standard against which to gauge profits because the earnings provided by such instruments depend on economic forces that have nothing to do with *veterinary* services. Indeed, at the time of this writing, such instruments paid approximately 3% annually—hardly an appropriate minimum profit level for veterinarians!

A range of fairness

It seems clear that if fees are to be fair, neither the time-based nor cost-plus methods can be utilized without supplementation. One must examine one's entire fee structure, and consider whether one has reached a fair fee for each service or product. Because fairness is not susceptible to strict mathematical analysis, this need not be an insurmountable task. For example, if a fee of $50 seems fair for a certain procedure, it need not be the case that $40 is too little (for oneself) or $60 too much (for clients). Assuring oneself that a fee is fair will generally involve judging that the fee falls within an acceptable *range*. In principle, there is nothing to prevent using either a time-based or cost-plus approach in the general process of attempting to locate fees within such a range. Speaking of a range of acceptably fair fees might strike the mathematically-inclined as too soft, intuitive, or subjective. But this is the way fairness works. The fact that fairness can be imprecise or would allow different practitioners to charge somewhat different fees for similar services does not make fairness any less real or any less important.

The nature of one's work, training, and expertise

As has been discussed, a factor in determining a fair level of fees is one's educational background, training, and the nature of one's work. Veterinarians are more highly educated than tradespeople, and they deal with momentous matters of life, death, health, and happiness (both animal and human). Therefore veterinarians should not assume that a level of profits normal for television repairmen or house painters is reasonable for them. If such tradespeople can earn a certain percent profit in a given community, it would not be unfair for veterinarians to try to earn more. If a particular kind of service or procedure requires a great deal of expertise, or time, or unpleasantness, it may be appropriate to mark-up that service more than one would more routine procedures.

Salaries and overhead

It is incorrect to begin asking about the fairness of fees only after one's salaries have been assumed. One must ask whether one's own salary and those of one's associates and employees are appropriate (see Chapter 25). Moreover, there can be ethical issues regarding overhead. If, for example, one is the only doctor in a community of people of modest means, and wants to purchase expensive equipment that will be used on a tiny fraction of one's patients, it can be asked whether it is fair to clients to buy this equipment if all clients will have to pay higher fees to cover the purchase.

Connecting fees and services

A fee ought to bear some relationship to, and be connected with, the services for which this fee is paid. It is appropriate to mark-up certain items such as drugs to cover the general costs of the practice, for unless the practice can operate, it will be impossible to provide any services. The mark-up one client pays for a surgery may enable the pharmacy to be properly stocked and the hospital to employ good technicians, all of which can inure directly to the benefit of that client and his animal. However, there can be an ethical problem with charging a client or a kind of client more to make up losses incurred because of services to other clients. Suppose, for example, that one charges 10% more for each comprehensive dental procedure because a competing mobile clinic has forced one to reduce fees for spays and neuters. A client whose animal needs dental work might rightly ask why she must subsidize the sterilization of other people's animals.

Limitations on profits

Although it will often be difficult to determine precisely when this might occur, at some point mark-ups or profit percentages can become so high as to be exorbitant. This can be the case for an item (such as a drug) that even after a mark-up cannot be called expensive.

Uniformity in fees

Because fees ought to be reasonably related to services provided, one should aim at charging all clients the same amount for the same procedures. Exceptions can be made for people who might have difficulty with the bill. However, it is wrong to charge wealthier clients more for the same procedure because they can more easily pay for it. This conveys the appearance—and involves the reality—of being paid a certain amount not because *this service* is worth it, but because one can get away with charging it.

It's the client's choice…or is it?

Some ethical questions regarding fees can be answered with the response that clients are not forced to pay a particular doctor's fees and can go elsewhere if they want. Nevertheless, clients cannot always make completely knowing or voluntary choices regarding fees. As was noted above, clients are usually ignorant about what factors go into a doctor's fees. For example, they might go elsewhere if they knew their animal's root canal was subsidizing other patients' vaccinations, but they might not know. Second, there is often great pressure on clients to remain with a doctor even if they are uncomfortable about her fees: there might not be another veterinarian in the vicinity; the current doctor might be familiar with the animal and its medical needs; the client might find it difficult to refuse a procedure on the grounds that it is expensive after the doctor has recommended it; or the patient might require immediate care. Often clients do not have the same bargaining power with their veterinarians as consumers have with, say, a department store. One can usually live without a television set, and buying it later elsewhere will not be a great sacrifice. But finding, or even thinking about finding, another veterinarian when one's animal needs care can be much harder.

Veterinarians, therefore should not take advantage of situations in which clients have a restricted choice of whether to accept their fees. If, for example, a course of treatment cannot be halted until it involves some expense, the client must be informed at the very start about the required fees and given the opportunity to decide whether they are acceptable. Under no circumstances should one take advantage of an emergency to raise a fee or urge unnecessary procedures, for here also the client might be in a weakened state and easy prey to manipulation.

Making Exceptions for Certain Clients

The ideal situation, both from a management and ethical standpoint, is to have firmly in place a fee schedule that applies across the board to all clients and patients. If one's fees are generally fair, one can ask clients for them confidently and without guilt.

Sometimes, however, a doctor will find it impossible not to consider whether one should reduce the fee for a client unable to pay it. Clearly, if the usual fee for a service is fair, one can first insist on exploring various ways of paying that fee. But sometimes, even this will be too burdensome for a client with an animal in need of one's services.

In considering the issue of reduced fees for certain clients, it is useful to keep in mind the distinction between obligations (actions one must morally do) and supererogatory acts (behavior that is not obligatory but morally praiseworthy) (see Chapter 5). I do not want to suggest that veterinarians are never morally obligated to reduce a fee for a needy client. However, it seems to me that a much stronger general argument can be made for saying that reducing a fee can be a supererogatory act—and should be encouraged in certain kinds of circumstances without justifying moral condemnation if it is not done. Private practitioners are not charities, and many are far from wealthy. Reducing fees can be a sacrifice. However, like other kinds of sacrifice, it can be morally praiseworthy. Moreover, there might sometimes be ways of reducing the sacrifice, such as budgeting a small amount for fee reduction, or instituting a fund to reduce fees for certain kinds of cases.

Taking Responsibility for One's Fees

There is no reason to feel guilty about one's fees if they are fair to clients and to oneself. And if fees are fair, it should usually be possible to explain to clients why they are fair. Evading responsibility for one's own fees makes it impossible to explain to clients why they are receiving value for their money.

Some practice management consultants believe that the process of setting and collecting fees can be made easier by not acknowledging or accepting full responsibility for fees. I once attended a practice management seminar, which considered the question of how to prevent young, nonowner veterinarian employees from reducing fees for clients for whom these doctors felt sympathy. The solution advised was to have all doctors in the practice utilize a check-list of services. This list would not include the fee for each procedure. Doctors examining a patient would simply check off which services should be provided, and the client would learn the cost for each service and the total bill after taking the list to the receptionist. This, it was suggested, would prevent guilty feelings about the practice's fees because doctors would not even be thinking about (and might not even know) what the client's bill will be.

One practice management text suggests utilizing the practice's computer to conquer fear of one's own fees:

> A clinician can team up with his clients versus the machine. 'Look how much the computer has charged us today (note the 'us') Mrs. Smith. Still for that price you can be satisfied that Charlie is getting the best care.' However, be judicious in invoking the editorial 'we' or you may be convinced by a persuasive client to override the decision of the electronic brain![5]

Neither of these approaches treats clients as mature, autonomous beings who are entitled to all relevant information before deciding what shall be done with their animals. Among such information is, clearly, how much it will cost and why. Veterinarians who are afraid to provide such information may think that if they were the client they would not find the fee acceptable. There are at least two possible messages in this application of the Golden Rule: either a client would be correct in objecting to the fee, or a client might need information to understand why the fee is appropriate.

Explaining Fees

There are many ways of explaining one's fee structure to clients who ask or need to know. One should always be prepared to describe the specific procedure one is recommending, including the nature of the materials and expertise required. However, the best way of convincing clients that one's fees are reasonable and fair is to encourage in them a general, high regard for one's talents and for the profession of veterinary medicine. As argued throughout this book, an important way of doing this is behaving with dignity, professionalism, and as a member of a healing profession interested in helping its patients and clients. Additionally, more specific ways of informing clients about one's worth as a doctor can include the following:

- Making available to clients brochures and hand-outs explaining the training and experience veterinarians possess and the kinds of sophisticated medical and surgical procedures they perform
- Distributing client newsletters explaining animal health conditions and veterinary procedures in ways that reveal the background and abilities of veterinarians
- Informing clients about one's educational background and attainments, in printed material and by displaying one's veterinary school diploma or diploma of specialty certification
- Conducting individual or general tours of one's facility, to explain the nature and sophistication of one's equipment and services
- Before performing a surgical procedure, asking a client if she might be interested in looking at one's surgery suite and learning more about the procedure
- Displaying photographs of the practice's doctors and support staff with their names, educational backgrounds, and distinctive professional accomplishments
- Displaying photographs of the practice's professional staff performing certain procedures

Legal and Official Approaches to Setting Fees

American law treats the matter of an appropriate fee differently, depending on whether there has been an agreement (either explicit or implicit) between a client and veterinarian that the client will pay the doctor's fee. Where there is such an agreement, one is usually free to charge as much or as little as one wants. In rare cases, where a businessperson exerts undue pressure on a disadvantaged consumer to charge an outrageously high price, the law will overturn even an agreed-upon price as unconscionable. However, the legal doctrine of unconscionability has been developed in the context of consumer purchases of goods, and it is not clear how it would apply (if at all) to veterinary services.

Where there has been no meeting of the minds about a fee, the law allows veterinarians a reasonable fee. What is reasonable is an issue for a jury and will depend on the doctor's training and skills, the nature of the work, the time and expense involved, and what other doctors in the area with similar qualifications would charge for similar services. In almost all jurisdictions, the client's wealth or ability to pay is not a relevant factor in determining the reasonableness of a fee. In this regard, the law reflects the ethical principle that the fee should be related to the nature of the work performed. However, the law does permit a doctor to take into account a client's ability to pay in determining a fee to which both parties then mutually agree.

The *Principles of Veterinary Medical Ethics* state that in determining fees, veterinarians "may be expected to consider the nature of the condition, the time, the expense of other resources applicable to the case, and the client's ability to pay."[8] Hopefully, the last part of this statement is not intended to encourage doctors to charge a different fee for each client rather than for each procedure, and then to vary this fee depending on each client's economic resources. As has been noted earlier, fairness in fees requires that a fee be for a particular service and the fee for that service be proportionate to the service provided.

⮑ COLLECTIONS

Collecting fees is another area that raises a myriad of difficult ethical problems. Different situations present varying problems. What approach is morally appropriate often depends on particular facts relating to the practice, doctor, client, and patient.

Among the many ethical questions that arise in the area of collections are the following:

- Does a veterinarian sometimes have a moral obligation to permit a client to be billed or to pay in installments?
- If postponed payment is permitted, may the doctor add a finance charge, and if so, what is the measure of a fair charge?
- Can the use of credit cards be demeaning to the veterinarian-client relationship?
- If credit cards are accepted, is it fair to cash-paying clients to build the additional costs of credit card transactions into the fees of all clients?
- How far may a doctor attempt to intrude into the personal lives of clients by asking specific questions about their financial situations and lifestyles before deciding whether to extend credit or to allow special payment arrangements?
- Should practitioners share information or impressions about the financial reliability of particular clients? Is it appropriate to circulate "deadbeat lists" containing the names of problem clients?
- Is it proper for a medical professional to accept items of personal property as collateral for payment? Are there ethical limits to the kinds or value of property that may be accepted?
- Is a doctor ever morally obligated to treat a client's animal when the client already owes a certain amount and seems unable to pay it? To what extent are the kind of the animal, the gravity of its condition, and the amount of money still owed relevant factors in approaching this question?
- How many reminder statements is it appropriate to send to a delinquent client and at what frequency?
- What are the moral limits to the kinds of language that may appropriately be included in such statements, or in other communications with the client intended to effect payment?

- Is it morally permissible to contact persons other than the client (such as family, friends, or employer) in order to effect collection?
- When is it appropriate to step outside the professional-client relationship and refer collections to a collection agency? Does a doctor have moral obligations regarding the choice of an agency to service his accounts?
- Is it morally appropriate to threaten a delinquent client with the sale or destruction of his animal? Is it morally appropriate to carry through such threats?

Threatening the Sale or the Killing of a Patient

In light of the current battle between more traditional views of veterinary practice and the model of the veterinary practice as a business (see Chapter 16), one of the most interesting ethical issue regarding collections concerns whether veterinarians have more stringent moral obligations in the collection area than do ordinary commercial enterprises. Television repair shops and department stores routinely threaten delinquent customers with bad credit ratings and other nasty actions by collection agencies or the courts. I would argue that because veterinarians should be viewed as medical professionals, certain kinds of actions are appropriate, if at all, far less often for them than for ordinary businesspeople.

The question whether veterinarians may threaten clients with the sale or destruction of an animal in their possession unless the bill is paid is especially important. The latter issue arose in a landmark decision of the Tennessee Supreme Court.[9] A client brought her dog to the doctor after it had been hit by an automobile. The doctor accepted and treated the patient. However, according to the client, the doctor demanded that she pay the $155 bill "in cash and in full" by a specified date and refused her request to pay in installments. The client alleged that a hospital employee telephoned her repeatedly and threatened that the hospital would "do away with the dog" as the doctor saw fit unless the bill was paid in full by the specified date.

The Court held that if the plaintiff could prove that her allegations were true, she would be entitled to a judgment for intentional infliction of emotional distress. The Court acknowledged the existence of a state statute permitting a veterinarian to turn over an animal to a humane society for disposal if a client does not fulfill his contractual obligations after a period of 10 days. But the Court pointed out that nothing in the statute justifies a veterinarian's *threatening* to do away with a client's animal. The Court held that the conduct alleged to have been committed by the veterinary hospital would be "outrageous and extreme and is not tolerable in a civilized society."

The Tennessee Court did not analogize the alleged behavior of the defendant to a human hospital's threatening to kill a baby in its care if the parents do not pay the bill. Nevertheless, clearly implicit in the Court's reasoning was a recognition that certain kinds of behavior that might be tolerated from ordinary commercial establishments concerning inanimate pieces of property are unacceptable when done by a veterinarian. The Court appeared to recognize that it is profoundly immoral for anyone to taunt someone with threats to kill a beloved animal—and that this is even worse if done by a veterinarian with a general commitment to saving animal life and assisting animal owners.

The Court's distinction between disposing of a delinquent client's animal after giving the client notice of one's legal right to do so and intentionally inflicting emotional distress by threatening such disposal is an important one. Even if the former might sometimes be morally (and legally) justified, the latter is not.

Equally important, however, is the issue of whether it is consistent with a veterinarian's commitment to patients and clients for him to kill, without threats, an animal wanted by a client. Some people would condemn such a course of action on the grounds that a veterinarian should never take the life of a wanted, healthy animal. (Some people believe that a veterinarian should never kill any healthy animal, wanted or unwanted.) However, one often can raise less radical arguments against killing the healthy animal of a delinquent client, as opposed to giving it to a shelter for adoption, or even returning it to the client. Killing the animal will usually accomplish very little for the doctor at potentially great cost to the client and animal. Charges might cease to accumulate, but this will itself not get the bill paid. Indeed, a client whose animal has been killed might be less willing to pay. Even if veterinarians are sometimes morally justified in killing a wanted animal, it does not seem terribly radical to suggest that if this is to occur, there must be at least some benefit in it for someone.

Sometimes, the only real rationale for killing a delinquent client's animal is a desire to punish the client or to prevent him from further enjoyment of the animal. However, it is far from clear why taking the life of an innocent animal is an appropriate way of punishing or withholding satisfactions from an errant human being—or why a veterinarian committed to saving animal life should want to have any part of this kind of punishment.

The same sort of argument can also often be made against putting the animal of a delinquent client up for sale and applying the proceeds to the client's bill. The process often will not be in the doctor's interests. It can cost a great deal of time, aggravation, and legal fees, and often will bring in less than the amount of the client's obligation. And selling the animal can involve a deprivation to an innocent creature that might more justly be imposed upon the real culprit through other means such as reports to credit bureaus or legal action to collect the fee.

Legal Issues

Veterinarians contemplating various approaches toward collecting a fee must be attentive to applicable laws. Federal and state statutes protect debtors against certain kinds of harassing behavior by or on behalf of creditors. Veterinarians who go overboard in criticizing delinquent clients or in pressuring clients to pay can find themselves liable for defamation of character or intentional infliction of emotional distress. Although a number of states do have laws permitting practitioners to sell or dispose of a delinquent client's animal under certain circumstances, these laws contain specific requirements regarding how long a bill must be unpaid before action can be taken, what kind of notice must be provided to the client, and precisely what the doctor must do. Failure to abide by these specific requirements can be disastrous. A veterinarian's scrupulous attention to the law might be the only protection he has against a judge's or jury's underlying opposition to one's killing or selling the animal. To be sure, the fact that a doctor does follow the law in having a delinquent client's animal killed or sold does not necessarily guarantee the morality of one's actions.

～ LOYALTY TO CLIENTS
Fee-splitting, Commissions, Rebates, and Kickbacks

As discussed in Chapter 14, veterinarians have an obligation of loyalty to clients, which requires that they not compromise the interests of a client in favor of their own interests or those of other clients. It is therefore unethical, as the *Principles of Veterinary Medical Ethics* once stated (see Chapter 9) and many state veterinary practice acts still insist, for veterinarians to split fees or to receive or to give a commission, rebate, or kickback in connection with referrals. Nor should a doctor receive such moneys as a result of a recommendation that a client purchase nonveterinary goods or services such as cremation, livestock supplies, and ordinary commercial pet food.

A rebate, commission, or kickback is not restricted to the actual transfer of money. Many creative forms of kickbacks are possible. For example, a doctor who agrees with Company X to dispense its products instead of Company Y's in return for a special extra discount on the normal cost of certain Brand X products is accepting no less a monetary benefit than if Company X passed cash to the doctor under the table.

Some doctors might object to a prohibition of kickbacks in circumstances in which they would make a certain referral or sell or prescribe a certain product anyway. In such a case, it might be argued, the only party that loses is the provider of the kickback. Such an approach is unsatisfactory because it raises unnecessary temptations that can intrude into doctors' independent exercise of their own best judgments on behalf of clients and animals. There may come a time when, for example, Company Y can provide a better product for certain patients. A doctor who is receiving a kickback from Company X has a strong motive for ignoring, or deluding himself about, the superiority of the better product. A client who comes to a veterinarian expecting his absolutely undivided loyalty should be able to rest assured that there is not present, even in the most remote part of the doctor's psyche, the slightest temptation to abandon the dictates of independent professional judgment.

Pharmacy Issues

One ethical controversy now facing human medicine concerns the growing practice by physicians of selling prescription drugs. Opponents of this practice believe that physicians who sell drugs face a conflict of interest between the needs of their patients and their desire to profit from the sales. It is feared that physicians will choose drugs and brands that will bring them the greatest profits or that can be most conveniently kept in stock, rather than those that are best for patients.[10]

The *Principles of Veterinary Medical Ethics* state that "in the choice of drugs, biologics, or other treatments...[veterinarians] are expected to use their professional judgment in the interests of the patient."[11] A practice's pharmacy, in which prices can be changed with the stroke of a pen, may provide some doctors a temptation to make decisions based primarily on their own monetary interests at the expense of the interests of clients. The following reminders therefore are appropriate:

1. Unlike most human medical patients, who still purchase pharmaceuticals at a pharmacy and can compare prices at different establishments, the majority of veterinary clients cannot or do not want to obtain a recommended drug other than from the doctor who has seen their animal. Because these clients are at the mercy of their veterinarian, one must be especially careful to dispense an appropriate drug at a fair price.

2. It is proper to factor into decisions about what drugs and dosages to keep in stock the usual needs of one's patients as well as one's financial requirements. However, when the best drug for a patient cannot be stocked routinely, it is morally as well as medically wrong to dispense a less-effective drug just because one has it and can turn a sale. In such cases, one's duty of loyalty to clients and patients requires one to obtain or refer clients to a place where they can obtain that drug. Sometimes, a doctor may afford a client the choice between a drug in stock and one that must be ordered specially; but this should be done only when the drug in stock is adequate for the job and the client is permitted to make a fully informed and voluntary choice. Clients are by and large unsophisticated about drugs and biologics. They are likely to agree with whatever is suggested by veterinarians.

In-practice Laboratory Testing

One service that is being recommended as a source of increased revenues,[12] but which can create a conflict of interest for doctors, is in-practice laboratory testing. In-practice testing can offer enormous potential for taking unfair advantage of clients. Unnecessary, redundant, or overpriced testing is a violation of a veterinarian's obligation of loyalty to clients.

I believe that many veterinarians are not adequately explaining to clients why, for example, they must take additional x-rays or do further blood work after similar tests have already been done by a referring or previous doctor. Physicians and human hospitals have done a wonderful job convincing the public that laboratory tests are sometimes unnecessary, are frequently done to protect physicians rather than patients, and are always overpriced. Veterinary testing will come to be perceived in the same way unless practitioners recommend testing only when it is required medically, explain the need for tests clearly, and price the service fairly.

Pet Health Insurance

Although pet health insurance plans appear to promise great benefits to many patients, clients, and practitioners, they can also create situations that test a doctor's loyalty to clients. Although no insurance plan can guarantee that a subscriber will save money in the long run, the attraction of insurance is that by paying a premium now, people have a possibility of saving money later. Veterinarians who run their own pre-paid health plan must be careful to price options so that they give clients a fighting chance of saving money in the long run. Doctors would also compromise the best interests of clients if they took commissions or kickbacks in return for their participation in a company's plan or for their display of its promotional literature. It would also be unfair to clients to raise fees just because insurance will now cover them. Ultimately, this will cost all subscribers more in premiums and out-of-pocket expenses than the legitimate worth of services provided would justify. To serve the interests of patients and clients, insurance programs must also permit referrals to and from other doctors.[13]

Admitting Mistake or Fault

Another kind of situation in which a doctor's loyalty to a client can conflict with one's own self-interest occurs when a mistake has been made. Clients are not legally obligated to pay for negligent services and are entitled to be compensated for certain kinds of damage caused by such services. Therefore it will sometimes be in a client's interest to be told that a mistake was made or that an injury to the patient was the fault of the doctor or an employee. On the other hand, admitting mistake or fault is almost never in a doctor's interest, because it can result in loss of the fee, loss of the client, a complaint before a professional or government body, or a lawsuit.

Two inappropriate responses

One response to the issue of admitting fault that I have found to be expressed by some veterinarians is the claim that at least when the patient is not injured or can be returned to the client in a healthy state, there is no issue regarding admission of fault. In such a case, it is said, the client is not harmed.

Aside from overlooking what might have happened to the unfortunate patient, this approach ignores the fact that clients are not legally obligated to pay for negligent or incompetent services. Therefore failure to tell a client that a mistake was made can sometimes harm the client, if the fee is demanded or retained for incompetent services. Indeed, it can be argued that retention of a fee in such circumstances is tantamount to theft.

A second common response to the issue of admitting fault involves an attempt to insist that "the truth has been told." Suppose, for example, that a doctor performs an unnecessary intestinal biopsy upon an animal with digestive problems, that he performs this procedure in a negligent manner, and that his negligence causes peritonitis and death of the patient. The client asks what happened, and the doctor responds that the animal died from uncontrollable peritonitis. This was a real case, and I use it regularly to evoke the moral intuitions of my veterinary students. Many of them are inclined to say that this doctor need not worry about admitting fault because he is not lying to the client. He is not lying, it is claimed, because he was not asked whether he was at fault, and what he told the client was literally true. Such a response refuses to address the issue of whether fault ought to be admitted, and it does so by employing a questionable concept of "telling the truth."

Arguments for admitting fault

There are very strong moral considerations that often appear to argue in favor of a veterinarian admitting mistake or fault. First, if a doctor does not admit fault or indicate to the client that something was amiss, one sometimes will demand or retain a fee that one does not legally or morally deserve. Second, in failing to admit that a mistake was made, a doctor will sometimes be lying to the client, if the client inquires about what really happened or asks whether any mistake was made. Third, failing to admit fault will often be a violation of the Golden Rule and its admirable implication that veterinarians should treat clients as they would want to be treated if they were clients.

The arguments against admitting fault

The strongest argument against admitting mistake or fault is that doing so can have bad consequences for the doctor. To the doctor, this is an important consideration. But if one looks at the matter from an objective standpoint, it is far from clear why a client's interest in knowing the truth should be subordinated to a doctor's interest in keeping a fee or not being criticized or sued. It is the client who is paying the fee and for whom the doctor works.

Morality in the light of prudence

Realistically, it is usually impossible to ask any professional person to admit a mistake or fault to a client. Therefore the task of normative veterinary ethics in this area will probably be to formulate the best guidelines that can feasibly be put into action. The following are intended as suggestions toward this goal. These suggestions all presuppose that a doctor already knows a mistake has been made, something that might not always be obvious.

1. Sometimes, failing to admit mistake or fault will not result in retaining a fee to which one is not legally entitled. In the eyes of the law, a practitioner is entitled to one's fee if one provides substantially the service for which the client agreed to pay. Moreover, a veterinarian's negligence alone does not excuse a client from his obligation to pay. Any negligence must also have been the cause of an injury that the law recognizes as compensable. Pain caused to an animal by a doctor's negligence is not among the kinds of compensable injury. In general, clients may recover only for physical or economic injury veterinary negligence has caused to them.

Suppose that a doctor removes a tumor successfully, but carelessly leaves the patient with a minor cosmetic disfigurement. Moral considerations might argue in favor of reducing the fee. However, in the eyes of the law, the doctor will be entitled to the fee and will not be liable for damages to the client, if the disfigurement does not cause the client economic damage (or the doctor did not guarantee there would be no disfigurement). If an error made by a veterinarian does not extinguish the client's obligation to pay the fee, where the doctor fails to admit such an error, at least one will not be retaining moneys that lawfully belong to the client.

2. Even when a mistake is significant enough to affect a doctor's legal right to all or part of the fee, one can sometimes employ means other than admitting fault to lessen the harm to the client. The fee can be reduced or waived, or the client can be offered reduced fees or gratuitous services in the future. To be sure, such actions might not compensate the client for additional damage caused by one's mistakes, and failure to admit the mistake can prevent the client from taking appropriate action to obtain compensation for these losses. Moreover, reducing or waiving one's past or future fees will sometimes be a signal that something went amiss, and for that reason might not seem a feasible approach.

3. Even if a doctor is unable to admit a mistake to a client, she owes it to all clients and patients to admit to herself when she or one of her staff erred or was at fault for injury to a patient. Every professional learns from mistakes. Such learning (and any consequent improvement in the quality of services one can provide to all clients) is impossible if one engages in self-deception regarding one's own mistakes or those of one's staff.

Serving Clients with Conflicting or Potentially Conflicting Interests

A veterinarian's loyalty to clients can also be tested by situations in which one is asked to serve clients with conflicting or potentially conflicting interests. Loyalty to one client might provide temptations to compromise the interests of another. This can happen when a doctor is asked by both the buyer and seller of an animal to examine it for soundness or some other feature of interest in a transaction. Each party needs the doctor's complete loyalty. But if the doctor is financially tied to both, one might not be completely honest with either, or both.

The *Principles of Veterinary Medical Ethics* condemn accepting a fee from the seller of an animal when one is employed by the buyer to inspect it for soundness.[14] However, the code does not discuss in general terms the problem of serving clients with conflicting or potentially conflicting economic interests. The following are but a few situations in which this issue can arise:

- Examining an animal to be purchased from a breeder by a member of the public when one's fee for the examination is paid by the breeder
- Examining for a fee to be paid by the purchaser an animal bought from a breeder who is a regular client, after the purchaser has been referred by the breeder
- Providing regular veterinary services at a racetrack for owners whose animals compete against each other
- Serving two competing local show dog breeders
- Providing theriogenology services for competing sellers of dairy cows

In these situations, a doctor might be able to help one client at the expense of another, by revealing to the former some vital piece of information about, or indeed by doing something to, the latter's animals. Although one might strive conscientiously to be impartial, financial or personal considerations can sometimes make complete impartiality impossible. Even if one remains impartial, if one's clients have a falling out, there could be blame (or a lawsuit) by either or both clients.

"Serving" two persons with potentially conflicting interests does not necessarily mean being paid by each. The following kind of situation, reported by a doctor who learned about conflicts between parties the hard way, is not uncommon. The seller of a horse informed a potential buyer that it had the heaves. The buyer stated that he did not wish to retain his own veterinarian. The seller told the buyer that he should feel free to talk to his veterinarian about the animal. The buyer called the seller's veterinarian after purchasing the horse and after the animal came down with a serious case of the heaves. The buyer then sued the seller to undo the sale, alleging that the seller did not disclose all the relevant facts about the animal. During the trial, the veterinarian was required to testify about what he said, or had not said, to both his regular client (the seller) and the buyer about the animal's condition.

It is unrealistic to prohibit all veterinarians from ever serving clients with potentially conflicting interests. Sometimes, there are not enough veterinarians or veterinarians qualified in a particular kind of practice to go around. Sometimes, the service a doctor provides to competitors is so routine that it will not involve the opportunity to compromise any of them. Sometimes, a doctor's serving an owner in competition with an existing client might be necessary to save the life of an animal belonging to the former.

There is certainly a moral obligation (and one recognized by the *Principles*[15] and many state practice acts) to protect the professional confidences of clients, unless one is required to reveal them by law or unless revealing them is necessary to protect the health or safety of animals or the public. However, although such a rule might be helpful in assuring confidentiality and loyalty to clients, the best way of promoting these values is usually to avoid situations in which they can be compromised. For their own safety and to assure the protection of clients, as a general rule, veterinarians ought to try to avoid serving clients with potentially conflicting economic interests. In the absence of an immediate medical emergency, they ought to avoid serving clients altogether when there is a substantial potential for loyalty to one client being compromised by loyalty to another. I would suggest that among the latter situations are the following: (1) being asked by both buyer and seller to examine an animal that is the subject of a sale; (2) serving competing clients after one client has asked for information regarding the animals or general business operations of another client; (3) serving competing clients after being exposed (even accidentally) to information that is essential to one client's competitive position and that could harm this client if revealed to another client; (4) serving competing clients after being asked by one not to serve any of his competitors because of the confidential nature of information that might be obtained during the provision of veterinary services; and (5) serving clients who are, or are likely to be, opponents in a lawsuit concerning animals that have been or are likely to be examined or treated by the doctor.

∼ COMMUNICATING WITH CLIENTS

Perhaps the most important area of client relations with ethical overtones is that of communication with clients. A client's problems or dissatisfaction can often be avoided or solved quickly by clear and respectful communication. If one has difficulty communicating with a client, it can be impossible to learn all the relevant facts required to decide on an approach that is medically and ethically proper.

Doctor-client communication is an area that has largely been ignored as a serious field of study by the profession. A few veterinary schools now offer formal instruction in communication skills.[16] Most students tend to pick up practical pointers from some of their instructors as they proceed through their clinics. However, such exposure tends to be spotty and inconsistent. Some of my students look at how differently their various instructors handle client communication. They conclude that how one deals with clients is just a feature of one's own personality, and is an individual matter that cannot be changed substantially.

Communication skills can, however, often be improved. Law schools routinely videotape students in simulated or actual settings with clients or judges so that they can see how their physical mannerisms, tone of voice, and ability to listen and convey their ideas affect their capacity to serve clients. I believe that even some of the most experienced veterinarians would be astonished if they viewed themselves on a tape replay as clients see them.

A serious discipline that would investigate veterinarian-client communication does not yet exist. Those who develop such a field must be careful not to view communications skills as a mechanistic set of behaviors than can be easily learned and routinely applied. A recent call for course work in communication by several veterinary school educators states that the:

> ...time has come when veterinarians should be expected to graduate from all veterinary schools with a reasonable understanding of the basis of communication, perhaps with a communications skills list checked off in the same way as a series of surgical skills might be checked off.[16]

There are, surely, routine basic skills and mannerisms that can be taught, mastered, and "checked off." At the same time, much of communication with clients involves *ethical* attitudes toward them, their animals, and the medical, financial, and psychological issues they face. A veterinarian who knows how to communicate effectively, but is communicat-

ing something that ought *not* to be communicated, or is influencing a client to do something it is *wrong* to try to influence the client to do is, if anything, worse than a veterinarian who communicates poorly. Put another way, communication skills are a technique or
tool, which, like any tool, must be employed in the service of good ends. Unfortunately, it
is not as easy to promote ethical attitudes as it is to assure that a proper suture technique
has been mastered. Without serious courses in ethics, veterinary schools cannot claim to
offer serious courses in communication. And any veterinary school instructor who claims
to possess a list of ethical principles that can be easily learned and "checked off" has
accomplished something which has eluded philosophers for centuries!

The relevance of ethics to communicating with clients becomes evident when one
considers that central to respectful and effective communication are certain moral
virtues. Among these virtues are the following:

Ability to listen: Veterinarians must keep their minds open to what clients are saying. They should not be too busy formulating their own statements when they
should be listening to the client.

Empathy: It is often necessary to put oneself in a client's place. A client who is
afraid of treating her pet with cancer chemotherapy might be transferring to the
animal memories of cancer treatment of a relative or friend. A doctor must be able
to understand why there might be such an impediment to the client's understanding of the treatment options. The doctor, who sees illness every day, must be able
to appreciate how strange and frightening the illness of an animal can be to an
owner accustomed to its good health.

Sympathy and compassion: A doctor must try to be sympathetic regarding a
client's worries or distress, even if one finds these concerns trivial or unreasonable.

Patience: Doctors must understand that clients sometimes might be unable or
unwilling to comprehend the facts or treatment options. Clients must be given
adequate time to appreciate the facts and to make decisions.

Sincerity: Few things are more offensive than a practitioner whose behavior
reflects insincerity, lack of interest, or downright hostility.

Clarity: A doctor must be able to speak clearly in language that the client can
understand, without treating the client in a condescending manner.

Tactfulness: A doctor must be able to be honest with clients while remaining tact-
ful and courteous. Sometimes, it might be necessary to make clear to a client that
he is the reason the animal is ill or is not recovering. This often can be done in a
way that encourages rather than criticizes.

Professionalism in appearance and demeanor: Effective communication requires
that the client be able to confide in the doctor and trust the doctor's information and
recommendations. This will be impossible if a client believes the doctor does not
really care about her and her problems. Regard for personal appearance and
demeanor is important in conveying to clients that one does care. Dirty or disheveled
clothing, or coarse and disrespectful behavior toward or in the presence of clients,
can create a wall between doctor and client that makes communication impossible.

REFERENCES

[1]There may be an exception to this long-standing legal principle. Included in the regulations of the Massachusetts
Board of Registration in Veterinary Medicine is the statement that "a veterinarian shall not refuse to provide
treatment to an animal unless such refusal is based on reasons such as the inadequacy of the facilities then avail-

able or the unavailability of all-night veterinary medical care for the animal." 256 *Code of Massachusetts Regulations* § 7.01(22). The only other approved reasons for refusing a case specifically enumerated in the regulations are the failure of an animal to be currently vaccinated (*Id*, § 7.01[29]), or a client's engaging in "physical or verbal abuse" towards the veterinarian or one of his employees (*Id*, § 7.01[31]). These regulations (which apply only in Massachusetts) appear to prohibit, among other things, declining a case because a client cannot afford to pay the fee or refuses to leave a deposit. Such an approach is objectionable on moral grounds because it sometimes is justifiable to decline or withdraw from a case when a client cannot or will not pay. It is also highly doubtful whether a state veterinary board has the legal authority to enforce a regulation that could have the implication of compelling doctors to provide free services for all or most clients.

[2]American Veterinary Medical Association: *Principles of Veterinary Medical Ethics*, 1993 Revision, "Guidelines for Professional Behavior," paragraph 6, *1994 AVMA Directory*, Schaumburg, IL, The Association, p 42.

[3]Tannenbaum J: Ethics: The why and wherefore of veterinary law, *Vet Clin North Am Small Anim Pract* 23:921-935, 1993.

[4]Nelson DA: Setting surgery fees based on actual cost, *Vet Econ* April 1990: 42-48.

[5]Sheridan JP, McCafferty OE: *The Business of Veterinary Practice*, Oxford, UK, Pergamon Press, 1993, p 29.

[6]Kay WJ and others: Fee setting and collection. In McCurnin DM, editor: *Veterinary Practice Management*, Philadelphia, 1988, JB Lippincott, p 191.

[7]Kay WJ and others: Fee setting and collection. In McCurnin DM, editor: *Veterinary Practice Management*, Philadelphia, 1988, JB Lippincott, p 196.

[8]American Veterinary Medical Association: *Principles of Veterinary Medical Ethics*, 1993 Revision, "Fees for Service," *1994 AVMA Directory*, Schaumburg, IL, The Association, p 43.

[9]*Lawrence* v. *Stanford*, 665 S.W.2d 927 (Tenn. 1983).

[10]Robertson JD: Doctors vs. pharmacists: Conflict of interest, *Med Malprac Law Strat* 4(6):5, 1987.

[11]American Veterinary Medical Association: *Principles of Veterinary Medical Ethics*, 1993 Revision, "Drugs, Practitioner's Responsibility in the Choice of," *1994 AVMA Directory*, Schaumburg, IL, The Association, p 45.

[12]Roth DF: In-clinic diagnostics bring profits and client appreciation, *Vet Econ* April 1986:45-52.

[13]*See*, American Veterinary Medical Association: *Principles of Veterinary Medical Ethics*, 1993 Revision, "Guidelines on Pet Health Insurance and Other 3rd Party Animal Health Plans," *1994 AVMA Directory*, Schaumburg, IL, The Association, p 82.

[14]American Veterinary Medical Association: *Principles of Veterinary Medical Ethics*, 1993 Revision, "Frauds," *1994 AVMA Directory*, Schaumburg, IL, The Association, p 44.

[15]American Veterinary Medical Association: *Principles of Veterinary Medical Ethics*, 1993 Revision, "Confidentiality," *1994 AVMA Directory*, Schaumburg, IL, The Association, p 44.

[16]Prescott J and others: Letter, Communications skills in veterinary education, *J Am Vet Med Assoc* 204:189-190, 1994.

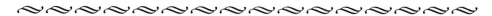

CHAPTER 21

Ethical Issues in Companion Animal Practice

One reason veterinary ethics is so interesting is that there is great variety in the value people place on veterinary patients. Some are treated as members of the family and for which no effort or expense is to be spared. Others are destined for the dinner table.

This chapter considers ethical issues in companion animal practice the difficulty of which results at least in part from the high regard many people have for pets. Although the discussion focuses on small animal practice, human-animal companionship (or the human companion-animal bond, which is not the same thing) is not limited to dogs, cats, and birds. Equine veterinarians, as well as other large animal doctors, can engage in what is rightly considered companion animal practice. Many of the issues developed here within the context of small animal practice are relevant to these veterinarians and indeed to noncompanion animal practitioners as well.

∾ IMPORTANT ISSUES OF LANGUAGE
"Pets" or "Companion Animals?"

Recently, the English language has been criticized by people who find some of the words it has traditionally employed offensive, derogatory, or demeaning. From the use of the masculine gender as a generic referent to all persons, to such terms as "spokesman" or "handicapped," the language is being changed to avoid burdening or offending various segments of society.

Some of these changes are, doubtlessly, appropriate. One word presently being subjected to *unjustified* attack is "pet." A term that millions have used for generations to refer to animals they deeply love, respect, and value has recently been discovered to reflect a demeaning attitude toward animals. We are now urged to avoid the word "pet" and to speak instead of "companion animals."

For example, Ingrid Newkirk, Chairwoman of People for the Ethical Treatment of Animals, has declared that "pet" is "speciesist language."[1] In other words, the term reflects an underlying, and for Newkirk, unacceptable view that people are more valuable than dogs, cats, and other animals they keep as companions. Dr. Michael Fox associates the term "pet" with the view of animals as "emotional slaves and status symbols."[2] He finds the term "demeaning,"[3] and declares his preference for "companion animal."[4]

Some might think that the issue of whether the word "pet" should be abandoned is unimportant. After all, it seems *clearly* incorrect to claim that the word is inherently derogatory to animals. There are many people who call their animals "pets" and who do not treat them with disrespect. Surely, it might be argued, their regard for their animals will not be diminished if everyone spoke only of "companion animals." And although this may be improbable, it is at least conceivable that some people who do treat what they call "pets" in demeaning ways will improve their behavior by speaking of them only as "companion animals." So, it can be asked, how could it possibly be harmful if use of the word "pet" disappeared?

It would in my view be a serious mistake to take the issue of the appropriateness of the term "pet" so lightly. By itself, it would not matter whether people spoke of "pets" or "companion animals." In fact, this book uses the two terms interchangeably. The problem is that assaults on the word "pet" are typically part of a larger program the underlying aims of which are neither value neutral nor insignificant. For Ingrid Newkirk, termination of the "speciesist" word "pet" is part of a plan that includes eventual termination of the "speciesist" practice of keeping companion animals. She would temporarily restrict animals in the home to:

> ...refugees from the animal shelters and the streets. ...But as the surplus of dogs and cats (artificially engineered by centuries of forced breeding) declined, eventually companion animals would be phased out, and we would return to a more symbiotic relationship—enjoyment at a distance.[1]

Dr. Fox would allow possession of "companion animals," though like Newkirk, he appears to think that the perpetuation of dog and cat breeds reflects the same degradation of animals inherent in the term "pet." For Fox, elimination of the word "pet" is part of a larger sanitation of language, which would include insistence on the use of personal pronouns to refer even to noncompanion animals:

> ...even though they, like we, do have gender, [they] are rarely referred to as 'she' or 'he' but rather in an epicene way as an 'it.' They are deanimalized further by such terms as 'that' rather than 'who' or 'whom.' English teachers, writers, journalists, and others might also help clean up our vocabulary where demeaning references are made about fellow creatures in describing essentially human traits and shortcomings: swine, sloth, bitch, brute, and beastly. ...
>   Our use of language does not serve only to distance us from animals but also tends to reduce them to the level of insensitive objects. It gives an aura of respectability to ethically questionable forms of animal treatment—even sanctioning the 'sacrifice' of animals in laboratories and the poisoning of 'pests.'[3]

Fox's statement indicates what is for some activists really behind the "clean up" of language of which elimination of the term "pet" is a part. Current syntax requires speaking of "the dog *that* walked into the room" or the "cow *that* gives milk," rather than "the dog or cow *who...* ." However, the point of such usage is not to question the status of these creatures as animals, but to assert that they are animals and not people. Dr. Fox's goal, indeed, is not to have animals regarded more like animals but more like people. He writes that the:

> ...principle of reciprocity brings us closer to a relationship with animals based not only on empathy and altruism, but also on respect and recognition of their interests (analogous to filial piety toward our own kind), thus laying the foundation for a transspecies democracy. The rights and interests of humans then would not take precedence over those that our common-sense morality recognizes in animals, nor would their rights and interests take precedence over ours.[5]

The term "democracy" derives from the Greek word *demos*, which means "the people," and a democracy is a political organization of equal persons. It is to personalize rather than to "animalize" animals that Fox insists on the use of personal pronouns, and only personal pronouns, to refer to them. Many who use only such pronouns (including writers in animal activist periodicals) do so precisely because they believe that animals have the same moral worth and value as persons. Some want the law to classify to certain kinds of animals *as* persons.[6]

I have first-hand evidence of the deleterious effects of such attempts to "clean up" language. Some of my veterinary students use such verbiage as "the cat who needed an operation" or the "snake who was euthanized." When I ask why, some will say that use of the personal pronoun reflects their belief that animals should not be considered property and should not be capable of ownership. (This is an interesting position for a future veterinarian to take.) Some respond that they have been told (by whom they cannot recall) that it is "better" only to use personal pronouns because it is more respectful of animals, as is the term "companion animal." When challenged further, some express a view that those who urge the "cleanup" of language want to hear—that some animals "are not just animals, but people, or just like people, sort of."*

Anyone who wants to believe that dogs, cats, or birds are more like people than animals, are really little people, or belong with humans in some kind of "transspecies democracy" (whatever that is), is free to do so. However, any such view is not intellectually respectable if (as in the case of some of my students) it results not from careful deliberation but from the unthinking use of a new kind of language. The criticisms of language by Fox and Newkirk hardly reflect a complaint that language should not embody ethical positions. Their protest is that current usage does not embody their ethical positions, and they would like language changed to do so.

There can be a problem with terminology that embodies particular ethical positions. Such language can automatically and unconsciously color one's thinking and lead one toward moral views about which one has not carefully thought.† The use of such verbiage as the "the animal who…" can do this, as some of my students demonstrate. However, both the terms "pet" and "companion animal" present no such danger. There are people who have called their animals "pets" and have treated them in demeaning and degrading ways, and there are people who have not subjected "pets" to such treatment.

---

*I am well aware that although, at the time of this writing at least, correct syntax frowns upon the use of the word "who" to refer to animals, there is no shortage of this usage in spoken and written parlance. The time may soon come (indeed, it may be already upon us) when speaking about animals "who" ceases to strike many people as odd or inappropriate. At such a point, the rules of syntax will doubtlessly be broadened to accept such usage. Some people may feel compelled to speak of animals "who" because they believe that animals are more than inanimate objects, more than mere things, more than just "its." However, speaking of animals "who" does not make them into persons. Nor, indeed, do most people who speak of animals "who" appear to think they are persons. It is interesting that some people appear to believe that our language gives us only two choices: speaking of animals as mere things or as "whos". There is, of course, an intermediate approach: using names to refer to animals, and referring to them as "he" or "she." As I note in Chapter 12, people tend to use language as they want to, objections of philosophers, veterinarians, or animal activists to the contrary notwithstanding. One can only hope that those who do insist upon speaking about the "dog who" or the "cow who" at least do not move, without the most careful consideration, from this usage to the position that animals are really people, or just like people.

†Thus I would agree with Dr. Fox that speaking of the "sacrifice" of laboratory animals is inappropriate because it does seem intended to sanitize, make less graphic, and perhaps even gloss over, what happens to these animals. Animals are "sacrificed" in certain pagan religious rites, but in laboratories, they are killed. To say this, however, is not to say that it is wrong to kill research animals.

There are people who have spoken only of "companion animals" and who have treated their animals well, and there are people who have not treated "companion animals" well. Both "pet" and "companion animal" are compatible with all varieties of ethical positions regarding the animals these terms denote. However, as part of a linguistic program that implies animals are people or are as valuable as humans, the recommendation that the term "companion animal" should replace "pet" is *not* value neutral.

"Animals" or "Nonhuman Animals?"

The word "pet" is not the most important linguistic target of animal activists. At the top of their list is the word "animal" itself. They do not want us to refer to members of animal species other than *Homo sapiens* as "animals" at all, but as "nonhuman animals." As philosopher Peter Singer puts it:

> We commonly use the word 'animal' to mean 'animals other than human beings.' This usage sets humans apart from other animals, implying that we are not ourselves animals—an implication that everyone who has had elementary lessons in biology knows to be false.
>
> In the popular mind the term 'animal' lumps together beings as different as oysters and chimpanzees, while placing a gulf between chimpanzees and humans, although our relationship to those apes is much closer than the oyster's.[7]

Singer believes that speaking of "animals" reflects and reinforces prejudices against them. These prejudices lead people to do to animals things Singer finds objectionable, such as using them for food, entertainment, and in scientific research.

The demand that the word "animal" should be replaced has become so commonplace, and has been acknowledged by so many in the academic community,[8] that it may be easy to overlook how pointless the demand really is. English (and, as Singer concedes, other languages too) has a term for nonhuman as distinguished from human animals. This is not an accident. Speakers of many languages have for centuries perceived there to be important differences between *Homo sapiens* and other animal species, even if science has discovered that these differences are not as extensive as some people may have thought. These animals (even chimpanzees) look different from us. They do not have the kind of language most people have (even if some might have some kind of language). They do not construct cities and roads; work in an economy as employees or employers; manufacture and trade goods; invent things; tell their history; read books and newspapers; create and enjoy works of music and art; practice religions; enact and obey laws; engage in scientific investigation; become veterinarians; become philosophy professors; or do any of a myriad of things the vast majority of humans not only do but also accomplish with ease.

Nor can it seriously be supposed that if Singer and others could somehow wipe the word "animal" from the lexicon, society would treat animals as Singer thinks they should be treated. Certain uses of animals are based on deep-seated factual, religious, and ethical views about what these animals are and deserve. Doing away with the term "animal" will do absolutely nothing to change these views. People will not, for example, stop eating meat if meat begins to come from "nonhuman animals." Moreover, use of the term "animal" does not bear responsibility in leading people to adopt incorrect scientific or ethical views about any kind, species, or individual "nonhuman animal." Someone who does not know, for example, that *Homo sapiens* and certain other nonhuman species belong to the animal kingdom is ignorant and needs knowledge—not different language. Use of the term "animal" does not imply, and is not inconsistent, with any particular view about how chimpanzees, oysters, or any other kind of nonhuman animal ought to be treated.

None of this is to say Singer is wrong about how animals should be treated. Nor is it of itself to dispute Singer's contention that it is indefensible to treat humans better than nonhumans simply because they belong to the species *Homo sapiens*. The real issue is how members of other species in the animal kingdom should be treated by members of the species *Homo sapiens*. This issue can be discussed thoroughly without jettisoning a distinction between humans and "animals."

Two examples show why ingrained distinctions in language need not preclude a wide range of views regarding the attributes and moral claims of beings to which these distinctions are applied.

For centuries, speakers of languages have had separate terms for male and female humans. Yet, over time, many different views have been held about how men and women might (or might not) differ physically and psychologically and whether men and women should be treated equally or differently. All these views have been consistent with use of the words as "woman" and "man" (and equivalents in languages other than English). Has it been inappropriate to distinguish between "men" and "women" because some people have made inappropriate judgments about women? If we spoke only of "people" (or perhaps, "male people" and "female people," "male people" and "nonmale people," or "female people" and "nonfemale people") instead of "men" and "women," would inappropriate judgments about women or men cease? If men and women ought to have equal ethical and legal rights, does this mean we should stop distinguishing between men and women? Would it be *possible* for speakers of any language to do so?

The most telling demonstration of why the word "animal" is both useful and inevitable comes from animal activists themselves. Most activists who object vehemently to the word have no problem advocating "animal rights" or "animal liberation"—instead of "nonhuman animal rights" or "nonhuman animal liberation." The reason for this, I submit, goes far beyond the fact that the latter terms are cumbersome and unlikely to have much effect in polemic or debate. Nor is Singer correct in stating that his continued use of the term "animal" in his own writing "is a regrettable lapse from the standards of revolutionary purity but...seems necessary for effective communication."[7] Animal liberationists like Singer *need* to use the word "animal," because the rest of us need to use the word, and always will. As noted above, the distinction between "humans" and "animals" will remain because there will remain enough differences between humans and animals to make the distinction seem natural, indeed unavoidable. Those who would argue that people should treat *them* in ways commonly thought appropriate to *us* will just have to accept that speakers of all languages do so distinguish between them and us. Even if the distinction between humans and "animals" could somehow be sanitized from the language, there would, as the history of so many different languages demonstrates, quickly appear a synonymous distinction to take its place.

Those who urge replacing the distinction between humans and animals with one between human animals and nonhuman animals themselves underscore the pointlessness of the change. Their own terminology merely restates, though in decidedly more cumbersome verbiage, the distinction between: *Homo sapiens* and *all* other species in the animal kingdom! This is, of course, *precisely* what the traditional distinction between humans and animals does. It seems odd to object that the distinction between humans and animals "sets humans apart from other animals" and propose another distinction that does exactly the same thing. Indeed, although some activists appear to think that repeating the word "animal" in both sides of their distinction somehow draws humans closer to other animal species, if anything their distinction between human animals and *non*human animals sets us farther apart. The logical operator "non" is the strongest and most uncompromising separator that can be used in any language. "*Non*human" animals must, necessarily, be *other than* human. Put another way, the traditional distinction between "human" and "animal" at least allows us to say that we humans are animals also. (In this respect the traditional distinction is exactly like the new.) However, the new, supposedly enlightened distinction between human animals and nonhuman animals does not allow us to say that we human animals are nonhuman animals. So much for linguistic improvement.*

∾ EUTHANASIA
Appropriateness of the Terms "Euthanasia" and "Putting an Animal to Sleep"

Other terms to which animal activists routinely object include "euthanasia," "putting an animal to sleep," or "putting an animal down." Philosopher Tom Regan notes that as the word is applied to human beings, "euthanasia" requires more than killing painlessly or with a minimum of suffering. If, Regan observes, I kill someone painlessly to inherit his money, that is not euthanasia, but murder. Regan asserts that the term "euthanasia" can be applied to people, or animals, only if killing them is in their interest. He objects to describing the killing of healthy animals with an interest in living as "euthanasia, properly conceived" because in his view one rarely helps an animal by killing it.[9] "To persist in referring to acts that culminate in the untimely death of these animals as 'euthanasia' is as inaccurate as the acts are regrettable."[10]

Regan is correct that the word "euthanasia" would not be applied to the killing of a healthy person for someone else's benefit. But his claim that it is therefore "improper" or "inaccurate" to speak of the euthanasia of a healthy animal for its owner's benefit is just incorrect. Veterinarians and most other people do use the word "euthanasia" to refer to killing an animal painlessly or with as little pain as possible, whether or not the animal is healthy or killing it can be said to be in its interest. This use of the word is too widespread to be called improper. The usage reflects what the word "euthanasia" now means in our language when it is applied to animals.

Clearly, Regan recommends a certain definition of the word "euthanasia" because he disapproves of many of the acts the word is currently used to denote. He would prefer a

*The inadvisability of replacing the term "animal" with "nonhuman animal" can be further appreciated by considering other changes in language the replacement would require. We would have to speak not of "animal welfare" but of "nonhuman animal welfare." Veterinarians would not practice animal medicine but nonhuman animal medicine, and would not be animal doctors but nonhuman animal doctors. Companion animals would become companion nonhuman animals. The human animal bond would be replaced by the human nonhuman animal bond. The human companion animal bond would become the human companion nonhuman animal bond, or perhaps (if people found this way of speaking too much to take) the human nonhuman companion animal bond. These locutions are as unnecessary as they are clumsy.

world in which the word "euthanasia" is applied to animals much as it is applied to human beings because he believes that human beings and many animals are in certain respects equal in worth and value. However, it is one thing to argue for such equality (which Regan does) and another to accuse those who oppose it of speaking inaccurately.

I have yet to find a veterinarian who does not know that "euthanizing" an animal involves killing it. I have yet to find a veterinarian who would not inquire about the morality of killing a patient or who would take a certain position regarding killing it *because* he or she uses the terms "euthanasia," "putting an animal to sleep," or "putting an animal down." It is also silly to suppose that only by enforced, unremitting use of the word "kill!" will veterinarians or anyone else pay attention to moral issues concerning the killing of veterinary patients. If a mere word or phrase can insulate someone from these issues, surely taking the word away will not cause him or her to engage in serious moral deliberation.

We all know what we are talking about: veterinarians sometimes kill their patients. They sometimes kill healthy patients the interests of which are not served thereby. They sometimes kill patients that ought not be killed. The current way in which the word "euthanasia" is applied to animals reflects the fact that most people do *not* regard the painless killing of animals as akin to murder. Whether things ought to be otherwise is a matter for moral argument and not definition of terms. In this book, the term "euthanasia" will therefore be used regarding animals as it is by most persons: to refer to the killing of animals painlessly or with minimal pain if such is unavoidable under the circumstances.

"Active" versus "Passive" Euthanasia

In human medical ethics, a distinction is sometimes made between "active" euthanasia, the taking of actions to end a patient's life, and "passive" euthanasia, withholding treatment and thereby allowing the patient to die. This distinction is the subject of much controversy among philosophers and theologians. Some contend that there is no sensible distinction because the motivation and result are the same.[11] Others maintain that only active euthanasia is morally prohibited, on the grounds, for example, that life is a gift of God and cannot be taken by people, or that physicians who commit active euthanasia will lose the confidence of patients if they cease to be viewed as vigorous battlers for life.[12]

The options of not resuscitating an animal or withholding treatment must sometimes be considered by veterinarians and clients. Nevertheless, in veterinary medicine, the distinction between killing ("active" euthanasia) and letting die ("passive" euthanasia) is of much less importance than it is in human medicine. In veterinary medicine, euthanasia is characteristically active. Indeed, veterinarians typically do not apply the term "euthanasia" to letting a patient die as distinguished from taking its life.

One reason the distinction between active and passive euthanasia is so significant in human medicine is that many human patients can be kept alive long after they cease to enjoy a significant quality of life. Veterinary medicine is beginning to approach the abilities of human medicine in this respect, which may or may not prove a blessing. However, at least at present, few veterinary clients have the inclination or financial means to prolong an animal's life when it has reached a vegetative state. Nor do most veterinary hospitals find doing this a reasonable utilization of limited resources.

Additionally, the vast majority of veterinarians and animal owners consider it inhumane to keep alive an animal that is moribund, especially if it is also in pain or distress. This ethical principle has prevented passive euthanasia from becoming a widespread approach in veterinary medicine. As discussed in Chapter 22, the reluctance of practitioners to keep animals alive after their time to die has come may be changing. It might be time for the profession to reassert the value of active euthanasia as a way of quickly and compassionately ending hopeless suffering.

The Choice of a Euthanizing Agent: The AVMA Panel Report

The choice of a euthanizing agent can be an ethical as well as a technical decision. If an inappropriate agent is used or an appropriate agent is used improperly, the animal can suffer needlessly, and ending its life might not be described properly as an instance of euthanasia.

The preeminent source of information regarding proper methods of performing euthanasia on animals is the *Report of the AVMA Panel on Euthanasia.* This document, which is updated periodically, surveys the most common methods with regard to such factors as safety for personnel, ease of performance, rapidity of death, efficacy, and species suitability. The *Report* contains detailed data about dosages, routes of administration, and ancillary techniques to assure animal comfort. It discusses at length the euthanasia of companion animals as well as farm and laboratory animal species. The 1993 *Report* lists several general criteria for determining the acceptability of a euthanizing method:

> ...(1) ability to induce loss of consciousness and death without causing pain, distress, anxiety, or apprehension; (2) time required to induce unconsciousness; (3) reliability; (4) safety of personnel; (5) irreversibility; (6) compatibility with requirement and purpose; (7) emotional effect on observers or operators; (8) compatibility with subsequent evaluation, examination, or use of tissue; (9) drug availability and human abuse potential; (10) age and species limitations; and (11) the ability to maintain equipment in proper working order.[13]

An important statement in the 1993 *Report* concerns the importance of scientific research regarding animal pain, distress, and consciousness in evaluating the ethical appropriateness of any method of euthanasia. The document complains that "many reports on various methods of euthanasia are either anecdotal, testimonial narratives, or unsubstantiated opinions" and "strongly endorses the need for well-designed experiments to more fully determine the extent to which each procedure meets the criteria"[14] for an acceptable euthanasia method. In short, we need to know much more about what animals do or do not experience as a result of various methods of euthanasia to assure that they experience no more pain, distress, or discomfort than is absolutely necessary. Thus the *Report* reflects one of the fundamental principles of normative veterinary ethics—that good ethics must rest on good science and that whenever knowing how to improve animal welfare requires the acquisition of empirical data, the search for such information is an ethical as well as scientific imperative.

Euthanasia as a Focus of Conflicting Interests

Veterinarians face ethical and psychological issues raised by euthanasia frequently. According to one study, a veterinarian:

...can expect to perform approximately one euthanasia for every fifty patients seen. An additional 1.2% of patient contacts involve discussion of euthanasia and alternatives where euthanasia was not performed. The veterinarian can therefore expect to encounter euthanasia and euthanasia alternatives in 3% of patient contacts.[15]

Few issues facing normative veterinary ethics present more problems regarding the balancing of conflicting interests than euthanasia. It is not always in the common interests of the patient, client, and doctor that euthanasia be performed. Even when an animal is suffering desperately and euthanasia seems clearly in its interest, killing the animal can place tremendous burdens on its owner. The situation can become even less clear where the animal has a serious disease that diminishes its quality of life without causing constant suffering; in some of these cases, the client's interest in keeping his companion alive as long as possible might seem weightier than the animal's interest in a superb quality of life. There are cases in which a client mistakenly thinks that his animal's best interests would be served by euthanasia. Sometimes, the animal can do quite well, and euthanasia might be intended less as a favor to the animal than as a way of preventing the client from experiencing unpleasantness or inconvenience. At the other end of the spectrum are those clients who have little concern for their animals and want them killed just to be rid of them.

Companion animal doctors are sometimes caught in the middle of these conflicts because they typically want to serve both the client and patient. They also might have their own conflicting interests in approaching the situation. They might have an economic interest in euthanizing the patient if another doctor will do it. They might have an economic interest in convincing the client to proceed with treatment first, and a professional interest in attempting to see whether their skills are up to the patient's malady. Their interest in serving and satisfying clients might incline them not to make too big a fuss when clients request euthanasia. On the other hand, their interest in elevating their own professional status might be served by encouraging a view of companion animals as beings that should not be killed until treatment alternatives are attempted.

Into this cauldron of competing interests must sometimes be stirred additional ethical, psychological, and social issues that go to the heart of how people view animals. For example, as is noted in Chapter 11, some people think that the only strong interest animals have is an interest in not experiencing "unnecessary" pain or discomfort. To these people, moral questions that assume animals can have an interest in a good life or in life itself seem illusory. There is also the troubling question of when attachment to a sick animal might become unreasonable or even pathological—so that keeping it alive cannot be viewed as a legitimate interest of its owner. Whether one finds a client's attachment to an animal reasonable will sometimes turn on whether one approves of certain kinds of attitudes toward animals. People who view pets as filthy nuisances will find no amount of attachment to them reasonable. Those who value companion animals highly might find trying to hold on to a desperately ill pet understandable or even mandatory. Given the wide range of attitudes toward animals in our society, it sometimes will be difficult to reach agreement about whether a client's reluctance to have his animal killed is "reasonable."

Euthanasia for Good Reasons: General Considerations Regarding the Process of Euthanasia

In thinking about the morality of euthanizing veterinary patients, it is useful to begin with situations in which the end result of euthanasia is appropriate. In this way, one can appreciate that there are ethical considerations regarding the *process* of euthanasia. The weight of these considerations can differ, depending on the precise circumstances and justification for euthanasia. (For example, when an animal is already near death, questions regarding the proper time to mention euthanasia and the proper timing of euthanasia will probably be less difficult than when the patient is in the beginning stages of a debilitating disease.) Nevertheless, these considerations tend to apply in all cases of justifiable euthanasia. As the following discussion demonstrates, they can be as important ethically as the decision about whether euthanasia is justified.

Among cases of clearly justified euthanasia are those in which all of the following elements are present: (1) the patient is suffering from a condition for which veterinary medicine cannot offer a cure or solution at any cost; (2) the condition is already causing the animal severe pain for which palliative measures short of inducing virtual unconsciousness are not available; (3) the client is psychologically able to make a voluntary and rational decision regarding euthanasia; and (4) the client is able to request euthanasia, understanding that the animal's interest in freedom from suffering ought to take precedence over his own impending grief or sense of loss. Euthanasia would be appropriate in such cases because putting the patient out of its misery clearly would be in the legitimate interests of patient, client, and doctor. Nor could it harm the profession or other companion animals by encouraging an attitude of disrespect for or lack of concern about companion animals in general.

Mentioning euthanasia

Even when an animal is in desperate need of euthanasia, simply hearing the word "euthanasia" or being told about the option of ending the animal's life can be a terrible shock to a client. The client might not appreciate the seriousness of the animal's condition or might have an initial (or continuing) resistance to the thought that euthanasia is really required.

Whenever possible, doctors should not begin their conversation with a client by mentioning euthanasia. Rather, the animal's condition should be described and explained first, and the topic of euthanasia introduced only when the client appears ready to confront it. If the animal is in pain or distress, one might consider an analgesic or sedative if possible to afford the opportunity of introducing the subject of euthanasia with due regard for both animal and client. If doctors are callous or inconsiderate in their first mention of the euthanasia option, the entire process of euthanasia can be a disaster for everyone.

Permitting the client to make, and to feel as comfortable as possible about, the decision

Although there might be limited exceptions to this rule, generally a veterinarian must permit clients to make their own knowing and voluntary decision whether to proceed with euthanasia. The client has a moral right to make such a decision. It is her animal, and it is she who must live with the decision after it is carried out. Veterinarians who manipulate a client's decision toward euthanasia or who quickly accept from a client the option of deciding what ought to be done also risk the possibility of great aggravation for themselves later. If the client has second thoughts, and appreciates that the doctor moved her forcibly to the decision, she might blame the doctor for making the wrong decision.

Allowing a client to make the decision requires that a doctor speak and act as objectively as possible. Even in cases when euthanasia is the only humane option, the likely results of prolonging the pet's life must not be dressed up in exaggerated or frightening terms.

Allowing clients to make the decision also requires providing them an environment in which they can make the decision rationally. In my view, although most veterinarians are extremely good in giving objective information and helpful advice regarding euthanasia, many provide their clients with terrible surroundings in which to make and reflect upon the decision. Some doctors remain in the examining room or hover over the client while she is supposed to make a decision, not realizing the kind of pressure such behavior can exert. Some veterinarians will indicate that the examining room must be used again soon or will disappear suddenly, unaware of how difficult it can be for the client to search one out for further advice. The typical examining room, with its clean but stark environment, can itself be an awful place to make a life and death decision.

Veterinarians are morally obligated to pay serious attention to the surroundings in which the euthanasia decision sometimes must be made. Ideally, there should be a place in which clients and members of their families can sit and think, unhurried and away from the hustle and bustle of the practice. The client should have access to a comfortable chair, a beverage, and the reassuring presence of support personnel or the doctor if needed. The client should be given the opportunity to be alone with the patient so that a final good-bye can be said. A comforting environment should also be available after euthanasia is completed.

Among the alternatives that should be discussed with clients is the option of being present during euthanasia. Some clients prefer this, but might feel uncomfortable about asking. What might be done with the animal after death may also appropriately be discussed before euthanasia is performed.

Postponing euthanasia

One sometimes can assist clients to make the right decision by suggesting that the decision be postponed. When an animal is near death, this might not be possible. But sometimes it will be feasible to encourage clients to go out for a cup of coffee, or to return home for a few hours or even longer so that they have time to think. Sometimes, encouraging clients to take the animal home when this is possible can give further assurance of the wisdom of euthanasia and can allow them to begin to accept their impending loss.

Performance of euthanasia

Dr. William Kay summarizes a doctor's ethical obligations regarding the performance of euthanasia succinctly: "the veterinarian and staff must respond with skill and concern."[16] As Dr. Kay explains, this can mean among other things (1) not allowing interruptions during the procedure; (2) discussing the client's decision to be present during or after the procedure; (3) making available to clients trained support personnel; (4) explaining the significance of body movements during euthanasia and emphasizing the absence of consciousness or pain; (5) providing a quiet place where clients can remain with the body should they so desire, and (6) using an intravenous catheter when possible to assure a smooth, quick injection.

Handling the body and remains

The patient's body must be treated with dignity and respect. This must be done not just to avoid unnecessary upset for clients but out of consideration for the being that is no more. To respect a dead patient is to affirm and celebrate the value of its life. This is why companion animal doctors and their staffs should treat the remains in a dignified and solemn manner even if no one else will ever know of it. Dr. Kay recommends that one close the eyes and place the tongue within the mouth, and clean the body carefully; that the body be wrapped in a clean blanket or other suitable material; and that its condition be explained to clients if they wish to view the body after euthanasia.

Doctors must never consider it a nuisance or something above and beyond the call of duty to assist clients in the decision about how to handle the remains. The doctor should assure that the client is aware of all the options available in the community. A client must not be pressured into making a decision the doctor would find preferable, and must be given adequate time to make a decision. The doctor should make every reasonable attempt to assist the client in making arrangements for cremation or burial, should one of these options be the client's choice.

Comfort and counsel

The doctor must stand ready to comfort the client before and after the animal is euthanized. Reassuring the client of the correctness of the decision can be most important. Telephoning, writing, or visiting the client after a pet's passing can provide further support. When appropriate, the doctor may mention the possibility of some day having another pet.

As Dr. Kay observes, many veterinarians feel uncomfortable about becoming involved in the psychosocial dynamics of euthanasia. They "consider this role to be outside their domain of knowledge, experience, influence, and responsibility."[17] Veterinarians traditionally have not been trained to deal with these matters, and some might prefer not getting involved to getting involved badly. Nevertheless, veterinarians do have a moral obligation to offer comfort and counsel to clients whose animals they euthanize.

First, there is usually no one else but the veterinarian to provide support; it is inhumane to end the life of a client's animal and then to bid a hasty good-bye, leaving her hanging in mid-air with her grief.

Second, quite often the best comfort a client can receive is reassurance that euthanasia was necessary for medical reasons. There is no one who has greater knowledge of the medical necessity for euthanasia or whose opinion will count more with the client than the doctor.

Finally, and most importantly, veterinarians are justified in defining *veterinary practice* to include ministering to the needs and interests of the patient's human companions. Physicians are as scientifically trained and devoted to their patients as veterinarians. But few people would argue that physicians should not comfort the relatives or friends of a sick or dying patient. What makes physicians doctors rather than just "human disease experts" is (ideally) their concern for the entire life of the patient—which includes the people who are important to the patient. This is part of what it means to say that the physician is interested in the whole person and not just the mechanics of the patient's body.

Veterinarians may well have a stronger claim to be able to minister to their patients' close companions than physicians. For a veterinarian can never communicate with and comfort a patient to the exclusion of the patient's human companions. It has always been the patient's human companion with whom companion animal doctors communicate and through whose eyes they see much of the patient. Veterinarians who maintain that they cannot become involved in the psychosocial dynamics of their clients' emotions are fooling themselves. They are already involved. They might as well be involved skillfully and compassionately.

Settling the fee

Doctors must avoid making clumsy or insensitive requests for payment after euthanasia is completed. Some clients will not be prepared to interrupt their grieving by stepping up to the receptionist's desk to write a check. Doing this can be even more difficult if the death of their pet was unexpected. On the other hand, a doctor sometimes will have a legitimate concern about whether the fee will be paid, especially if there are outstanding charges for services preceding the euthanasia and the client shows signs of dissatisfaction with these services. Although circumstances vary, doctors should try to be flexible in the manner in which the fee for euthanasia is settled. A polite indication from the receptionist that there is no need to worry about the bill now can go a long way in helping distraught clients through their ordeal. They might remember this thoughtfulness when it comes time to seek veterinary care for another animal.

Issues Concerning the Appropriateness of Euthanasia

Even when a doctor feels comfortable about euthanizing a particular patient, it can be a major effort to pay sufficient regard to one's moral obligations to patient and client. The situation can be complicated substantially when it is not clear whether euthanasia is appropriate, or when one disagrees with a client's decision or the client's reasons for that decision.

The following discussion presents typical situations in which questions about the *justification* of euthanasia must also be raised. In all these situations—as indeed always in one's approach to clients—a veterinarian must not confuse the question of what would be best for patient and client with the issue of who has the moral and legal right to make the decision (see Chapter 10).

When a client mistakenly believes euthanasia is necessary for the animal's welfare

Sometimes, a client will request euthanasia with the intention of serving the animal's interests but is mistaken in believing that euthanasia is necessary for this purpose. This can be a relatively easy kind of case to handle, if in fact the client has the animal's interests in mind. For example, some clients believe that euthanasia of their dog is preferable to amputation of one leg because they think that a three-legged dog cannot be active and happy. Likewise, some clients assume that a pet that has lost its eyesight is necessarily condemned to a life of misery. In many such cases, one can serve the interests of both the patient and client by explaining that such animals sometimes do quite well with a bit of patience and effort from their owners. The doctor might not have to challenge the preferences of the client because one might be able to provide information that will permit clients to satisfy their own preferences.

When the animal is at beginning stages of a progressive illness or can live comfortably for some time

Clients sometimes want to consider euthanasia when an animal is at the beginning stages of a progressively debilitating illness or has a condition that is not yet distressing the animal or with which it can live comfortably at least for some period of time. Once again, if the client's concern is the animal's welfare, one sometimes will be able to point out that euthanasia might be advisable some time in the future but is not yet necessary. The situation becomes stickier when part of the client's motivation for preferring euthanasia is his own fear of seeing the animal grow progressively worse, or his reluctance to experience sadness and grief as the animal deteriorates. Although it would be presumptuous for a doctor to underestimate or belittle such emotions, there sometimes is a role in assisting the client to make sure that euthanasia would indeed serve the client's underlying preferences. For example, one might be able to determine that the client is really afraid of watching the animal suffer, and in some cases, one will be able to show the client that this need not happen in the short term and can be addressed appropriately later. Or, the client might be overestimating the amount of effort required to maintain the animal.

A doctor can also often further the client's own preferences and assist the patient by being sensitive to any anthropormorphizing that might be responsible for a misapprehension of the facts. If the client is trying to put himself in his pet's position and is imagining how he would feel if he knew he had a terminal illness, one should be able to point out that the animal will have no such understanding, and in the short term at least, might do quite well. Sometimes, this is exactly what a client wants to hear.

When keeping the animal alive will cause unwanted inconvenience

The situation can be extremely difficult where a client wants an animal euthanized because taking care of it is an unwanted inconvenience. There is a wide range of possibilities here. The client might be ill or infirm, so caring for the animal might be a major burden. At the other end of the spectrum are people for whom more than opening a can of pet food is a major inconvenience. Even if one supposes that a veterinarian should serve patients as well as clients, it is sometimes far from clear that euthanasia is the wrong approach. Where a client is infirm or incapable of taking proper care of the animal, and the animal cannot be placed elsewhere or would do poorly if placed with another owner, the argument that keeping the animal alive is in its best interests might not be very strong. Where clients have little concern for their animals, it might be questionable whether they can ever be persuaded to provide what their animals need for a satisfactory life.

I would suggest that the profession take two general approaches to clients whose animals can live a decent life but who prefer euthanasia to inconvenience.

In the long term, veterinarians can encourage a more caring attitude toward pets. Clients must be educated about not only the pleasures of animal ownership but also its responsibilities. The profession should not be bashful about proclaiming that companion animals are beings of great worth entitled to love, respect, and first-class veterinary care. As such an attitude becomes more prevalent, veterinarians should see fewer clients for whom inconvenience is a reason for euthanasia.

In the short term, doctors can approach clients who prefer euthanasia to inconvenience by doing what they can. Where appropriate, one can point out that the inconvenience might not be so great. Perhaps the client can take the animal home for a while to see how things work out. One might also explore the possibility of placing the patient elsewhere, perhaps with a relative on a temporary basis until the client is capable of caring for it. Some veterinarians tell me that they would like to suggest such things but are afraid of appearing too pushy. If a client cannot at least understand why a *veterinarian* would want to suggest ways of saving an animal's life, that person will probably never be worth much in monetary terms to the practice.

When an alternative to euthanasia will cost clients more than they are willing or able to pay

Adequate care is sometimes beyond the economic abilities of some clients. However, ethical analysis is not served unless one speaks carefully before asserting that a client is "unable" to pay for or "cannot afford" treatment. In our society, many people purchase goods and services for which they cannot pay in full at the time of purchase. Yet, they can "afford" to purchase these things because they undertake to purchase them. Many clients who say, or have convinced themselves, that they "cannot afford" an alternative to euthanasia can afford it in the sense in which they would literally be able to pay for it if they made financial arrangements to do so. What they really mean is that they do not regard saving the animal to be worth the economic burden.

There surely are clients who cannot afford an alternative to euthanasia, or who are justified in concluding that they should not undergo the economic sacrifice helping their animal would entail. Nevertheless, in one's approach to the issue of euthanizing animals capable of being helped, a doctor must distinguish clearly between cases of true economic inability and of unwillingness to pay. This is so for the following reasons:

1. Because the problem is often unwillingness to pay and such an attitude is often beyond the ability of doctors to change when a client is in the office, the most effective way of challenging the attitude that a pet is not worth the economic sacrifice is probably to prevent this attitude from forming in the first place. The best way of accomplishing this is to promote throughout society the view of the companion animal as a member of the family entitled to first-class medical care.

2. The profession might be less motivated to fight for such a view of companion animals if doctors overestimate the occurrences of cases of true inability to afford treatment.

3. Although veterinarians generally must avoid coercing or pressuring clients into making decisions, doctors are not obligated to lift the burden of decisions from clients' shoulders. When a client wants to euthanize the animal because treating it is not worth it to him, the client should know that this is the reason behind the decision. Some clients could care less about such a realization, but it might stimulate others to rethink their choices. When a doctor suspects that the decision is not really one of affordability, it is not inappropriate to say to the client politely, but firmly, "Mr. Jones, we can save your pet. It could take us some time to figure out how we can do this consistent with your cash flow situation. But I want you to know that I think we can do it, and I am willing to sit down with you and try if you are willing." If such a client chooses euthanasia, at least he will know it is his choice and not the doctor's.

4. Clients tend to conclude that they "cannot afford" an alternative to euthanasia the higher the cost of the alternative. If the profession wishes to reduce the number of medically unnecessary euthanasias, it must try to help clients reduce the burden of cost (though not necessarily the cost) of treatment options as much as possible. Many veterinarians extend credit when doing so is necessary to save a patient's life. Pet health insurance programs could reduce the number of euthanasias performed because of client inability or unwillingness to pay for treatment.

5. Sometimes, it will be appropriate to refuse to euthanize a patient. Suppose an animal could be brought back to health for just a few dollars more than it would cost to euthanize it and the client requests euthanasia to save the money. Here, a veterinarian would be within one's rights to tell the client that one's personal and professional values prohibit one from killing animals that can be helped with minimal additional expense and that one considers euthanasia under such circumstances to be no different from killing a perfectly healthy animal simply because its owner wants to be rid of it. I do not mean to minimize the problems that can arise once one concedes the appropriateness of refusing to euthanize if one considers that the financial burden to the client does not justify it; for then, one must think about how high a financial burden may be expected of a client. Nevertheless, it seems clear that companion animal doctors who include among their values the saving of animal life and the promotion of animal health must at least be open to the possibility of refusing to kill an animal when euthanasia is requested for trivial reasons.

Euthanasia of healthy, well-behaved patients

Although many veterinarians do euthanize animals because their owners no longer want them, there are strong moral arguments against this practice.

NOT IN THE INTERESTS OF THE PROFESSION. First, it is not in the general interests of the profession to perpetuate an image of itself as willing to kill any companion animal on demand. As I argue in this book, companion animal doctors will be able to meet their full earning potential only if society comes to view pets as beings entitled to love, respect, and first-rate veterinary care. Veterinarians who kill on demand are sending a message to clients and the public that their patients are not worth much at all. Clients will not believe the pleas of the profession that their animals are worth excellent and sometimes expensive care if individual doctors do not endorse this attitude themselves.

To promote an image of their patients as beings of importance, veterinarians need not always oppose the euthanasia of unwanted animals. Sadly, euthanasia seems the only way of dealing with some of these animals. What I am urging is that *veterinarians should not be involved in their private practices in this tragic process*—except in the most unusual and compelling kinds of cases, such as when it is clear that a client will kill an animal himself if the doctor does not do it. Doctors can tell clients that it is against their ideals to kill healthy, well-behaved animals on demand. They can tell clients that they believe in the value of their patients' lives and they believe that if a healthy animal is not wanted, at least it should be given a chance at being adopted. They can tell clients who insist on euthanasia that it must be done at an animal shelter or humane society, not by the doctor.

Some veterinarians might protest that economic pressures compel them to euthanize a healthy animal when a client requests it, because if they do not do it, someone else will, and they will lose the fee. This attitude is shortsighted. In the long run, this approach prevents the community of companion animal doctors from meeting the economic challenges of the day with the most potent weapon at its disposal: the image of the kind and compassionate healer dedicated to the interests of one's valued patients.

NOT IN THE INTERESTS OF CLIENTS. It often is not even in the interests of clients to have their unwanted animals killed by a veterinarian. For this can cost the client more than surrendering the animal to a shelter, which usually costs nothing. To be sure, some clients might prefer to have a veterinarian euthanize their animal because they might view this as approval of their decision by the doctor. Although veterinarians should not be discourteous to owners who seek euthanasia for healthy animals, they have no obligation to make these people feel comfortable about the decision.

NOT IN THE INTERESTS OF THE PATIENT. It is not in the interest of a healthy companion animal that could do well with another owner to be killed. But neither is it in the interest of companion animals in general. For it is in the interest of all companion animals to be afforded good veterinary care by their owners. Insofar as the killing of healthy animals by veterinarians hinders the full development of the image of companion animals as beings entitled to respect and care, the killing of individual healthy animals will have some effect in preventing members of the public from giving the very best veterinary care to their animals.

When euthanasia is contemplated because of behavioral problems

It has been estimated that 40% of pet owners who are not satisfied with their animals are unhappy about perceived behavioral problems, and that between 35% and 50% of all euthanasias of companion animals are performed because of behavioral problems.[18]

Euthanasia for behavioral reasons presents difficult ethical and technical issues for the profession. Sometimes, an animal's behavioral problems are attributable at least in part to its owner. Nevertheless, even when this is so, the animal can be so vicious or intractable that returning it to the owner's home or placing it elsewhere is unfeasible. Doctors are sometimes faced with the apparently unfair, but unavoidable, situation of having to kill an animal because of the misdeeds of its owner.

The profession in general is not yet equipped to stem the tide of medically unnecessary euthanasias resulting from behavioral problems. Important work is being done by some veterinarians and behavioral scientists to establish verifiable empirical knowledge in the area of companion animal behavior.[19] However, many pet owners who seek advice about behavioral matters from a veterinarian are likely to receive the same kinds of homespun suggestions they can obtain from friends, relatives, or a local book store. Many veterinary schools still regard behavior as a "soft" subject that merits at best a sprinkling of (usually elective) class hours when students desire some diversion from the rigors of the "real" curriculum.

As is the case when a client inclines toward euthanasia because he believes keeping his animal will be too inconvenient or costly, a veterinarian can perform a useful function in clarifying for the client his own preferences, by making it clear if a behavioral or combination of a behavioral and a medical approach might solve the problem. Likewise, doctors can tell clients when, in their view, euthanasia is unjustified or at least premature, and may refuse to euthanize when they believe that the animal might be helped or placed with another owner.

Nevertheless, it seems clear that if the number of euthanasias of pets with behavioral problems is to be reduced significantly, the profession as a whole must wage a two-front attack. It must place in the hands of doctors as much useful knowledge as is available regarding approaches to behavioral problems. The profession must also promote better education of pet owners about the causes of common behavioral disturbances and about the personalities and behavioral problems of various kinds and breeds of animals. If clients can be educated about behavioral matters before they bring a pet into their homes, the likelihood of certain kinds of predictable problems will be reduced.

A major burden rests squarely on the veterinary schools. They must have on their faculties behavioral experts who will do research applicable to situations faced by practicing doctors. Students must be required to take meaningful course work in behavioral issues. Behavioral studies—like ethics—must be recognized as a legitimate intellectual endeavor of crucial importance to the mission of the schools.

When the alternative to euthanasia might cause the patient to suffer or to experience a diminished quality of life

The most complex ethical issues regarding euthanasia tend to arise when the alternative to ending a patient's life can involve its suffering pain or experiencing a diminished quality of life. In such situations, the interest of the patient in a continued life can conflict with its interest in not suffering and in not living a life of greatly reduced quality. The client might have an interest in keeping the animal alive that can conflict with his desire that it not suffer, as well as with his interest in not undergoing undue inconvenience and expense. The doctor might be torn between one's interest in serving the patient and one's interest in serving the client. All this can be complicated by that fact that it is sometimes unclear what the results of a given noneuthanasia approach will be. Clients must sometimes weigh the uncertainty of the success of a treatment option against the potential benefits and harms to their animals and themselves.

In considering how to approach situations in which alternatives to euthanasia might cause discomfort to the patient, it is useful to appreciate the variety of possible different kinds of cases. This can be done by listing some of the more important morally relevant considerations and the possible different permutations of these factors. Clearly, the following are among such morally relevant considerations: (1) the probability that a given approach will meet with success; (2) the nature of such "success" in terms of the likely quality of life to be experienced by the patient; (3) the probable duration of this quality of life before grave illness occurs and euthanasia must be considered again; (4) the likely amount of pain or discomfort that will be experienced by the patient as a result of the approach; (5) the likely upset or inconvenience the approach will cause the client; and (6) the likely expense of the approach.

Table 21-1 presents several possible ways of categorizing these considerations and can be used to generate a large number of possible permutations taking just these factors into account. The table also lists four of the possible situations. A doctor should want to consider with the client all feasible noneuthanasia approaches. These approaches should then be compared with euthanasia in terms of their effects on the patient and client.

Because of the large number of possibilities, it is difficult to set forth brief guidelines that will do justice to all possible situations. However, the following suggestions emerge from the table and the realities it reflects.

1. Because there are, in the abstract, so many different possibilities, one important ethical function of the doctor is to provide the client accurate information. Each medically feasible noneuthanasia approach and its likely effects on the patient and client must be presented clearly. The doctor must view it as the first order of business to help the client restrict the universe of discourse to the truly appropriate choices by making sure that the client understands the facts about each alternative.

2. A doctor has a moral obligation to treat a client as an intelligent adult capable of understanding all sides of the situation. Some doctors find it helpful to put themselves, in turn, in the place of the client and the animal. For example, suppose the alternative to euthanasia involves loss of the patient's ability to urinate. The doctor can describe how the animal is likely to live, and then explain what its continued life entails for the client. There is great potential in relating the facts to abuse one's position of trust. It is one thing to explain to a client what it is to express an animal's bladder. It is quite another to twist one's face into a contorted appearance and exclaim with great horror, "Do you know what you will have to do day in and day out? You really don't want *that*, do you?"

3. Part of a doctor's obligation to present the facts is making sure that the client truly understands the facts. Some clients will try to insulate themselves from their animals' suffering by leaving them in the hospital, unvisited, until the worst is over. The doctor must make it clear to the client how the animal is doing. This will sometimes require insisting that the client see what is happening.

4. A doctor's general obligation to permit a client to make the decision about care for the patient does not preclude the doctor from presenting oneself as an advocate for the animal and offering on its behalf arguments against the apparent tendencies of the client. Although clients must be presumed more knowledgeable about themselves and their own needs, the veterinarian is more knowledgeable about what is likely to happen to the patient. It is sometimes appropriate for a doctor to state, for example, that it is inhumane and unfair to keep the patient alive. At times, it will be appropriate to state that if the client insists on keeping the animal alive, she must take it to another doctor. One problem with this approach is that it can be so forceful that it might exert undue influence on clients' ability to make their own voluntary decision.

5. One way of dealing with the situation in which a client insists on a course of treatment that is clearly not in the patient's interest is to suggest that the client consult another doctor (perhaps, another doctor in the practice) for a second

TABLE 21-1

**Some morally relevant considerations
bearing on the appropriateness of euthanasia**

Probability of reaching intended quality of life if given noneuthanasia approach is taken	Intended quality of life	Probable duration of intended quality of life	Likely pain or discomfort to animal resulting from approach	Likely upset or inconvenience to client of treatment and continuing care	Likely expense to client of treatment and continuing care
high	excellent	long	great	great	great
moderate	good	medium	moderate	moderate	moderate
low	fair	short	minimal	minimal	minimal
uncertain	poor	uncertain	uncertain	uncertain	uncertain

Selected possibilities:
- A treatment (or nontreatment) alternative to euthanasia has a high probability of giving the animal a long and excellent quality of life. The animal likely will experience minimal pain, and there likely will be minimal upset and expense to the client.
- A treatment (or nontreatment) alternative to euthanasia has a low probability of giving the animal a short and fair quality of life. The animal likely will experience moderate pain, and there likely will be minimal upset and expense to the client.
- A treatment (or nontreatment) alternative to euthanasia has a low probability of giving the animal a short and fair quality of life. The animal likely will experience moderate pain, and there likely will be great upset and expense to the client.
- A treatment (or nontreatment) alternative to euthanasia has an uncertain probability of giving the animal a good but short quality of life. The animal likely will experience moderate pain, and there likely will be great upset and expense to the client.

opinion. This can sometimes help to convince the client that the requested approach is indeed inappropriate. Suggesting a consultation with another doctor can also help when the client is under the misapprehension that a perfectly appropriate procedure (such as amputation of a leg) will ruin the animal or its relations with the client.

6. Just as speaking up for the patient will sometimes mean presenting the arguments for euthanasia, so will it sometimes mean advising against euthanasia. As is the case when a client is inclined toward euthanasia for reasons of inconvenience or expense, even when treatment might entail some discomfort for the animal, a companion animal doctor should try whenever possible to think life rather than death. Getting into the habit of agreeing to clients' requests for euthanasia can put one in a frame of mind in which alternatives might not be explored vigorously.

Is there always a right time?

One of the worst aspects of the euthanasia of a beloved animal is the tendency to assume that there must be one right time for euthanasia, and that if one waits beyond this time one will act wrongly. This assumption may come from feelings of sorrow or guilt in deciding to put one's animal down. "Did we wait too long, or not long enough? Did we do it at the *right* time?" If such questions result from sorrow or guilt, they may never be resolved, for the sorrow or guilt may never disappear.

To be sure, it is sometimes possible, as when a pet is in terrible and incurable agony, to know with certainty that it is wrong to allow it to live a moment longer. However, more typical is the case in which an animal's discomfort, disability, or diminished quality of life progresses too slowly to compel the conclusion that any particular moment marks *the* right time. Nevertheless, the heart may persist in thinking that one waited too long, even if the brain knows—or rather, sometimes knows—otherwise.

The reader will forgive a personal illustration. Shortly after the publication of the first edition of this book, my own dog was euthanized. I found that all the writing and thinking I had done about euthanasia had not prepared me for the inevitability and brutal difficulty of agonizing about the *right* time. At the age of 18, blind for 2 years, slowly losing weight for 6 months from an undiscoverable cause, and experiencing infrequent mild seizures for 3 months, Phillip collapsed suddenly one morning. My wife, a veterinarian, and I still worry years later about whether we waited too long. Should we have put him to sleep when he lost his eyesight? He seemed happy, but were we being selfish in supposing so? Perhaps the right time came when his gait became a bit unsteady or fatigue began to cut down on the length and vigor of his walks, or the loss of a number of teeth meant he could no longer chew on his favorite crunchy biscuits. Did we begin to behave wrongly after the first seizure, which may not have seemed a watershed event because we were unwilling to recognize it as such?

In the typical kind of case, in which immediate euthanasia is not obviously required, veterinarians must not coerce clients into a prompt decision to euthanize. If, as is surely the case with many owners, it will take time and effort to become reconciled with the decision even after one has made it by oneself, there is far greater potential for even more distress, anxiety, and guilt—and anger at the veterinarian—if a client thinks the doctor forced the decision.

However, the most important lesson I try to take from the passing of my little friend is that there often will *not* be one right time. It probably would not have been wrong to have put Phillip to sleep at any number of times during his slow decline. He would have been spared additional distress. At the same time, I cannot say with any degree of certainty that, except in the last few hours, his life was on balance more distressful or painful than it was pleasurable. I cannot say that he did not want to continue on. Indeed, I know that he did.

For many elderly, declining, or ill animals there will be some time, sometimes a significant length of time, during which euthanasia would be acceptable but not ethically mandatory. Moreover, in deciding when the final decision should come it is appropriate for owners to consider their own feelings of impending separation and their need to adjust to the terrible reality. A human-companion animal bond is, after all, a relationship between both human and animal members (see Chapter 15). So long as an animal is not in such desperate condition that it must be euthanized immediately, the feelings and needs of the human partners in such a relationship also count for a great deal in the acceptable timing of euthanasia. This is a fact that veterinarians who are attendants to a human animal bond must never forget.

Making a Difference

Some of my veterinary students become extremely upset by cases in which clients choose euthanasia because they do not want to incur the inconvenience or cost of treatment or because they are just tired of their animals. These students wonder if it makes sense to study for years to learn how to save life if they are going to be asked time and again to take life.

I suggest to them that it is far better to be depressed about such situations than to be unfeeling, because those who feel nothing are unlikely to work for change. On the other hand, one cannot take upon oneself the burden of the world's mistakes. One must realize that we live in a society in which many companion animals die needlessly. Yet, change is possible. Slowly but surely, as the profession promotes the value of companion animals and individual doctors make sure that clients understand when treatment is available, fewer medically unnecessary euthanasias will be performed.

It is sometimes easy to lose sight of how much attitudes toward companion animals have already changed. To students who despair of the possibility of change, I quote an 1897 decision of the United States Supreme Court. In that case, the Court expressed strong reservations about dogs and indeed about other animals people now treasure deeply. According to the Justices, dogs cannot be:

> …considered as being upon the same plane with horses, cattle, sheep and other domesticated animals, but rather in the category of cats, monkeys, singing birds and similar animals kept for pleasure, curiosity or caprice. …Unlike other domestic animals, they are useful neither as beasts of burden, for draught (except for a limited extent), nor for food. They are peculiar in the fact that they differ among themselves more widely than any class of animals, and can hardly be said to have a characteristic common to the entire race. While the higher breeds rank among the noblest representatives of the animal kingdom, and are justly esteemed for their intelligence, sagacity, fidelity, watchfulness, affection, and, above all for their natural companionship with man, others are afflicted with such serious infirmities of temper as to be little better than a public nuisance. All are more or less subject to attacks of hydrophobic madness.[20]

Today this view of the dog, cat, and "singing bird" seems a curious reflection of a time long gone. Of course, one reason it is gone is that veterinary medicine can now provide first-rate medical care for these animals. Some day, clients who request euthanasia when their pets can be helped might be no less a thing of the past. In the meantime, veterinarians committed to health and life may do what they can to urge against every medically unnecessary euthanasia. In a lifetime of practice, this can add up to many lives saved.

⮂ EUTHANASIA: VETERINARY MEDICINE AND HUMAN MEDICINE

The medical profession is engaged in heated controversy regarding the acceptability of euthanasia. The stimulus of much of this debate has been Dr. Jack Kevorkian, whose activities in helping terminally ill patients to kill themselves led his opponents to call him "Dr. Death." Although some physicians support physician-assisted euthanasia, most physicians, medical ethicists, and theologians condemn it strongly.

Several arguments are made against physician-assisted euthanasia. It is claimed, for example, that it is almost always unnecessary for patients in pain to have themselves killed, because there are pharmaceutical means of alleviating even the most horrible pain.[21] It is asserted that if physicians are permitted to take lives, they will sometimes kill persons who are incorrectly diagnosed as terminally ill.[22] It is claimed that, while it may or may not be appropriate for terminally ill people to kill themselves, it violates the role of the *physician* to participate in the process, because physicians are obligated to save life.[22] The argument raised most often against euthanasia, and especially against physician-assisted euthanasia, is that the practice will eventually lead to much killing of people who should not be killed, and of people who do not want to die:

> ...society might gradually move in the direction of nonvoluntary and perhaps involuntary euthanasia—for example, in the form of killing handicapped newborns to avoid social and familial burdens. There could be a general reduction of respect for human life as a result of the official removal of barriers to killing. Rules against killing in a moral code are not isolated fragments; they are threads in a fabric of rules, drawn in part from nonmaleficence, that support respect for human life. The more threads we remove, the weaker the fabric becomes.[23]

From the perspective of veterinary medicine one feature of the debate about euthanasia in human medicine can only be characterized as astonishing. Discussions of euthanasia by prominent medical ethicists do not mention veterinary medicine or the euthanasia of veterinary patients. This apparent lack of interest is startling because many objections to euthanasia in human medicine stem from the fact that human medicine has had little experience with it. Many people fear that society may be unable to predict its consequences. Some of the possibilities seem so terrible that allowing euthanasia by physicians does not appear to many people to be worth the risk.

However, there is a healing profession with extensive experience relating to the euthanasia of its patients. These doctors have long had to worry about when (if at all) euthanasia is justified, how to perform it, and what effects it can have on those close to the patient.

It is beyond the scope of this discussion to speculate about why connections have not been made in the bioethics literature between euthanasia in human and veterinary medicine. Nor is it possible to consider here all the ways in which physicians and veterinarians might learn valuable lessons about euthanasia from each other. The following observations are intended to stimulate consideration of these issues.

1. The experience of veterinary medicine shows that a profession allowed by law, its own official ethical standards, and societal attitudes to kill its patients may well kill too many patients. Euthanasia sometimes occurs in veterinary medicine when it is not ethically defensible.

2. However, the practice of euthanasia in veterinary medicine may also indicate that fears about *who* might be responsible for any overutilization of euthanasia in human medicine may be misplaced. Some medical ethicists raise the specter of physicians, or government, imposing on people the decision whether they or a loved one should be euthanized. Veterinarians know all too well that the impetus for euthanasia often comes not from the doctor but the client. Few veterinarians enjoy killing an animal because its owner is tired of it, cannot afford treatment, believes mistakenly that it will not have a decent quality of life, or is unwilling to expend the effort required to assist it. If euthanasia in human medicine leads to unnecessary and unjustified killing, perhaps the problem will come not from physicians but from those they serve: patients or their families. If this is the case, society should be looking more closely at its own values, rather than fearing the medical profession.

3. Veterinarians also know that practitioner-induced euthanasia is not inevitably associated with disrespect for and devaluation of the patient. Veterinarians know that the decision to euthanize is often made by clients out of the highest respect, regard, and value for the patient. To euthanize an animal in a terminal state, suffering horrible and unremitting pain and with no chance of even a brief tolerable quality of life, is usually an act of kindness and love. Biomedical ethicists Tom Beauchamp and James Childress argue that because of the potential dangers of physician-induced euthanasia, and the profound changes it would make in the medical profession, those who object to physician-assisted euthanasia should not bear the burden of proving why the practice is wrong. Rather, Beauchamp and Childress insist that those who defend physician-assisted euthanasia should bear the burden of proving that it is appropriate.[24] These ethicists ask legitimate questions about the potential dangers of physician-assisted mercy killing, but there is one question they do not ask. This question suggests that the burden of proof may well rest on those who oppose physician-assisted euthanasia. This question is: How can we in good conscience put ourselves and our loved ones through suffering and torment we find intolerable for our pets?

4. At the same time, the experience of veterinary medicine confirms the view of human medical ethicists who see a link between the value people place on a being (or kind of being) and their willingness to choose euthanasia for it. Veterinarians know that just as some people choose euthanasia for their animals out of love, respect, and regard, others have their animals euthanized out of disregard and lack of concern. Veterinarians also know that there is a correlation between their unwillingness and that of their clients to choose euthanasia instead of treatment, and a general elevation in society of the value of companion animals. As more people value pets more highly, they are demanding treatments that prolong these animals' lives and are agonizing more often and more intensely about the euthanasia of their animals.

Thus widespread euthanasia of people might be associated with a lack of regard for human life. However, the experience of veterinary medicine raises questions about the claim that the availability of euthanasia in human medicine will cause a lowered regard for human medical patients and for human life. Rather, the experience of veterinarians appears to suggest that the causal arrow might point in the *other* direction—that a low regard for patients would lead to widespread euthanasia. Because euthanasia is freely and lawfully available in veterinary medicine,* to those who regard their animals highly and to those who do not, it is difficult to argue that the availability of euthanasia has much to do with the degree of regard people have for their animals. Surely, few veterinary clients think less of their animals because they can have them killed. Rather, those who come to the veterinarian with high regard for their animals will likely choose euthanasia because of such

---

*Indeed, it is worth emphasizing for the benefit of physicians and other nonveterinarians that euthanasia is *always*, in *every* situation, a lawful option in veterinary medicine. Provided a client has the legal authority to request euthanasia, veterinarians may lawfully perform it, whether or not the animal is terminal, curable, or completely healthy.

regard, in situations in which euthanasia is truly in their animal's interests. Those who come to the veterinarian with low regard for the patient will more likely opt to have it euthanized for less than adequate reasons. The potential lesson here is that if euthanasia in human medicine is associated with a lowered regard for human patients, much of this lowered regard might be attributable not to the availability of euthanasia but to other causes.

5. Many veterinarians have seen situations in which it would be in the best interests of a patient to be euthanized, where the client refuses to authorize euthanasia, and where euthanasia could be done without the client knowing how the animal really died. Although some students and practitioners admit they might sometimes be tempted to euthanize an animal contrary to a client's wishes, it is my firm conviction, based on years of probing veterinarians on this issue, that unauthorized euthanasia by veterinarians almost never occurs. Some opponents of physician-assisted euthanasia cite "horror cases" in which well-meaning physicians or nurses have run amuck killing terminally ill or elderly people.[25] However, if veterinary doctors are loathe to kill *animals* without authorization—even when they could get away with it—fears that physicians will begin performing widespread nonvoluntary euthanasia on *people* may be highly exaggerated.

6. In fact, the experience of veterinary medicine indicates that a major cause of euthanasia is economic. Many clients do not want to kill their animals, but do so because they cannot afford treatment. If the human medical establishment truly fears the overutilization of euthanasia, it might do well to assure that the availability of medical procedures is not rationed severely by government or providers of insurance. If such rationing occurs, physicians may find themselves in a quandary veterinarians often experience, torn between the desire to help and the economic necessity to kill.

7. Finally, the experience of veterinary medicine raises questions about the claim that, however justified euthanasia may sometimes be, it should never be performed by physicians because taking life is inconsistent with their status as *medical* professionals. The fact that veterinary doctors perform euthanasia demonstrates why the concepts of "medicine" or "doctor" are not inconsistent with performing euthanasia. Most people insist that veterinarians should euthanize sick animals to assure that the task is performed as quickly and painlessly as possible. One can only wonder why, if euthanasia of sick people is ever acceptable, we could allow anyone other than physicians to do it, so that people could have the same protection we demand for our pets.

⤳ COUNSELING CLIENTS: THE VETERINARIAN'S TASK?

Veterinarians must be sympathetic to clients who are considering difficult choices. Several veterinary school teaching hospitals and large practices have social workers on staff to counsel clients. Some of these people do much good, helping clients through difficult decisions, and consoling and supporting them through their grief.[26] Some clients might benefit from a referral to an outside mental health practitioner. Some veterinarians might benefit from expert instruction about how to approach upset or bereaved clients. Nevertheless, serious questions must be asked about the advisability of assigning, within a veterinary hospital, routine counseling of clients to social workers.

Will this encourage some veterinarians to define themselves as technical experts, whose function is to deal only with the mechanics of the patient's body? Will such a definition render some veterinarians less sensitive to clients' interests when medical options are discussed? For some veterinarians, will the availability of a social worker provide an easy rationalization for not engaging in difficult ethical deliberation, and for quickly moving on to the next appointment? Are social workers really better at counseling clients about animal medical issues than veterinarians? Do social workers possess special expertise in dealing with the many *ethical* questions that can arise when clients must contemplate various alternatives for their animals? In general, would the routine use of social workers encourage, or discourage, veterinarians from viewing attention to ethics as part of their professional role? Will the models of the veterinarian as a healer and friend (see Chapter 16) be furthered or undercut by the notion that veterinarians require another profession to assist them in approaching their patients and clients?

I am not suggesting that social workers cannot provide assistance to veterinarians, but only that important questions must be addressed before veterinarians relinquish to another profession one of their most important traditional functions.[*]

∾ DEALING WITH CLIENTS WHO ARE UNABLE TO MAKE RATIONAL DECISIONS

As I have argued, whether or not one of the alternatives to be considered includes euthanasia, a veterinarian should always strive to permit clients to make their own informed, rational, and voluntary decisions about what will be done with their animals. Sometimes, however, clients are unable to make such a decision. They can be physically or psychologically infirm. They can be unable to understand the facts and options the doctor is attempting to relate. They can be so emotionally overwrought that they cannot understand the nature and consequences of treatment options or appreciate what some of these options could do to them or their animals.

Some doctors tell me that in such cases they believe they are justified in forcefully guiding the client toward a particular decision, especially when failure to make that decision will cause the animal to suffer. (This might be done by bullying the client into a decision, or more subtly, by shading the truth or characterizing the alternatives so as to make the option decided upon by the doctor the inevitable "choice" of the client.) In my view, such approaches might be appropriate in very rare instances, perhaps when immediate action is required to prevent or alleviate a patient's suffering. However, as a general approach, forcing one's own decision upon an infirm or irrational client confuses the moral right of a veterinarian to speak for the patient with the right to speak for the client as well. Veterinarians rarely have better knowledge about their clients than clients possess about themselves. Moreover, even in instances in which a doctor might

---

[*]Determining proper and safe boundaries within which veterinarians may counsel clients will not be easy, and may require assistance of the legal system. Some states license clinical psychologists, psychiatric social workers, and psychotherapists. Veterinarians in these jurisdictions must take care not to engage in activities that would require a license. Moreover, even when veterinarians may counsel clients without a license, if they counsel badly or incompetently they might be held liable by courts to clients or members of their family for negligence. It is therefore important for legal as well as ethical reasons to refer clients who require the assistance of a mental health professional to such a person. To preserve its ability to deal effectively with human-animal relations, the veterinary profession needs to expand its knowledge in this area. It may also need to convince government and the mental health professions that veterinarians have a legitimate role to play in dealing with emotional responses of clients within the practice of veterinary medicine.

know more about a client's needs than the client, there usually will be other people who not only know more than the doctor about the client but have a much stronger moral claim to speak on the client's behalf. I am referring to relatives of clients, who do have a moral right that supersedes that of someone outside the family to make a decision for a loved one. Others who have a stronger moral claim to speak on a client's behalf than a veterinarian are close friends of the client.

It follows that when clients do not appear able to make a voluntary and rational choice regarding care for their animal, and when the animal's condition allows time for postponing an immediate decision, the doctor should attempt to contact a family member or friend who can assist the client in making a decision. Ideally, such a person should come to the practice to confer with both the client and doctor. This approach will not only assure that the client's needs will be spoken for. It can help to protect the doctor against a potential legal claim that the doctor violated the client's right to make the decision regarding treatment of the patient.

~ PROTECTING A PATIENT FROM AN IGNORANT, NEGLECTFUL, OR ABUSIVE CLIENT

Practitioners sometimes see clients whose decision about a particular treatment, or whose general care for their animal, is harmful to the animal. In such situations, a doctor's inclination to speak out in the animal's behalf can conflict with one's desire to keep the client or the realization that the chances of changing the client's behavior are negligible.

Veterinarians occupy a different position in circumstances involving abuse or neglect of patients than do physicians. In various kinds of situations, state laws require physicians to report to public health or law enforcement authorities injuries or conditions that appear to have resulted from neglect, abuse, or certain kinds of criminal activity. This can afford physicians protection from complaints by patients because they can respond that they were compelled by the law to report a problem. Veterinarians, on the other hand, are rarely, if ever, required by law to report cases of abuse of their patients, even those so serious as to amount to the crime of animal cruelty. Moreover, there is often no assurance that an abused animal will be cared for properly when abuse is reported to the authorities; some humane societies are more likely to euthanize such animals than to try to rehabilitate and adopt them out.

In short, in many cases in which clients are harming their animals, the only person who will be able to speak up for that animal is the veterinarian—and if the doctor does speak out, there probably will be no one to shield one from the consequences.

Possible responses to cases of ignorance, neglect, or abuse vary widely. When clients seem genuinely concerned about their animals, but are harming them out of ignorance, a doctor can make a significant contribution to the interests of both animal and client by educating the client. In such cases, contacting the client periodically or scheduling regular follow-up visits might be helpful. When the problem is laziness on the client's part to attend to the animal's needs, some enthusiastic exhortation and encouragement might do the trick. The difficulties become greater when a client has a positively bad or abusive attitude toward the animal. In some cases, careful criticism of the client's behavior might be possible, but criticism can be pointless when a client seems incapable of really caring about the patient. Some doctors sometimes will suggest that a client think about giving up the animal for adoption and even volunteer to take it from the client to assure that adoption will be attempted. In extreme cases, sparing the animal further suffering might require reporting the matter to the local government body authorized to deal with animal cruelty.

Sometimes, the only self-respecting and ethical approach will be to oppose the client's requests and to insist on a particular course of action if the client wants to retain one's services. In one case, a client came to the hospital with a desperately ill and suffering cat. The client was about to leave for a weekend trip with his family. He understood that his animal faced certain agony if permitted to live a moment longer without pain-deadening drugs. But he did not want to ruin the weekend for himself and his family by having the animal euthanized right away, and asked the doctor to keep the animal going under intensive care, no expense spared, until the following Monday when the family returned and could cope with the situation. There seemed to the doctor only two humane approaches: to agree to the client's request, to euthanize the animal, and to tell the client that it died of natural causes over the weekend; or to advise the client that keeping the animal alive was wrong and to use all means at his disposal to persuade the client to agree to prompt euthanasia. The former approach would bring the advantages of a larger fee and the possibility of retaining the client. The latter approach would be consistent with the high moral ideals that motivated the doctor's dissatisfaction with the client's request in the first place.

～ LYING TO HELP PATIENTS OR CLIENTS

The last example raises another important ethical question: Under what circumstances might a veterinarian be justified in lying to clients to protect the interests of patients or clients?

Lying is a controversial subject among philosophers and medical ethicists. Some maintain that one should never lie, whatever the consequences.[27] Others believe that we have a strong obligation to tell the truth but that this obligation is sometimes outweighed by an obligation not to hurt people unnecessarily, or to help them.[28] Some recommend liberal use of lying in the medical context to benefit patients.[29]

The following are among the kinds of lies veterinarians can tell to clients to protect the interests of patients:

- Telling the client that the animal's suffering is much worse than it is in order to induce the client to agree to euthanasia so that the patient will not suffer needlessly
- Telling a client who asks if there is a noneuthanasia alternative that there is no such alternative, when in fact there is, in order to induce the client to choose euthanasia rather than the alternative, which will cause the animal to suffer and has a low probability of success
- Telling a client that one will euthanize his healthy animal when in fact one has no such intention and will attempt to place the animal in a suitable home
- Deliberately underestimating the cost of a proposed procedure to get the client committed to the procedure to a point where he will feel obligated to pay the additional costs once they become necessary
- Deliberately overestimating the cost of a noneuthanasia alternative that is not likely to succeed in order to induce the client to choose euthanasia

The following are some of the kinds of lies a doctor can tell to clients to benefit them:
- Telling a client that her animal died peacefully and without suffering, when in fact it suffered considerably
- Assuring a client who chose euthanasia prematurely that putting the animal to sleep was medically necessary at the time
- Telling a client that there are no alternatives to euthanasia, when in fact there are, to spare the client the considerable upset or expense such an alternative would entail
- Deliberately overestimating the costs or underestimating the probability of success of a noneuthanasia alternative to spare the client the upset or expense of such an alternative
- Assuring a client that her animal died from unavoidable natural causes, when in fact its death was caused by the owner's neglect or abuse

It is beyond the scope of this text to offer a theory of lying in the veterinary context. I offer the following observations to assist readers in formulating their own approach to the issue.

1. To lie is to make an assertion that one knows to be false with the purpose of inducing someone else to believe that it is true. Lying is only one form of deception, and that a deception might not be termed a lie does not make it morally correct. Failing to tell a client that a member of one's staff was responsible for a patient's death might not be properly called "lying." But whatever one calls it, it certainly can be a deception that raises moral issues, for it can involve withholding information from a client with the intention of preventing him from knowing something he might want to know. Sometimes, the moral issue for a veterinarian will be whether it is justifiable to withhold or manipulate information even though doing so might not, strictly speaking, be termed "lying."

2. One must avoid any temptation to think that lying is justified if it produces more happiness than unhappiness for all concerned. Lying is inherently evil. It involves a manipulation, indeed in a very real sense, a possession of the person to whom one lies. This is so even when a lie is intended to benefit the person who is told the lie. As philosopher Charles Fried explains, lying:

> ...violates the principle of respect [for persons], for I must affirm that the mind of another person is available to me in a way in which I cannot agree my mind would be available to him—for if I do so agree, then I would not expect my lie to be believed. ...When I do intentional physical harm, I say that your body, your person, is available for my purposes. When I lie, I lay claim to your mind.[30]

When a veterinarian lies to a client, she violates the implicit understanding between the two that the doctor serves the client, who is an autonomous adult capable of making his own choices. Therefore if lying to a client is ever justified, it can only be justified for the gravest of reasons, and only in the most extreme and infrequent of circumstances.

3. As Fried argues,[31] a case *can* be made for lying when one is being forced into either lying or violating a very important moral duty, and lying to a potential wrongdoer is the only way of acting in accordance with the duty. Fried imagines a situation in which someone is forced by an assassin to tell the whereabouts of the assassin's would-be victim. Here, Fried maintains, lying is justified because the assassin has no right to the truth, telling the truth would violate one's duty not to cause great harm, and the lie would be told to someone attempting to perpetrate a greater wrong. Although lying normally involves great disrespect for the person who is told the lie, the assassin in Fried's example forfeits the right to this respect because he is attempting to use the institution of truth-telling to enable him to act in a way that is fundamentally disrespectful of others.

Fried's principle does not justify lying when it would result on balance in more happiness than unhappiness. A veterinarian might be able to maximize happiness by telling a client that one will euthanize a healthy patient, intending all the while to give it to someone else, or by lying to a client about the availability of treatment to spare the client unnecessary upset or expense. However, such clients would not be forcing the doctor into a choice between lying or causing great harm. In these, and many other kinds of cases, the doctor is not being asked to lie, and even if he were, he could continue to tell the truth knowing that he is not responsible for the fact that someone would be more upset by the truth than a lie.

On the other hand, one can imagine circumstances in which a client's demand for the truth would put a veterinarian in a position in which she must lie to avoid being an integral part of a heinous moral offense. Suppose a race horse will suffer irreparable injury and great pain if it is run, the client requests a medication that the doctor knows will enable it to run, but the client makes it clear that the horse will be scratched only if the doctor (and no one else) says it will literally break down if it is run under any circumstances. Here, I would argue, the veterinarian may lie about the horse's ability to run because she is being placed in an unavoidable position in which her telling the truth would be part of a great moral wrong.

To be sure, this last example is somewhat fanciful—a fact which illustrates that Fried's principle justifies lying by a veterinarian (or anyone else) only in the most unusual circumstances. For if the doctor in the example knows that she routinely must lie to spare the client's animals great suffering, she will probably be able to extricate herself from the professional relationship. When this is possible (as it often is) or when there is another doctor who will do a client's unsavory bidding, it is difficult to characterize the situation as one in which the veterinarian is being coerced by the client into a choice of either lying or doing great harm.

～ VETERINARIANS AND BREED STANDARDS

The standards of breed associations raise ethical problems for companion animal doctors. They might be asked to euthanize a healthy animal, the only "failing" of which is that it does not meet such standards. Veterinarians routinely perform surgical procedures required by certain breed standards. Some doctors are asked to remove or conceal breed standard "defects."

A Professional Approach to Breed Standards

To a large extent, the existence of these problems stems from the breed standards themselves. If breed standards were more inclusive, there would be fewer animals for which euthanasia or fraudulent cosmetic procedures are sought.

Breed standards can play an important role in assisting people to choose an appropriate animal. Different breeds provide different physical and psychological characteristics, which can be matched to the needs and proclivities of owners. Additionally, the various appearances and personalities of the breeds are often intrinsically interesting and pleasing. Although breed standards are all, to a certain extent, accidents of history, given the breeds as they have emerged, some standards can make esthetic and behavioral sense and need not in themselves involve a denigration of the value of the animal. For example, it is not unreasonable to restrict show quality Yorkshire Terriers to a weight of 7 pounds and their distinctive range of colors.[32] A 20-pound Yorkie is quite a different kind of critter. There seems nothing wrong, given the way this breed has developed, to ask that people who prefer a small white dog consider the Maltese, which have their own delightful appearance and personality.

Unfortunately, some breed standards make no sense from an esthetic standpoint. Yorkies are "disqualified" if they have an albino toenail, even though it can take some effort to find any nails under all the hair. Some breed standards cause animals discomfort because they require the surgical procedure of ear-cropping. Other standards involve or have resulted in physical characteristics or genetic predispositions that range from the uncomfortable, as in the case of the many-wrinkled Shar-pei prone to skin problems, to the fatal, as in the case of the Manx cat which has a high incidence of spinal and neurological anomalies.[33]

There are several reasons veterinarians must take an active interest in the promotion of rational breed standards.

First, the profession already plays an important role in supporting breed standards: some veterinarians euthanize or sterilize animals that do not meet these standards, and they often acquiesce in the judgments of breed associations that certain animals are only "pet quality." If veterinarians are supporting breed standards, they should support morally defensible standards.

Second, as healers and protectors of companion animals, veterinarians should not tolerate standards that cause such animals significant pain, discomfort, or disease for no other reason than that some people find traits associated with these problems pleasing.

Third, as professionals who serve the interests of their clients, veterinarians have a moral obligation to help clients avoid unnecessary expense and emotional distress. Some esthetically foolish breed standards result in greatly higher fees that owners must pay for "acceptable" animals. Other standards can bring clients significant heartache and veterinary bills when the time comes to cope with a breed-associated disorder.

Finally, as we have seen, veterinarians have a strong self-interest in elevating the image of their companion animal patients. Clearly, some breed standards degrade and devalue companion animals. An animal is not regarded as something of great value if it is subjected to painful procedures or can suffer a debilitating disease simply because some people find a certain trait esthetically pleasing.

It follows from these considerations that the profession should, at the very least, work to eliminate breed standards that (1) are esthetically superfluous given the general appearance of a breed and that are used as a justification for the killing of healthy animals; (2) require veterinary procedures that cause significant discomfort to patients and expense to clients; and (3) are associated with significant discomfort or disease. Some breeds might be associated with so many problems, infirmities, and diseases that they should probably be ended altogether.

The AVMA has recognized in principle the legitimacy of efforts by the profession to promote rational breed standards. Its official position on ear trimming recommends "that action be taken to delete mention of cropped or trimmed ears from breed standards for dogs and to prohibit the showing of dogs with cropped or trimmed ears if such animals were born after some reasonable date."[34] Unfortunately, the AVMA has not sought aggressively to eliminate ear trimming or other medically harmful breed standards that unnecessarily plague pets, clients, and veterinarians.

Is the perpetuation of pure breeds ethically acceptable?

Some people oppose the breeding and ownership of purebred dogs and cats. If, as these people claim, it is wrong even to have such animals as pets, it would be inappropriate for veterinarians to seek changes in breed standards that would still allow the breeds to continue. Three different arguments are commonly raised against the propagation of pure breeds.

BREEDS INVOLVE SICKNESS AND INFIRMITY. The least radical of these arguments is that the perpetuation of pure breeds leads to sick and infirm animals, either through the intentional breeding of traits that cause medical problems or by progressive debilitation associated with continuing in-breeding of similar genetic stock. This argument is not very radical because, as a condemnation of *all* pure breeds of dogs and cats, it is factually incorrect. No one should underestimate the amount or difficulty of the work that needs to be done to spare animals and their owners breed-related disorders and infirmities. However, it is just not the case that perpetuation of pure breeds must always be associated with serious or intractable medical problems. Some breeds are quite hardy and long-lived. Others are associated with certain medical problems that are not present in all members of the breed, and are minor or quite manageable when present. Although the problem of genetic inbreeding may be difficult to address with breed fanciers unwilling to allow new stock into the gene pool, there seems no reason in principle why progress along these lines cannot be made.

IT IS WRONG TO PERPETUATE BREEDS WHEN OTHER ANIMALS ARE AVAILABLE. A somewhat more radical view condemns the breeding and possession of purebred dogs and cats as long as there are unwanted or formerly stray animals available at shelters and pounds. According to this argument, it is wrong to bring another dog or cat into the world when millions of others are killed each year because no one wants them. This argument can be characterized as radical because, although consistent in principle with the perpetuation of breeds, it would preclude propagation of pure breeds until there are no available shelter animals—something that probably will never happen. A variant of the argument holds that people who buy or breed purebred dogs and cats are themselves responsible for the death of surplus animals that would otherwise not be killed.

This second kind of objection to purebred animals enjoys considerable popularity, especially among humane societies that face the terrible burden of killing millions of unwanted animals each year. Indeed, some find this second objection so obviously correct that it is often no longer deemed worthy of supporting argument. Dr. Michael Fox, for example, states that "it is *surely* wrong to deliberately breed any dog when there are so many homeless ones in the shelters in need of a good home, waiting to be adopted. But that is almost like telling people not to have children!"[35]

The force of Dr. Fox's contention is blunted by some hard facts. First, many animals in shelters are not good candidates for adoption, because they are ill, old, or have serious behavioral problems.[36] Second, many potential pet owners are reluctant to adopt a shelter animal because they cannot observe its parents or obtain other reliable information (of the sort that often comes from knowing that the animal is of a certain breed) about its medical history, and likely size, longevity, and personality. Third, many potential pet owners will forego having an animal if they cannot have a purebred dog or cat, or a dog or cat of a certain breed. Insisting that such people adopt shelter animals will therefore not reduce the number of adoptable shelter animals, will deprive potential owners of the benefits of the human-animal bond, and will reduce the demand for veterinary services. Finally, a moratorium in the propagation of pure breeds until the shelters are emptied of adoptable animals would surely end these breeds because it would take generations of animals before the overpopulation problem can be solved. Not surprisingly, supporters of pure breeds sometimes suspect that the real motivation of this second (supposedly temporary) objection to the breeding of purebred dogs and cats is the desire to end pure breeds altogether.

These facts aside, there remain many dogs and cats in shelters that would make fine pets. However, the claim that it is immoral to breed or purchase a purebred dog or cat as long as other animals are available for adoption remains misguided because it makes a fundamental ethical mistake. The claim rests on the faulty principle that people who want a purebred dog or cat have an obligation to alleviate the effects of a problem they had no role in causing—simply because they might be capable of alleviating these effects. If I want a purebred dog because I find that its characteristics are best suited to my family's needs (or just because I prefer such an animal) why should I be deprived of it because *other* people have acted irresponsibly by allowing their dogs to breed? We do not always hold ourselves responsible for alleviating the wrongs of others, even when we can lessen misfortune or unhappiness thereby. Most people do *not*, for example, believe that they should avoid having children while there exist unwanted children to adopt. Nor does it seem reasonable to posit, as this second objection to pure breeds appears to, a general moral obligation to save animal life when one has had nothing to do with putting such life in jeopardy. Otherwise, we should all be searching our back yards, neighborhoods, and wilderness areas for animals to save.

To be sure, it is morally admirable to adopt a shelter animal. But, I would argue, people who have not contributed to pet overpopulation have no moral *obligation* to do so. All owners are obligated to assure that their animals will not produce unwanted or stray animals. However, this is quite a different obligation and one that applies equally to those who have purebred animals and those who do not. The assertion that people are not obligated to adopt shelter animals is not hard-hearted nor does it denigrate the need to address seriously the problem of surplus and stray animals. However, there is little to be gained, either in solving this problem, or placing blame for it where it belongs, by casting a general, society-wide net of guilt or responsibility.

PERPETUATING BREEDS IS INHERENTLY IMMORAL. The third and most radical argument against the propagation of pure dog and cat breeds that it is inherently wrong to perpetuate breeds. On this view, selective breeding of pets is no different from deliberate or forced breeding of people for favored traits.

It is difficult to understand how one could accept the keeping of animals in the home without conceding the appropriateness of *some* genetic manipulation. For if animals can be kept at least in part for human enjoyment and benefit, it is important (for the animals as well as their owners) to assure that such animals have traits that are compatible with such an existence. The notion that it is inherently disrespectful or harmful to pets to breed any kind of characteristic pleasing or useful to people appears to follow from the view that it is unethical to use any animal for any human purpose. This is indeed a radical position. As demonstrated in Chapter 12, this position requires the elimination not only of companion animals but also the veterinary profession.

Euthanasia and Sterilization of "Defective" Animals

As I have argued, it is a denigration of the value of companion animal patients and of veterinarians as medical professionals to kill, on client request, healthy animals that can make good and loving pets. Killing healthy animals that can make wonderful pets but that deviate from purely esthetic breed standards is no less a devaluation of the patient and veterinarian, regardless of whether these standards are defensible from an esthetic standpoint.

It is certainly better to sterilize a "defective" healthy animal than to kill it. However, if a particular standard is one veterinarians ought to oppose, sterilizing animals that do not have a required trait in order to "protect the breed" is to engage in further support of an improper standard. Nevertheless, a doctor who can convince a client who wants a so-called "defective" animal killed to sell it as "pet quality" on condition that it be sterilized, has done a good deed given the world as it is. (Of course, sterilization of companion animals can often be recommended on the grounds of convenience to owners and prevention of unwanted strays.) Surrender of a "defective" purebred animal to a shelter can often allay a client's fear that the breed will be "polluted" and can save the animal's life, because many shelters now require sterilization of adopted animals.

Ear-cropping and Tail-docking

In recommending the elimination of nontherapeutic ear-cropping,[34] the AVMA has determined that whatever benefits might result from the process do not merit the costs to patients and clients. The correctness of this judgment is, I submit, beyond dispute. The procedure requires general anesthesia, as well as substantial knowledge of the surgical technique and meticulous attention to detail on the part of the doctor. Even then, it is associated with hemorrhage, difficulty in keeping supporting braces in place, self-trauma, and adverse psychological effects. These problems tend to be worse in older animals subjected to the procedure.[37] Commonly, the ears fail to stand, necessitating further intervention.[38]

One veterinarian concedes in a discussion instructing doctors how to trim ears that some veterinarians are opposed to the procedure. He justifies his discussion by claiming that if veterinarians "refuse to do it…others who are less qualified will do it much less humanely."[39] This is a terrible argument. The fact that some people might treat animals more inhumanely than veterinarians does not justify their being treated inhumanely. Indeed, if anything, it is worse if veterinarians treat them inhumanely, because veterinarians are committed to the prevention of unjustifiable animal suffering.

Some animal welfare advocates also call for elimination of docked tails from breed standards on the grounds that this is an immoral "mutilation" or "disfigurement."[40] These terms are not so much an argument as a conclusion, and in the case of tail-docking, they appear to me to be highly overblown. Few people would argue that sterilizing an animal for the convenience of its owner or to prevent unwanted strays is a "mutilation," even though it involves invasive surgery and might be of no direct benefit to the animal. The question is whether the possible detriments are serious enough to outweigh the benefits.

British veterinarian Dr. David Morton provides a meticulous scientific and ethical analysis of the various alleged benefits and detriments of tail-docking. He concludes that a persuasive case cannot be made that docking generally promotes hygiene or prevents damaged tails in the home. Dr. Morton also rejects docking to improve an animal's appearance on the grounds that veterinarians:

> ...take an oath...which states that they will do their best to protect the welfare of animals in their care. Welfare can be interpreted in many ways but many would take it to include an obligation not to inflict unnecessary suffering. In the event of any uncertainty, it could be argued that the primary responsibility of a veterinary surgeon is to be the animal's advocate and to give the benefit of any doubt to the animal. Veterinary surgeons, particularly, therefore should not cause animals to suffer pain, distress, discomfort or lasting harm without good reason. ...
>
> When justifying docking for the sake of the animal's appearance it is the author's belief that human pleasure is being balanced against animal suffering. ...
>
> But if docking is claimed to be justified on these grounds, might not the same argument be used to sanction ear-cropping and even dog fighting?[41]

Dr. Morton's treatment of this issue is instructive in appreciating the importance of fundamental value judgments in ethical argument. He concedes that there have been no carefully conducted scientific investigations of the effects of tail-docking on puppies. His claim that the procedure is painful rests on the observation that puppies "usually squeal and squeak when the tail is cut off," and a single "study" carried out by a family that breeds Cocker Spaniels. This study consisted of the observation of one litter of puppies several hours before and after their tails were docked. It was found that "0.29 puppies cried per hour before, compared with 3.8 puppies after docking." "There was a decrease in the amount of time puppies spent feeding (4.86 versus 4.0 puppies per hour) and sleeping (8.57 versus 5.56 puppies per hour after docking)." Although, as Dr. Morton admits, this was an observation of one litter without control animals that were not docked, he concludes that the study "provides obvious evidence for pain at the time of docking."[42] Morton concludes that because this pain is not associated with a procedure that benefits the animals, and because docking ordinarily has no more than esthetic value to owners, tail-docking is ethically inappropriate.

I do not wish to criticize the manner in which Dr. Morton constructs his discussion, which carefully addresses all the arguments that could conceivably be made for and against tail-docking. The most interesting feature of his article, I believe, is the foundation of his disapproval of the practice: the pain puppies experience. Morton demonstrates conclusively that tail-docking is not generally a therapeutic procedure, although in certain instances it might be. It is also a fact (which is not contradicted by his "data") that when performed early in a puppy's life, tail trimming can be accomplished quickly without anesthesia and does not appear to cause great or long-lasting distress.[43] But is such temporary squealing and squeaking, or even an hour or two of slightly diminished sleep or eating sufficient to justify ethical condemnation and even legal prohibition of tail-docking? One can concede that the esthetic enjoyment of a short tail by people is not a momentously important benefit. But one can also maintain that the detriments of the procedure need not be serious either. I myself would say that, given the impact on the animals, the procedure is not morally prohibited. On the other hand, a respectable argument can be made that because tail-docking is useless and not of significant benefit to either patient or client, it would be better if veterinarians did not do it. I would suggest that the issue of docking is illuminated by the distinction, explained in Chapter 5, between acting in a way that is morally obligatory and doing something that is not required but may still be morally desirable.

All this shows that those who disagree about such procedures as tail-docking, ear-trimming, and declawing may not disagree about what these procedures actually do to the animals—but about whether, in their view, what is done to the animals is of sufficient *value* to justify the practice. The ethical conclusion may rest on value judgments that have nothing to do with the facts.

Interestingly, there appears to be a cultural aspect to views on whether tail-docking, for instance, inflicts unjustifiable pain. In talks with American veterinarians about tail-docking, I have found quite a few who are completely comfortable with the practice, many who do it but would be happy not to, some who find it inappropriate, and very few who would characterize it as evil. A 1989 survey of Australian veterinarians found that 86% of respondents opposed nontherapeutic docking and described it as "archaic," "barbaric," and "pointless."[44] The European Convention for the Protection of Pet Animals, signed by 12 countries as of 1992, also prohibits nontherapeutic tail-docking as well as ear-trimming and "de-barking of dogs," and nontherapeutic declawing of domestic cats.[45] Shortly after the publication of Dr. Morton's article, the Royal College of Veterinary Surgeons decided to prohibit tail-docking by veterinarians in the United Kingdom except for therapeutic reasons. The Royal College had already prohibited ear-trimming. Veterinarians in the Scandinavian countries have long been forbidden to perform nontherapeutic ear-cropping or tail-docking.

Concealment of Breed Defects

One unacceptable approach to sensible or indefensible breed standards is concealment of traits that violate these standards. To do this is to deceive or defraud those for whom buying, breeding, or showing animals with genuine traits is important. Doctors who find certain breed "defects" to be insupportable or who do not regard sterilization of animals with such traits to be reasonable can behave ethically by opposing the relevant standards openly, instead of engaging in behavior that could deceive someone down the line.

∼ DE-CLAWING AND "DE-BARKING"

The removal of the claws of domestic cats raises ethical issues because the procedure can have a definite negative impact on the animals. There is the discomfort and normal risks associated with the surgery, and the fact that a de-clawed cat can suffer serious injury or lose its life if it escapes from the house. The AVMA has attempted to strike a balance between the problems this procedure can cause for the animals and the fact that for some owners, de-clawing is necessary for preventing destruction of their possessions. The AVMA believes that "de-clawing of domestic cats is justifiable when the cat cannot be trained to refrain from using its claws destructively."[46]

Few pronouncements of official veterinary ethics are ignored more frequently than this one. De-clawing is a very common procedure. It is, surely, far more common than the number of cats that cannot be trained to refrain from destructive use of their claws. If doctors are to follow the official standard and pay due regard to the interests of feline patients, they should attempt to help clients address the problem of destructiveness by all available nonsurgical means. If de-clawing still appears to be necessary, clients must be informed clearly about what must be done to safeguard the animal.

According to one veterinary surgeon, surgery on the vocal cords to suppress barking is "often done when dogs are kept alone in apartments during the day or whenever their barking becomes a nuisance."[47] This procedure poses significant risks to the animal. It is associated with long-term complications that are difficult to correct, including stricture or webbing of the glottis.[48] Routinely, the animal continues to make a noise that is described by the veterinarian quoted above as "a coughlike sound."

Some veterinarians chastise objections to de-barking as unscientific and sentimental. The dogs, they claim, do not know the difference, and people who criticize the procedure are merely imagining the unhappiness they would experience if they were unable to talk.

Whether de-barked dogs experience frustration or unhappiness is not the only issue. Most dogs make an enormously wide range of sounds. Barking and more subtle kinds of vocalizations can be used to ask for or demand food or a walk, to gain an owner's attention, warn off intruders, signal that the dog does not wish to be annoyed, express anger or frustration, and in play. Clearly, to take such behaviors away is to prevent the great majority of dogs from doing many things they would ordinarily do. Their lives and experiences will be less. Indeed, because barking seems so much a part of the nature of most breeds, many people would be inclined to say that de-barking these animals makes them less of a dog.

Moreover, although we have limited access to the canine mind, there seems more reason to conclude that dogs do feel frustrated by being unable to bark than that they do not. Dogs are sophisticated in their mental apparatus, which is constructed in most of them to include vocalization. Few things that are so much a part of such a being's life would not cause discomfort or frustration if removed or severely restricted. I have seen de-barked dogs that appeared to be trying in vain to warn their owners of an approaching stranger. They seemed to know that they were not quite making it work. To dismiss this interpretation as sentimental is to close one's eyes to the facts.

Given the potential medical complications of de-barking, its clear deprivation of a range of behaviors, and its likely result of frustration or discomfort, there must be very strong reasons for de-barking a dog. It is not enough that the barking is a nuisance to the owner or his neighbors. It is not enough that addressing the problem by nonsurgical means will require behavioral training or expense. Surely, no weaker showing should be made for de-barking a dog than for de-clawing a cat. If one were to apply the AVMA's position on de-clawing to de-barking, one would have to insist that before de-barking is justified, the problem must be serious enough to be called destructive, and behavioral or other nonsurgical means cannot work. Veterinarians who perform this procedure just because a client finds his dog's barking to be a nuisance are participating in a serious denigration of the value of their canine patients and their profession.

∿ VETERINARIANS AND PET OVERPOPULATION

It is estimated that between 10 and 20 million unwanted and stray dogs and cats are euthanized in animal shelters each year in the United States.[49]

Because the overpopulation problem affects various segments of society different-ly, it has aroused predictably different responses. Some animal activists, for example, believe that legislation is required to prohibit any breeding as long as there are surplus animals,[50] and some breeders and breed clubs maintain that they are not a major cause of the problem.[51] Veterinarians see the problem at close hand. They attempt to repair countless dogs and cats that are strays, or are injured by strays. They see the results of botched or inhumane attempts by owners to rid themselves of animals. Some veteri-narians participate in the euthanasia of unwanted animals. The profession can enhance its role as the guardian of animal welfare by taking an active role in pursuing the causes and solutions of the overpopulation problem.

The AVMA has official policies regarding pet overpopulation. Its 1981 Position on Animal Population Control and Ovariohysterectomy Clinics[52] and 1984 Guidelines for Veterinarians Participating in Ovariohysterectomy-Orchiectomy Clinics[53] encourage doctors to participate in neutering clinics as a means of control-ling the number of unwanted animals. The 1992 AVMA Animal Welfare Forum was devoted to the overpopulation issue. The proceedings of this forum address develop-ments ranging from medical research into new techniques of preventing and termi-nating pregnancy;[54] working with breeders to reduce the number of unwanted pure-bred animals;[55] early age neutering of dogs and cats;[56] and practical ways individual doctors can make progress educating the public and encouraging clients to sterilize their animals.[57] In 1993 the House of Delegates passed a landmark resolution, recog-nizing the work of Dr. Leo Lieberman, supporting early (8-16 weeks of age) ovario-hysterectomies and gonadectomies in dogs and cats as a means of preventing the birth of unwanted animals.[58]

Although much can be said about various suggested technological approaches to preventing pet overpopulation, the distinguished author, journalist, and animal welfare advocate Roger Caras has, I believe, put his finger on the fundamental problem. The problem is not technological, but ethical. Too many people have an underlying attitude that allows them to treat pets as throwaways. Because this attitude comes from within, and is often deeply ingrained by the time people are old enough to own animals, it is not sufficient to attempt to control the attitude's effects. Caras believes that:

> We are one generation away from having a humane and kind world that really takes animal wel-fare into account. Teach one generation of American and Canadian children what it means to care, what it means to be responsible, what it means to accept responsibility, what it means to look outside themselves, and they will train their children the same way. What are veterinarians doing about that? Do you have programs in your clinic, and bring in high-school students to see what you do, to see what mercy is like, to see what it is to help and share in this life? Do you go out into the schools or have the classes come to you, or work with boys' clubs and girls' clubs and church groups? ...The solution to the problem is not going to come about because of spay-

ing or neutering or because of any technologic device that bans conception; it is going to come about because we got to the hearts and souls of one generation of people and turned them around.[59]

These wise words are relevant not just to the issue of pet overpopulation but to many ethical problems faced by veterinarians. Too often, when a veterinarian confronts an ethical issue it is too late to deal with it satisfactorily because the client already has a deep-seated attitude that caused the problem or makes its solution more difficult. People want healthy animals euthanized, they refuse to make reasonable economic and personal sacrifices for the medical care of their animals, they acquiesce in foolish or harmful breed standards, for the same reason they abandon animals to the streets. They care only about themselves and do not have sufficient regard for helpless beings that have become so dependent on them. Can a veterinarian change such an attitude in the office, during a 10- or 15-minute appointment? It is highly doubtful. The attitude must be prevented in the first place. Caras observes that much of the burden of encouraging proper attitudes toward companion animals must be borne by the veterinary profession because no one else is capable of speaking more knowledgeably or effectively about animal welfare.

Caras' statement that we are a generation away from inculcating proper attitudes toward pets and other animals is both hopeful and pessimistic. The fact that we are only a generation away means that great changes are possible if we work for them. The fact that we are a generation away means that it will take significant time and effort to effect these changes.

REFERENCES

[1]Quoted in: Just like us? *Harper's Magazine* 277:50, August 1988.
[2]Fox M: *Inhumane Society: The American Way of Exploiting Animals*, New York, 1990, St Martin's Press, p 156.
[3]*Id*, p 21.
[4]*Id*, p 14.
[5]*Id*, p 235.
[6]*See*, Tischler J: Rights for non-human animals: A guardianship model for cats and dogs, *San Diego Law Rev* 14: 484, 1977; Cavalieri P, Singer P, editors: *The Great Ape Project*, New York, 1994, St Martin's Press.
[7]Singer P: *Animal Liberation*, ed 2, New York, 1990, Avon Books, p vi.
[8]For example, in his ground-breaking study of views of animal mentality in ancient Greek thought, philosopher Richard Sorabji states that "for ease of reading, despite my sympathies, I shall not call [animals] 'other' animals, nor substitute 'humankind' for mankind." Sorabji R: *Animal Minds and Human Morals: The Origins of the Western Debate*, Ithaca, NY, 1993, Cornell University Press, p 1. It is a measure of the effect of animal activism that an outstanding scholar believes readers might not appreciate his sympathy for "animals" unless he apologizes for using the word.
[9]Regan T: *The Case for Animal Rights*, Berkeley, 1993, University of California Press, p 109.
[10]*Id*, p 119.
[11]Rachels J: Active and passive euthanasia, *N Engl J Med* 292:78-80, 1975.
[12]Louisell D: Euthanasia and bioeuthanasia, *Linacre Q* 40:307, 1973.
[13]*1993 Report of the AVMA Panel on Euthanasia, J Am Vet Med Assoc* 202: 232-233, 1993.
[14]*Id*, pp 244-245.
[15]McCullough MJ, Harris JM, McCullough WF: Human-animal bond and euthanasia—a special problem. In Ettinger SJ, editor: *Textbook of Veterinary Internal Medicine: Diseases of the Dog and Cat*, ed 2, vol 2, Philadelphia, 1989, WB Saunders, p 243, citing McCullough M, Bustad L: Incidence of euthanasia and euthanasia alternatives in private practice. In Katcher A, Beck A, editors: *New Perspectives on Our Lives with Companion Animals*, Philadelphia, 1983, University of Pennsylvania Press, p 366.
[16]Kay WJ: Euthanasia, *Trends* 1(5):52-54, 1986.
[17]*Id*, p 52.
[18]Schwabe CW: *Veterinary Medicine and Human Health*, ed 3, Baltimore, 1984, Williams & Wilkins, p 624.

[19]*See*, for example, Hart BL: *Behavior of Domestic Animals*, San Francisco, 1983, Freeman; Houpt KA, Wolski TR: *Domestic Animal Behavior for Veterinarians and Animal Scientists*, Ames, IA, 1982, Iowa State University Press.

[20]*Sentell* v. *New Orleans and Carrollton Railroad Co.*, 166 U.S. 698, 701 (1897).

[21]Beauchamp TL, Childress JF: *Principles of Biomedical Ethics*, ed 3, New York, 1989, Oxford University Press, p 144.

[22]*American Medical Association Principles of Medical Ethics and Current Opinions of the Council on Ethical and Judicial Affairs—1989*, Section 2.20, "Withholding or Withdrawing Life-Prolonging Medical Treatment." In Gorlin RA, editor: *Codes of Professional Responsibility*, ed 2, Washington, DC, 1990, Bureau of National Affairs, p 201 (stating that the "social commitment of the physician is to sustain life and relieve suffering. ...For humane reasons, with informed consent, a physician may do what is medically necessary to alleviate severe pain, or cease or omit treatment to permit a terminally ill patient to die when death is imminent. However, the physician should not intentionally cause death. ...").

[23]Beauchamp TL, Childress JF: *Principles of Biomedical Ethics*, ed 3, New York, 1989, Oxford University Press, p 141.

[24]*Id*, pp 146-147.

[25]Pross C: Nazi doctors, German medicine, and historical truth. In Annas GJ, Grodin MA: *The Nazi Doctors and the Nuremburg Code*, New York, 1992, Oxford University Press, p 40.

[26]Cohen SP: The role of social work in a veterinary hospital setting, *Vet Clin North Am Small Anim Pract* 15:355-363, 1985.

[27]For example, Kant I: *The Doctrine of Virtue*, Philadelphia, 1964, University of Pennsylvania Press (translated by MJ Gregor), pp 428-430.

[28]For example, Beauchamp TL, Childress JF: *Principles of Biomedical Ethics*, ed 2, New York, 1982, Oxford University Press, p 223.

[29]For example, Leslie A: Ethics and the practice of placebo therapy. In Reiser SJ, Dyck AJ, Curran WJ, editors: *Ethics in Medicine*, Cambridge, MA, 1979, MIT Press, p 242 (stating that "deception is completely moral when it is used for the welfare of the patient"); Collins J: Should doctors tell the truth? In Reiser *et al*, p 221 (maintaining that "every physician should cultivate lying as a fine art").

[30]Fried C: *Right and Wrong*, Cambridge, 1978, Harvard University Press, pp 69-78.

[31]*Id*, 67.

[32]Munday E: *The Yorkshire Terrier*, New York, 1967, Arco, p 17.

[33]For a list of breed-associated diseases and disorders, *see* Kirk RW, Bistner SI, Ford RB: *Handbook of Veterinary Procedures and Emergency Treatment*, ed 5, Philadelphia, 1990, WB Saunders, pp 843-864.

[34]American Veterinary Medical Association: "Positions on Animal Welfare," "Companion Animals, Horses, and Wildlife," paragraph 4, *1994 AVMA Directory*, Schaumburg, IL, The Association, p 56.

[35]Fox M: *Inhumane Society: The American Way of Exploiting Animals*, New York, 1990, St Martin's Press, p 167, emphasis added.

[36]Caras R: One generation away from humanity, *J Am Vet Med Assoc* 202:910, 1993.

[37]Smith KW: Cosmetic ear trimming. In Bojrab MJ, editor: *Current Techniques in Small Animal Surgery*, ed 2, Philadelphia, 1983, Lea & Febiger, pp 90-93.

[38]Smith KW: Surgical correction for faulty carriage of trimmed ears. In Bojrab MJ: *Current Techniques in Small Animal Surgery*, ed 2, Philadelphia, 1983, Lea & Febiger, pp 93-96.

[39]Smith KW: Cosmetic ear trimming. In Bojrab MJ, editor: *Current Techniques in Small Animal Surgery*, ed 2, Philadelphia, 1983, Lea & Febiger, p 90.

[40]Association of Veterinarians for Animal Rights: Cosmetic Surgery or Surgery to Correct "Vices," Position Statements, Greenwich, CT, undated, The Association, unpaginated.

[41]Morton D: Docking of dogs: practical and ethical aspects, *Vet Rec*, October 3, 1992:306.

[42]*Id*, p 303.

[43]Cawley AJ, Archibald J: Plastic surgery. In Archibald J, editor: *Canine Surgery*, ed 2, Santa Barbara, 1974, American Veterinary Publications, p 139.

[44]Morton D: Docking of dogs: practical and ethical aspects, *Vet Rec*, October 3, 1992:301.

[45]*Id*, p 302.

[46]American Veterinary Medical Association: "Positions on Animal Welfare," "Companion Animals, Horses, and Wildlife," paragraph 5, *1994 AVMA Directory*, Schaumburg, IL, 1993, The Association, p 56.

[47]Leighton RL: Soft tissues, tonsils, pharynx, larynx, and trachea. In Archibald J, editor: *Canine Surgery*, ed 2, Santa Barbara, 1974, American Veterinary Publications, p 350.

[48]Kagan K: Devocalization procedures. In Bojrab MJ: *Current Techniques in Small Animal Surgery*, ed 2, Philadelphia, 1983, Lea & Febiger, p 264.

[49]Nassar R, Talboy J, Moulton C: *Animal Shelter Reporting Study 1990*, Denver, 1992, American Humane Association.

[50]Sturla K: Role of breeding regulation laws in solving the dog and cat overpopulation problem, *J Am Vet Med Assoc* 202:928-932, 1993.

[51]Strand P: The pet owner and breeder's perspective on overpopulation, *J Am Vet Med Assoc* 202:921-928, 1993.

[52]American Veterinary Medical Association: "Position on Animal Population Control and Ovariohysterectomy Clinics," *1994 AVMA Directory*, Schaumburg, IL, 1993, The Association, pp 55-56.

[53]American Veterinary Medical Association: "Guidelines for Veterinarians Participating in Ovariohysterectomy-Orchiectomy Clinics," *1994 AVMA Directory*, Schaumburg, IL, 1993, The Association, p 89.

[54]Olson PN, Johnston SD: New developments in small animal population control, *J Am Vet Med Assoc* 202:904-909, 1993.

[55]Cloud DF: Working with breeders on solutions to pet overpopulation, *J Am Vet Med Assoc* 202:912-914, 1993.

[56]Theran P: Early-age neutering of dogs and cats, *J Am Vet Med Assoc* 202:914-917, 1993.

[57]MacKay CA: Veterinary practitioners' role in pet overpopulation, *J Am Vet Med Assoc* 202:918-921, 1993.

[58]Spaying/neutering comes of age, *J Am Vet Med Assoc* 203:591, 1993.

[59]Caras R: One generation away from humanity, *J Am Vet Med Assoc* 202:910-912, 1993.

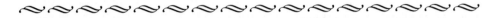
Ethical Challenges of High-tech, Innovative, and Academic Veterinary Medicine

*V*eterinarians are rightly excited about technological developments in medical care for animals. New diagnostic techniques, surgical procedures, and treatments now enable doctors to help animals that once had no chance for survival or a decent quality of life. However, the use and search for advanced procedures raise serious ethical issues. So does the academic clinical environment in which much of the development of new procedures takes place.

∾ ETHICAL ISSUES IN HIGH-TECH MEDICINE
What is "High-Tech" Veterinary Medicine?

Whether a procedure or treatment is classified as "high-tech" depends largely on who is doing the classifying. What seems high-tech or advanced to clients might not appear so to veterinarians. What the public views as high-tech turns largely on its familiarity with veterinary medicine and its level of regard for animals. For example, few people would regard blood banking and transfusions as "high-tech" for human medicine. However, many animal owners are astonished when informed that transfusion medicine is available for animals, and they marvel that veterinary medicine has advanced so far. For some people, such an attitude can result from lack of knowledge about what veterinarians do. For others, surprise about the sophistication of veterinary medicine can come from a low regard for the veterinarian's patients, and disapproval of "how much some people are willing to do to for *animals*."

Clearly, what is regarded as advanced or "high-tech" will change. Given the eagerness of many people to provide their animals the best the profession can offer, today's "high-tech" procedure can quickly become routine. For purposes of discussion, I want to suggest that we classify as "high-tech" procedures or treatments that (1) typically involve scientifically or technologically complicated activities, equipment, or drugs; (2) are typically (but not necessarily) costly; (3) are often (but not necessarily) innovative in the sense that they are not yet a part of ordinary veterinary practice; (4) often require a significant commitment of time and energy from clients; and (5) would appear to most members of the public as an advance or breakthrough in providing to animals care similar in kind or quality to that available to people.

Table 22-1 lists some procedures that, following this working definition, could be considered "high-tech" or advanced.

Overview of the Issues

In one sense, there is nothing distinctive about ethical issues raised by high-tech veterinary procedures. These issues are all presented somewhere and to some extent by more common and less-sophisticated kinds of veterinary care. Nevertheless, high-tech medicine tends to make standard ethical issues more difficult because it tends to require greater sacrifices from patients and clients. It follows that as advanced procedures filter down from academic veterinary centers and the specialties into the day-to-day work of general practitioners, there will be an increase in the intensity and difficulty of ethical issues faced by all veterinarians.

For example, as has been discussed in Chapters 20 and 21, two sources of ethical problems are the inability of some clients to pay for procedures that can help their animal and the insistence by some clients that an animal be kept alive when euthanasia would be in its best interests. The dissemination of high-tech veterinary procedures throughout the profession will increase the number and difficulty of both kinds of cases. Many advanced procedures are considerably more expensive than more typical kinds of care—and so there will be even more clients who can afford a more traditional kind of service but who cannot pay for a high-tech procedure. Likewise, some advanced procedures will allow

TABLE 22-1

～

Some "high-tech" or advanced veterinary procedures

• **Radiology**	• **Dentistry**
Ultrasonography	Root canal therapy
Computer tomography (CT scanning)	Orthodontics
Magnetic resonance imaging (MRI)	Periodontics
Radiation cancer therapy	• **Neurology**
• **Orthopedic surgery**	Hearing aids
Bone pinning	• **Gastroenterology**
Hip replacement	Endoscopy
Disc and vertebral surgery	Laparoscopy
• **Soft tissue surgery**	• **Ophthalmology**
Skin flap reconstructive surgery	Advanced diagnostic procedures
• **Transplantation surgery**	Use of medicated contact lenses
Kidney transplants	Cataract surgery
Bone tissue transplants	• **Equine medicine**
• **Hematology/Oncology**	Computer-assisted gait analysis
Blood banking and transfusion medicine	Neonatal foal intensive care
Cancer chemotherapy	• **Emergency and intensive care**
Cancer immunotherapy	Advanced monitoring of bodily functions
• **Cardiology/Cardiac surgery**	Total parenteral nutrition
Telephonic cardiac diagnostics	Maintenance of animals on respirators
Echocardiography	• **Behavioral medicine**
Pacemaker implantation	Use of psychotropic drugs, such as Prozac® and
Angioplasty	Valium®
Open heart surgery	
• **Dermatology/Allergy**	
Allergy skin testing	

clients and doctors to keep alive animals that formerly had to be euthanized—and so there will likely be even more animals that ought to be euthanized but are not.

Because ethical problems in high-tech or advanced procedures tend to present ethical issues that have already been discussed in this book, this chapter proceeds differently. Each issue raised here will be illustrated with one or more cases.* Following each case are questions readers are invited to consider in their approach to the case. I also discuss some of the ethical dilemmas posed by the general issues the cases illustrate and offer suggestions about how to approach these dilemmas.

We will consider the following general issues:

- **Affordability:** Can clients pay for an advanced service that is medically appropriate or advisable, and if they cannot, what ethical burdens, if any, should be borne by the practitioner?
- **Humaneness to patients:** When is it unfair or inhumane to patients to subject them to high-tech procedures?
- **Humaneness to clients:** When might it be unfair to clients to perform high-tech or advanced procedures?
- **Nonuniversal affordability:** Is it fair that only some clients can afford advanced procedures, and if so, what ethical problems might this create for practitioners?
- **Limited resources:** What ethical problems are raised if an advanced procedure, service, or product cannot be provided to all patients that would benefit from it?
- **Animal "donors:"** What ethical problems are raised by the fact some resources utilized in high-tech procedures come from other animals, which sometimes must be killed to provide such resources?
- **Professional definition:** How might the ability to provide, and the resources necessary to maintain, high-tech or advanced procedures affect how veterinarians define their professional role?

Affordability

Case 22-1 Chemotherapy. You are a generalist with a small animal practice. You are presented with Sylvia, a 3-year-old intact female Golden Retriever. The dog has enlarged lymph nodes, a slight cough, and some pleural effusion. Sylvia appears alert and happy. The clients, Mr. and Mrs. Brown, are a couple in their late 60s. They are of modest means, but have shown themselves to be very dedicated to the animals they have brought to you over the years.

You conduct a physical examination of Sylvia and, suspecting lymphoma, persuade the clients to authorize blood work, chest and abdominal radiographs, lymph node biopsies, and urinalysis.

The results of the tests confirm a diagnosis of early stage lymphosarcoma. Among the options are (1) immediate euthanasia; (2) doing nothing until Sylvia's quality of life deteriorates, probably in several months, and then euthanasia; or (3) chemotherapy.

Chemotherapy would have to be performed by a colleague at a nearby specialty facility. Her current chemotherapeutic regimen has allowed her to achieve an approximately 75% to

---

*These cases, like all those presented in this book, are intended to raise ethical issues. They do not purport to reflect the latest medical knowledge or techniques. It is especially important to keep this fact in mind regarding cases involving advanced or innovative procedures, for such procedures are characteristically in a continuous state of development and change. The fact that doctors would at this or some future time come to conclusions or employ approaches different from any presented in these cases would itself be of ethical significance. As explained in Chapter 10, an approach cannot be good ethically if it is inappropriate medically. Readers should nevertheless find it useful to accept as stated the facts presented in these cases and to ask what ought to be done given these facts.

80% probability of remission lasting from 5 to 17 months, time during which Sylvia could have a good quality of life. Almost 20% of such dogs on which she has used this regime have survived for 2 years.

Dogs like Sylvia differ in their response to such treatment, which consists of cyclic adminis-trations of vincristine, cyclophosphamide, asparaginase, and prednisone. Side effects are not uncommon. They can include perivascular irritation, constipation, neurologic problems, myelosuppression, hemorrhagic cystitis, and vomiting. Palliative measures can be given to alleviate side effects.

The cost of the therapy, including diagnostic tests, would be approximately $1500 at the specialty hospital. Additionally, the treatment would require a substantial commitment from the clients, who would have to transport Sylvia to the hospital for the therapy and assist in helping the animal through possible side effects.

The clients are extremely nervous in the office setting and appear puzzled and frightened. They tell you that they desperately want to proceed with the chemotherapy but do not think they can afford it.

What do you say to them?

Questions

FOR THE GENERAL PRACTITIONER. In approaching this case, it is useful to consider dif-ferent questions that can be asked by the generalist and the specialist. As discussed in Chapters 20 and 21, veterinarians often have enormous influence in determining what clients will choose by tailoring how alternative approaches are (or are not) revealed and discussed. Clearly, the generalist here has a legal obligation at least to inform Mr. and Mrs. Brown about the chemotherapy option, for this is regarded in the profession as a medically acceptable approach to such cases. Generalists have an especially important role to play before a referral is made to a specialty facility. Once specialty care is begun, it can sometimes be too late for clients to turn back. They may then be prepared or eager for advanced care. It may also be difficult to terminate treatment once it has begun, especially if it shows signs of success. The following questions are among those the generalist might ask in Sylvia's case and which I invite readers to consider:

- If I believe chemotherapy is not the best option for these clients, because of its cost and likelihood of providing only temporary relief for Sylvia, would it be right for me to attempt to influence them not to choose chemotherapy?
- Should I dissuade the Browns from choosing chemotherapy by emphasizing the negative aspects of this choice, including the cost, the uncertain probability of success, and the amount of time and energy they would have to expend?
- Is it appropriate to tell the Browns that I will speak to the specialist to see if some-thing could be done by her either to reduce her customary fee or to make special payment arrangements?
- Is it even appropriate for me to consider or worry about their ability to pay for chemotherapy? Shouldn't that be their concern and decision alone?
- Would it be appropriate to consider my own economic interests?* If the Browns face a large bill from the specialist, would they be unable to provide medical care for another animal they might want after Sylvia dies?

---

*Some readers may find this or other questions raised in this chapter offensive. My purpose here is not to suggest approaches that are morally defensible but to stimulate readers to formulate their own views. Sometimes, this is effectively done by asking questions some people might (and might rightly) find offensive.

FOR THE SPECIALIST. Once Sylvia and the Browns are referred to the specialist, the issue of affordability, as well as certain other ethical problems, are out of the generalist's hands. The specialist can ask different questions regarding the cost to these clients, including the following:

- Do I ever have, or do I have here, an ethical obligation to reduce my customary fee for clients who may not be able to afford the best care I can provide for their animal?
- Do I ever have, or do I have here, an ethical obligation to tailor arrangements for payment of the fee, such as installment payments, that will lessen the burden on the clients to pay either my customary or some other fee?
- To what extent would it be appropriate for me to ask the Browns to prove their inability to pay my customary fee or to demonstrate that they are capable of keeping up with a special payment plan? After all, when some clients say they "cannot" pay, what they really mean is that they do not want to pay. Why should I jeopardize my economic position and my ability to assist really needy clients unless I know that these clients need assistance?
- If I do sometimes have a moral duty to help certain clients with a fee, given that I cannot afford to help all clients, how do I decide which clients to help? To what extent might the following factors be relevant?
  –The patient's prognosis
  –The importance of the patient to the client
  –The client's financial ability to provide future veterinary care for the patient
  –The financial burden upon my practice of helping this client
  –The other kinds of cases and clients that might merit some kind of help
- Should I even be concerned about a client's ability to pay my fee? I am not a general service veterinarian but a specialist. If clients cannot afford a fee I believe to be reasonable and fair, that is unfortunate, but why is it my problem?

Ethical headaches

Sylvia's situation illustrates many of the ethical headaches (I use this term advisedly) that the availability of high-tech treatments raises for the profession. Some of these dilemmas result from high-tech medicine itself, others from the interplay between advanced veterinary procedures and the value clients place on their animals.

The inability of some clients to pay for advanced procedures will raise the problem and consequences of the affordability of veterinary care to a new level. It is not just that many such procedures are more expensive than older approaches and are therefore more difficult for many clients to afford. This greater expense is often coupled with previously unavailable prospects for a successful outcome. Therefore the reactions clients have to not being able to afford a procedure will often be intensified when they cannot afford a new advanced procedure—after they are presented with something new and special and are then told that their animal cannot have it.

Among these unpleasant consequences is, of course, unhappiness at not being able to help one's animal. Another is guilt about not being able to pay for such help. For many clients, guilt may soon turn to resentment against their veterinarian and perhaps against the veterinary profession. The phenomenon of resentment is one that many veterinarians have seen in more mundane circumstances when a client cannot afford a procedure. In any area of life, many people tend to want something even more after being told that it is now available for the first time. Moreover, many who are offered something at a higher price than they can afford tend to direct their frustrations at the person who offers the service and demands the price.

However, the problem of resentment of veterinarians by people unable to afford the best the profession can offer goes deeper than wanting something they cannot afford. Today, many clients place great value on their animals, either as members of the family in the case of pets, or as valuable economic assets in the case of some agricultural and performance animals. The veterinary profession has encouraged this high valuation of animals, especially in its promotion of the human-companion animal bond (see Chapter 15). As animals come to be regarded as essential to people's happiness and security, it is inevitable that more people will come to view medical care for these animals as a *right*, as something to which they and their animals are *entitled*. (I want to make clear that I am not defending such an attitude, but only describing it.) This is why many people today believe that medical care for people is a right. It is so important a condition of existence that to many, it seems something deserved simply by virtue of needing it so badly.

Of course, it follows from the principle that medical (or veterinary) care is a right, that someone else has an obligation to provide it. Many practitioners have encountered clients who believe that they are entitled to veterinary services and that it is the veterinarian's duty to provide it. This fact was illustrated dramatically by a 1994 *Boston Globe* article, which criticized one of the world's most famous veterinary hospitals for forcing clients to pay for lifesaving veterinary care. The front-page article, subtitled, "Some say money drives decisions of which animals to treat," reported, with astonishment and indignation, that at Boston's Angell Memorial Animal Hospital:

> ...a frequent occurrence ... is the ordering of a 'financial hold' just before surgery on an animal. In these cases, which occur several times a day, the financial office cancels surgery if a pet owner has not paid the bill upfront or agreed to a required financial plan.
>
> The employees [of Angell Memorial] also said on a number of occasions pet owners have opted to have their animals euthanized, in part because they cannot afford to pay a bill.[1]

The article did not mention that some of the advanced surgical procedures for which the Angell requires payment agreements cost hundreds or thousands of dollars. Although the article reported that the hospital offers $100,000 in subsidized care to needy clients each year, it lambasted the Massachusetts Society for the Prevention of Cruelty to Animals, which operates the Angell, for giving its busy executives raises at the same time some pet owners are unable to afford certain services. The article fairly seethed with anger that a veterinary hospital, especially one owned by a public charity, could even think of refusing services to clients who cannot pay for them.

This article illustrates how the option of euthanasia, which has always been available in veterinary medicine, can work together with the problem of affordability of advanced procedures to bring criticism upon veterinarians. Previously, clients may have had no choice other than to euthanize a beloved animal because there was nothing veterinary medicine could do. However, if there is a new or advanced procedure that can now help but is withheld because of clients' inability to pay for it, some of these clients will think they are being forced to kill their animal by greedy and heartless veterinarians.

Complaints against veterinarians for not subsidizing care for animals will increase as more advanced and expensive procedures become available. Thus the development of high-tech procedures will place the profession on the horns of a terrible dilemma. On the one hand, if veterinary medicine does not encourage the development of new, high-tech techniques, it will restrict its scientific and technological potential, and it will limit the ability of practitioners to gain income from advanced procedures. On the other hand, by developing expensive high-tech procedures, the profession may engender unhappiness, guilt, and resentment by people who cannot afford these procedures. The profession may also stimulate responses that can counter the profession's desire to elevate the images of its patients and itself, such as the retort that people who cannot afford expensive veterinary care should not complain because "having an animal is a luxury."

Approaches to these dilemmas

I do not mean to suggest that veterinarians never have an ethical obligation to assist clients who cannot afford care for their animals, high-tech or otherwise. However, people who think that veterinarians can or should generally subsidize services are in serious need of education—about both the economic pressures on veterinarians and the responsibilities of animal ownership. The following are some of the approaches individual doctors and the profession can take to the problem of the cost of high-tech care.

- One should never tantalize clients with high-tech or advanced procedures but should present these procedures as objectively and with as little emotionalism as possible.
- In discussing such procedures, one must give clients an accurate prediction of:
  –the cost of the procedure.
  –its likely effects on the animal, including a realistic appraisal of the probability of success.
  –the likely effects of the procedure on the clients, including the emotional commitment required to see the patient through the procedure and necessary follow-up care.
- One should not hesitate to explain to clients who have difficulty with the cost of an advanced procedure or treatment the reasons for this cost, including the expense of equipment, medicines, and support staff.
- One should allow clients sufficient time to make the decision regarding whether to undertake a high-tech or advanced procedure and make certain they understand if, once such a procedure is begun, fairness to the animal will require that the treatment not be terminated before completion.
- In general, it is not advisable to reduce one's fee for particular clients, as this can make managing one's practice difficult, threaten one's ability to serve other animals and clients, and diminish the perceived worth of a procedure and of one's services in general.
- One may consider ways of alleviating the burden of one's fee on certain clients, such as installment payments, but one should do so in a way that does not endanger one's economic position and assures that deserving clients and animals can be extended such an accommodation.

• The profession should attempt to educate the public regarding the responsibilities of pet ownership, through public relations campaigns and in classroom contact with primary and secondary school students. From an early age, people must be encouraged to understand that:

–Animals get sick and grow old.

–Veterinary medicine can provide new treatments for once intractable conditions, but owners must be prepared to pay for such treatments.

–People should not even consider owning an animal unless they are prepared for the possibility of advanced and expensive veterinary care.

–People should plan ahead for such an eventuality, by purchasing pet health insurance, or where such insurance is not available or does not cover advanced procedures, by taking other steps to assure they have sufficient funds to provide veterinary care. (For example, clients can open a savings account when they purchase an animal and contribute regularly to it.)

Such approaches may not remove entirely the pain and resentment some clients will feel at not being able to provide the best care for their animals. However, these approaches could prevent an onslaught of bad feelings against the profession and might at least encourage people to understand that veterinary care is a responsibility *they* must accept.

Humaneness to Patients

Sylvia's case also raises another important issue that is often intensified in high-tech veterinary medicine: whether an advanced procedure is humane to the patient. For reasons discussed in Chapter 21, Mr. and Mrs. Brown are morally obligated to consider the possible effects of the chemotherapy on their dog, and to ask whether these effects justify the likelihood of a temporary remission. Each aspect of the factual situation is critical. In Sylvia's case, a 75% to 80% chance of remission for 17 months seems quite promising. However, a low probability of success of a much shorter period of remission would make chemotherapy less justifiable. Table 21-1 presents some of the permutations and combinations of factors that are relevant in determining whether treatment or euthanasia is the appropriate approach. The following case amplifies these issues still further.

Case 22-2 Heroic measures. You are a clinician at a specialty facility. Your hospital has a state-of-the-art intensive care unit with the latest equipment and highly trained support staff.

You have been treating Samantha, a 6-year-old female Siamese cat referred by her local veterinarian for treatment of lymphosarcoma. From the time you have seen her, she has been anemic, extremely lethargic, and anorexic. Chemotherapy was begun 4 weeks ago, but Samantha has been unresponsive to it. Her condition is worsening daily. Her prognosis is extremely grave.

The clients tell you to "do everything possible" and that "cost is no object." You inform them that Samantha could be admitted to your intensive care unit, where chemotherapy might be continued. Additionally, it might soon be necessary to install a total parenteral nutrition (TPN) catheter so that she can be fed intravenously when she becomes unable to eat on her own. You tell the owners that, even in intensive care and with TPN, Samantha could die at any time, and probably will not survive for more than a week or two. The cost of Samantha's intensive care could exceed $1000.

The owners express enthusiasm about putting Samantha in intensive care because their son's life was saved in an intensive care unit after an automobile accident.

What do you do now?

Questions

- To what extent is it relevant for me and the clients to consider Samantha's likely quality of life, as distinct from any pain or distress she might experience? Put another way, if we can control her pain, could it still be wrong to place her in intensive care if she would exist in a vegetative or semivegetative state, in which she does not behave even remotely like a cat?
- Does it make sense to speak of an animal's "dying with dignity," and if it does, can it be argued that allowing, or forcing, Samantha to continue on is unseemly, undignified, or unfair to her?
- To what extent are the clients' interests in coming to terms with Samantha's inevitable death relevant to the appropriateness of maintaining her in intensive care? How strong a consideration is this in light of their apparent optimism? How should one respond to their enthusiasm and their comparison of Samantha's situation to that of their son?
- If I believe that it is unfair—to Samantha—to place her in intensive care, how strongly may I attempt to persuade the clients to have her euthanized?
  –May I browbeat or berate the clients if they insist on intensive care?
  –May I lie to them about Samantha's prognosis, making it appear even worse than it is to encourage them to choose euthanasia?
  –May I *insist* that Samantha be euthanized?
  –May I refuse to treat Samantha any further and tell the clients to take her elsewhere, or let her die at home?
  –May I insist that they visit Samantha frequently in intensive care, so that they will consent to euthanasia when they see how poorly she is doing?
- Would it be appropriate to "negotiate" a compromise with the clients, according to which, for example, Samantha would be admitted to the ICU but euthanized at my option when it is clear she is near death or in distress?
- If Samantha is admitted to the ICU, would it be appropriate to have her euthanized, to spare her further suffering, and then tell the clients she died on her own?
- To what extent, if any, is the fact that placing Samantha in intensive care and utilizing TPN will bring my facility needed revenue relevant to what I say to the clients?

Ethical headaches

Samantha's case illustrates additional ethical headaches the increasing availability of high-tech procedures will cause the profession. One of these dilemmas relates to the attractiveness of euthanasia. The veterinary profession's ability to euthanize hopelessly ill and suffering patients has enabled it to prevent much unnecessary suffering. However, as techniques such as TPN or the maintenance of animals on respirators become more readily available, many animals that surely ought to be euthanized or allowed to die without treatment will be kept alive. There are at least two ways in which high-tech medicine will contribute to increased unnecessary suffering of patients. First, as it becomes possible to treat more animals or keep them alive, many clients who previously consented to euthanasia because there was nothing else will choose treatment or maintenance. Second, the very existence and increasing availability of high-tech procedures will surely create a "technological imperative" for more and more veterinary hospitals to provide it. If advanced equipment and techniques are perceived as "state-of-the-art," veterinarians who want to remain "on the cutting edge" will feel compelled to offer them. This compulsion will be fueled in part by the demands of clients for these procedures. The effects of such a technological imperative can already be seen in intensive care units, which all veterinary schools and many large specialty practices now view as mandatory. Although these units undoubtedly do much good, some contain animals that are terminally ill, suffering, or subsisting in a vegetative state—animals veterinarians have no business keeping alive.

There is, then, a decidedly dark side to high-tech veterinary medicine that will be as inevitable as its wonderful ability to help animals. Because more and more clients will want to keep alive animals that ought to be euthanized, the role of the veterinarian in objectively counseling what is in the patient's interest will take on added importance. This role may not be easy to assume, especially if one has an intensive care unit or can provide advanced procedures. When a practice offers revenue-generating, high-tech medicine, or its doctors just feel the understandable professional duty to provide the very best medicine possible, how will one assure that patients' interests are protected?

Approaches to these dilemmas

There are many ways veterinarians can seek to protect their patients' interests when advanced and potentially stressful procedures are being considered, among them the following:

- In discussing and explaining a high-tech or advanced procedure, make certain to explain fully the likely effects on the patient and encourage the client to consider whether the likely benefits are worth the risks to the patient.
- Consider asking the client to seek a second opinion, from another doctor in the practice, or from another veterinarian, especially regarding a complex or experimental high-tech procedure.
- If other patients have undergone the procedure, consider asking the client whether she would want to meet with another client whose animal has received the treatment to verify how it is likely to affect the patient.
- Do not allow the medical challenge of an "interesting" case to divert your attention from your obligation to serve the patient's interests.
- When clients are so eager to proceed with an advanced treatment that they are not giving due regard to the patient's interests, it is appropriate, indeed often mandatory, to assume the role of the animal's advocate.
- It is often beneficial for a specialist recommending a high-tech procedure to have the clients speak first with their family veterinarian, who may know them and their animal better than the specialist, and who may be able to provide objective and compassionate advice.
- The *Principles of Veterinary Medical Ethics* state that "Veterinarians should consider first the welfare of the patient for the purpose of relieving suffering and disability while causing a minimum of pain or fright. Benefit to the patient should transcend personal advantage or monetary gain in decisions concerning therapy."[2] This rule is intended to discourage not just the administration of therapies that benefit practitioners at the expense of patients but also procedures that cause patients unjustifiable suffering or disability.

Humaneness to Clients

Cases 22-1 and 22-2 raise another issue commonly raised by high-tech or advanced procedures: the importance of treating clients humanely. In both cases, the advanced procedure risks harm to the clients as well as the patient. The potential for acting against a client's interests cannot be approached with the simplistic statement that a veterinarian "serves the animal and not the client." As argued throughout this book, veterinarians typically serve *both*, and have moral obligations to *both*.

Questions

The cases of Sylvia and Samantha, like many situations in which clients can choose an advanced procedure that risks harm to themselves, pose many ethical questions, including the following:
- To what extent, if any, am I obligated to protect clients against an emotionally or economically harmful procedure, if this is what they want?
- Is it ever appropriate to shade my discussion of the options or not mention certain options to assure that clients make a choice that does not harm them economically or psychologically?
- Is it ever appropriate to refuse to perform an advanced procedure that might be beneficial to the patient in order to protect clients economically or psychologically?
- Is it ever appropriate to lie about the costs of a procedure or its effects on the animal to protect a client?
- Is it ever appropriate to deny the client a special payment option, or a reduced fee, not because such steps are necessary to protect one's own economic position, but to protect the client's economic interests?
- To what extent, if at all, should one attempt to learn more about clients' personal or economic affairs to determine how they will tolerate a high-tech procedure?
- Once one agrees to perform a procedure one knows will be difficult for a client, to what extent is one obligated to try to help the client through the difficulties, for example, by comforting or counseling the client, or referring the client to a mental health professional?

Ethical headaches and approaches to these dilemmas

Another ethical dilemma intensified by advanced procedures is faced by any profession that must allow its clients to make their own decisions. Allowing clients to determine the course of events will sometimes harm them because clients will sometimes make bad decisions. This dilemma is often intensified by high-tech or advanced veterinary procedures, which can result in significant economic and psychological burdens for clients.

As is the case with all the ethical dilemmas posed by high-tech procedures, there are many ways of approaching questions that force one to consider how to protect the interests of clients. Among these are the following:
- In discussing and explaining a high-tech or advanced procedure, make certain to explain fully the likely effects on the client and the client's family, including:
  – the economic costs.
  – the time and energy that will be required to see the patient through the procedure.

—the effects having the animal undergo the treatment may have on other family members, especially children and the elderly.

—the likelihood that the treatment will succeed and of the eventual need for terminating treatment or for euthanasia.

• If other clients' animals have undergone the procedure, and this client voices concern about how he or his family will be affected by it, consider asking the client whether he might want to meet with one or more of these other clients to learn about how the procedure affected them.

• Do not allow the medical challenge of an "interesting" case to divert your attention from your obligation to serve the client's interests.

• As always, give the client time to make a decision whether to authorize a procedure.

• As always, be very careful how you respond to the question "What would you do if this were your animal?" It is not always possible to know precisely what the animal means to the client, and you may be blamed later for making a decision the client claims she would not have made.

Nonuniversal Affordability

Another set of issues long present in veterinary practice but intensified by high-tech and advanced medicine is raised by the fact that only some clients can afford a procedure that will help their animal. This is not new. However, as advanced procedures become available, there will likely be many more clients who cannot afford the best the profession can provide because the best will more frequently consist of advanced and sophisticated treatments, which tend to be more expensive than less sophisticated procedures.

> *Case 22-3 Radiotherapy for Winston.* A 1989 article in the Toronto Globe and Mail *told about Winston, a 14-year-old male Standard Poodle.*[3] *Winston had a walnut-sized malignant tumor in his foot, and underwent radiation treatment for it at Canada's first animal cancer radiation clinic at the University of Guelph's Ontario Veterinary College.*
>
> *Winston's therapy, which cost his owner $375, went well, but the treatment stirred considerable controversy. As the article reported, the Guelph cancer clinic treats approximately 100 pets a year at an average cost of $1,000 per animal. At the same time, according to the article:*
>
>> *"...the country's biggest cancer centre, the Princess Margaret Hospital in Toronto, declared a crisis: two of its 10 radiation machines are shut down, and 280 new patients are waiting up to seven weeks for treatment. ...The main problem is a severe world-wide shortage of trained technologists to run the radiation machines."*
>
> *The article related that the physician of Winston's owner, and others, were furious that animals like Winston could be treated expeditiously for owners able to pay for it, while people throughout Canada were waiting weeks for similar kinds of therapy. The article noted that the Guelph radiation unit was donated by a human hospital that had purchased more advanced equipment. However, the article raised several questions, which were stated in a manner not entirely sympathetic to animals, pet owners, or veterinarians:*
>
>> *"Why should animals be treated ahead of humans? Why do we deliberately cause cancer in experimental animals, yet spend thousands of dollars to treat it in others? Will pets suffer at the hands of owners who want to keep them alive for selfish reasons? What can be said about a society that places pets on an equal footing with people?"*
>
> The Globe and Mail *piece closed with a lament from a medical ethicist that "We're treating animals better than some people."*

Questions

This story is useful in considering problems raised by the inability of some clients to afford advanced services. The issue of a perceived disparity between some lucky animals and many unlucky humans usually arises in discussions of expensive high-tech veterinary procedures. People who cannot afford to help their animals while others can, often move from the complaint that "It isn't fair *she* can afford to help her animal" to "It's unfair that an *animal* gets help when so many people need medical care." The *Globe and Mail* article also illustrates that there are people who will criticize or ridicule high-tech veterinary medicine because of problems in the human medical care system.

The following are among the questions veterinarians can ask when contemplating an expensive advanced procedure affordable only to some clients:

- Should I feel guilty because only some clients can afford high-tech procedures?
- Do I have an ethical obligation to assist clients who cannot afford to pay for such procedures, either by reducing my fee or making it easier for clients to pay the fee?
- If I do sometimes have such an obligation, what factors might be relevant in determining when I have it? For example, should I be more willing to extend financial assistance if the advanced procedure has a higher probability of success? Is sought by clients more dedicated to their animal than others? Is not as expensive as others?
- How should I respond to the inevitable question whether it is right for animals to be treated in ways that many people cannot afford for themselves and families?

Ethical headaches

The limited affordability of certain high-tech procedures raises many of the same dilemmas for the profession as the inability of some clients to afford more standard procedures, but with potentially more unpleasant consequences.

If veterinarians seek to develop and offer high-tech procedures, they will enable a continuing elevation of the regard many clients have for their animals. People who want to value their animals highly will be more able to do so if they can help these animals live longer and better lives. On the other hand, by offering even more procedures many people cannot afford, the profession risks resentment from an increasing number of people who will not be able to pay for these procedures. This resentment can harm not only the good name of veterinarians and their ability to convince clients that their recommendations are generally trustworthy. Resentment fueled by the limited affordability of high-tech procedures can diminish the image of the veterinary patient, which in turn, can result in more general reluctance by clients to seek veterinary services. Some people who cannot afford to pay for advanced veterinary care may turn against animals, thinking that they are just not worth the expense. Others who cannot afford high-tech veterinary services may feel better supposing that having a pet is "just a luxury," like having an expensive car or piece of jewelry—something one can do very well without.

Approaches to these dilemmas

The following are among the approaches the profession can take to issues raised by the nonuniversal affordability of advanced procedures.

- Clients and the public should be educated about how much advanced procedures cost veterinarians.

- Clients and the public should not be tantalized with any new high-tech procedure unless it has been established to have a reasonable degree of success.
- Once an advanced procedure is shown to be effective, efforts should be made to reduce its cost. For example, the manufacturer of a drug or appliance might be encouraged to increase production to reduce unit cost, donations of used equipment from human hospitals can be sought, and groups of veterinarians can refer clients to a single facility that has an expensive piece of machinery or offers a costly procedure, rather than incurring unnecessary expense by investing in such equipment themselves.
- The profession should encourage the development of animal health insurance plans that cover high-tech procedures.
- The profession should avoid telling those who cannot afford the most advanced procedures that having an animal is "a luxury," but should rather stress that animals are worth the responsibilities necessary to care for them.
- Veterinarians should be prepared to explain why caring well for animals is not inconsistent with caring well for people.

Limited Resources

Another set of ethical challenges raised by high-tech and advanced veterinary procedures relates to the fact that some of these procedures are in short supply and sometimes cannot be offered to all clients able to pay for them. Scarcity of resources can result from different factors such as the expense of equipment that allows only certain practices to possess it, a shortage of practitioners with sufficient training to do a procedure properly, the difficulty or expense of procuring or maintaining advanced equipment, or a larger population of animals requiring an advanced procedure than veterinarians can accommodate. Intensive care units illustrate how the demand for high-tech procedures can exceed its supply. As in human medicine, there may often be more patients that can benefit from these facilities than the facilities can help. As in human medicine, the limited number of available intensive care beds sometimes compels the facility to decide that only certain patients will gain entry and that some intensive care patients should no longer be maintained, so that other patients can be treated.

Case 22-4 To transfuse or not to transfuse? Ashley, a 4-year-old spayed female domestic cat is brought to your hospital. A year ago she was diagnosed as feline leukemia positive. She remained asymptomatic until several months ago when she began to lose weight and became somewhat lethargic. Blood tests done at that time indicated moderate anemia, neutropenia, and lymphocytosis. You informed the client that Ashley was beginning to succumb to the disease and that she should be brought back as soon as she started feeling worse.

On this visit, Ashley looks terrible. She is very weak. Her mucous membranes are pale. Blood is drawn again. The hematocrit has fallen to 11% and the hemoglobin to 3.0 gm/dl. Neutrophils are 3.9×10^3/ml and lymphocytes 7×10^3/ml.

It is now clear that unless something is done soon, Ashley will deteriorate rapidly. She can be euthanized now. However, you can order blood for a transfusion, which will likely improve her condition temporarily, but not affect the underlying disease. Subsequent transfusions would be possible, but eventually the leukemia will progress to the point where transfusions will be useless.

One specialty hospital in your area maintains a blood bank, but refuses to release any blood for transfusion to leukemic cats because of the short supply of blood and a policy decision to provide blood only for patients with a good ultimate prognosis. A hospital maintained by a humane society also has a blood bank but will allow only one transfusion per feline leukemia case to allow owners to come to terms with the necessity of euthanasia while providing temporary alleviation of symptoms. A nearby veterinary school hospital blood bank provides blood on a first-come first-served basis, even to feline leukemia patients, if it is available.

The client does not know about any of these options. What do you tell and advise her?

Questions

This case, like others discussed in this chapter, illustrates how a situation in which an advanced treatment or technique can be offered raises ethical issues relating to fairness to patients and clients. Among such questions are the following:

- Is it appropriate not to mention the option of a transfusion if I believe that this is not in the best interests of Ashley or the client?
- In deciding whether to mention, or how strongly to advise, a transfusion, is it appropriate to consider the needs of other patients, of mine or of other veterinarians, that might benefit more from blood and might be denied blood if it goes to Ashley?
- Is it appropriate for an animal blood bank to refuse to supply blood to a specific animal that can benefit from it:
  –based on a shortage that might exist for subsequent potential patients, even if blood is presently available?
  –based on its view that it is ethically wrong to allow any or any more than a limited number of transfusions even when blood is available?
- If it is appropriate to ration limited resources, what criteria for doing so should be utilized? To what extent, for example, is the ultimate prognosis relevant? The importance of the animal to the client? The age of the animal and its likely life span even if the procedure is successful? The ability of the client to pay?
- In discussing with a client the advisability of providing a limited resource, to what extent, if any, is it appropriate to mention the need other animals might have for the resource?

Ethical headaches

Companion animal veterinarians, like physicians, are accustomed to focusing on the needs of one patient at a time. They are not accustomed to considering the interests of other current or potential patients in deciding how to treat the patient at hand. If veterinarians must allocate or ration resources, how should this be done? Is it acceptable for different facilities to have differing approaches, as in Case 22-4? Will veterinarians who ration advanced procedures or treatments arouse resentment from clients who want to obtain the resource for their animals? If veterinarians allow clients (or clients' ability to pay) to decide which patients receive a scarce resource, will they risk treating unfairly other animals and clients that might be more deserving of the resource? If hospitals allow individual doctors discretion in allocating scarce resources, how can they assure that appropriate criteria are used, and used correctly, in deciding which patients receive these resources? As Ashley's situation illustrates, the best response to a scarce resource might not always be increasing its supply.

Approaches to these dilemmas

• It is important for facilities that do offer advanced procedures to institute consistent policies regarding the allocation of such procedures if they are in limited supply (see Chapter 10). If scarce resources are distributed inconsistently or arbitrarily, some deserving patients and clients will be deprived unfairly, others will benefit unfairly, and many clients are sure to complain.

• Without violating antitrust laws, veterinarians should attempt to work together to prevent methods of providing limited resources that can unnecessarily lead to scarcity or maldistribution. For example, some practices consider it a badge of pride to maintain their own blood bank. What is in short supply at one blood bank may be in ample supply at another, and it would be unfortunate if some animals were denied blood because the resource from the latter is unknown or unavailable to a patient at the former. This possibility argues for the establishment of regional or even national centers for blood or other kinds of resources and treatments from which availability could be maximized.

• Great sensitivity must be exhibited toward clients when resources are too limited to provide for their animal. Policies regarding the availability of such resources should be explained clearly and sympathetically, without giving clients the impression that their animal is less important than another.

Animal "Donors"
Animals kept as living donors

The case of Ashley is useful in considering issues raised by limited affordability. It illustrates that treatment resources are sometimes scarce because these resources must come from other animals. Consider the following case:

> *Case 22-5 Is there any way out of here?* *You have recently joined a small animal practice as an associate doctor. Six months ago, the practice obtained a 50-pound 1-year-old male mixed breed dog from the local animal shelter for use as a blood donor. The dog, named "Donordog" is housed in a pen in the hospital's boarding facility. Donordog is taken outside the hospital for a walk several times a day by hospital staff and is occasionally placed in one of the facility's outdoor runs when one of these is not being used by a boarded dog. Aside from these times, Donordog never leaves his pen. This is the second Donordog. The first served as the hospital's blood donor and lived under the conditions in which the current Donordog lives for 8 years, when he was euthanized after becoming ill.*
> *Are there any ethical issues here? If so, what should you say or do?*

Questions

There are many questions one can ask about the case of Donordog and the general issue of keeping dogs and cats as blood donors. Among these are the following, which I invite readers to consider.

• What, if anything, is owed to animals kept in veterinary facilities as blood donors?
 –May they be kept in cages or pens, or should they be afforded a more natural or enjoyable life? For example, should some of these animals be taken home evenings or allowed to roam in parts of the facility?

–How much expense is a practice morally obligated to incur to provide "donor" animals satisfactory conditions? To what extent is a practice entitled to consider the costs to owners of recipient animals in determining how much to spend on "donor" animals?

–To what extent, if any, are veterinarians obligated to provide "donor" animals medical care and treatments, in return for the service provided by these animals?

• Should cats and dogs kept as blood donors be retired after some period of time, that is, adopted out to members of the public or staff in return for their service, rather than kept as donors until they are no longer useful, and then euthanized?

• Is it appropriate to use as donors cats or dogs from shelters, if this means taking from these institutions young or healthy animals that might be adopted by members of the public who would provide them with a better life?

• Greyhounds are excellent blood donors because they have long necks suitable for venipuncture and have a greater percentage of red cells than most dogs.[4] Is it appropriate to use former racing greyhounds, which have already done considerable service to people, sometimes under less than optimal conditions? (See Chapter 23.) If so, does one owe to such animals something over and above what one would owe to other kinds of "donor" animals, such as even better living conditions and attempts to adopt them out after some period of time if kept as inhouse donors?

• One innovative program coordinates the adoption of greyhounds to families in an area and utilizes these dogs as donors for small, regional blood banks.[4] To what extent are facilities that maintain blood banks ethically obligated to seek blood from animals owned by clients rather than keeping dedicated blood donors?

Use of animals for organ and tissue transplants

Animals employed as blood donors usually remain alive, at least for a time. Some high-tech procedures require that donors be located when about to die, or more typically, these procedures can involve the killing of these animals. Organs and tissue for transplantation also tend to be a limited resource in part because of the need to find or euthanize animals with usable organs or tissues.

There is already a tendency, in both the popular and veterinary literature, to focus on the animal receiving a transplant and to overlook or minimize what must sometimes be done to another animal to make the transplant possible. For example, a 1994 article on the cost of veterinary care in *Money* magazine, described an Oregon family whose 8-year-old cat received a kidney transplant:

> Two months later, the fortunate feline returned home with a functioning kidney and a bill for $6,000. Twice-daily doses of cyclosporine capsules (to prevent tissue rejection) and regular blood tests currently cost … about $2,500 a year. Next year, when testing is reduced, annual expenses will become $2,000 for as long as the kidney lasts—an estimated three to five years … [The family] together agreed to forego fancy vacations for a few years to meet the expense. 'This drew us together tremendously. It's made us more of a family,' [stated one of the cat's owners].[5]

The article did not mention the source of this fortunate feline's new kidney.

A more scholarly discussion of bone grafting and banking illustrates how veterinarians can become focused on medical issues raised by a high-tech procedure. This paper considers how to set up a bone bank in one's practice "as a convenient place to store cortical allografts for multiple recipients."[6] The article discusses conditions for which such allografts are indicated, selecting and removing bone tissue from a "euthanized donor dog," methods of fixation, potential complications, "donor" selection, methods of preserving banked bone tissue, and the preparation of preserved bone for transplantation. Regarding the advantages of bone banking, the authors of this paper write:

> ...it may be difficult to find a healthy animal of the appropriate size when a cortical allograft is needed. By establishing a bone bank, the clinician can be prepared for allograft transplantation in advance of surgery. When a bone bank is established, donor dogs can be used more efficiently because a single dog can provide grafts to multiple recipients. The need for a concurrent surgical procedure is eliminated; therefore, the total cost of surgery is reduced.
>
> Because one donor can potentially provide bone to many recipients, careful selection is important to prevent transfer of infectious disease. Donors must undergo complete physical examination and complete blood cell count and must test negative for *Brucella canis*. Young, adult, large-breed dogs with a documented vaccination history are ideal candidates.[7]

Nowhere does this article mention where such healthy "donors" might be obtained. Nowhere does the article acknowledge ethical questions that must be faced by clinicians seeking to maintain a bone bank.

There are three potential sources for bone, kidneys, corneas, or other kinds of organs or tissues veterinarians might want to transplant: client-owned animals, shelter animals, and purpose-bred animals. Each source raises ethical questions.

OWNED ANIMALS. It would be ideal if transplantable body parts could all come from animals that are brought to a facility near death or in need of euthanasia. However, as the article on bone grafting illustrates, medical requirements sometimes dictate the use of young or healthy animals. These animals must sometimes be killed to provide the needed resources. It would appear that a fertile source of such "donors" among client-owned animals would be candidates for what I have termed "convenience euthanasia": healthy animals, the owners of which simply no longer want them. Other potential "donors" may be animals with minor medical problems that can be cured, but the animals' owners either do not want or cannot afford treatment. In Chapter 21, I argue that convenience euthanasia is not in the interests of patients, clients, or the profession. Will a doctor who needs transplantable tissue be so interested in the needs of the recipient that she will overlook the ethical problems in convenience euthanasia and will quickly accede to a client's wishes to be rid of an animal—not because doing so would benefit *this* patient, but because tissue is needed for *another* patient? There are various ways of overlooking or minimizing the interests of one patient to smooth the way for obtaining body parts for another. One might be tempted not to disclose all possible treatment options, or exaggerate the severity of the patient's condition or the cost of treatment, to assure that the client will choose euthanasia and provide transplantable tissue. One might be less interested in working out financial arrangements with clients who want to help their pet but would have some economic difficulty doing so, so that transplantable tissue can be offered to clients who are eager to pay for it. In sum, obtaining transplantable organs or tissues from *any* of one's current patients raises a conflict of interest for a veterinarian: one can be tempted to sacrifice the needs of some patients and clients to satisfy the needs of other patients and clients.

SHELTER ANIMALS. Obtaining donors from shelters or pounds also presents ethical problems. Many shelters do not want to release, and many are prohibited by law from releasing, animals for purposes other than adoption. Will some practitioners (or more likely, unscrupulous animal dealers from which donors might be purchased) pose as adopters to obtain "donor" animals? Even where obtaining a "donor" from a shelter is done openly and lawfully, there is a danger that animals capable of being adopted by people who want them as pets will become "donors" instead—if veterinarians scour these facilities for healthy young specimens and get to them before members of the public can. One could argue that most animals in shelters have gone through enough already and that it is therefore preferable to offer those capable of being adopted by loving owners continuing life as a pet. Why, it can be asked, are these animals' interests any less important than those needing transplants?

PURPOSE-BRED "DONOR" ANIMALS. Using animals bred and kept specifically to provide transplantable body parts would obviate conflicts of interest that would arise from obtaining donors from clients. Nevertheless, this approach also raises ethical questions. Who will breed and keep these animals? Can one assure they will be treated properly, and not be subjected to the kinds of neglect or abuse characteristic of some so-called "puppy mills?" How will one assure that animals certified as purpose-bred do not come from shelters or are not people's pets, stolen off the streets? Is it seemly for veterinarians to maintain facilities in which animals are bred and kept for body parts, while at the same time presenting themselves to the public as healers of animals? Is it reasonable to breed dogs and cats for body parts when so many unwanted animals are in shelters and could provide transplantable tissue for considerably less cost than would be associated with purpose-breeding?

Approaches to these dilemmas

Enthusiasm for the "miracle" of transplantation must be accompanied by serious consideration of these and other ethical questions relating to the use of animal parts. The following principles are offered to stimulate discussion:

- No client-owned or shelter animal should be euthanized with the primary purpose of obtaining organs or tissues for transplantation. Veterinarians can avoid a conflict of interest only if tissue is obtained from animals the euthanasia of which is advisable or unavoidable for other medically or ethically appropriate reasons.
- Any owner whose animal will be used for transplantable tissue must exercise a fully informed consent to such use. Owners have not only a moral but also a legal[8] right to know about and control the disposition of their animals' remains. They must be told before authorizing euthanasia whether and how their animals' body parts will be used. Incomplete or incorrect representations about what will be done with transplantable tissue are unacceptable.
- The profession should pay sustained attention to ethical issues raised by various sources and uses of transplantable animal tissue.

Professional Definition

One of the most important ethical choices veterinarians must make is how they, individually and as a profession, want to define their role. As discussed in Chapter 16, there is currently a battle between a model of veterinary practice as a business and more traditional images of the veterinarian as a healer of patients and a friend of clients. I have argued that these traditional images are in the long-term best interests of clients, patients, and veterinarians.

Ethical headaches

At first glance, the advent of high-tech and advanced procedures might appear destined to strengthen the model of the veterinarian as healer. High-tech procedures seem clearly directed at healing. They seem to raise the level of concern for animal health to new heights. Indeed, not only is high-tech veterinary medicine similar to human medicine, much of high-tech veterinary medicine is *identical* to human medicine, utilizing the same kinds of equipment, drugs, and techniques. Surely, it might be argued, high-tech procedures will not only enable, but also require, veterinarians to convince the public that veterinary medicine is a healing profession, capable of dedicating the most scientifically sophisticated medical tools to helping patients.

There is, however, much in high-tech medicine that could draw practitioners toward a less patient-oriented, more entrepreneurial approach. High-tech veterinary medicine is expensive. It can require costly machinery and drugs and highly paid staff. Although veterinary school hospitals, most of which are owned by state governments, might be able to justify such expenditures without attendant profits, this will not be possible for private practices. Some practices with expensive high-tech facilities may feel compelled to keep these facilities filled and used, even if doing so is not always in the best interests of patients and clients. Some practices may turn to aggressive promotional behavior to sell, sell, and sell again to pay for the high overhead of high-tech. Some practices faced with high-tech expenses could find it necessary to accept ownership by capital-rich nonveterinarians or nonveterinary companies (see Chapter 16).

Another possible unfortunate consequence of high-tech medicine could be a take-over of the market for veterinary services by enormous "mega-practices," whose larger incomes might be necessary to provide high-tech services. Large veterinary hospitals have a great deal to offer, but so does the one-, two-, or three-doctor practice, which is sometimes capable of more personalized attention and is preferred by some clients.

Potential legal problems may also result from the trend toward high-tech medicine. The increased use of advanced procedures will surely lead to more, and more expensive, malpractice lawsuits. Clients who spend a good deal of money are more likely to sue to recover their expenses if something goes wrong. More importantly, treatments resembling those in human medicine may motivate courts to allow clients to recover damages for their emotional distress caused by a veterinarian's negligent care of their animals. It seems incongruous for the profession to maintain animals in intensive care units, to treat their cancers with chemotherapy and radiotherapy, to mend their broken bones with surgically implanted pins, to save their teeth with root canals, to manage a range of medical maladies with the latest miracle drugs, and to claim—when mistakes are made—that clients should not be allowed to sue for emotional distress because their animals are just pieces of property like televisions sets or sofas (see Chapter 15).

∾ ETHICAL ISSUES IN INNOVATIVE AND EXPERIMENTAL VETERINARY MEDICINE

High-tech and advanced procedures do not arrive from nowhere. They must be developed and tested before they can be utilized in the general patient population. This process of development itself raises important ethical problems.

"Innovative" and "Experimental" Procedures

Medical jurisprudence has traditionally used the term "experimental" to refer to procedures, techniques, appliances, or drugs that have not gained sufficient general acceptance or use to be considered a standard part of general or specialty practice. It is in this sense, for example, that some medical insurance policies deny coverage for heart or bone marrow transplants on the grounds that these procedures are "experimental."

This is not a useful way of speaking about "experimental" procedures. It lumps together nonstandard procedures that are part of what can rightly be called an experiment or experimental trial with those that are tried in less formal ways by individual doctors or groups of practitioners.

I find it more helpful to classify as "innovative" rather than experimental any procedure or technique that is not, or is not yet, considered standard in general or specialty practice but is nevertheless within the bounds of medically accepted approaches. "Innovative" is not synonymous with "new." There can be innovative procedures that were first conceived or tried some time ago, but have not yet gained general acceptance. In contrast, I shall reserve the term "experimental" for procedures being developed or tested in a scientific experiment, which in veterinary or human medicine usually involves studying the effects of a technique on a number of subjects, including appropriate controls, to verify its efficacy or safety.[9] As will be discussed, "experimentation" in this sense raises distinctive ethical issues not presented by nonexperimental innovative procedures.

It is often difficult to determine whether a procedure is "innovative." A procedure ceases to be innovative when the profession begins to regard it as sufficiently established to be considered whenever certain circumstances or conditions arise. There can be a significant period of time when a procedure remains in a "gray area," in which some doctors regard it as a standard approach and others do not. For our purposes, the most important issue is not whether a procedure is clearly "innovative," but whether it gives rise to ethical issues of a kind that are typically raised by innovative procedures.

Ethical Issues Raised by Innovative Procedures

Case 22-6 Hormone therapy or ovariohysterectomy? You are a general practitioner.

On the staff of a nearby specialty hospital is a board-certified theriogenologist. She has been using PGF2α, a prostaglandin, in the treatment of pyometra in dogs. There are several reports in the literature that injections of PGF2α can be beneficial in the treatment of pyometra, and the theriogenologist has been successful with it in about half the cases in which she has tried it. PGF2α causes contractions and drainage of the uterus as well as increased blood flow. Common side effects include vomiting, diarrhea, hypersalivation, and rapid breathing. Even when PGF2α is beneficial for the treatment of pyometra, recurrence may occur at the next estrus.

Hannah, a 5-year-old intact female Standard Poodle presents with a severe pyometra. She is in great discomfort. She has never been pregnant before, despite efforts to breed her. The owners tell you she is a "show dog" and that they want puppies to sell. During the past 4 years, Hannah has had several episodes of pyometra.

You would prefer to perform an ovariohysterectomy. This treatment, unlike the prostaglandin, precludes breeding, but also eliminates the possibility of recurrence of pyometra. It would also avoid the side-effects of the PGF2α.

The owners want your advice. They say that unless Hannah can be bred, they have no use for her and want her euthanized. Money is no object.

What do you advise?

Questions

This case evokes many of the same questions as do the others discussed thus far in this chapter. However, Hannah's situation raises in a sharper way the general question of how much a veterinary patient's interests count. In our other cases, the client appeared eager to help the patient at least in part for the patient's own sake. In Hannah's case, one does not have to turn to a high-tech or innovative procedure to help the patient. A standard, routine treatment will cure her malady. An innovative procedure is under consideration because it might satisfy the client's wishes, but in a way likely to cause the patient discomfort and distress.

Fortunately, not all innovative procedures are done primarily, or solely, with the intention of benefiting clients at the expense of patients. However, Hannah's case illustrates ethical issues that do tend to arise from innovative procedures more often than from more standard techniques. Because innovative procedures are not generally accepted or available, clients are less likely to know about them and to appreciate their effects. (Indeed, doctors may still be learning about their effects.) Therefore one can probably get away with not informing a client about a possible innovative procedure more often than one could with a standard procedure because the client would otherwise not know of it. (Veterinarians are generally not obligated legally to inform clients about procedures that are not generally accepted within the profession.) Second, because an innovative procedure is likely to be sophisticated, a practitioner may have little trouble convincing a client to agree to it by impressing the client with scientific hypotheses and data to support doing it. Finally, a practitioner who is likely to perform an innovative procedure such as prostaglandin therapy for pyometra will almost certainly have a scientific interest in determining whether the therapy is effective. Such an interest sometimes can seem more important than the patient, which can become a means toward the testing of a hypothesis rather than the object of one's loyalty. When, as in Hannah's case, the innovative procedure can be associated with some harm to the patient, there may be a tendency to look away from this harm toward a potential scientific advance.

The following questions relate to the key ethical issue raised by Hannah's case: under what circumstances, if any, may a veterinarian subject a patient to a procedure that is less beneficial, indeed potentially harmful, to it to serve the client's needs when there exists a proven technique that would serve the patient's needs?

- To what extent is Hannah's value as a show dog relevant in deciding whether to mention, recommend, or perform prostaglandin therapy? Would the procedure be more justifiable if she were truly champion quality than if she were more ordinary show quality? Than if she were not even show quality? Would the procedure be more justifiable if the owners were experienced and successful breeders who could well make a great deal of money on Hannah's puppies than if they were less successful "backyard breeders?" Would the procedure be justifiable if they in fact have had no experience breeding and selling puppies?

- To what extent, if any, is the fact that Standard Poodle puppies, and many other kinds of puppies, are readily available to potential owners, relevant in determining the appropriateness of this therapy on Hannah?

- To what extent, if at all, is it important that Hannah is a dog? Would one have the same reaction if this case involved administering a potentially distressful therapy to a cow to facilitate its being able to produce valuable offspring?

- Should one let a client's threat to put an animal down motivate one to approve a procedure less beneficial to it? How strong is the argument that Hannah is better off alive suffering through PGF2α than dead? What steps, if any, would be appropriate to try to save Hannah if one decided one could not recommend or offer prostaglandin therapy?

- If the probability of the success of the prostaglandin therapy improved (say to 75% or 95%), would the therapy be more justifiable if it still causes distress and discomfort?

- To what extent is it relevant that performing the therapy on Hannah might lead to advances in knowledge and eventually improvement in the success of the therapy?

- Should one tell the clients about the prostaglandin therapy if one believes that it is wrong to do it in Hannah's case and knows that telling them will make the therapy inevitable?

Case 22-7 Amputation or preoperative chemotherapy? You are board-certified in internal medicine and practice at a large specialty hospital. George, a 7-year-old intact male Boxer, has been referred to you by George's regular doctor. George has been limping on his right hind leg for several weeks and is not eating well. There is a slight swelling over the proximal right tibia with some muscle atrophy.

You ordered blood work, radiographs, and a bone scan. Blood results were within normal ranges, but the radiographs and scan revealed a probable primary tumor in the proximal tibia, without visible bone metastasis. Radiographs of the chest did not indicate pulmonary metastases. You then had a biopsy done, which confirmed early stage osteosarcoma.

Standard therapy for George's condition is amputation of the limb followed by chemotherapy with cisplatin. Approximately half of your patients like George have survived for longer than 1 year with a good quality of life. You have every reason to believe that George will do fine without the leg.

When visiting a colleague at your state's veterinary school you heard a presentation on the use of preoperative chemotherapy for osteosarcoma that was based on a treatment used for human osteosarcoma. This approach utilizes several injections of an antitumor antibiotic followed by either bone resection or amputation and further chemotherapy if indicated. The treatment is utilized frequently in human medicine.

At the presentation, case studies were reported, and literature cited, indicating that in early stage osteosarcoma such as George's, the new therapy is as effective on dogs as immediate amputation and cisplatin. However, one study done at another veterinary school reported that the new approach has a slightly lower probability than the standard therapy of resulting in 1 year survival.

You would like to try the new treatment on George because you think he is a good candidate for it and because your veterinary school colleagues would like to know more about how the treatment works when administered in other facilities. You are however, aware that this is not standard therapy, and there may be a greater risk of metastases if amputation and cisplatin chemotherapy are not done now.

What do you tell and advise George's owner?

Case 22-8 **Surgery or radiotherapy for Goliath?** *You are a second-year resident at a veterinary school. Your educational program requires that you have three clinical reports accepted by refereed journals.*

You are presented with the Gleasons, and Goliath, their 11-year-old intact male Pomeranian. Goliath has a large (for Goliath) perianal gland adenoma. The growth is ulcerated and bleeds frequently. Defecation is difficult and uncomfortable.

The standard treatment for Goliath's condition is surgical excision of the adenoma and castration. Castration, by removing the testicular hormones, is sometimes utilized alone for this benign condition because it can result in regression of the tumor. In Goliath's case, excision of the adenoma is advisable because of its size. Castration will also decrease the probability of new tumors.

Goliath is a good candidate for the standard therapy. He is in good general health. Surgery is unlikely in his case to damage the anal sphincter or cause nerve damage that would lead to incontinence.

There are reports in the literature that radiotherapy has been effective in the treatment of perianal adenomas, but the major publications on this procedure appeared several years ago. A more recent text relates a survey in which two veterinary schools reported a 70% to 89% probability, and one a 90% to 100% probability of a 2-year cure for perianal gland adenoma using radiation alone.[10] Among the possible side-effects of this therapy are severe radiation proctitis and stricture of the anal canal.

Radiation could be an attractive option where surgery might cause incontinence or where the patient is a valuable breeding animal. Goliath is not such a patient, but more recent data on the procedure might prove useful.

What do you tell and advise the Gleasons?

Questions, dilemmas, and suggestions

The cases of George and Goliath illustrate some of the ethical issues raised by innovative procedures. One dilemma presented by both cases pits the interests of the profession in developing new and more effective techniques against the loyalty of a doctor to patient and client. Unless new procedures are tested, their effectiveness and safety cannot be verified. It is often impossible to develop and test without using client-owned animals. Even if clinicians wanted to do so, it is often impossible to produce conditions in research animals to test a new approach. Many conditions only occur in sufficient numbers in animals owned by clients. At the same time, clients bring their animals to the doctor to help these animals. Many may not be interested in subjecting their animal to a procedure that might be less effective than the best approach available so that animals in general might be helped in the long run. Clients expect undivided loyalty to them and their animal. They would rightly regard it as a violation of the assumptions of *their* veterinarian-patient-client relationship for a doctor to recommend an approach based not on the needs of their animal but on the interests of the profession in developing new treatments for other animals.

Both cases also illustrate the power a veterinarian often has to influence a client's decision, and the importance of a doctor's honesty and trustworthiness—of being completely truthful even when clients cannot subject one's judgments to scrutiny. In many cases it probably would be easy to persuade a client not to have a pet's limb amputated or testicles removed. A doctor who wanted to perform the innovative approaches in these cases would probably get his way. This will often be true of innovative or untested procedures, for there will probably be no reason even to think about developing or testing such a procedure unless there were *something* about it that, under the best of circumstances, would make it more attractive than a standard approach.

Both the obligation of loyalty to the client and patient, and one's power to influence the client's decision, suggest the following approaches to innovative procedures.

1. One should not advise an innovative procedure if (a) there already exists a standard procedure that is effective in alleviating the patient's condition, and (b) it is not clear that the innovative procedure will be at least as effective as this standard procedure. Where one can already achieve an acceptable result with a standard approach, one is morally obligated to use that approach. It appears to follow from this principle that treating Goliath's perianal adenoma with radiation would be unethical, even if one could get the clients to agree to it.

2. In cases like George's, where the standard therapy does not promise great probability of success, one may consider an alternative innovative approach. However, one may recommend such an approach only if there exist reliable data or information that provide reasons to believe the innovative procedure would benefit the patient, and is no less likely to benefit the patient than a customary procedure or another innovative procedure. This principle appears to argue against using the innovative procedure on George without more compelling evidence of its likely benefits to him.

3. When an innovative procedure is morally acceptable, it is appropriate to attempt to gain from the procedure data relevant to its scientific soundness and effectiveness. However, an innovative treatment should never be performed to obtain such data. The primary motivation must be to benefit the patient.

4. An innovative procedure should be done only by someone qualified to do it and capable of gaining from it whatever useful knowledge it may present. In general, this means that only specialists or practitioners working closely with specialists should attempt innovative procedures. If a generalist is contemplating an innovative approach because she is unaware of any other effective approach, it is possible that a specialist will know of an effective approach or an approach that is more likely to succeed than the one the generalist is considering. Moreover, a specialist is likely to have greater knowledge than a generalist about the kind of condition for which the generalist is contemplating an innovative treatment and may be better able to evaluate the treatment.

5. When an innovative procedure is medically and ethically acceptable, the client should be informed clearly about the nature of the procedure, the nature and likely consequences of any other available procedures, the potential known risks of the procedure to the life and quality of life of the patient, the possibility of unknown risks if the consequences of the procedure are unpredictable, and the fact that this is an innovative procedure.

Ethical Issues in Experimental Procedures

The use of an innovative procedure on a particular patient can lead to a clinical trial to test the procedure more rigorously by employing a statistically significant number of animals. More typically, practitioners begin to use an innovative approach after one or more experimental trials of the approach are published in the literature or are reported by colleagues. Successful innovative procedures in turn can become standard approaches.

There is sometimes a gray area in which it may not be clear whether to classify a procedure as innovative or experimental. There are different kinds of protocols that could legitimately be viewed as experimental, ranging from clinical trials utilizing a large number of animals, to modest pilot studies to determine whether a larger trial would be useful, to treatment of a series of individual patients in a manner suggested by a larger trial to verify the results of that trial. In general, experiments are characterized by (1) a pre-arranged plan or protocol that (2) utilizes a statistically significant number of animals and (3) compares the results obtained from a group receiving a tested procedure or procedures against the results obtained from controls, or from a group or groups receiving another procedure or procedures.

This chapter focuses on client-owned animals. Experiments or experimental trials on animals owned by a research facility or a granting agency supporting an experiment raise distinct ethical issues, some of which are discussed in Chapter 24. Relatively few veterinarians conduct true experimental procedures. However, it is useful here to consider briefly the most important ethical problem raised by experimental veterinary procedures because this problem is inherent in innovative treatments, which are done by a significant number of practitioners.

Experimental procedures, especially randomized clinical trials (RCTs) in which subjects are assigned randomly to experimental and control groups, have stirred controversy in human medicine.[11] The following are among the many ethical questions that can be asked about clinical trials in veterinary medicine:

- When is it appropriate to begin an experimental trial? Can a trial ever be justified if there already exists an effective treatment for a condition?
- How far should a trial proceed when it becomes apparent that the procedure being evaluated will not work? Is it fair to subject patients to such a procedure in the interest of obtaining a complete, scientifically acceptable, demonstration of the procedure's ineffectiveness?
- Should a patient be removed from a study if it becomes apparent that the procedure being tested will not help it or if there is another procedure that will but removing the patient from the study will confound its results?
- Should patients in a control or nontreatment group be removed from it and treated with the procedure being tested if it becomes clear that this treatment would be more beneficial to these patients?
- To what extent, if any, are placebos ethically appropriate in clinical experiments?
- To what extent should a client be allowed to decide that the patient would benefit from withdrawing from the study or receiving another kind of treatment?
- To what extent is it appropriate to charge clients for a tested procedure, or medical care necessitated by it?

These are all important ethical issues, but none is the most important ethical problem raised by experimental trials, especially RCTs. The most critical ethical problem in all experimental procedures with owned animals is that the patient is no longer solely an end in itself. The patient is also a means toward another goal, the evaluation of a scientific hypothesis or the testing of a procedure or product. The doctor is not interested solely in the patient and cannot promise to follow whatever course is in its best interests, for this could invalidate the entire experiment. The more a clinician focuses on the requirements of the trial, the less he may focus on the needs of any individual patient in it. Indeed, at some point in some trials it may not be appropriate to describe what is essentially the subject of a research project as a "patient" at all.

As philosopher Charles Fried has argued,[12] human RCTs, in which the medical problems of patients are not considered in determining to which treatment or control group they are assigned, deprive patients of one of the central values in the doctor-patient relationship: the "good of personal care." Medical patients assume that their doctor will exhibit complete loyalty to their needs and expect that the trust placed in their doctor will not be complicated or diverted by the need to generate data. This undeviating devotion to the patient, Fried observes, must be lacking in RCTs by their very nature even in the presence of laws requiring patients' consent to participate. The danger in even innovative care that is not part of a larger clinical trial is that the interests of science, the desire to obtain even a small piece of useful data, can intrude into the unswerving loyalty assumed by the client. This danger is intensified in full-scale clinical trials, where the doctor's interest is in multiple patients simultaneously, which all serve to some extent as means to gain benefits for others.

The typical veterinary client, like the typical human medical patient, enters the professional relationship assuming the doctor's single-minded and uncompromising loyalty (see Chapters 14 and 20). It follows that an experimental procedure cannot be utilized unless all the following conditions are satisfied.

- The procedure is as likely to benefit this patient as any other available procedure, and there exists no procedure that will effectively cure or alleviate the patient's malady.
- The client is given full and honest disclosure that the procedure is experimental.
- The client is informed about the nature and amount of evidence regarding the effectiveness of the procedure being developed or tested.
- The client is told how the experiment is justified by its potential wider benefits.
- The client is told about the likely and potential consequences of the procedure to her animal.
- The client is informed about the kinds of procedures that will be done in the experiment, and the kinds of experimental groups into which her animal could be placed.
- The client is informed about what will happen if the animal does poorly or if it appears that another procedure will benefit it more. If the animal will not be withdrawn from the study or given treatment appropriate to its needs, the client must be told this explicitly.
- The client is told whether she will be financially responsible for medical consequences of the procedure and for veterinary care for conditions not attributable or related to the procedure.
- The client is given the time and opportunity to exercise an informed consent. Whenever it might be unclear whether a procedure is "experimental" or "innova-

tive," one should not attempt to classify it as the latter, hoping thereby to avoid the necessity of full disclosure to the client. Disclosure would also be obligatory for innovative procedures.

• All experimental procedures must adhere to the most basic ethical principle of animal experimentation, which is discussed in Chapter 24: No experiment on an animal can be justified ethically unless it is justifiable scientifically. If the aims or methods of the experiment (including the number of animal subjects) are insupportable from a scientific standpoint, that experiment cannot justify any infliction of pain, suffering, distress, stress, or discomfort.

• To assure that the experiment is justified scientifically and ethically, it should be reviewed and approved by a group of persons, including at least one veterinarian who is not participating in the experiment and is not beholden to anyone who is a participant, and including at least one member whose function would be to advocate the interests of experimental subjects. This committee would function like an institutional animal care and use committee required by federal law for various kinds of animal experimentation (see Chapter 24).

∼ SOME ETHICAL ISSUES IN ACADEMIC VETERINARY MEDICINE

Most high-tech, innovative, and experimental procedures emerge from a common source: the clinical and research facilities of the veterinary schools. A small proportion of the profession practices at these institutions. However, normative veterinary ethics must attend to distinctive ethical issues raised in academic practice. If high-tech, innovative, or experimental procedures raise ethical problems, they will often be apparent during the development of these procedures by academic veterinarians. Moreover, the veterinary colleges are charged by the profession with leading the way in technical as well as ethical standards. Finally, and most importantly, every practitioner must pass through one of these institutions. The lessons about ethical (or unethical) behavior learned during this time can last for a professional lifetime and can spread doctor by doctor throughout the profession.

Veterinary schools are fascinating places. Vibrant and complex institutions, they can present a wide range of ethical questions. Some of these issues reach beyond the interests of patients and clients, and relate, for example, to how various groups in an academic clinical environment (senior faculty, junior faculty, students, and support staff) deal with each other. This discussion focuses on several ethical issues that involve patients and clients. Limitations of space permit mention of only some of these issues, and in a manner that highlights their importance rather than offering definitive guidance. For background discussions, the reader is referred to treatment of appropriate topics throughout this book.

Academic Justification

The most important distinctive ethical principle relating to academic practice is that certain behavior, which would not be appropriate if done by a veterinarian in a nonacademic setting, may be justified in a veterinary school. Veterinary school hospitals have two tasks that go beyond the treatment of current patients. They develop and test new procedures for the benefit of other patients and clients. They also train future veterinarians and specialists. Both the research and teaching functions of veterinary schools sometimes permit subjecting patients and clients to procedures that would be wrong in private practice.

When do research interests justify burdens on a patient or client?

Several years ago, a neonatal foal intensive care unit was begun at Tufts University, the school at which I am privileged to teach. Its aim was to develop ways of saving foals that would otherwise die. At first, the success rate of this unit, like that of similar facilities at other schools, was not great. Some students would ask whether it was ethical to attempt to save animals that did not have a great probability of pulling through, especially if they were in distress. The response of the clinicians was that by having the opportunity to test and refine various techniques of maintaining neonatal foals, procedures might be improved.

The clinicians were correct. Today this unit and others like it achieve a much higher rate of success. Through better equipment and training of doctors and support staff, foals that formerly would die or be euthanized are surviving. Part of what justified this endeavor was that it was done at a veterinary school with a long-term commitment to the project and the financial means and clinical staff to offer a reasonable chance of success. In contrast, an individual doctor who was not part of such a clinical development program might well have acted wrongly in attempting to keep such animals alive.

It is difficult to provide general principles that will satisfactorily determine whether a procedure that ought not to be done in ordinary circumstances is acceptable in an academic clinical context. There are many different possible academic reasons for doing a procedure and innumerable different fact situations. A beginning principle, identical to that applicable to any innovative or experimental procedure, is that any treatment or therapy done in an academic setting must be done with the aim of benefiting the patient, and a procedure may not be done if there already exists an approach that would achieve satisfactory results. A second incontrovertible rule is that the client must be told about any wider possible justifications for a procedure done in an academic setting and must be given the opportunity to exercise an informed consent to it. Third, nothing should ever be done to an animal, even—indeed especially—in an academic context unless doing so makes for good science, medicine, or teaching. After this point, however, one may only be able to list a number of factors that are relevant in determining whether a procedure that might be questionable in another context is appropriate in academic practice. Among these factors are the following:

- Is this patient's condition life-threatening? If the patient is in danger of dying or suffering a serious infirmity, there may be a stronger justification for trying something with potential wider benefits, provided, again, that no effective approach now exists.
- How serious a condition does the academic procedure aim to illuminate? The more detrimental the condition to an animal's health, the more justifiable an academic procedure directed at that condition may be.
- How many future patients might knowledge about the procedure be likely to help? If a significant number of animals might benefit, an academic procedure might be more justifiable than if very few patients would benefit.
- How much pain, distress, stress, or discomfort will the procedure involve? It is a fundamental ethical principle that one must always attempt to avoid causing an

animal unnecessary pain or distress (see Chapter 11). However, a small or even moderate amount of distress might be justified if caused by an academic clinician developing a procedure with broader applications.

• What is the probability of success of an academic procedure on this patient? All other things being equal, the less likely a new procedure will work the less justified it would appear to be, and such a procedure will be even less justifiable the more pain or distress it will cause.

These principles fare well when tested against cases presented in this chapter. One cannot appeal to an academic justification in support of radiation therapy for Goliath's perianal gland adenoma (Case 22-8) because the interests of this patient clearly require that the effective standard therapy be used. Goliath does not need a special academic approach to be helped, and any benefits that could be obtained from the proposed study simply do not justify the potential risks to him.

The problem with treating George's osteosarcoma with preoperative chemotherapy (Case 22-7) is that, as assumed by the case, this therapy has not been established to be at least as effective as the standard approach. However, it might be appropriate to administer the same preoperative chemotherapeutic regimen to George if he were part of a carefully conducted experimental trial at a veterinary school. Under such circumstances George would be treated by doctors with some experience performing the therapy. Moreover, his progress could be monitored against that of other patients; part of this monitoring could (and I would argue should) involve amputation and standard chemotherapy as soon as any metastases might be suspected. Third, the expense of the therapy and ancillary medical care could be borne by the veterinary school. A critical fact about George is that he has life-threatening cancer and that the standard therapy, while sometimes successful, is not always so. In evaluating the appropriateness of placing George in an experimental study of the new therapy one would, of course, need the best possible information relating to the probability that the therapy could work in his case.

In contrast, the principles stated above appear to argue against prostaglandin therapy for Hannah (Case 22-6) even in an academic context—a fact, I would argue, that lends further credence to these principles. It might be desirable to have an effective prostaglandin therapy so that certain dogs with pyometras can breed. However, this aim is not of great medical, social, or economic significance. It is typically not very important, except to its owner, that *any* bitch unable to breed because of pyometra be rendered capable of bearing puppies. There are already enough purebred puppies of any breed for those who wish to own them. It is therefore difficult to maintain that the hardships caused by the therapy are outweighed by its importance, even if caused by an academic clinician attempting to develop the therapy. What makes the procedure even worse is that there is a way of helping such animals once and for all.

THE DONATION ISSUE. If an animal's condition seems hopeless and euthanasia inevitable, or a client cannot afford an expensive treatment, some veterinary schools will accept (or solicit) donation of the animal to the school for research purposes. By itself, accepting such a donation need not be unethical. However, I have spoken with clinicians at a number of veterinary schools who appear to believe that once an animal has been donated, things that would be inappropriate to do to an owned animal can now be done to it. Some academic clinicians tell me that because a donated animal will no longer be owned by its former client, there is no need to inform the client prior to the donation what will be done to it.

It is, I would argue, a violation of a client's moral and legal rights not to disclose fully what would be done with her animal. Clients do not necessarily lose concern about their animal once they donate it for research or teaching. They must be given the option of choosing euthanasia, or some other approach, if they cannot accept their animal's future role. Moreover, it would be highly unethical to demand any less justification for a procedure because an animal is no longer owned. Such animals feel no less pain or discomfort, and they are entitled to no less concern, after they are donated. Perhaps those who believe that a freer hand can be taken with donated animals suppose that once there is no longer an owner, there will be no one to fuss, bother, or object to what a clinician wants to do. This is not an acceptable attitude in anyone, much less in a veterinarian. It would also be unethical to manipulate a client to make a donation by inflating or exaggerating the fee or overstating the burdens of future treatment on the patient or client.

When do teaching interests justify burdens on patients or clients?

A veterinary school's job of training future doctors, interns, and residents also sometimes justifies imposing upon animals and clients burdens that would be ethically unacceptable in private practice.

Perhaps the most routine and harmless of such sacrifices involves subjecting an animal to a physical examination by a somewhat inexperienced student, whose hands may not be the steadiest in inserting a thermometer and whose auscultatory attempts may make up in intensity what they lack in efficiency. Clients can also be unnerved by listening to students reciting their impressions of the patient's condition to a clinician. Such activities are appropriate when supervised closely by faculty and done within an acceptable range of comfort for patients and clients.

Important ethical issues arise, however, when procedures that involve distress or discomfort are undertaken to educate students or clinicians-in-training. This can occur, for example, when an animal has a terminal illness such as feline leukemia or lymphosarcoma, some palliation or treatment is possible, the client decides that he does not want or cannot afford further procedures, but the veterinary school subsidizes the treatment to provide students learning experiences regarding these procedures. As in the case of research-oriented activities, it is difficult to prescribe in the abstract a set of principles that will determine whether any given pedagogical use of a patient is ethical. In general, I would urge clinicians never to base a decision on whether to do a procedure upon its potential benefits to students. Any procedure must be justified itself, both medically and ethically, and if it is, students may then observe or participate. This approach appears to follow from the ethical principle that clients are entitled to a veterinarian's complete and undivided loyalty to them and their animals. Thus if it would be inappropriate to transfuse a feline leukemic cat or to treat an animal for lymph cancer with chemotherapy, that students could observe such treatment would not render it more justifiable. If a veterinary school is unable to provide students sufficient experience in a range of diseases, it needs to work on its caseload. It should not tolerate or manufacture for pedagogical reasons situations that unnecessarily burden patients or clients.

The case of Goliath's perianal gland adenoma (Case 22-8) illustrates an issue regarding which clinicians who supervise the training of interns or residents may sometimes need to exercise firmness. Educational requirements of veterinary schools and specialty boards often require interns or residents to find something new or "interesting" that demonstrates their diagnostic, therapeutic, or scientific prowess. Clinical faculty must supervise these junior clinicians to assure that an educational requirement never affects what options are disclosed to clients or what procedures are performed on animals. It would be appropriate to recommend an approach based on a student's or clinician's educational interests, only if there is no other approach that would be more advisable and only if the client has the opportunity to decide whether she wishes her animal to be a subject in the inquiry.

Quality of Care

There are several kinds of ethical problems to which administrators and clinicians in academic veterinary hospitals must be sensitive. One such issue concerns the earnestness and efficiency with which uniformly high standards of medical care are maintained. Veterinary schools represent themselves to the public as offering the most advanced care available, and generally, they do. Many clients bring their animals to these hospitals relying on this representation. They assume their animals will be diagnosed and treated by specialists and cared for by the best available support staff.

In fact, a good deal of the care that patients receive is provided by people—students in various stages of their program, interns, residents, and board-eligible doctors—who have significantly less expertise than clients may be expecting. This is acceptable in light of a school's function to train practitioners. However, it is essential for veterinary schools to maintain the level of care they claim to provide, by assuring that people with various levels of background perform tasks appropriate to their skills. It is not sufficient to state in brochures or consent forms that clients "understand some services will be provided by veterinary students, interns, or residents." Clients who assume that a specialist is attending to their animal should not be served by a resident, unless they are told that a resident is handling their animal's case and this is acceptable to them. Students should not be doing what is appropriate only for interns or residents. I have received reports from students and residents at a number of veterinary schools that, especially at nights and on weekends, some animals are not receiving the quality of care assumed by clients, because students (sometimes exhausted by 24- or 36-hour shifts) are providing the bulk of medical care. This is not fair to students, patients, or clients.

The Coerciveness of the Academic Setting

As I argue in this book, a doctor should enable, indeed encourage, clients to decide for themselves, free of pressure or coercion, what should be done to their animals. Those who practice in an academic hospital and are accustomed to the facility may not appreciate how frightening and highly pressured such a place can seem to clients. Some clients travel great distances to bring their animals to these hospitals. In unfamiliar surroundings, and having already made a substantial investment of time or money just to get to the facility, some clients may find it difficult to resist a clinician's recommendations. Many clients who come to academic hospitals have been referred by their local veterinarian or a specialist because their animal's condition is so difficult that only a veterinary school hospital would have any chance of dealing with it. These clients, many of whom already want to learn that something can be done *here*, may also be vulnerable to a clinician's arguments. The ability of clients to think calmly and clearly can also be impaired by an environment unlike any they may have seen before in an animal hospital: large facilities, impressive high-tech equipment, and scores of clinicians and students attending to a large number of patients. It is therefore especially important for veterinary school hospitals to assure that clients have the opportunity to exercise an informed consent to any procedure.

Communication and the Problem of Multiple Clinicians

Another problem that probably occurs with greater frequency in veterinary school hospitals than in typical private practices results from the fact that at teaching hospitals clients are likely to encounter a large number of professional staff. One or more students or residents, technicians, the patient's primary clinician, a doctor on staff to whom the patient may be referred for diagnosis or specialized treatment, all these and more may have the opportunity to speak with the client. If some of these people tell the client different or conflicting things, the client can become confused, upset, or angry. It can be difficult enough for clients to absorb everything they are told and to ask the right questions. This process can be made easier if doctors decide beforehand who will be speaking with a client on behalf of the medical staff.

Criticism of Colleagues and Professional Improvement

As discussed in Chapter 19, one of the most difficult issues in professional ethics relates to whether or under what circumstances doctors may criticize the performance of another veterinarian to clients. This is an especially important issue in academic practice. Many patients at academic hospitals are referred by other veterinarians or are brought by clients after they have taken their animal to another doctor. Academic clinicians are therefore in a position where they frequently can evaluate the performance of other practitioners. Sometimes, they find mistakes made by these doctors. Chapter 19 offers suggestions for approaching situations in which one faces the possibility of criticizing another doctor's behavior. Although these suggestions also apply to academic clinicians, veterinary school practitioners have distinctive ethical obligations relating to criticism of colleagues.

Because part of the mission of the veterinary schools is to improve the quality of care offered by the profession as a whole, it is especially important that an academic clinician who has questions regarding a previous doctor's performance attempt to speak with that doctor. If there is a technique or procedure about which the doctor should know, the academic clinician should impart this information. Hopefully, this can be done in a way that does not threaten or intimidate the doctor or discourage her from making further appropriate referrals.

I would also urge academic clinicians to be particularly careful before judging that a referring doctor or general practitioner has erred. One should always be cautious before criticizing a colleague, in part because the case one now has may well be different from that seen previously by the other doctor. Academic clinicians, most of whom are board-certified specialists, should keep in mind that both the law and the profession hold specialists to a much higher standard of care than generalists.[13] It does not follow that if specialists in a veterinary teaching hospital would have made a different diagnosis, done a different procedure, or reached a different conclusion, the first doctor acted incompetently or improperly. As bad as it is for a specialist to conclude that a generalist performed poorly because she did not do what the specialist would do, it is still worse to state or imply to a client that the previous doctor therefore acted improperly.

Setting an Example

Academic clinicians are role models for future doctors. Students who are impressed by the high ethical standards of admired teachers may be motivated to emulate these standards in their own professional life. Academic clinicians, students, interns, residents, and support staff set an equally important example to the public. Clients who pass through these institutions are likely to associate their virtues or failings with the profession itself. Few things can sour clients more on veterinary medicine than a bad experience at a veterinary school. Few experiences can be more impressive than being served by an institution that matches its medical prowess with the highest standards of honesty, loyalty, compassion, and respect.

REFERENCES

[1]Armstrong D: Pet owners rip MSPCA: Some say money drives decisions of which animals to treat, *Boston Globe* February 2, 1994, p 1.
[2]American Veterinary Medical Association: *Principles of Veterinary Medical Ethics*, 1993 Revision, "Guidelines for Professional Behavior," paragraph 2, *1994 AVMA Directory*, Schaumburg, IL, The Association, p 42.
[3]McLaren C: Cancer treatment for pets, *Toronto Globe and Mail* September 9, 1989, pp D1-D2.
[4]Kahler S: Banking on greyhounds, *J Am Vet Med Assoc* 204:1295-1299, 1994.
[5]Smith MT: The wild new world of health care for your pet, *Money* 23:149, April 1994.
[6]Kerwin SC, Lewis DD, Elkins AD: Bone grafting and banking, *Compend Contin Educ Pract Vet* 13:1558-1566, 1991.
[7]*Id*, p 1562.
[8]*Corso v. Crawford Dog and Cat Hospital*, 97 Misc.2d 530 (Civ. Ct. Queens Cty. 1979).
[9]Both "innovative" and "experimental" procedures must be distinguished from "unconventional" or "alternative" treatments or approaches. The law recognizes the existence of "schools" of medicine—general approaches that are endorsed by significant portions of a healing profession. A kind of treatment will be regarded as ordinary and customary if it is accepted by a school that is itself generally accepted as legitimate within the profession. In contrast, an "unconventional" approach is one that is not accepted by the profession as a whole or by a school or group accepted by the profession. A 1988 AVMA policy statement declares both holistic and homeopathic veterinary medicine to be "unconventional" and states that there is "no scientific evidence" demonstrating the safety or efficacy of the latter. American Veterinary Medical Association: "Guidelines on Alternate Therapies," *1994 AVMA Directory*, Schaumburg, IL, 1993, The Association, p 54. Unconventional or alternative approaches can become accepted schools or modalities. The 1988 AVMA statement states that acupuncture and acutherapy are "valid modalities" although it warns against "the potential for abuse." "Innovative" procedures exemplify or are based upon generally accepted approaches and employ a novel modality that would, if effective, not constitute so radical a departure from generally accepted approaches to be classified as unconventional. Utilizing in animals a new cancer chemotherapy drug just approved for use in humans might constitute an innovative approach, but might not be classified as unconventional because chemotherapy is an accepted mainstream modality in cancer therapy.
[10]Feeney DA, Johnston GR: Radiation therapy: Applications and availability. In Kirk RW, editor: *Current Veterinary Therapy VIII*, Philadelphia, 1993, WB Saunders, pp 428-434.
[11]Levine RJ: *Ethics and Regulation of Clinical Research*, ed 2, Baltimore, 1986, Urban & Schwarzenberg.
[12]Fried C: *Medical Experimentation: Personal Integrity and Social Policy*, New York, 1974, American Elsevier Company.
[13]Tannenbaum J: Benefits and burdens: Legal and ethical issues raised by veterinary specialization. In Dodds WJ, editor: *Specialization: The Bridge from Science to Veterinary Practice*, Orlando, in press, Academic Press.

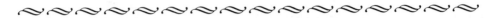

CHAPTER 23

Farm, Food, and Performance Animal Practice
The New Frontier of Veterinary Ethics

Normative veterinary ethics can rely on a growing consensus regarding the nature of companion animals and their importance to clients. An increasing appreciation of the value of these animals prompts many of the questions that must be asked about companion animal practice and points the way to certain answers.

In contrast, there is as yet little general agreement about the nature or value of farm, food, or performance animals. The overwhelming majority of people believe that it is morally permissible to use certain kinds of animals for food, draft, or fiber, and in sporting events. However, few people know very much about the lives of these animals. It is far from obvious what they would say about ethical issues relating to such animals if these animals received greater public attention. Indeed, there is significant uncertainty and disagreement among those who study and work with agricultural and performance animals about what scientific and ethical principles should govern people's behavior toward them.

The very fact that most companion animals are so highly regarded raises difficult issues for agricultural and performance animal doctors. Some of these animals are not markedly different in their mental capacities from many companion animals. At a time the profession seeks to promote companion animals as members of the family, to what extent must it also advocate the interests of its food, farm, and performance animal patients? In general, what should be the role of practitioners who serve economic interests of *owners* of agricultural and performance animals in a profession whose increasing proportion of companion animal doctors has a strong stake in the promotion of *animal* interests?

These issues are complicated by the severe economic pressures faced by many large animal doctors. Normative veterinary ethics must recognize the legitimate interests of these veterinarians and of their clients. Nevertheless, due regard also must be given to the interests of the animals and the public. There can be no guarantees that ethical deliberation will always make life easier for beleaguered large animal practitioners.

The primary aim of this chapter is to identify important issues relevant to assessing the profession's moral obligations regarding agricultural and performance animals. Several general principles and specific recommendations will be advanced. However, the central thesis of the chapter is that normative veterinary ethics stands barely at the frontier of serious consideration of many issues raised by food, farm, and performance animal practice. There is need for much scientific and ethical investigation. In the meantime, we must avoid premature and superficial solutions to hard questions.

∼ SETTLING UPON BASIC PRINCIPLES

One task for an acceptable approach to ethical issues in agricultural or performance animal practice is to establish certain basic premises from which practical moral deliberation can proceed. The following are offered as examples of such principles.

1. People may use and benefit from agricultural and performance animals. A fundamental premise upon which all farm and performance animal practice rests is that people may sometimes use animals for purposes such as food, fiber, and entertainment. This view is so widely and deeply held that one can assert it not just as a fact of life which any realistic approach to veterinary ethics must accept as a given, but also as a correct moral principle.

To be sure, some people believe that it is inherently immoral for human beings ever to use animals for our own benefit. Some of these people think they are owed a demonstration of why the human use of animals is permissible. Several arguments for weighting human interests more heavily than animal interests are presented in Chapter 11. But to engage here in an attempt to refute animal-use abolitionism would be a hopeless task. Those who endorse abolitionism are no more likely to accept refutations of their point of view than the rest of us would be disposed to agree that an animal farmer is the moral equivalent of a slave owner, or that a meat-eater is no better than a human cannibal.

Articulating the objections to animal-use abolitionism is a legitimate task for animal ethics, which as a branch of philosophical ethics seeks theoretical completeness. However, for the veterinary profession, its clients, and the vast majority of the public, abolitionism is a fringe position espoused by a hardy, but nevertheless tiny, few. It has almost always been so. This is not just a historical fact, but important moral evidence. Through the centuries, in diverse places and cultures, the overwhelming majority of humankind has consulted its basic moral intuitions—and has concluded that it is proper to use animals for food, fiber, draft, entertainment, and companionship. Abolitionists may prefer to think that this belief has been a giant, horrible prejudice. However, the fact that most people who have lived and toiled on this earth have arrived at the same general conclusion is powerful evidence of its correctness.

2. Agricultural and performance animal clients are entitled to a fair profit and may factor economic considerations into management decisions. Because people may morally have certain animal products and services, producers of these goods and services are entitled to a fair profit. Otherwise, these items could not be provided. Because producers are entitled to a profit, they may sometimes factor economic considerations into decisions about what will be done with their animals, even though such decisions sometimes might have a negative impact on the animals. This is not the end of the matter. The animals also have legitimate needs and interests, which place limitations upon how they may be used or treated.

3. The role of public demand in the determination of how agricultural and performance animals are treated must not be underestimated. People who are critical of the treatment of agricultural and performance animals tend to focus on owners, veterinarians, and others involved in the production process as the source of alleged problems. In fact, the ways in which agricultural and performance animals are treated rarely flow from some immutable value system or mind-set of producers or veterinarians. The *public* is the preeminent force in the determination of how agricultural and performance animals are used. I have met few producers who would object to more extensive facilities for swine, or greater growing space for broiler chickens, or spending the resources to try to save every sick animal—if consumers were willing to pay the higher prices such measures would entail. The fact that producers cannot make a living unless they provide what the public wants at an acceptable price does not, of course, make all means toward this end morally acceptable. Moreover, producers can be mistaken in thinking that a given husbandry method is more profitable than others which might be better for the animals. Nevertheless, public expectations set many of boundaries within which deliberations about agricultural and performance animal welfare operate. Success in promoting the welfare of these animals will depend substantially upon an educated and compassionate public.

4. Agricultural and performance animals have interests that must be taken into account. Although animal interests need not always prevail when a farm or performance animal client is faced with a management question, these interests exist nevertheless and must be given the attention and weight they deserve. This seems obvious. Nevertheless, discussions devoid of attention to animal interests are appearing with frequency in the literature espousing the model of the veterinarian as herd health consultant (see Chapter 16).

4A. Profit is not enough.

A central claim of this emerging model is that maximization of profit should be the overriding aim of producers and that noneconomic concerns should be considered only after the likelihood of maximum profit is assured. One discussion recommends computing the "expected value" of each alternative approach to an animal health question by:

> …weighting the value (in dollars) of each potential outcome with the probability that the outcome will occur, given a particular decision, and then summing the weighted values for all potential outcomes for a given branch of the decision tree. If the decision maker chooses the branch with the highest expected value, then he can expect to maximize his profits over a series of such choices.[1]

To illustrate this method, the authors ask whether a dairy cow in early lactation with a left displaced abomasum should be given an omentopexy or should be rolled. They calculate that the probable net profit for the operation exceeds that for rolling and therefore recommend the operation. On the other hand, the probable outcomes for omentopexy and percutaneous fixation using a bar suture are calculated as identical. "Since the expected values are equivalent," the authors conclude, "the decision about which approach to use can be made on other than economic grounds."[2] The discussion does not mention the animal's present or future welfare as a relevant consideration in decisionmaking.

A paper on the effects of *post partum* disease on milk production in dairy cows reports that certain conditions (for example, cystic follicles and milk fever) are associated with increased production, while other diseases diminish production.[3] The discussion sets forth *post partum* disease incidence rates, goals and "action levels" for a number of common diseases. It is stated, for example, that there should be a goal of less than 3% of lactations affected by milk fever, and action to address the disease should commence when this level rises to 10%.

The discussion does not identify the actual or potential discomfort experienced by the animals as an independent variable in determining whether or at what point veterinary treatment ought to be administered. "Veterinary service" is included as a cost to be factored into a farmer's decision. However, there is no indication that animal pain or distress—insofar as these are evils for the animals themselves, as distinguished from potential problems for producers—are relevant to determining the need for veterinary care. It is urged that "(b)efore making recommendations regarding nutrition, disease prevention, or reproduction, the veterinarian should compare the losses incurred from the disease problem with the cost of reducing or alleviating that problem."[4] Such a statement need not be objectionable, provided attention is given somewhere to the animals as objects of concern in their own right. However, the authors state that "the cost" of disease:

> …may include the following major components: (1) decreased milk production, (2) milk withheld from market following antibiotic therapy, (3) direct veterinary services, (4) medications, (5) reproductive inefficiency, (6) extra labor, (7) disease preventive and control programs, and (8) loss of animals by death or involuntary culling.[4]

Detriments to the animals are not included explicitly as an independent "cost" of disease or relevant criterion in decision making.

4B. The concept of an ethical cost

The notion that all management decisions can be made solely on the basis of probable maximization of profit is ethically unacceptable. Sometimes, profit may appropriately be the deciding factor. If, for example, two approaches to animal husbandry are equally acceptable from an ethical standpoint (say, because neither causes more distress to the animals than the other), a farmer might be justified in choosing the more profitable approach. Sometimes, economic considerations may justify a somewhat diminished level of animal welfare, provided that at least an acceptable welfare level is maintained.

However, one should not assert as a general principle that noneconomic considerations can be entertained only after probable profit maximization is calculated. Farm and performance animals are not machines or plants, but sentient beings. They can feel pain, distress, stress, and discomfort. As argued in Chapter 11, all animals capable of experiencing negative mental states have an interest in not experiencing such states. One must always give some consideration to the impact upon this interest of any production method or course of veterinary care. This is owed to farm and performance animals in return for what is taken from them.

An "ethical cost" can be defined as a detriment, not solely expressible by or reducible to monetary terms, of some behavior or enterprise that must be considered in determining the moral appropriateness of that behavior or enterprise. Ethical costs are not restricted to (although they may sometimes include) such negative mental states as pain, suffering, distress, or discomfort. An ethical cost of a certain course of action can be the fact that it would violate a moral right not reducible to utilitarian cost-benefit analysis. Ethical costs in veterinary practice are not limited to detriments to animals. Among the potential ethical costs of certain ways of treating animals may be the failure of certain animals to experience positive goods. Ethical costs can also include human noneconomic costs such as insensitivity to animal welfare that might result from certain ways of treating animals.

It does not follow from the concept of an ethical cost that profit may never justify animal distress. The concept of an ethical cost does not preclude taking into consideration quantifiable economic costs associated with attempting to lessen or remove some ethical cost. The concept of an ethical cost is consistent with deciding not to provide a certain kind of veterinary care in the service of general herd productivity, if ethical analysis should determine that such an approach is justified under given circumstances. It may be difficult to identify relevant ethical costs in herd management practices and to assign these costs their proper weight. But ethical behavior in agricultural or performance animal practice requires that *ethical* costs be considered together with economic costs and benefits.

4C. Is due regard for animal interests consistent with a completely quantitative approach to herd management?

Many discussions of cost-benefit analysis in herd management appear to assume that making decisions can be reduced to calculating and comparing numbers. However, if animal interests must also be factored into decision making, it is doubtful whether completely quantitative approaches are achievable either in theory or in practice.

Animal mental states, like human mental states, are not precisely quantifiable. Although some researchers are attempting to find measurable behavioral or physiological signs of states such as stress,[5] the states themselves are not capable of exact measurement. We do not have, and we surely will never have, units of pain so that we can say that one animal is experiencing, say, twice the pain as another—although we can often determine that one appears to be in more or less pain than another. (We do not even have precise pain units for people, who can communicate their mental states to others.) Nor is it clear how we should quantify and compare across different mental states. Does an hour of moderate discomfort equal 5 minutes of moderate pain in the same animal? In different animals of the same species? In animals of different species? I do not mean to suggest that it is foolish to try to estimate and compare animal pain or distress. It sometimes seems appropriate to do so, and it is often possible to do it roughly. Rather, it seems impossible to engage in precise quantification of the sort that mathematical models of herd management would require to place animal interests into their formulae.

Moreover, even when one can reach an intuitively plausible comparison involving animal mental states, there will often remain an independent ethical element not reducible to quantitative comparison that must be factored into the decision about how one ought to act. Suppose it seems reasonable to say that by raising veal calves in total confinement in 60 cm-wide crates a farmer can achieve a certain level of profit and can produce a level of satisfaction in the public that taken together "exceeds" any pain or distress experienced by the animals. There still remains the question of whether the profit and public satisfaction provides sufficient *ethical justification* for the practice. Sometimes, simply comparing benefits with detriments might seem appropriate. But it will not always be so.

4D. Verbal Maneuvers: Redefining "disease"

Some advocates of the model of the veterinarian as herd health manager admit that they will tolerate disease under certain circumstances to promote productivity.[6] However, other proponents of this model want to redefine the concept of disease so that a dilemma between choosing between productivity and health does not arise. Dr. Thomas Stein suggests that "disease" should not be identified by the presence of such things as fever, diarrhea, or cough in individual animals:

> Rather, problems are identified as inadequate performance. In dairy herds this might be measured by calving-to-conception interval, days in milk at first breeding, or rolling average for annual milk production. … Disease in populations describes a deviation between what is happening and what is expected to happen … This redefinition of disease implies that health and production are identical.[7]

In other words, one should not speak of "disease" in, or the "health" of, individual members of a herd or population. The presence of individual animals with cough and fever caused by some microorganism would not indicate the presence of "disease" if the whole herd or population functions as a whole to maximize expected profitability.

It is not surprising why such a redefinition of disease might appeal to some veterinarians. As I suggest in Chapter 16, many people would doubt whether someone who always subordinates decisions about disease to questions of economic productivity ought to be called a "doctor," or a practitioner of veterinary *medicine*. By redefining health and disease in terms of productivity, some proponents of the model of the veterinarian as economic manager may be asserting that they are rightly classified as medical practitioners.

In any event, Dr. Stein's proposed redefinition has little to recommend it. His definition certainly would have a hard time coexisting with the concept of disease utilized in companion animal practice, where disease is a condition of individual animals and productivity is rarely an issue, much less is considered synonymous with absence of disease. Most important, the ethical issue is not whether something called "disease" may be tolerated to maximize production. The issue is whether or to what extent some of the physical states currently seen as components or signs of disease (such as fever, diarrhea, and cough) and the mental accompaniments of these states may be tolerated to promote production. This question will not disappear if the word "disease" is redefined to mean lack of expected productivity.

4E. Thought substitution: "Animal welfare goes without saying."

"When one challenges producers and veterinarians who do not include explicit reference to animal welfare in their discussions, one often receives the response that "of course, animal welfare goes without saying." This is so, it is claimed, because methods that are productive are also good for the animals. Productivity and animal welfare, it is said, are necessary and invariable correlates: "A productive animal is a happy animal."

There is impressive evidence that productivity is often associated with animal welfare. Certain husbandry practices clearly protect animals from the vicissitudes of weather, disease, predators, and the animals themselves. From a pragmatic standpoint, the frequent link between productivity and welfare may be the most important tool veterinarians and animal welfare advocates possess to improve the lives of farm and performance animals. The argument that profits can be improved by attention to animal welfare should be accepted readily by producers.

However, there are several reasons it is *obvious* that productivity and welfare need not always go hand in hand. First, as farm animal scientist Stanley Curtis observes, animal welfare is not an absolute. One can often say that there are different possible levels of welfare, ranging from conditions so slightly beneficial that one would want to say there is a minimal level of welfare, to conditions that approach or constitute optimal welfare.[8] Although certain methods of production may yield minimal welfare or a higher level of welfare than other methods, they may still be far from producing optimal welfare. This does not necessarily make such methods ethically wrong. The judgment must sometimes be made to sacrifice some degree of welfare to achieve a certain level of productivity. However, once one recognizes that this is sometimes a possible choice (even if it can be a correct choice) one cannot simply assume that productivity and welfare always converge. One must at least entertain the possibility that they diverge, so that one can then justify an approach that does not yield optimal welfare, or that yields a lower level welfare than another possible approach.

Second, economic forces contributing to profitability often have nothing to do with animal welfare. The fact that consumers may refuse to pay more than a certain amount for pork or want lamb or turkey during certain holiday seasons puts economic pressure on producers to institute certain kinds and schedules of production. However, there is no reason in principle why such economically induced husbandry methods must also result in any particular level of welfare.

Third, it is beyond question that some production methods either cause animals some distress or produce a level of welfare at least somewhat lower than optimal. Among common examples are dehorning calves without anesthesia, total indoor husbandry of swine, and intensive battery cage confinement of laying hens. It is worth emphasizing again that a given husbandry method is not rendered impermissible just because it might not produce optimal welfare. However, the issue of whether a given level of welfare is morally justified cannot be raised at all if one blindly proclaims an identity between productivity and welfare.

I am not maintaining that economic cost is an irrelevant or unimportant consideration in determining what producers and veterinarians may do. My target is the view that attention to animal interests is irrelevant or is relevant only insofar as it is a means of furthering the interests of farmers, veterinarians, or the public. Economic analysis of food and farm animal management is still in its infancy. It is premature to conclude that no mathematically rigorous decision procedures will seem ethically as well as economically acceptable for certain kinds of management situations. Nevertheless, there is a growing theme in the herd management literature that attention to the interests of individual animals is old-fashioned, soft-headed, and ignorant of the facts of life.[9] Animal interests, and moral obligations in veterinary practice that reflect the existence and importance of these interests, are as much unavoidable facts of life as anything else. Animal welfare is too important to "go without saying."

5. Individual animals count. Another basic premise for normative veterinary ethics is that individual agricultural and performance animals count. Herds or groups do not feel pain or undergo distress. Individual animals do. Therefore even insofar as it might be appropriate to apply utilitarian considerations to animals in herds, attention must still be paid to the mental states of individual animals. Individual animals also count in the sense that the interests of one or of a few can take precedence over some interest of producers, veterinarians, or the public. This can happen if the price of bringing trivial enjoyments to a large number of people is the imposition of grave suffering upon a smaller number of animals. Individual agricultural and performance animals also count in the sense that pain, distress, and discomfort can be as much an evil to them as to other kinds of animals.

6. Agricultural and performance animals have certain basic moral rights. I argue in Chapter 12 that animal interests are sometimes sufficiently important to give rise to moral rights. According to the concept of "rights" endorsed in that discussion, because agricultural and performance animals are sentient beings, they have some basic moral rights. For it is impossible to suppose that they may be subjected to the most severe pain or the most deprived conditions even if this would bring great pleasure to someone or a large number of people. At some point, the line of permissible treatment will be overstepped.

It is considerably easier (for some people, at least) to say that agricultural and performance animals have some moral rights than to demonstrate what rights they have or to determine the strength of these rights relative to human interests and rights. Perhaps normative veterinary and animal ethics can suggest preliminary or interim principles regarding the rights of agricultural and performance animals, while further necessary ethical and scientific investigation proceeds. One famous statement of minimal basic animal rights was offered by the British "Brambell Committee" to Enquire into the Welfare of Animals Kept under Intensive Livestock Husbandry Systems. (As discussed in Chapter 12, a similar list was adopted, more generally and for all animals, by the World Veterinary Association.) The Brambell Committee proposed "five freedoms" for agricultural animals: "sufficient freedom of movement for an animal (1) to get up; (2) lie down; (3) groom normally; (4) turn around; and (5) stretch its limbs."[10] These demands relate not just to the fact that animals deprived of certain basic natural movements are likely to experience negative mental states. The "freedoms" also reflect the intuitively appealing notion that certain aspects of an animal's nature are entitled to at least a modicum of respect.

6A. The relevance of domestication

Dr. Fred Jacobs argues that domesticated animals cannot have moral rights. He states that they "have been created by man rather than by nature and hence are, through necessity, subject to the control of man from cradle to grave. Were man to relinquish control of these animals, both man and the domestic animals would suffer catastrophe as biological species." Jacobs criticizes those who think that domesticated animals have "inalienable rights to a perfect existence," or a "right to existence," or must be left free to "roam the countryside and backwoods and damage the environment."[11]

Jacobs' objections to obviously extreme positions are reasonable, but his objections do not count against the view that domesticated animals have moral rights. As explained in Chapter 12, the concept of animal rights does not entail any particular claim about what rights animals have. To say that animals have rights is to say that they have some very strong interests and claims upon people, the weight of which claims cannot be reduced to utilitarian calculation of detriments versus benefits. One can say that domesticated animals have a right not to be treated inhumanely and deny that they have the right to roam freely, or a right to life.

The fact that certain characteristics of farm and performance animals, including parts of their temperaments, have been affected by domestication is a relevant consideration in determining the nature and weight of their interests. However, at least at present, domesticated animals are capable of experiencing pain and distress. They also have other interests domestication has not extinguished. Moreover, because domestication often produces animals that cannot fend for themselves, we are obligated to protect them from certain conditions they cannot manage without human help.

7. Although assessment of mental states is an important consideration in the determination of animal interests, one must avoid exaggerated claims about these states. One of the most difficult tasks faced by animal welfare science is determining what mental states animals actually experience. Strict behaviorists either deny the existence of animal mental states or refuse to talk about these states because they cannot be observed and measured "objectively." Such behaviorists have little to contribute to animal welfare discussions, which proceed from the eminently reasonable view that animals do have sensations and experiences.[12]

On the other hand, there is no shortage of grossly exaggerated attributions of sophisticated mental states to animals. If one underestimates or overestimates the mental lives of animals, one cannot assign proper moral weight to their interests. Even a cursory look at the literature regarding the assessment of animal mental states reveals that a great deal of conceptual and scientific work remains to be done before a morally satisfactory approach to animal interests can be fashioned.

7A. Mental states and physiological processes

Some investigators proceed on the assumption that if certain chemicals or physiological processes are associated with specified mental states in human beings, the presence of such chemicals or processes in animals would demonstrate the existence of the *same* mental states in the animals.[13] This approach may involve redefinition of the concepts we now apply to human beings, resulting in attribution of something quite different to the animals. For example, "fear" as people ordinarily speak of it, involves not just an unpleasant mental state but also the perception of an object or state of affairs (that which is feared) which is seen as dangerous or threatening. If chemical or physiological process X was to be found in the brains of human beings when we experience fear and in the brains of cows when these animals appear to be avoiding or reacting negatively to some condition, it would not follow that the cows are experiencing fear. It is far from obvious that cows are sophisticated enough to perceive something as an object distinct from themselves and to perceive *it as* dangerous or threatening—although we may be able to say that they have some kind of negative mental experience akin or analogous to fear. Nor does the mere presence of a chemical or physiological process in an animal's brain seem sufficient evidence of such mental activity, except to someone who is already disposed to ignore the criteria people normally demand before we say that someone or some being is experiencing fear.

7B. The dangers of premature definition

In 1987 the AVMA held a Colloquium on Recognition and Alleviation of Animal Pain and Distress. The *Proceedings* of this meeting[14] demonstrate that the profession stands ready to take the lead in the scientific study of animal pain. But there was also evidence of a tendency of some investigators to engage in superficial definitions of extremely complex mentalistic concepts.

A *Colloquium Panel Report* offered definitions of the terms "pain," "anxiety," "fear," "stress," "suffering," "comfort," "discomfort," and "injury." "Anxiety," for example, was defined as "an emotional state involving increased arousal and alertness prompted by an unknown danger that may be present in the immediate environment." It was asserted that fear "can be defined similarly, except that fear would refer to an experienced or known danger in the immediate environment." The *Report* surmised that a dog trembling in a veterinarian's office during its first visit may be experiencing anxiety while such behavior during the second visit may better be described as "fear of a remembered event."[15]

These definitions of "anxiety" and "fear" depart from what people ordinarily mean by these terms. They also reflect substantive views of animal mental states that are, at the very least, premature. People commonly speak of fear of the unknown, and of anxiety about a known event that is distant from the "immediate environment" temporally or spatially. One can also feel anxious about a past event (for example, about whether a relative was harmed in a natural disaster), provided there is something one does not yet know about that event. It is also incorrect to refer to either anxiety or fear as "an" emotional state. Our concepts of these states include ranges of different, but related experiences. Anxiety can involve feelings of uncertainty, fear or dread about one's self. To say that you are anxious about your veterinary licensing exams or an impending hospitalization is to say that you see yourself, your plans, your happiness, and your state of mind threatened by some event or contingency. Experiences of anxiety often require a highly developed sense of the future because being anxious typically involves an appreciation that one does not know what the future will bring. The term "anxiety" is frequently applied to deep and brooding uncertainty relating to life's more important experiences.

It has been determined that receptors for benzodiazepines are found in all vertebrates except the cartilaginous species,[16] and that such substances appear to have calming effects on animals as well as people we would describe as anxious.[17] Yet it simply does not follow from these facts that dogs in veterinarians' offices—much less cows, sheep, chickens, or laboratory animals—have a sufficient sense of self or of the future, or are capable of sufficient dread about their own predicaments to justify the attribution of anxiety.

Defining "anxiety" and other mental states without including the sophisticated experiences these concepts ordinarily encompass, will lead some people to think that the task of describing animal mental states is much easier than it is. These people may find (some may be assuming this from the beginning) that animals are more like human beings than they really are. They may conclude that the presence in animals of some chemical or some part of the complex behavior we view as evidence of certain mental states shows that animals, too, experience these very same states. And they may conclude this not because scientific evidence demonstrates that animals experience these states but because new concepts are being employed that can be applied more easily to animals.

As the AVMA Panel recognized, it is important that investigators have some commonality of definition, lest they talk and argue about different things. However, the fact that animals have real mental experiences does not justify going overboard in ascribing mentalistic concepts to them. These concepts have important moral implications. For example, if a certain husbandry method really causes cows to experience *anxiety*, the argument against this method would be stronger than if it merely causes slight discomfort. If these concepts are not applied with care, we risk mischaracterizing both the mental lives and moral claims of the animals the welfare of which we seek to promote.

8. All other things being equal, a husbandry method or course of veterinary care that causes animals less pain, suffering, distress, or discomfort is preferable to one that causes them more. Some pain or distress is beneficial either as a way of assisting an animal to protect itself or to counter other negative states. Nevertheless, all other things being equal, pain and other negative states are bad for animals just as these mental states are bad for people. Therefore if several alternative approaches are equally profitable but one would cause the animals less pain, suffering, distress, or discomfort than the others, it would be wrong not to pursue the less painful (distressful, etc.) approach. To do otherwise would cause the animals unnecessary pain or distress, something even the anticruelty position (see Chapter 11) regards as wrong.

9. All other things being equal, a husbandry method or course of veterinary care that gives animals more positive mental states or greater well-being is preferable to one that gives them less. Many people believe that animals are entitled to freedom from "unnecessary" negative states and conditions, but they deny that animals are entitled to positive benefits such as pleasure, happiness, or general well-being (see Chapter 11). Nevertheless, it does not seem terribly controversial to suggest that if several management or veterinary approaches are equally profitable, but one would bring more positive benefits to the animals than the others, the more beneficial approach ought to be chosen. Doing otherwise would be ungenerous and uncharitable for no apparent reason. The premise that, all things being equal, one ought to promote animal benefit is far from trivial. It requires farmers, the profession, and animal behavior scientists to support efforts to determine how positive animal mental states might be promoted.

10. It is often unhelpful to maintain that animals should be spared "unnecessary" pain, suffering, distress, or discomfort, or that they should be treated "humanely."

10A. "Necessity"

As observed in Chapter 11, typically, to claim that a given amount or kind of animal pain or distress is "necessary" is to make two judgments: (1) that a human aim for which the pain (distress, etc.) is imposed is legitimate or sufficiently important to justify the pain; and (2) that the amount or kind of pain in question is in fact required for the achievement of that aim.

For example, some veterinarians, farmers, and animal welfare advocates argue about whether total confinement rearing of veal calves is really "necessary." (This husbandry method is discussed in greater detail below.) Although they seem to be discussing the same thing, they may be talking about two quite different matters. Some people will assume the legitimacy of tender, white veal meat as a goal and are arguing about the possibility of a confinement method that will produce such meat but will not cause the animals undue distress. For others, the issue is whether such meat is a legitimate goal to begin with or a sufficiently important goal to justify any amount of animal distress.

Debates about the "necessity" of a given kind of animal treatment often bog down in confusion and disagreement. One reason this can occur is that people arguing about "necessary" pain or distress tend to shift back and forth between the issues of the legitimacy of the goal and whether a given means toward that goal is in fact required for achieving it. When agreement seems possible about whether a certain amount of animal pain is in fact required for a certain goal, suddenly there will be disagreement about whether that goal is legitimate or sufficiently valuable to justify the animal pain. And if agreement about the legitimacy of a goal seems likely, someone will ask whether a proposed treatment of animals is really required to achieve that goal. This process of shifting between the two very different questions encompassed by the notion of "necessity" can repeat itself endlessly. The notion of "necessity" contributes to this process, because those engaged in argument may think that they are still discussing only one issue, namely the "necessity" of some animal pain, distress, or discomfort.

The best way of avoiding such confusion is to stop talking about the "necessity" of pain or distress associated with various ways of using or treating animals. It is far better to address directly the two questions encompassed by the current notion of "necessity": (1) whether a human aim for which some animal pain or distress is imposed is legitimate or sufficiently valuable to justify the pain; and (2) whether the amount or kind of pain in question is in fact required for the achievement of that human aim. Such issues can be difficult enough. The chances of resolving them will only be diminished by the ambiguous and distracting concept of "necessity."

10B. "Humaneness"

It is difficult to object to the assertion that people ought to treat animals humanely. As most people ordinarily use the term, treating animals "humanely" means treating them as they ought to be treated, in accordance with the moral obligations we human beings have regarding them. Thus saying that people should treat animals "humanely" is like saying that people should act rightly. Each statement is obviously correct. But by itself, each tells us nothing. We need to know what, more precisely, it is to act rightly or to treat animals humanely. An animal farmer and an animal-use abolitionist will almost certainly agree that "all animals ought to be treated humanely." However, to the farmer, humane treatment is consistent with raising animals for food, while to the abolitionist it is not. They will disagree about what constitutes the humane treatment of animals because they disagree about how animals ought to be treated.

There is nothing inherently wrong with applying the terms "humane" or "inhumane" to various ways of treating animals. But to assert that a given way of treating them is humane or inhumane typically is to express one's conclusion about whether such treatment is or is not morally appropriate. Statements about "humaneness" and "inhumaneness" therefore belong at the very end of arguments, after reasons for one's conclusions have already been given.

∼ THE IMMENSITY OF THE TASK
A Host of Conceptual, Empirical, and Ethical Issues

The 10 basic principles developed earlier cut against some views regarding how agricultural and performance animals may be treated. However, these principles only lay preliminary groundwork for many difficult questions.

Some of these issues are conceptual: they involve the definition of terminology used in factual and ethical claims about animals. Among the concepts that require further analysis before normative veterinary ethics can make substantial progress in the farm and performance animal area are animal "welfare," "pain," "suffering," "distress," "discomfort," "pleasure," and "benefit." As discussed in Chapter 13, there are significant differences among animal scientists and veterinarians about how to define the term "welfare," in part because of differences about what animals used in agriculture ought to be provided.

Other difficult issues are empirical: their resolution requires investigation into factual matters. Among such issues are determining what mental states farm and performance animals do experience, what husbandry methods promote or hinder such states, and whether certain methods result in productivity as well as animal welfare.

Empirical investigations can also raise ethical questions. For example, two people might agree that pigs do in fact experience boredom and are happier with visual stimulation. Yet they may still disagree about whether a producer has a moral obligation to make his pigs happier. Another important ethical issue concerns the extent to which diminutions in levels of animal welfare are justified by the interests of producers and the public.

∼ AGRICULTURAL ANIMALS
∼ Current Welfare Issues in Husbandry and Production

Tables 23-1 and 23-2 present an overview of welfare issues relating to food animals. Table 23-1 focuses on swine as an example and presents (without supporting arguments) some of the major issues and claims made for or against certain practices. Table 23-2 relates several current debates relating to the welfare of other species. Many of the positions taken regarding these issues are similar to those that are raised in discussions about swine.

The tables illustrate many, but by no means all, of the questions that currently occupy the attention of producers, veterinarians, and animal welfare advocates. Inclusion in the tables does not indicate a view on my part that an issue points to major deficiencies in current husbandry methods. Nor am I suggesting that the opposing sides on each of these issues always have equal credibility. In the interest of brevity, many of the topics in the tables are presented in general terms. For example, it is not enough to talk about "concrete flooring" for pigs. There are different kinds of concrete, and some concrete floors can be coated or padded so as to change effects of the concrete on the animals. Some investigators believe that great improvements in animal welfare can sometimes be achieved not by abandoning a general kind of technique, but by making subtle modifications.[18] Nor is the presen-

TABLE 23-1
⁓

Some animal welfare issues relating to the production and care of swine

MANAGEMENT METHOD OR TECHNIQUE	CLAIMED BENIFITS	CLAIMED PROBLEMS
Total confinement rearing (in enclosed buildings)	productivity disease control protection from weather management efficiency	joint diseases decreased weight gain infertility improper ventilation leading to discomfort, disease management inefficiency violation of "telos"
Concrete flooring	improved sanitation durability	joint disorders violation of "telos"
Slatted flooring	eliminates need for bedding reduced labor costs improved sanitation improved disease control efficient waste management	injuries, lameness, arthritis (concrete slats) decreased weight gain nipple necrosis
High stocking density during finishing	reduces heating expense management efficiency	insufficient ventilation "social confusion" aggressiveness injuries infection buildup
Dark or semidark lighting conditions	reduced aggression decreased expense	depression stress boredom inspection/supervision problems violation of "telos"
Nonpelletized (dry, sandy) feed	reduced expense	esophogastric ulcers
Accelerated fattening (for example, *ad libitum* feeding)	meat productivity	joint and leg weakness
"Skip" (alternate day) feeding of sows	obesity prevention	hunger, discomfort violation of "telos"
Tail-docking	prevents cannibalism, injuries	unnecessary mutilation ignores underlying causes of aggression
Castration	eliminates meat odor offensive to some consumers	great expense, no real benefit unnecessary mutilation
Continuous tethering/confinement of sows	efficient use of floor space efficient monitoring	lameness behavioral problems violation of "telos"
Farrowing stalls/crates	efficient use of floor space improved waste management protection of piglets	increased disease longer labors, dystocia greater incidence of stillborn and mummified piglets nipple necrosis abnormal behavior, stress violation of "telos"

Continued.

TABLE 23-1 CONT'D

Some animal welfare issues relating to the production and care of swine

MANAGEMENT METHOD OR TECHNIQUE	CLAIMED BENIFITS	CLAIMED PROBLEMS
Early weaning of piglets	quicker breeding of sows improves dietary management	growth delay violation of "telos"
Raising of piglets in elevated battery cages	efficiency improved waste management protection of piglets	inferior health of piglets contamination by dropping wastes violation of "telos"
Subtherapeutic antibiotics in feed	prevents disease promotes growth	masks underlying causes of disease
Long-distance transportation to slaughter	necessary in some areas	dramatic "shrinkage" in body weight stress

TABLE 23-2

Some animal welfare issues regarding the production and care of ruminants and poultry

Dairy Cows and Calves
Open (outdoor) feed-lot rearing
Separation of calves from cows 1 to 3 days following birth
Tying of calves to barn walls
Rearing of calves in single-animal pens
Housing of cows in "comfort stalls" restrained by neck chain without freedom to enter or leave at will
Total indoor confinement of cows and calves
Flooring in indoor systems (for example, slatted versus nonslatted; hard flooring without bedding; elevated
    metal-rod flooring for calves)
Dehorning without anesthesia
Castration without anesthesia
Surgical alteration of bull penis to aid in estrus detection

Veal Calves
Single-animal stalls or crates
Flooring (slatted versus nonslatted; oak versus other materials)
Cleanliness of stalls or crates, waste removal
Ventilation, light
Feeding of low-iron, low-fiber liquid diets
Use of antibiotics in feed

Beef Production
Open (outdoor) feed-lots
Total (indoor) confinement systems
Allegedly stressful transition of animals to feedlot
Proper density of animals in feedlots and enclosed barns
"Bulling" of males by other males in feedlots
Dehorning without anesthesia

Table 23-2 cont'd

Some animal welfare issues
regarding the production and care of ruminants and poultry

Beef Production (cont'd)
Castration without anesthesia
Hot-iron (versus freeze) branding
Use of subtherapeutic antibiotics, growth stimulants, and reproductive regulators
Methods of shipment to slaughterhouses
Humane handling of animals in slaughter plants
Ritual (kosher) slaughter

Sheep Production
Total (indoor) confinement systems
Outdoor feedlots lacking shelter or windbreaks
Early shearing to stimulate appetite
Use of subtherapeutic doses of antibiotics
Castration without anesthesia
Tail-docking without anesthesia
Allegedly cruel, ineffective methods of predator control

Broiler Chickens
Cage (versus floor) systems
Stocking densities
Low illumination systems
Heat, ventilation, removal of ammonia and other air pollutants
Killing of unwanted chicks, poults, and pipped eggs by suffocation, volatile liquids, or simple disposal
Beak trimming
Concentrated, low fiber diet
Use of vaccinations and medicated feeds
Losses and injuries during catching and loading of poultry for shipment
Effectiveness of electrical stunning prior to killing

Laying Hens
Intensive battery cages (stocking density per cage, degree of cage slope, wire-bottomed cages)
Size of colony
Forced moulting (use of starvation/water deprivation, lighting reduction, or low-sodium/calcium diets)
Beak trimming
Declawing
Enriching the internal environment to prevent "boredom" and "boredom"-related vices
Dubbing (partial removal of comb)
Extension of laying periods through manipulation of lighting
Heat, ventilation, removal of ammonia and other air pollutants
Killing of unwanted chicks, poults, and pipped eggs by suffocation, volatile liquids, or simple disposal

Turkeys
Use of slatted floors (versus deep litter)
Stocking densities
Proposed cage systems for breeder hens
Control of lighting to regulate egg production
Heat and ventilation
Desnooding
Wing clipping
Toe clipping

tation by Table 23-1 of conflicting arguments in terms of claimed benefits and problems intended to suggest that these issues should all be resolved by utilitarian or "cost-benefit" analysis.

The tables illustrate the formidable task faced by normative veterinary ethics and animal welfare science in assessing and promoting farm animal welfare. Embedded in many of the issues are hard conceptual, empirical, and ethical questions only the surface of which has yet been scratched. What mental states do these animals experience? How should we conceive of varying levels of welfare for them? How are their interests in these levels to be weighed against legitimate human interests? What methods of production and veterinary care might now improve welfare while having minimal impact on productivity, so that animal welfare can be enhanced while animal welfare science goes about determining how welfare can be promoted in the long term? To what extent must profits be decreased so that certain levels of welfare can be assured? What is an animal's nature or "*telos*" and to what extent and for what reasons might it be entitled to respect? To what extent should the law attempt to assure certain levels of animal welfare? What, more precisely, should be the role of the veterinary profession in advocating farm animal welfare?

Dehorning Cattle without Anesthesia

One of the central arguments of this chapter is that in approaching agricultural and performance animal practice, normative veterinary ethics and animal welfare science should avoid premature conclusions that are not justified by current factual and ethical knowledge. Nevertheless, I want to illustrate the application of principles developed in this book to some specific issues. I shall discuss briefly (and by no means exhaustively) two of the more controversial topics in agricultural animal welfare: the dehorning of dairy and beef cattle without the use of anesthesia and total confinement rearing of so-called "milk-fed" veal.

Some people condemn the dehorning of calves without anesthesia because the practice causes the animals pain. The fact that pain is imposed certainly provides moral weight in opposition to the practice. However, there are important considerations on the other side. On balance, these considerations show that although dehorning young calves with anesthesia might be an ideal, it is still not the case that all farmers who dehorn these animals without anesthesia are acting wrongly.

Dehorning often is required to prevent the animals from injuring themselves and their human handlers.[19] When performed properly on younger animals, dehorning without anesthesia does not appear to cause long-lasting pain or discomfort. The anesthesia process may itself cause some distress because it requires the injection of a nerve-blocking agent, which prolongs the length of the entire procedure. Finally, dehorning with anesthesia can be time-consuming and expensive. For many farmers, anesthesia of calves would cause a major drain on already scarce resources. This would compromise their ability to provide their animals more important things, including veterinary care to prevent or cure serious illness.

Although dehorning young calves without performing a nerve block often seems justifiable, dehorning adult animals without anesthesia is another matter. This practice can not only impede productivity (of lactating dairy cows, for example) but also result in pain that appears to be much greater and longer-lasting than that experienced by calves dehorned without anesthesia. Here, I would urge, one crosses the line between what can be imposed on animals in the name of economic cost.

An important moral ideal of veterinarians is to spare all patients as much pain as possible. Accordingly, the AVMA has called for research to develop "improved techniques for painless, humane castration and dehorning" of cattle and supports "the use of procedures that reduce or eliminate the pain of dehorning and castrating of cattle. These procedures should be completed at the earliest age practicable."[20] If cost-effective ways of painlessly dehorning calves become available, their use will no longer be praiseworthy, but morally obligatory.

Total Confinement Raising of "Milk-fed" Veal

Total confinement production of formula-fed veal often involves calves "chained in single stalls 56-61 cm $\times$ 1.5 m on raised wooden slats to facilitate cleaning. No bedding or freedom of movement is provided. The calves can neither turn nor lie down with ease in these stalls."[21] They are also fed a liquid low-fiber, low-iron diet that, together with the restrictions in locomotion, are said to produce the characteristic light-colored meat.

Interests of the public

It is difficult to maintain that the public has a strong interest in the kind of pale meat that results from this husbandry practice. It is not clear that most people can discern any difference between the color of "milk-fed" and non–"milk-fed" veal, once it is cooked. Milk-fed veal is an expensive, luxury product. It is substantially different from dairy products, eggs, chicken, pork, and beef, which are staples of the American diet. A significant decrease in the supply or increase in the price of these products would cause great hardship across the economic spectrum.

Interests of the animals

It is beyond question that some veal calves are subjected to terrible conditions. There exist facilities (which, producers often say, are smaller, less profitable operations) that are filthy, smelly, dark, and are constructed of materials on which the animals can injure themselves. But there are problems even with more "modern" facilities. In many, there is continuous medication with antibiotics to suppress infection and illness. The low iron and roughage diet has led to cases of general weakness, excessive sucking and licking, and fur balls resulting from licking of the coat to obtain roughage.[22]

Additionally, there is the inability of the animals to move about in a variety of ways normal to the species and to come in contact with other animals. Aside from the common-sense conclusion that such confinement must be distressing (and evidence that it sometimes is), these animals are being deprived of certain freedoms that impartial reason declares they have a great interest in experiencing. Part of the problem with confining veal calves in small enclosures for the whole of their existence is that they are deprived in their short lives of a semblance of what it is like to be themselves. This problem remains even if the animals do not experience significant pain, suffering, or distress.

Objecting to total confinement and formula-feeding of veal calves does not imply condemnation of all husbandry methods that restrict animal movement or diet. Each kind of case must be considered on its own terms with due regard for the importance of the public's interest in inexpensive and safe food products. The problem with total confinement of veal calves is that it serves such an inessential human interest at such an enormous cost to the animals.

Interests of producers

Some producers argue that it is possible to produce satisfactory veal at a profit with far less deprivation to the animals than that associated with total confinement methods.[23] If correct, such contentions argue strongly against more restrictive methods. Moreover, the fact that total confinement raising of veal calves is profitable or may be more profitable than other methods is not a conclusive argument in its favor. The facts that one can make money at some enterprise and that elimination of the enterprise would bring great hardship to those already engaged in it do not render it morally acceptable. Likewise, there is little force to the claim that producing "milk-fed" veal provides a market for dried skim milk which would otherwise go into government stockpiles.[24] It hardly seems fair to address the problem of what to do with surplus milk by causing misery or deprivation to innocent animals. Another argument often raised in favor of total confinement husbandry is that it provides an outlet for many unwanted dairy calves that would otherwise simply be killed. This may provide an argument in favor of some use of these animals, but it does not demonstrate the appropriateness of total confinement veal production. Indeed, we sometimes think it is better to end the lives of certain animals (such as unadoptable stray dogs and cats) than to permit them to suffer terrible conditions.

Interests of the farm community and veterinarians

I believe that some farmers and veterinarians who are not engaged in veal production express support for total confinement husbandry because they view opposition as the first stage of a general attack on animal agriculture. Some animal activists hope that abolition of total confinement raising of veal calves will lead to ending the use of animals for food. However, opposition to certain husbandry methods does not entail opposition to animal agriculture. Nor does the fact that certain people take a stance against a husbandry method make that stance wrong or unworthy of support by veterinarians. Opposing certain reforms because activists endorse them can only harm farmers and the veterinary profession in the long run, because it assists opponents of animal agriculture to present themselves to the public as the only people who care about the animals.

The official position

The AVMA's official view is that "veal calf production is well established, can be humane, and can improve the welfare of calves."[25] The AVMA *Guide for Veal Calf Care and Production*[26] permits confinement rearing, with limitations. For example, "animals should be able to stretch, stand, and lie down comfortably and naturally. Calves may or may not be allowed to turn around, depending on management, housing and health." It is also urged that "veal calves kept in total confinement be kept on oak slatted floors" to permit ease of movement, ventilation, and waste removal. The *Guide* counsels proper construction materials and the seeking of professional advice in the event of injury or distress. The *Guide's* recommendations are clearly well-intentioned, and would improve the lot of many animals. As a document of official veterinary ethics, it is not surprising that the *Guide* attempts to reconcile existing competing interests. However, it seems to miss the intuitive appeal of the argument that calves do better, and live a more tolerable (if not happier) life if allowed to eat normal food, move about, and socialize with other animals.

At present the formula-fed industry in this country does seem "well-established." But things can change. Opposition to total confinement husbandry of calves appears to be growing among the public and veterinarians in the rest of the world.[27] Time will tell whether the American veterinary profession will be judged to have missed an important opportunity to establish its credibility in the farm animal welfare area.

Some Other Welfare Issues in Veterinary Care
To treat or not to treat?

Farm animal veterinarians sometimes must face the question whether to treat a sick or injured animal (as opposed to recommending that it be killed immediately or shipped for slaughter) when treatment may be economically unwise for the client.

Among the relevant considerations are, of course, the probable economic costs of treatment, slaughter, or immediate euthanasia. However, due regard must also be paid to animal welfare. This can mean among other things: (1) not delaying a decision whether to treat when delay would cause the animal unnecessary suffering; (2) taking into account the relative likely suffering as well as the relative expense associated with various treatment options; and (3) not permitting an animal to suffer for a prolonged period of time. Often the most cost-effective and humane course of action will be euthanasia or expeditious shipment.

An important issue in agricultural practice concerns the role of the doctor in the making of a client's decisions. Some large animal practitioners tell me that they are quite aggressive in recommending euthanasia or slaughter when one of these approaches is in the client's economic interest. They are especially forceful when a client balks at making a decision because of emotional attachment to an animal. It is surely appropriate for a veterinarian to point out economic aspects of various alternatives. Nevertheless, if a client makes a decision that the doctor finds economically imprudent, it is still the client's decision to make.

Another important aspect of the decision whether to treat concerns the administration of drugs that will keep an animal alive long enough to be shipped. Several veterinarians have admitted to me that they administer drugs even when not completely confident that at the time of slaughter the legally required withdrawal time will have passed. Among the justifications offered for such an approach are that it is the responsibility of a slaughterhouse inspector to condemn an animal that is too sick or drugged and that any drug residues in a particular animal will be "diluted" by other meat when it reaches the consumer's table. As discussed in the following, veterinarians can have legitimate, good-faith differences with government authorities about the proper use of drugs in food animals. But if a practitioner knows that an animal may contain drug residues at slaughter and pushes the determination onto someone else who may or may not make it, he is committing a great moral wrong upon the public. He also risks exposing the profession as a whole to condemnation for reckless drug use and to more vigorous government regulation than might be necessary.

Advocating animal interests

A veterinarian's status as a medical professional puts one in a unique position to speak for the interests of patients. The following are among the kinds of information that veterinarians can provide to clients when animal welfare considerations must be factored into decision making:

- Whether an animal is being overworked to the extent that it is threatened with acute or chronic injury or disease, and whether resting, euthanasia, or shipment for slaughter is the only feasible way of preventing short- or long-term suffering
- Whether an animal is too injured or infirm to be used for breeding without causing suffering or discomfort
- Whether an animal needs special nutritional treatment or care
- Whether a condition suffered by one or several members of a herd is likely to spread to other animals unless action is taken
- Whether animals require care from the veterinarian to be maintained at an adequate level of welfare

Underutilization of veterinary services

Many veterinarians and animal welfare advocates agree that there is far less utilization of veterinary services by farmers than animal welfare and productivity require.[28] The AVMA *Report on the US Market for Food Animal Veterinary Medical Services* stated that in 1985 beef producers spent 62% of their total animal health care expenditures with a veterinarian; dairy producers 75%; hog producers 47%; and sheep producers 54%.[29]

The AVMA *Report* suggested that the solution for veterinarian underutilization is the model of the agricultural doctor as herd health consultant (see Chapter 16). According to the *Report*, the veterinarian is the "logical person" to deliver advice focused on the entire "financial performance of the livestock enterprise." The *Report* was quite certain that the "fundamental task" for food animal doctors is to shift to providing such services.[30]

However, it is far from obvious that the profession should rush quickly to promote the model of the economic manager for all farm animal practitioners. The *Report* concedes that few veterinary students receive serious training in agricultural economics,[31] and that producers consider private practitioners less knowledgeable about agribusiness and economics than they themselves or agricultural extension agents.[32] The *Report* also admits that the "feasibility of improving veterinarians' knowledge and cost-effectiveness relative to other suppliers of information is a *critical question*" from veterinary educational and marketing standpoints.[33]

Descriptive veterinary ethics (see Chapter 6) should determine how many practitioners and students are suited—intellectually, aesthetically, and morally—to the model of the veterinarian as economic manager. Many veterinarians, surely, gravitate toward farm animal practice because they like the kind of life it traditionally has provided, including opportunities for hands-on interaction with large animals and farmers.

Many agricultural doctors have an abiding concern for the welfare of farm animals. Before the veterinary schools and professional associations set out to refashion the image of the agricultural practitioner, it might be wise to determine how many present and future veterinarians are interested in such a transformation. The profession should also consider more fully how due regard for animal welfare can be maintained by those veterinarians who might want to function as economic managers. Also relevant are the potential effects of management-oriented approaches upon the public's image of agricultural practitioners and the profession as a whole.

∼ AGRICULTURAL ANIMALS
∼ MIXED WELFARE AND PUBLIC HEALTH ISSUES
The Extra-label Drug Use Issue

After years of effort by the AVMA, the U.S. Congress enacted the Animal Medicinal Drug Use Clarification Act of 1994. This was an achievement the political, legal, and ethical significance of which cannot be overestimated.[34] Veterinarians who were using drugs on species, for conditions, or in dosages other than those indicated on the labels of these drugs were in violation of the Food, Drug, and Cosmetics (FD&C) Act, which declared "unsafe" any animal drug used other than as directed on its label.[35] The FDA, recognizing that compliance with the law would cripple the ability of practitioners to treat patients, issued guidelines that allowed extra-label use of animal and human drugs under certain circumstances. These guidelines were not successful. They were confusing and unclear. For example, one of several revisions of the policy on extra-label use in food-producing animals stated that the FDA would "*consider* regulatory action" against any veterinarian who engaged in such use, but then said that extra-label drug use "*may* be *considered* by a veterinarian when the health of animals is immediately threatened and suffering or death would result from failure to treat the affected animals." Having then allowed what it appeared previously to disallow, the policy seemed to take back the permission, occasionally. It warned that "in instances of this nature regulatory action would not *ordinarily* be considered," provided certain criteria were met, among them that there was no marketed drug specifically labeled to treat the condition diagnosed or that drug therapy at the dosage recommended by the labeling has been found clinically ineffective in the animals to be treated.[36]

Not only were the FDA's policies on extra-label use unclear, but also veterinarians who complied with them were still in violation of the FD&C Act. The Act still prohibited extra-label use of drugs: not just of animal drugs on animals, but also of drugs labeled for human beings (such as cancer chemotherapeutic agents) on veterinary patients. Because the FDA guidelines themselves ignored the statute they were supposed to enforce, any protection provided by the guidelines seemed flimsy and unassuring. The comfort level of practitioners was eroded further by the ability of the FDA to change or withdraw the guidelines without notice or input from the profession; by the declaration of the FDA Commissioner that "a veterinarian who uses a drug in an extra-label manner does so at his peril"[37]; and by the claim of a powerful congressman, intent on stopping all extra-label use, that the FDA policy put "the public's health at risk by exposing consumers to residues."[38]

The Animal Medicinal Drug Use Clarification Act specifically legalizes discretionary extra-label use of drugs by veterinarians. The Act allows extra-label use of

FDA-approved animal drugs only by or on the lawful written order of a licensed veterinarian, within the context of a veterinarian-client-patient relationship and in compliance with regulations of the Secretary of Health and Human Services. Unlike the former compliance guidelines, these are true regulations, which must be open to public review and discussion prior to adoption. The Act allows the Secretary to prohibit particular uses of an animal drug and to establish safe levels of residues for animal drugs where extra-label use may present a risk to public health. The Act prohibits extra-label use in or on animal feed, and when the labeling of another animal drug that contains the same active ingredient and is in the same dosage form and concentration provides for that intended use. The Act also permits extra-label use of human drugs by or on the lawful written order of a licensed veterinarian within the context of a veterinarian-client-patient relationship and in compliance with regulations of the Secretary of Health and Human Services.[39]

As Dr. Stephen Sundlof, Director of the FDA Center for Veterinary Medicine explained, enactment of the new law was not the end but the beginning of full exploration of the proper bounds of extra-label use by practitioners. The law:

> ...takes extra-label drug use out of the closet, and it allows us now to engage in free exchange of ideas without the threat that there's going to be litigation involved. And because of that, hopefully, there will be more activity, more scholarly discussion on the issue. From that scholarly discussion will come better ways of preventing extra-label drug use from becoming a food safety issue.[40]

Clearly, additional scientific data will be required about the effectiveness of various extra-label approaches and about the detection and prevention of drug residues in food products. Nevertheless, there will remain fundamental *ethical* questions about what to do with such information. The most important of these issues concerns the extent to which any verifiable risks associated with certain drug uses in food animals is justified by the benefits to society at large. In other words, if extra-label uses are effective in promoting animal health and producer profitability, and if such drugs are associated with risks to human health, how much risk is acceptable so that consumers may have safe and inexpensive foods?

Lying beneath this general issue are difficult ethical questions that require sustained consideration by government, producers, veterinarians, and the public. In balancing risks against benefits, how important are the interests of those involved in the production process? To what extent does the government have the right, or obligation, to protect the public against its own desire for cheaper foodstuffs, if such products also carry health risks from drug use? When evidence regarding the risks of a drug is inconclusive, should the government err on the side of safety and prohibit its use or on the side of productivity and allow it? To what extent does any individual citizen have a basic moral right to be free from risk from drug use and thus to be protected from utilitarian analysis of total risks versus benefits? To what extent do government and producers have a moral obligation to inform consumers about the risks of drugs used in the production of foodstuffs?

There are also ethical issues regarding the effects of drug use (whether or not extra-label) on the animals themselves. One must consider the extent to which drugs substitute for good hygiene and management, mask underlying animal stress or discomfort, or threaten the development of uncontrollable animal diseases.[41]

All these ethical questions must figure prominently in the scholarly and practical discussions about the proper role of the use of drugs in food producing animals generally and extra-label use in such animals in particular. Moreover, the Animal Medicinal Drug Use Clarification Act of 1994 places enormous ethical responsibilities on food animal veterinarians, responsibilities for which the present state of knowledge regarding extra-label use and drug residues may not provide sufficient guidance. The public will likely consider safe food more important than helping particular animals or assuring the profits of any particular producer. However, veterinarians—faced as they are with the actual animals and clients before them—may understandably focus on their ability to employ an extra-label use to treat their patients. The profession must accelerate the search for information about safe and effective extra-label drug use and assure that individual veterinarians will act ethically. Otherwise, the FDA (which is the same FDA that issued the problematic animal drug use compliance guidelines) could reimpose by regulation substantial restrictions upon extra-label use.[42]

Lay Administration of Animal Drugs

The FD&C Act explicitly creates a category of "veterinary prescription drugs," defined as animal drugs that are unsafe for animal use except under the professional supervision of a licensed veterinarian.[43] However, the FD&C Act also recognizes a category of FDA-approved animal drugs that need not be used under veterinary supervision and are available over-the-counter to laymen. Producers who administer such drugs to food animals are further protected by state veterinary practice acts, which typically exempt producers who treat or medicate their own animals from the general prohibition against practicing veterinary medicine without a license.

Today the great majority of drugs for food animals is purchased not from veterinarians or pharmacies, but farm stores, feed mills, and mail-order companies. The comprehensive 1987 AVMA *Report on the Market for Food Animal Veterinary Services* found that in 1985 only 24% of the total $949.4 million sales of food animal veterinary pharmaceuticals and biologicals (excluding feed additives) was made by veterinarians. Based on manufacturers' prices, it was estimated that veterinarians accounted for only 9% of the total $1,779.2 million sales of pharmaceuticals, biologics, and feed additives.[44] The *Report* documented widespread dissatisfaction among agricultural veterinarians about administration of drugs by farmers; sales of drugs and vaccines by feed and animal supply stores; dispensing of drug advice by lay feed and drug salespeople; aggressive marketing techniques by lay drug sales operations; roving lay salespeople who dispense from trucks; and mail-order operations conducted by laymen or veterinarians.[45]

Clearly, some farmers and self-styled "experts" do not know what they are doing. Animals suffer. Veterinarians sometimes are called when problems become so bad that producers can no longer pretend to be able to deal with them. As bovine practitioner Dr. Darryl Johnson observes, the open availability of so many drugs used in food animals has encouraged some inappropriate attitudes among producers:

> The current system has produced more than a generation of livestock producers, aided and abetted by marketing and advertising, who generally regard animal medicines much as other agricultural commodities used to optimize production. A dose of something was indicated for almost everything and specific label directions often gave way to expediency and complacency. A bottle,

bag, or syringe was, at times, used in an attempt to substitute for accurate diagnosis, management, changes, or capital improvements.[46]

Reliable data are needed regarding the effects of lay administration of various drugs and biologics on animal welfare, productivity, and public health. It would be unrealistic to require that all drugs always be administered by or under the direct supervision of veterinarians. In many cases, there are both economic and welfare justifications for administration of drugs by farmers. But because it is clear that there is far too much medication of animals by laymen, the profession need not fear research into welfare and productivity aspects of this practice. Whatever is learned cannot help but strengthen the economic position of agricultural doctors. Dr. Johnson, for example, argues that veterinarians "must be the hub for effective supervision of how animal drugs are to be used on the farm, and that is not synonymous with controlling the sale of all animal drugs."[47]

If factual analysis of the effects of lay medication warrants, government authorities ought to consider requiring *some* form of veterinary participation in the medication of food animals. At the very least, the states ought to prosecute laymen (such as drug salespeople dispensing veterinary advice with their products) who engage in the unlawful unlicensed practice of veterinary medicine as currently defined in these jurisdictions. State boards of veterinary medicine and professional associations should move decisively against any veterinarians who are involved in the indiscriminate supply of drugs to farmers, without adequate information about the animals that receive them.

Veterinarians and the Federal Accreditation Program

In 1912 the USDA established its program of accreditation of veterinary practitioners to assist the federal government in performing a wide range of responsibilities in protecting animal and human health. The program is administered by the Animal and Plant Health Inspection Service (APHIS). Accreditation permits veterinarians in private practice to inspect animals and apply tests for shipment and to issue official certificates to accompany such animals pursuant to state and federal regulations; to participate in cooperative state and federal programs for the control and eradication of animal diseases; and to perform various functions in accordance with the federal Horse Protection Act.

The federal accreditation program encountered serious problems, one of which was veterinarians who signed certificates without examining animals or who falsified information on these certificates.[48] Responding to these difficulties, in 1992 APHIS made significant changes in the regulations that govern the qualifications, duties, and supervision of accredited veterinarians.[49] The new regulations set forth lengthy and specific ethical standards for accredited veterinarians, including prohibitions against issuing or signing a certificate without personal and sufficient observation of animals, and issuing or signing any certificate or form without sufficient identification of animals and tests performed. The new regulations permit more efficient discipline of practitioners who violate the technical and ethical requirements. The regulations also establish accreditation on a nationwide instead of a statewide basis. The regulations illustrate how government agencies enforce ethical as well as technical standards, and how administrative ethical standards can result from perceived ethical problems.

~ BIOTECHNOLOGY, GENETIC ENGINEERING, AND TRANSGENIC ANIMALS

Much controversy has arisen regarding biotechnology, genetic engineering, and the creation of so-called "transgenic" animals. These issues involve the veterinary profession because veterinarians are major participants in the development and application of biotechnological techniques. More importantly, these techniques may affect how many veterinarians will treat their current patients and the kinds of conditions—indeed, the kinds of patients—they may be called upon to treat in the future.

The scientific, ethical, and political literature addressing animal biotechnology and related techniques is growing at a frightening pace. Many people see in the new scientific manipulation of animals a glorious millennium of human health and agricultural productivity. Others see dangerous challenges to traditional philosophical and religious values concerning the nature of humans as well as animals. Animal biotechnology raises very serious, and by no means easily answered, questions about the nature and value of technology, the relative importance of public safety and economic gain, the relative importance of animal welfare and corporate profits, and the proper role of government in the support and regulation of science and technology.[50]

Because of the enormous implications of animal biotechnology, this brief discussion can only scratch the surface of this challenging subject. I will offer a few basic tools that veterinarians and others who are interested in the potential effects of biotechnology on *animals* can use in approaching some of the ethical issues.

Biotechnology, genetic engineering, and transgenism are not limited to agricultural or large animals. To date, more work has been done on the genetic engineering of mice than on other species, and transgenic animals already play an important role in biomedical research. However, a discussion of animal biotechnology is appropriately placed in this chapter. Many of the more immediate effects of biotechnology on the public are likely to be seen in the agricultural area. Bovine growth hormone is already in use in the United States. Much work is being done on other products to improve agricultural animal productivity and on the development of vaccines for large animals. Because of their size, farm animals such as cows, sheep, pigs, and goats are being developed to produce pharmaceutical products in their milk. Insofar as veterinarians have direct contact with animals affected by biotechnology or genetic engineering, much of this contact is likely to be with farm animals.

Differing Definitions

In approaching ethical issues relating to animal "biotechnology" and associated techniques, it is essential to understand what one means by critical terminology. There appears to be virtually universal agreement that the terms "transgenism" and "transgenic animals" refer to "animals that have integrated foreign DNA into their germline as a consequence of experimental introduction of DNA, usually by microinjecting recombinant DNA into pronuclei of fertilized eggs."[51] However, there is no shortage of varied, and sometimes inconsistent, definitions of "biotechnology" and "genetic engineering." These definitions may sometimes be intended to further more fundamental goals of their proponents.

For example, one scientist defines "biotechnology" as "the application of biological organisms, systems, or processes to manufacturing and service industries."[52] This definition regards as examples of "biotechnology" such ancient (and by no means high-tech) activities as the baking of bread and the brewing of beer. Another definition restricts biotechnology to "manipulations at the molecular or cellular level that affect genetic material in a specific manner"[53]—that is, alternations that do not just affect biological processes, but do so through direct modification of molecules or cells. The former definition tends to be employed by those who argue that people should not fear such techniques as direct genetic manipulation or protein engineering because, they will then argue, genetic and protein manipulation is really no different from ancient techniques such as fermentation that use biological processes in manufacturing.

Likewise, according to one discussion "genetic engineering" refers to "the field of manipulating the DNA of a cell or an animal to alter the genetic information contained within the organism's genome. The standard techniques of recombinant DNA are used."[54] In contrast, philosopher Bernard Rollin speaks about "traditional genetic engineering," which "was done by selective breeding, over long periods of time."[55] Although a common argument in favor of genetic engineering is that it does not differ in principle from traditional kinds of selective breeding which also results in genetic change, this position may seem easier to make if one does not define genetic engineering to require direct manipulation of DNA.

Broad Characterizations and the Thesis of "Ethical Neutrality"

More important than divergent definitions of critical terms is the tendency of many in this area (mostly supporters of new scientific techniques) to speak very broadly about the subject matter. Frequently, one finds discussions of the potential benefits or dangers of "biotechnology," "genetic engineering," or the "creation of transgenic animals." Such ways of talking are unfortunate not just because they lump together very different kinds of processes and activities, but because they render the argument in favor of the new scientific manipulation of animals much easier to make than it really is.

This process may not be deliberate, in the sense of being intentionally designed to belittle arguments against scientific manipulation, but the effect can be the same. It happens as follows. The question put for debate (usually by advocates of "biotechnology" and so forth) is whether "biotechnology," "genetic engineering," or "transgenism" are inherently good or bad. Once the question is phrased like this, the answer is obvious, and skeptics must lose. For unless one believes that it is necessarily wrong to manipulate an animal's genetic material or to do so in ways that create new species or kinds of animals, "biotechnology," "genetic engineering," and "transgenism" *cannot* be considered *inherently* wrong. For there must, surely, be *some* potential good effects of these activities. Therefore "biotechnology," "genetic engineering," and "transgenism" are ethically neutral. Taken by themselves, they are neither good nor bad. The issue then becomes whether they are used for good or bad purposes, and to produce good or bad consequences. Philosopher Bernard Rollin expresses what I shall call this "thesis of ethical neutrality" as follows. His conclusion is entirely justified, given the very broad subject matter of his discussion: "the genetic engineering of animals."

> …[T]he genetic engineering of animals in and of itself is morally neutral, very much like the traditional breeding of animals or, indeed, like any tool. If it is used judiciously to benefit humans and animals, with foreseeable risks controlled and the welfare of animals kept clearly in mind as a goal and a governor, it is certainly morally nonproblematic and can provide great benefits. On the

other hand, if it is used simply because it is there, in a manner guided at most only by considerations of economic expediency and "efficiency" or by quest for knowledge for its own sake with no moral thinking tempering its development, it could well instantiate the worst rational fears... .[56]

Problems with the Thesis of "Ethical Neutrality"

Rollin's statement of the thesis of ethical neutrality should not be interpreted as a green light for genetic engineering. However, for some advocates of genetic manipulation of animals, the thesis of ethical neutrality is likely to seem the end, and not as it is for Rollin, the beginning of ethical assessment of a given biotechnological technique. When informed that "genetic engineering" ("biotechnology," "transgenism," or whatever) is ethically neutral, some scientists will in fact conclude that they can proceed with their research unencumbered by ethical questions. The thesis of ethical neutrality reaches a receptive audience of scientists, many of whom begin with the erroneous belief that science is value-free (see Chapter 13).

"Genetic engineering doesn't hurt people or animals, people do."

The major problem with the thesis of ethical neutrality is not that it is likely to be misinterpreted by advocates of biotechnology as support for research divorced from ethical deliberation about the appropriateness of the research. Rather, the thesis is at best a correct answer to a bad question. The thesis of neutrality misses the point many who have doubts about the new manipulation of animals are trying to make. It renders these doubts more difficult to raise by diverting attention toward the issue of whether such general activities as "biotechnology," "genetic engineering," or the "genetic engineering of animals" are inherently good or evil.

The thesis of ethical neutrality is identical in important respects to an argument sometimes made by opponents of handgun control. It is sometimes said that it is wrong and foolish to restrict gun ownership because "guns don't kill people, people do." This argument is both obviously correct and obviously beside the point. Guns do not jump by themselves out of holsters or cabinets and kill people. Guns can be used for good as well as bad purposes. Guns are therefore "ethically neutral." The point, I take it, opponents of handguns are attempting to make is that, given the background conditions in late twentieth century America, allowing private citizens to own guns is like lighting a match (itself an "ethically neutral" activity) in the midst of a cloud of escaping natural gas—something certain to result in trouble. Advocates of gun control claim that, in fact, guns are more likely to be used by bad people for bad purposes and that society would benefit if private citizens were not permitted to possess them.

My intention here is not to endorse this latter argument for gun control, but to observe that the argument must be assessed by consideration of *facts* relating to those who use or are capable of using guns. Likewise, when people assess certain kinds of biotechnology or genetic engineering, they need to ask not whether these activities are inherently ethically neutral, but whether, in fact, given conditions that now or are likely to exist in our society, *certain kinds* of scientific manipulation of animals are likely to do more harm than good. These are not foolish or easy questions. It is possible that consideration of the facts will require the conclusion that opponents or skeptics are grossly exaggerating the potential bad effects of certain biotechnological processes, just as it is possible opponents of gun ownership are mistaken in thinking that gun control is, in fact, an effective way of ending the carnage on our streets. However, to such factual issues, claims of "ethical neutrality" are irrelevant.

As a British Veterinary Association study group on biotechnology has observed, we must avoid generalities. Each biotechnological technique, process, or product must be considered on its own merits. "Any ethical analysis will have to weigh up the overall value of the product against any harms that may result from its production or commercial use, for example, either to the animals, or to the environment."[57]

Claimed Potential Benefits and Harms of Genetic Engineering of Agricultural Animals

Table 23-3 lists some of the potential benefits and harms that have been attributed by supporters and opponents to animal biotechnology, genetic engineering, and transgenism. The table does not list all the kinds of claims that can be raised on either side. The table is not intended to assert that the case against animal biotechnology is as strong as the case for it or that all of the listed arguments on either side are of equal merit. The table does indicate, however, the depth and breadth of the ethical, religious, social, economic, and political issues raised by animal biotechnology.

What Should Veterinarians Do? The Example of Bovine Growth Hormone

Veterinarians must ask what role they should play in the difficult issues relating to animal biotechnology. One answer to this question is suggested by something about which many veterinarians are already familiar: the use of bovine growth hormone, or bovine somatatropin (BST), to stimulate milk production in dairy cows.

A complete history of BST has not been written, and a satisfactory consideration of the scientific and ethical issues raised by the product is beyond the scope of this discussion. However, certain parts of the story can usefully be noted. BST is a protein that is naturally produced by the pituitary gland and regulates a cow's lactational cycle. The Monsanto Company discovered a way of producing large quantities of the hormone through genetic engineering and determined that daily injections of BST can significantly increase the production of milk.[58] In 1985 the FDA decided that BST was safe for human consumption and in 1986 that the hormone would not harm the environment. In November 1993 formal approval was given to Monsanto to market one of four forms of genetically engineered BST. Monsanto agreed to undertake a 5-year program of dairy herd monitoring to determine whether the potential labeled side effects of the drug on cows were manageable with current mastitis control programs and techniques. By late 1994 the Monsanto product, Posilac®, was in widespread use in the United States.

PUBLIC SAFETY. This brief outline greatly simplifies what has been a complex series of events. From the start, objections have been raised to BST by people who claimed (alternatively or in combination) that it is not safe for human consumption; that its long-term safety has not yet been demonstrated; and that there is no reason even to subject the public to the slightest possibility of risk in light of the fact that America's dairy cows already produce more milk than the public can consume. Perhaps because of the almost religious role cow's milk plays in American culture, some people found in BST an effective vehicle to promote among the general public general objections to biotechnology and genetic engineering. A number of farmers and grocery chains declared that they would not produce or sell "BST milk" or dairy products. Because the

Table 23-3

～

Examples of claimed potential benefits and detriments of biotechnology and genetic engineering in agricultural animals

Claimed Potential Benefits
For People
- Increasing the supply and availability of meat and animal food products by modifying animals so that they are no longer seasonal breeders; adding muscling and growth genes; increasing appetite to increase production relative to maintenance costs; genetically altering animals for earlier puberty and shorter gestation; controlling timing and rate of ovulation to produce twins in cattle, sheep, and goats, larger litters in swine, and daily ovulation in chickens; decreasing turnover of gut epithelium to decrease maintenance costs; rejuvenating hens by simulating molting[*]
- Genetically engineering animals to produce higher-protein and lower-fat meat, milk, and eggs
- Use of genetically engineered products to increase production of food products or growth rate
- Production of disease-resistant food animals that do not require administration of antibiotics, thus protecting people from consumption of drug residues
- Increasing adaptability of food animals to local environmental conditions such as high or low temperatures or disease
- Decreasing the cost of food products by developing disease and parasite-resistant animals, drugs, and vaccines
- Genetic engineering of farm animals to produce proteins for the prevention, treatment, or diagnosis of human diseases (such as human growth hormone, tissue plasminogen activator, and blood factors)

For Animals
- Creation of animals more resistant to disease and better able to tolerate husbandry conditions with minimal impact on welfare
- Development of diagnostic tests,[†] vaccines,[‡] and more effective drugs
- Genetic engineering of animals, such as blowfly-resistant sheep, naturally resistant to common parasites[§]

Claimed Potential Detriments
To People
- Creation and consumption of food products the long-term safety of which has not been or cannot be established
- Creation of animals that can carry zoonotic diseases for which treatments may not be available
- Unintended release of transgenic animals into the environment, where they can do unpredictable damage or can transfer their genetic material to wild or domestic animals
- Economic dislocations and hardships caused by the concentration of genetically engineered agricultural animals or by the use of genetically engineered products in the hands of larger agricultural entities and businesses
- Possession of the tools of biotechnology (especially, the patenting of transgenic animals) by private businesses, which will profit unduly from the technology and prevent their use by all farmers or at least those who cannot afford to pay
- Promotion of a general attitude that people can do as they like with nature, which will lead to a general disregard of nature and the environment, which will in turn harm people
- The violation of natural or religious law by those who manipulate genes or create new kinds or species of animals

To Animals
- Negative effects on animal welfare associated with the production effects of genetic engineering, such as pain or distress associated with accelerated growth, increased stress, or disease associated with increased

Continued.

[*]Seidel GE: Characteristics of future agricultural animals. In Evans JW, Hollaender A, editors: *Genetic Engineering of Animals*, New York, 1986, Plenum Press, p 303.
[†]Jackwood MA: Biotechnology and the development of diagnostic tests in veterinary medicine, *J Am Vet Med Assoc* 204:1603-1605, 1994.
[‡]Yilma T: Genetically engineered vaccines for animal viral diseases, *J Am Vet Med Assoc* 204:1606-1615, 1994.
[§]Headon DR: Biotechnology: Endless possibilities for veterinary medicine, *J Am Vet Med Assoc* 204:1597-1602, 1994.

TABLE 23-3 CONT'D

~

**Examples of claimed potential benefits and detriments of
biotechnology and genetic engineering in agricultural animals**

Claimed Potential Detriments (cont'd)
To Animals (cont'd)
    production (for example, claimed increase in incidence of mastitis in cows given BST)
  • Creation of deformed or incapacitated animals that require extensive monitoring and supervision and
    will suffer if careful supervision is not provided
  • Negative effects on animal welfare associated with the need to administer genetically engineered sub-
    stances (such as growth hormone), relating to the frequency of administration of such substances, and
    the improper administration by untrained personnel
  • Potential suffering experienced by genetically engineered animals that are part of experimental develop-
    ments, and are "failed" attempts at such development because they are deformed or have other problems
  • Promotion of the attitude that people can do what they like to animals, which will result in general dis-
    regard for the value of animals, which will in turn result in cruel and abusive treatment not just of
    genetically engineered animals but animals in general

opposition to BST on the grounds of public safety appears insupportable by scientific evidence, some commentators believe opposition reflects a generalized irrational fear of technology, ignorance of science, or opposition to science.[59]

ECONOMIC AND SOCIAL EFFECTS. Some people have opposed BST on the grounds that it will cause economic hardship, by driving out of business small dairy farmers who either might not be able to afford the product or cannot compete with larger producers whose use of the product would give them even greater competitive advantage.[60] Among the responses generated by this objection to BST are that small dairy farms would close independently of the use of the hormone; that small dairy farmers can use the product profitably; that our economy rewards efficiency and if BST enables the production of cheaper dairy products, millions more people would benefit from it than the relatively few farmers who might be harmed; and that government support of inefficient industries or means of production is in the long run bad for everyone because it stifles innovation and competition.

ANIMAL WELFARE. Questions have also been raised regarding the effects of BST on the cows. In 1994 Dr. David Kronfeld published an extensive review of reported results and regulatory actions.[61] Kronfeld maintains, among other things, that (1) BST can be associated with catabolic stress, which can be cumulative with stress caused by rough handling, poor housing, and disease; (2) more information is needed about the ability of cows to tolerate the increased body heat associated with the hormone; (3) exogenous BST increases mastitis incidence, duration per case, and days of antibiotic treatment per herd in one of every two or three treated herds; (4) mastitis-related effects are extremely variable and unpredictable so that it is possible to see no effects in some herds and significant effects in others; (5) increases in the incidence of mastitis are not attributable to the increase in milk production alone; and (6) unless producers and veterinarians develop support programs for cows on BST serious animal welfare questions will arise concerning its use. Other veterinarians have raised concerns about the potential effects of BST on cow welfare.[62] There have also been reports from veterinarians who have seen no welfare problems with the product,[63] and from farmers who have used it successfully.[64]

THE ROLE OF VETERINARIANS. It is clear from just this skeletal summary of events that the issues relating to BST (like the issues relating to genetic engineering of animals and animal products generally) raise considerations that go far beyond the expertise of any single profession. Veterinarians must allow experts in public health and human medicine to determine the effects of genetically engineered products on human health and safety. Veterinarians cannot assess the economic effects of animal technology. Veterinarians cannot structure or restructure government so that it engages in risk assessment that pays due regard for animal welfare, much less human economic and social considerations likely to be affected by biotechnology.

Veterinarians can, however, relentlessly raise questions about the effects of biotechnology on animal welfare. The primary engine of biotechnology will be profits. Moreover, those who benefit from animal biotechnology (including, it should never be forgotten, the general public) are likely to *want* to believe the old adage that a productive animal must be a happy animal. As one advocate of animal genetic engineering puts it:

> ...the driving force determining the kinds of animals on farms in 2025 will be profitability. This means producing animal products that meet consumer demands as efficiently as possible. In response to animal welfare concerns, there will be more attention paid to the way animals are kept; to some extent animals will be bred with personalities to fit their environments. Fortunately, in most cases the well-being of animals is closely related to efficient production.[65]

Because there are likely to be many economic advantages to increased agricultural production enabled by biotechnology, veterinarians must stand on guard for the animals. They should encourage the development of biotechnological techniques that can help animals resist disease and cope more successfully with husbandry conditions. But they must also raise questions if productive efficiency is *not* associated with animal welfare. The profession may be in a difficult situation. At least at present, the great bulk of American society is likely to be no more concerned about the welfare of genetically engineered farm animals than it has been about the welfare of traditional farm animals—which is not very greatly. At the same time, if something goes wrong, and even only a few animals are substantially harmed by biotechnology, the public may become immediately outraged and then will likely seek someone to blame. They might ask veterinarians where *they* were all this time.

To protect itself as well as its patients and clients, the profession must become a forum for animal welfare questions relating to agricultural biotechnology. This will not always be easy. Paychecks and grants can be involved. Veterinarians employed by companies developing genetically engineered products may have to exhibit courage in making the case that, in the long run, they are doing their employers a favor by raising welfare and ethical questions during product development, before problems with the public might arise. Veterinarians who work for universities with economic ties to biotechnology companies may sometimes have to argue that, as academics, they are morally as well as professionally obligated to ask uncomfortable questions. Farm animal doctors who receive financial inducements to use genetically engineered products, either from manufacturers or clients,[66] must carefully observe the effects of these products.

People who do not ask questions rarely formulate the best arguments for their positions. They may accept weak or indefensible positions. They can fail to see questions that should be addressed. Veterinarians like Dr. Kronfeld who tenaciously ask questions about animal welfare are doing everyone, including biotechnology companies and government a favor. Even if all of the questions can be satisfactorily answered, at least the questions will have been asked, and a better case will then have been made for the humaneness of a given technique. If appropriate answers to some of the questions indicate that more needs to be investigated or done to protect the animals, then animal welfare can be improved.

Should veterinarians welcome the genetic engineering of submoronic animal machines?

Some people believe that genetic engineering might be beneficial to farm animals by enabling the creation of animals that will not have unpleasant experiences or that will be positively happy under conditions of intensive production.[67] One might, for example, make calves that are content never to move or chickens that do not mind being kept in tiny cages. It does seem plausible to argue that producers have a moral obligation not only to improve husbandry methods to reduce animal stress but also to try to change animals to reduce the kinds of objectionable experiences they can have. Yet even such an argument has its limits. In *Brave New World*, the novelist Aldous Huxley imagined a society that genetically manipulates and clones humans to have different levels of intelligence so as to enhance the productivity and happiness of the population as a whole.[68] This society is fundamentally disrespectful to human beings. It makes many of them less than what people can be, even if most are too stupid to know it. Farm animals are beings of some worth and value in part because of their ability to perceive their environment. They are lucky, compared with plants, amoebae, and earthworms, because there is so much more of the world that they are capable of taking in. It is therefore not altogether foolish to ask whether too much engineering to extract distressful mental states would make of agricultural animals less than we ought to allow them to remain. The creation of submoronic farm animals capable of little more than ingestion, excretion, and production might not be a bother to these animals. But it would say something about the regard one has for these creatures, and perhaps for other animals as well. This may not be a view of animals veterinarians should want to encourage.

Beyond Specific Effects: Humankind's Relationship with Nature

It is important to understand and evaluate possible effects of specific biotechnological processes or techniques. However, one of the most interesting and potentially significant objections to biotechnology is that in the aggregate biotechnology may foster an attitude toward nature which, in the long run, will harm people, animals, and the environment. As philosopher Strachan Donnelly writes:

> If we come to see our world as solely our own human creation or artifice—if this becomes our ethical, philosophic, or religious horizon or worldview—then we will have become, against our own fundamental nature as living organisms, thoroughly denaturalized. We will have exacerbated the 'human-nature' split begun in earnest in the 17th century. This would be the end of us as seekers after 'living' natural norms and ways of being human and, given the press of our present technological powers, no doubt the end of much of nature's richness and goodness itself. …Here

is a crucial reason why animal biotechnology, amidst its great practical promise for human welfare, must find its ethics of interventions into nature: an ethics of limitations, the controlling of animal biotechnology's own Promethean powers.[69]

It is far from obvious that animal biotechnology will lead or contribute to the kind of world view about which Donnelly warns. However, the important concerns he raises tend to be ignored when scientists, regulators, and even ethicists argue about whether specific biotechnological techniques are "ethically neutral" or will have good or bad consequences. *Will* human beings, animals, and the environment benefit from a world view in which we humans intervene in nature to the point where we believe that every part of nature is ours for the shaping? All advocates of biotechnology—indeed all of us who are likely to be affected by biotechnology, which is of course all of us—*should* read Huxley's *Brave New World*. Here is a society every part of which is engineered by humans for human purposes. (Of course, genetic features that nature developed intrude from time to time in Huxley's "utopia," and cause problems for its engineers.) It is a dull, predictable, and ultimately unsatisfying world. It lacks complexity, diversity, and significance because nature left to its devices is wonderfully and some times terribly unpredictable, complex, and messy. It is a pale reflection of what life can be because it can be no better than the ideas of those who engineer it. Hopefully, Huxley's predictions will never come to pass. However, his "brave" world may be preventable only if people regard the potential impact of biotechnology on their general world view as important a matter as the production of vaccines and drugs, inexpensive milk, or long-lived tomatoes.

∾ PERFORMANCE ANIMAL PRACTICE: GENERAL CONSIDERATIONS

Performance animal practice can be defined as veterinary practice upon animals that compete or are an integral part of competition in events requiring athletic or physical prowess by animals, human handlers, or both. The following discussion focuses upon ethical issues relevant to veterinary practice on the most common performance animals: thoroughbred, standardbred, and quarter horse racing horses; show horses (including participants in combined training events); greyhound racing dogs; and rodeo animals. There are important ethical issues regarding other kinds of performance animals (for example, polo horses and competition sled dogs) and noncompetitive performance animals (for example, circus animals), but considerations of space do not permit discussion of these issues here.

Performance animal practice presents many of the same ethical issues that arise out of food and farm animal practice. Like agricultural animals, many performance animals are on the one hand economic assets expected to yeild income for owners, but are also sentient beings with legitimate interests of their own. As is the case in agricultural practice, there are important unresolved conceptual, empirical, and ethical issues that must be addressed before a satisfactory approach to performance animal welfare can be fashioned. For example, as equine athlete specialist Dr. Reuben Rose observes, "in comparison with the extensive body of information available on human athletic performance, the scientific study of the equine athlete is still in its infancy."[70] Regarding the analysis of locomotion and gait, researchers still lack much needed data, standardized nomenclature and recording systems, and critical analyses of pain, fatigue, and the causes of lameness.[71]

Performance animals, especially horses, play a significant role in the American economy and culture. In 1992 approximately 71 million people attended U.S. race tracks and wagered an estimated $14 billion. Wagering at these tracks has contributed over $600 million in state tax revenues and created hundreds of thousands of jobs. In 1993 there were approximately 10,000 sanctioned horse shows as well as thousands of unsanctioned events.[72]

Despite the economic and cultural significance of performance animal events, there is an important difference between using animals for agricultural purposes and using them in competitive sporting events. Performance animals do not furnish sustenance or products used to satisfy basic human needs. They provide entertainment. Although people surely require entertainment for their well-being, it is difficult to maintain that they must have entertainment involving animals. Society provides innumerable opportunities for diversion, including many sports that do not use animals. As I argue in this book, the more a given human use of animals has negative impact upon animal interests, the more weighty must be the legitimate human interests served by that use. Such sports as horse and dog racing provide many people enjoyment and profit. However, they (and other animal sports) are simply not, in the general scheme of things, nearly as important as feeding the population or conducting biomedical research aimed at the alleviation of disease and suffering. Some conditions that are acceptable for agricultural or research animals might be impermissible for performance animals, given the nature and weight of the human interests involved.

∾ RACE AND SHOW HORSES
Precompetition Administration of Drugs

No issue regarding performance horses has aroused more controversy than the question of the appropriateness of administering certain drugs prior to competition. The disputes differ depending upon what drug is involved. In general, there is disagreement about whether medication (1) is "restorative," that is, allows animals to perform more comfortably at their own levels, or is "additive," that is, significantly affects performance; (2) permits the racing of animals that ought to be rested or retired by masking pain or other debilitating conditions; (3) leads in the long run to pain, debilitation, breakdown, or shortening of an animal's competitive career; (4) really increases the number of horses capable of competition; and (5) adversely affects the breed by permitting lower quality animals to continue to compete. The drugs that arouse the greatest controversy are phenylbutazone, furosemide, and corticosteroids. Precompetition administration of phenylbutazone, for example, is characterized by some as a mild analgesic similar to aspirin. Others see it as a heartless way of extracting more profits from animals, by permitting them to compete without feeling pain caused by underlying disease processes. Furosemide is believed by many to reduce bleeding from the nose. Others dispute this effect and see its real purpose as adding to performance by reducing weight, stimulating the animal, or preventing the detection of other performance-affecting drugs.[73]

The controversies about these drugs and other medical treatments can be quite bitter. Opponents of premedication sometimes characterize veterinarians who administer drugs as not only ignorant, but cowardly and venal.[74] There is also a good deal of broad generalization from both sides about "track veterinarians," "horses," "owners," "trainers," and "state racing commissions"—even though all these participants in the equine competitive world can vary greatly.

An outside observer cannot fail to be impressed by the fact that there are highly competent and respected veterinarians with differing views regarding many of these issues. Such differences are also reflected in the variety of approaches that are taken by state governments, which regulate drug use in thoroughbred and standardbred racing horses. The following are among the matters about which states differ: restrictions on the ability of horses to race after bleeding episodes; criteria required for horses to be able to receive bleeder medication; detention requirements for horses receiving bleeder medication; maximum and minimum dose levels of furosemide; approved bleeder medications other than furosemide; the latest time of administration of nonsteroidal antiinflammatory drugs (NSAIDs) prior to racing; criteria for the use of such drugs; NSAID postrace test level limits; whether urine and/or blood are tested for NSAID levels; which horses are tested for NSAIDs after a race; whether there must be public notification of horses receiving NSAIDs; and whether bleeder medication or NSAIDs may be used in 2-year-old horses.

It is beyond the scope of an ethics text to settle heated factual disputes regarding the effects of precompetition medication. The following thoughts are offered to facilitate consideration of some of the moral issues that are included within these controversies. Some of these suggestions are applicable to issues that relate to other means of influencing the performance of horses, such as neurectomies, ice-packing of legs, injection of corticosteroids into the joints, and removing blood from a horse for transfusion prior to competition ("blood doping").[75]

1. **Ethical argument is not furthered by asking whether a drug merely permits a horse to do more comfortably what it is capable of doing anyway (and is therefore supposedly unobjectionable), or is improper because it "affects," "enhances," or "improves" performance.** Many things, including good nutrition and training, affect, enhance, or improve performance. If trainers did not think that certain medications improved performance, they would not use these substances. Whether a certain drug use is acceptable will depend upon whether it is sufficiently respectful of the interests of the relevant parties—not on whether a cliché such as "affects performance" is attached to it.[76]

2. **If one accepts the legitimacy of animal athletics, one has already conceded that performance animals may be used for human ends.** This, in turn, means that human interests also count, and may sometimes count enough to justify depriving some of these animals of optimal welfare. Regarding show and race horses, it seems obvious that there will sometimes be a departure from optimal welfare. Strenuous athletic activity is inherently associated with the possibility of pain and injury. We do not always prohibit human athletes from competing when they require medication to shield them from pain or discomfort or when immediate resting would help an underlying problem. But they are not permitted to compete under such conditions indiscriminately. We do not want them to suffer unduly during competition. Nor do we want them to risk being seriously injured or shortening their careers. With horses, also, the question one must ask is whether performing in some discomfort or assisted by palliative measures is justified in light of the potential costs.

3. Intuitively, the following questions seem appropriate in evaluating the acceptability of a drug prior to competition: (a) Will this drug lead the animal to experience significant pain or distress soon after competition? (b) Will the drug permit the progression of underlying disease processes, thereby causing pain, debilitation, or breakdown in the long run? (c) Does the drug give a horse an unfair competitive advantage? (d) Does the drug tend to mask other substances the use of which can result in pain, distress, debilitation, or breakdown, or that give the animal an unfair competitive advantage? (e) Is the drug being used at least in part with the intention of assisting the animal in the short or long term or simply to permit it to compete? (f) Are the effects of the drug sufficiently understood so that its impact on health and performance can be known by veterinarians and the public? (g) Is the drug detectable routinely and reliably?

4. Meaningful drug regulation requires that veterinarians cooperate with the letter and spirit of restrictions. Practitioners and trainers who constantly attempt to use new, as yet unregulated or undetectable substances to enhance performance seriously undermine the ability of authorities to protect the animals, owners, and the public. These tinkerers send the unmistakable message that they do not care about the animals or the public at large. For they are willing to experiment with substances the effects of which may not be known. The inevitable result of surreptitious use of even newer drugs will be more stringent restrictions on all drug use. An additional effect may be the regulation of horse racing by the federal government, which might be forced to step in if the states appear unable to control abuses.

5. It is in the long-term economic and professional interests of veterinarians that horses be viewed as patients of value entitled to first-class, respectful medical care. One thing that detracts from the value of patients is administering or selling drugs simply because trainers want them or a profit can be made. Another practice that undermines the value of equine patients is providing medications that allow horses to train or compete while permitting underlying disease processes to worsen so that proper treatment becomes more difficult, more painful, or impossible. Admittedly, there is considerable controversy about when this point might in fact be reached, and about the role, if any, of corticosteroids and other drugs in contributing to breakdowns.[77]

6. The veterinary profession has a serious image problem, which has been getting worse in recent years. More than a few observers of the equine competitive world (including a fair number of veterinarians) believe that the chemical "quick fix" is coming to replace good management and good medicine. Some practitioners do shoot up horses with drugs because they can turn a profit doing so, because they do not have the time to attend to their patients' needs, because they share American society's belief in chemical solutions to many of life's problems, or because they simply do not know enough about horses and the sports in which these animals compete. (G.E. Fackelman, equine surgeon: Personal communication). The problem need not be one of competence. Some veterinarians who overmedicate know precisely what they are doing.

The possibility that some veterinarians may be contributing to the alarming increase in the breakdowns of racing horses has not escaped public notice. A lengthy article in *Sports Illustrated* reported that in 1992, 840 horses, or 1 for every 92 races, suffered fatal racing breakdowns in 1992 on American tracks. A much larger number, 3,566, or 1 in every 22 races, broke down so severely that they were unable to finish the races in which they were injured.[78] The article concedes that "no one can say with precision why so many horses break down on the race track."[79] The author, distinguished sports journalist William Nack, explains that there are probably factors over which veterinarians have little or no control. Among these are the rise of the commercial yearling market and the breeding of horses primarily for sale—an emphasis that leads to breeding for price rather than soundness and that motivates some owners to raise horses that look good rather than those with sufficient toughness. Yet Nack returns repeatedly to a fact many veterinarians will concede, at least privately: there is too much medication of horses, and some of these animals are being raced with dangerous infirmities masked by painkillers. According to one prominent equine doctor quoted in the article:

> The horse owner is pressing the trainer to win at any cost. The trainer's trying to do everything he can. The veterinarian's the only one who has the knowledge, and *should* have the judgment to say, "This is enough. Don't go any further. We're crossing the line with this animal." He's got to have enough gumption to stand up and say, "No!" But they don't. They're under economic pressure themselves. ...I feel sorry for the young vet that comes on now, because he's almost obligated to cheat if he wants to earn a living. I don't understand how he can withstand the pressure.[80]

This practitioner believes that more than half the breakdowns at tracks are related to the legal or illegal masking of pain with drugs, and that for every veterinarian who refuses to administer drugs that are not good for the horse, there are another three who will. Even if both these claims are exaggerated, say, by a factor of 10, there would still be far too much drugging of race horses by veterinarians. Some equine practitioners whom I ask about overmedication—doctors who would not think of acting unlawfully or unethically—bristle at the question. They see hostility in such questioning to horse racing itself. Nothing could be further from the truth. Indeed, for their own self-interest the many decent and dedicated equine doctors must see to it that both laws and actual behavior protect these magnificent animals. As newspaper columnist George Vecsey warns, if the breakdowns continue the entire sport could be finished:

> Boxers and football players and racing-car drivers make rational decisions for money and fame and challenge. Horses are doing it for hay. Their legs shatter so people can bet on them, either at the parimutuel window or through ownership.
>
> Every time I see a horse go down, I wonder how long it will be before the animal-rights people take a look at racing. But I get around to the barns, and I know racing people tend to love their horses, and I only hope for their sakes there is a respite from this horror.[81]

Ethical Responsibilities of Attending Veterinarians

Administration of precompetition drugs is only one area in which attending veterinarians have important moral responsibilities. The following discussion highlights some other ethical issues in equine performance animal practice.

The attending veterinarian as an advocate of the patient's interests

There are many situations in which someone is needed to speak up on behalf of a horse. This can occur when an animal is worked very hard to earn money for its owner.

An advocate for the horse may also be required when an owner lacks sufficient knowledge about how to care for it. The world of horse owners is varied, and generalizations are dangerous. But these two situations occur with significant frequency among the owners of performance animals. Many owners are in it for the money, and some who are not hand their animals over to trainers who view success in monetary terms. Other owners are new to their sport, or may be attracted more to its glamorous aspects than to the moral responsibilities it imposes regarding care of the animals.

The client hell-bent on winning can raise difficult problems for a practitioner. Clients who seek only profits may want something that is not in the animal's interests. They may request things that are not even in their own long-term economic interests. They may view the veterinarian as little more than a legal source of drugs and procedures already decided-upon. Some will go elsewhere if a demanded service is not provided. Veterinarians who will do whatever a client requests, even while knowing that doing it may harm the animal, make it more difficult for all doctors to speak up for horses' interests. Ultimately, the rationalization "If I don't do it, someone else will" can disappear only when enough doctors refuse to do it.

When clients do not have sufficient knowledge about how to care for their horses, it can become the veterinarian's task to provide basic instruction regarding general management and preventive medicine.[82] From the purchase examination, to education about feeding, grooming, and sanitation, to instruction about first-aid, the doctor often may be able to best serve client and patient by assuming a role of general advisor. This, in turn, can enable prevention of problems before they arise and can assure that practitioners are called when their services are required.

Obligations to owners and trainers

Attending veterinarians have moral obligations to owners and trainers. Among these are the duties of honesty, loyalty and protection of confidences, trustworthiness, and respect (see Chapter 14). The primary foundation of an attending veterinarian's moral obligations to an owner or trainer is one's agreement with them to provide professional services. Whether or not it is stated explicitly, part of this agreement is to assist the client in furthering the client's own goals. If one disagrees with these goals or believes that they are incompatible with one's duties to the animal or to others (such as riders and the public), a doctor may attempt to convince the client to change his or her goals. The doctor may be justified in withdrawing from the professional relationship. But one may not surreptitiously substitute one's own priorities for those of the owner, for then one is serving under false pretenses, which is a form of deception. True loyalty to a client sometimes requires declining to provide a service or product even if the client wants it and it will not harm the animal. Some veterinarians sell drugs or special "home" remedies they know are useless, because a trainer or owner wants them. Such an approach may be profitable in the short run, but it is deleterious to the image of the veterinarian as a healer and as a friend of the client (see Chapter 16).

WHOM DOES ONE SERVE? Although veterinarians are obligated to serve clients loyally, it may sometimes seem unclear who the client really is. In the eyes of the law, the doctor almost always works for the owner, who ultimately pays the bills. But in actuality, it is often a trainer who engages one's services directly and requests treatments or procedures. Taking a course of action that displeases a trainer can result in loss of a patient or many patients, even if this course of action would benefit the owner. What should a doctor do when she finds something or is asked to do something that the trainer may be keeping from the owner or that the doctor believes is not in the interests of the owner or the animal? It is sometimes dangerous to presume that a trainer is not acting in accordance with the owner's instructions. I would argue that when a doctor is certain that the owner is not receiving important information or advice, she has a moral obligation to attempt to provide the owner with this information. This obligation flows from the fact that it is the owner who is paying for one's services, and is the person who owns the animal. This obligation is not always extinguished even if one has been told by the owner to deal exclusively with the trainer.

PURCHASE EXAMINATIONS. One of the most important areas in which the attending veterinarian's moral duties to the client come into play is in the conduct of purchase examinations. Because so much can turn on the results, a doctor must not only be thorough and honest but must also call relevant questions and issues to the client's attention even if the client does not raise them. As discussed in Chapter 14, generally, a practitioner should not work for both the buyer and seller. Nor should a doctor's decision about a horse's suitability be affected by a desire to curry favor or economic gain from someone else (for example, a trainer) who might have a stake in the sale.

Obligations to third parties and the public.

Attending veterinarians have moral obligations to persons who do not pay their fees. Practitioners who perform a procedure on a horse that can result in injury to riders or spectators commit a grave moral wrong. They also subject themselves to potential legal liability to those injured as a result of their wrongdoing. Practitioners who knowingly participate in attempts to gain an unfair competitive advantage for their clients by providing illegal substances or procedures also harm the betting public, owners, and trainers who rely on general adherence to the rules of fair competition.

INSURANCE ISSUES. It is immoral, and highly imprudent, for a doctor to be dishonest in completing documents relating to insurance applications or claims. One may think that it is helpful to a client to provide an incomplete or ambiguous statement about a horse's condition or history. One may think that the failure of an insurance company or client to pay adequately (or at all) for an insurance examination justifies a quicker, less careful approach. The result of dishonesty or carelessness may be denial of coverage by the insurer and legal action against the veterinarian by the company or client. Even when an insurance company can be fooled, others are victimized. "Successful" fraud eventually leads to higher premiums for all purchasers of insurance.

It is also profoundly immoral to help a client obtain an insurance payment by doing something to bring about or accelerate the illness or death of a horse. In addition to being fraudulent, such behavior can cause the animal unnecessary suffering. In the early 1990s the horse show world was rocked by reports of the killing of horses by or on behalf of owners to collect equine mortality insurance. The stories, involving electrocution and brutal clubbing of helpless animals, were grotesque and shocking.[83] In 1994 a federal grand jury indicted more than 20 people, among them prominent show jumpers and owners, for crimes ranging from insurance, mail, and wire fraud, to money laundering and income tax evasion. One of the defendants was charged with illegal racketeering, including conspiracy to murder, solicitation to murder, and the murder of candy heiress Helen Vorhees Brach. Two of the defendants were veterinarians.[84] At the time of this writing, trials have not yet begun, although several of the defendants (including the veterinarians) have pleaded guilty to various charges.[85] However, even before all the facts could be ascertained, the indictments set off a flurry of articles in the veterinary literature, some of which suggested that, while veterinarian knowledge of or participation in insurance fraud is not common, there is still the need to educate some practitioners about how to spot and react to shady behavior. One insurance lawyer believes that some veterinarians knowingly sign veterinary certificates that misrepresent whether a horse is sufficiently healthy to be insurable. Some owners bring in a veterinarian who has never seen the horse before, who is not likely to find a condition that is not immediately observable, and who honestly and to the best of his or her knowledge signs a certificate the horse's attending doctor would know is inaccurate and might refuse to sign.[86] An equine insurance adjuster suggests that some veterinarians may be too trusting of their clients, and do not look for foul play when a previously healthy horse is suddenly reported dead in its stall.[87] Among possible remedies are better education of veterinarians about their legal responsibilities pursuant to insurance law, drafting of specific laws prohibiting equine insurance fraud and the killing of horses, and better general education of practitioners about how they can help animal control officials and insurance investigators detect cruelty or fraud.[88]

One ethical problem that seems to arise with some frequency concerns an attending veterinarian's obligations when a horse needs to be put out of its misery, but permission for euthanasia cannot be obtained quickly from the insurance company. I have heard credible stories about insurance company representatives who delay returning telephone calls requesting permission or who attempt to speak with younger less experienced doctors in a practice to postpone euthanasia as long as possible. Insurers have a legitimate interest in avoiding making a payment on a mortality policy when euthanasia is medically premature or is motivated by fraud. But permitting a horse to suffer when there is no medical justification for doing so is intolerable. Several doctors have told me that the best way to avoid such a situation is to become known to insurance company representatives as someone who is honest, but who will not tolerate delay when euthanasia is necessary.

Ethical Responsibilities of Official Veterinarians

An official veterinarian at a race or competition works for the institution or organization under whose control or auspices the competition is being held. He or she may be a full- or part-time employee of the state or of a track, association, or competition organizer.

Many of the legal and moral responsibilities of official veterinarians flow from the regulations or rule books governing their actions. They must therefore know what their mandated responsibilities do and do not include.

Official veterinarians are called upon to serve many interests. They must attend to the interests of the horses and their riders. They also promote the interests of owners, bettors, and spectators by assuring that rules upon which all rely are followed. The official veterinarian also serves to support the credibility of the state government or association in their roles as regulators. How an official veterinarian performs these functions can vary with the nature of the competition. As equine practitioners Drs. M. Mackay-

Smith and M. Cohen observe, in combined training or distance riding events, "participation as a learning experience for the competitor is probably more stressed...than is the case in more traditional horse sports. The veterinary officer stands, therefore, in the role of teacher as well as practitioner." These authors urge that in such events, the veterinarian's first moral obligation is "to protect the horse's interests and his or her second duty is to assist the rider in the competition."[89] The official veterinarian at a racetrack is typically forbidden by law to attend to routine, nonemergency matters.

Official veterinarians also have moral and legal responsibilities to what William Nack calls "racing's other endangered species, the jockeys."[90] In 1992 a jury ordered a Florida track to pay a jockey $4.4 million in damages after a spill from his horse left him paralyzed from the chest down. Although the track veterinarian was not named as a defendant, the jury found the track negligent in not performing an adequate prerace inspection of the horse. According to the plaintiff, it was insufficient for the track to employ only one official veterinarian and to allow this doctor to conduct visual inspections in the paddock rather than hands-on examinations in the stalls.[90,91]

Official veterinarians must apply the rules impartially and consistently. They must not permit themselves to be influenced by their own economic interests. To preserve their ability to convince others that they are serving impartially, they should avoid any behavior that would give even the slightest appearance of impropriety. Therefore whenever competition or money is a major element of an event (which is almost always the case), the same doctor ought not to serve as both the official veterinarian and an attending veterinarian to some or all competitors. Those using another veterinarian may wonder whether the official veterinarian will side with owners whose animals he or she is attending. Even when an official veterinarian will attend to the routine medical needs of all competitors, some owners may ask whether she will be most loyal to those from whom she can gain the most remuneration. The AVMA and the American Association of Equine Practitioners have adopted a policy critical of horse shows which permit the same person to serve as official veterinarian and attending veterinarian. This policy recommends that a show select as official veterinarian a doctor from outside the local area who is "not closely familiar with the horses being shown and who has no clients among the exhibitors."[92]

Ethical Responsibilities of Government and Associations

Protection of the interests of horses, riders, owners, and the public requires vigorous activity by government and private groups charged with protecting these interests.

STATE GOVERNMENTS. State racing commissions and veterinary licensing boards have substantial authority to discipline attending and official veterinarians who violate these agencies' technical and ethical rules. Licenses to practice at tracks can be suspended or revoked by the racing commission. The state board can restrict the activities of a doctor who behaves incompetently or unethically at the track. Effective government supervision depends upon the willingness of those who encounter abuses to report them. Racing commissions and state boards must also have sufficient funding, personnel, and legal talent to make effective enforcement possible.

That state racing commissions call for vigorous monitoring by official veterinarians does not necessarily make it so. A study of thoroughbred racing at a state fair in Massachusetts conducted by Dr. G. E. Fackelman found that 72% of the horses permitted to race exhibited orthopedic, respiratory, or conformational unsoundness; 69% showed signs of previous injury or deformity of the musculoskeletal system; 6% were injured while racing; and 14 horses of the 296 entering the paddock could not complete the race because of already known orthopedic problems. The study documented injuries that worsened "as a direct result of the (sometimes successful) completion of a given competition." The mere presence of the veterinarians conducting the survey reduced the level of injuries. "When owners came to realize that our undertaking was serious and steady, they showed the tendency to eliminate their animals [from competition] and not even present them in the paddock."[93] The study also revealed questionable adherence to state regulations prohibiting official veterinarians from treating horses except in cases of emergency.

State racing commissions must assure that official veterinarians have sufficient knowledge, experience, and courage to be able to stand up to owners, trainers, and attending veterinarians when necessary. Required prerace examinations must be conducted thoroughly and competently. Periodic investigations should be undertaken by racing commissions to evaluate the performance of official veterinarians. Racing commissions should consider including animal welfare experts among their full-time staff. Such persons might be able to assure that the interests of the animals, as well as those of owners, the public, and the state revenue department, are advocated in commission deliberations.

Some state racing commissions have been accused of lack of knowledge about horses in general and equine veterinary medicine in particular. In a number of states, the relationship between practitioners and commissioners appears to be warm and cooperative, while other commissions are perceived as hostile adversaries who impose rigid rules. In some states, commission membership must include veterinarians or people actually involved in the industry, while in others such members are excluded on the grounds of potential conflicts of interest.[94] In my view, it is absolutely essential to have veterinarian representation on racing commissions, so that the interests of the horses and the legitimate concerns of veterinarians can be knowledgeably represented. It makes no more sense to exclude veterinarians from membership on racing commissions on the grounds that they cannot be impartial than it would to exclude veterinarians from serving on state veterinary licensing boards for the same reason. The primary function of both racing commissions and licensing boards is to protect the public and its animals. Veterinarians have served on both kinds of bodies conscientiously and impartially.

PRIVATE ASSOCIATIONS AND ORGANIZERS. Private associations under whose auspices show events are held are ethically obligated to monitor behavior by attending veterinarians. For example, the American Horse Shows Association (AHSA) has a drug testing program and a lengthy and specific list of prohibited drugs and medications.[95] The AHSA also states that "no veterinarian should be party to the administration of a drug or medication to a horse or pony for the nontherapeutic purpose of affecting its performance. This is unethical, and it encourages unethical conduct among trainers, owners, and exhibitors."[96] However, AHSA rules do not allow for the disciplining of attending veterinarians who might knowingly administer drugs in violation of the rules; the entire burden is placed on owners and trainers. Associations should be able and willing to discipline attending veterinarians who participate in prohibited procedures with the purpose of enabling animals to compete in violation of requirements. It is unrealistic for associations, which are closer to the situation, to expect state veterinary boards or federal authorities to bear the entire burden.

FEDERAL REGULATIONS. The Federal Horse Protection Act of 1970[97] gives the USDA Animal and Plant Health Inspection Service (APHIS) responsibility for enforcing rules to protect the welfare of show horses. APHIS regulations provide that no "chain, boot, roller, collar, action device, method, practice, or substance shall be used with respect to any horse at any horse show, horse exhibition, or horse sale or auction if such use causes or can reasonably be expected to cause such horse to be sore."[98] The regulations define the term "sore" and contain many specific prohibitions. They also impose inspection, detainment, and reporting requirements. Private practitioners can participate in inspections and enforcement through licensing as a "designated qualified person" (DQP). Veterinarian-DQPs must have general APHIS accreditation. In addition, they must be either members of the American Association of Equine Practitioners (AAEP), large animal practitioners "with substantial equine experience," or "knowledgeable in the area of equine lameness as related to soring and soring practices."[99] The regulations specify procedures DQPs must follow in making required visual and hands-on inspections.[100] DQPs are not licensed directly by APHIS, but by industry organizations or associations that have obtained general certification from APHIS for their DQP programs. Additional inspection and supervisory functions are carried out by APHIS veterinarians.

⟳ DOG RACING

Greyhound dog racing is an enormously popular sport with a substantial economic impact. Some 30 million people visit dog racetracks each year. The sport generates 100,000 jobs and contributes more than $230 million a year to state treasuries.[101] Yet many veterinarians will admit that they know very little about the sport or its impact on the animals. Even state authorities empowered to regulate greyhound racing can lack a complete understanding of the sport. For example, the Massachusetts state legislature appointed an advisory committee to determine what happens to greyhounds bred for racing that do not qualify for pari-mutuel races or reach the end of their racing career.[102] The committee could not answer the question. It found "an abysmal lack of official or authoritative data" concerning the number of greyhounds that race or end their racing careers in Massachusetts, are moved to other racing states, are adopted, or are utilized in medical research.[103]

Despite its popularity, in recent years, greyhound racing has received considerable unfavorable publicity. Many people associated with the industry, including many veterinarians, are attempting to improve the sport and its treatment of the animals. Nevertheless, unmistakable misdeeds of less reputable people have made dog racing easy pickings for animal activists. Indeed, even people who have no particular ax to grind often are so taken by abuses that they seem unable to resist giving problems greater prominence than the facts warrant. For example, in 1992 the *Boston Globe* published a series of lengthy articles on greyhound racing in New England and other parts of the country. Much of the series described people who care about the animals and are attempting to improve their lives: owners and trainers who invest substantial sums in their operations and who genuinely grieve when animals are injured or must be euthanized; track owners who maintain modern facilities; and groups that are succeeding in placing out for adoption an increasing number of dogs that can no longer be raced.

The articles also suggested that many of the problems faced by the sport are caused by less professional owners and trainers who have little money or expertise. However, the series uncovered enough problems—including dogs suffering from malnutrition and parasites, backyard breeders who do not know what they are doing, poor and ramshackle tracks, and cases of outright torture—to allow the presentation of the bad as a counterweight, almost an equal counterweight, to the good. Typical of the resulting "balance" of the series was its conclusion that "although abuse of greyhounds is isolated, emaciated and sore-ridden dogs recently were found at one New England track while at another, two animals' penises were wired to prevent them from masturbating."[104] Although the series (which was titled "Running for their Lives") was careful to state specifically that "instances of abuse seem to be few and diminishing,"[104] the general characterization of the industry was quite different. The articles claimed to "probe the strange world of greyhound racing—a world populated by devoted dogmen and conniving capitalists, by trainers and breeders clinging to outmoded, sometimes cruel techniques, and those forging state of the art solutions."[105] Perhaps because dog racing involves *dogs*, many people may always attribute even the most isolated abuses to the sport in general.

Objections to the Sport

There is considerable opposition to greyhound racing among humane societies and animal welfare advocates. Objections typically are based on one or more of the following positions: (1) a belief in animal-use abolitionism, which implies condemnation not just of dog racing but also of all animal sports; (2) the view that it is wrong to use *dogs* for sport and wagering; (3) opposition to the manner in which racing dogs are treated during breeding, training, or racing; and (4) opposition to the fact that the sport results in the killing of many surplus dogs or their use in research.

Animal-use abolitionism is not a plausible position and need not be discussed again here. The view that it is disrespectful to use the beloved dog in a wagering performance does have intuitive appeal to some. However, I have found that when people who express a general opposition to dog racing are challenged to explain their feelings, they usually invoke the third objection listed above. For it seems unreasonable to single out dogs as inappropriate beings for performance and wagering events. It makes little sense to concede (as almost everyone will) that it is not inherently degrading or demeaning for human athletes to run around tracks or to compete in sporting events on which bets may be placed, but that it is so for dogs.

It is more plausible to try to object to dog racing on the grounds that the animals are not treated as well as they ought to be. Such an objection usually takes one of two forms. Some people believe that the dogs are subjected to bad conditions, which cause them suffering or distress, such as poor living conditions, inadequate veterinary care, difficult training and racing schedules, inadequate opportunities for socialization, and so on. Other people assert that however well-cared-for racing dogs may be, they will never be treated as they deserve to be treated because they cannot live the kind of life a valued family pet would enjoy.

The contention that some greyhounds live unpleasant lives is undoubtedly true. In any group of animal owners there will be some who do not treat their animals properly. One hears stories of greyhound operations that do not have adequate heat or light or where animals are not given good care. But there are also greyhound breeding and training facilities in which the animals are treated well and are genuinely liked by their owners and trainers. As I shall indicate below, there are a number of issues that must be explored regarding promotion of the welfare of these animals. However, the fact that some owners may not treat their animals properly or that more sometimes can be done to treat them better does not mean that all greyhounds are condemned to an unacceptable life.

It is more difficult to counter the objection that dogs used for racing, even when treated as well as can be expected within the context of the sport, just do not live the kind of life that can be enjoyed by a typical family pet. As a statement of fact, this is surely correct. Racing dogs are kept in a kennel environment, they are trained and run in ways family dogs are not, and few experience the same measure of human companionship as do typical pet dogs. It would certainly be better for racing dogs if they had such a life. But this does not make the life they do lead morally intolerable, any more than it is wrong to race horses because these animals might have a better life as companion animals. Animals are not people. Therefore most of us will sometimes accept treating different animals of the same species in varying ways. We believe this is sometimes appropriate because we do not regard all animals of a given species as entitled to the best life that can be provided to them. It is interesting to speculate whether dog racing would be as much the target of objections as it is today if dogs (like horses) were primarily working and sporting animals rather than pets.

The Adoption Issue

In my view, the most difficult ethical issue in greyhound racing concerns what happens to the animals when they are no longer useful. This question cannot be addressed just by improving racing dog welfare. The problem is generated by the sport itself and requires hard decisions by the industry and government.

The first source of the problem is the number of dogs needed to maintain the sport. In a state like Massachusetts, each greyhound race will have 8 animals. On average, a track will offer 12 races per performance, and on some calendar days, a track will have more than one performance. Some dogs are raced as often as twice a week. The number of dogs used in pari-mutuel races is therefore substantial. In 1986 there was in Massachusetts alone a total of 11,760 races involving some 95,000 entries.[106] But the number of dogs that actually reach the betting races may represent only the tip of the iceberg. Dogs must first qualify in official schooling races. Not all make it, and some require so many attempts that they are not profitable for owners to keep. Moreover, the search by breeders for speedy animals results in the birth of many dogs that are not promising enough even to enter qualifying races. Dogs that do make it to the pari-mutuels may have brief careers if they do not do well, and few dogs race after they are $3^1/_2$ to 4 years of age. Dogs weeded out of the process (and eventually all are) may be euthanized, sent to another state in which competition is less severe, adopted as pets, or sold or donated for medical research. Although the number of animals generated each year around the country is substantial, it is not yet possible to determine accurately how many there are or what becomes of them. Estimates of how many greyhounds are euthanized annually vary. The Humane Society of the United States places the number at 50,000. The National Greyhound Association, an industry group, believes the figure is approximately 20,000.[104] Although both figures are considerable, they are dwarfed by the total number of dogs killed in shelters and pounds, by some estimates perhaps as many as 10 million annually.[107]

The second source of the problem is that many racing greyhounds are far from useless when their role in the sport ends. Many can make wonderful pets. The time required to acclimatize healthy, uninjured greyhounds to people and the life of a family pet can be quite brief, sometimes just a few days. Many of these animals are near the beginning of their natural lifespans. They are no more expensive or burdensome to keep than most other breeds.

The present system discards many animals that perform, or are an integral part of a system that performs, a profitable service. This is wrong. Greyhounds were all once valued companion animals. The breed has been appropriated, refined, and trained for racing. This process earns millions of dollars for owners, trainers, tracks, associations, bettors, veterinarians, and state governments. In return, those who benefit—including states whose treasuries share the bounty—have a moral obligation to give something back to as many animals as possible.

What can be done?

The following approaches are suggested for consideration by the industry, government, and veterinarians. Some of these suggestions are already being tried or contemplated in several states.

1. Information should be gathered in each racing jurisdiction regarding the number of animals bred and their disposition, including transmittal out of state, adoption, euthanasia, and receipt by research facilities. Racing states must therefore require rigorous record-keeping of such occurrences by owners, tracks, track veterinarians, attending veterinarians, adoption services, animal shelters, and research facilities. Reliable information would enable state authorities to ascertain what is happening and would assist in the monitoring of programs to promote adoption or humane euthanasia.

2. Each racing jurisdiction should establish a fund to assist in the adoption of retired and surplus greyhounds. Moneys for such a fund should come from owner winnings and track and state shares of the racing handle. Proceeds from the fund would be distributed to greyhound adoption services (including individuals such as veterinarians) approved by the state. Consideration might also be given to providing rewards to owners who transmit animals to adoption organizations or new owners.

3. Standards ought to be established for greyhound adoption services to assure that animals are properly socialized, receive adequate veterinary care, are cared for properly, and are placed in appropriate homes.

4. The industry ought to publicize the availability of greyhounds so that bettors and the general public become aware of adoption possibilities.

5. A concerted effort should be made by all beneficiaries of greyhound racing to counter the image of the breed as vicious and intractable. This view of greyhounds may make some people feel better about the fact that so many surplus dogs are killed. But the image is false and unnecessary. It also makes placing surplus animals more difficult.

6. State and local veterinary medical associations can encourage their members to publicize nonprofit greyhound adoption services in their waiting rooms. VMAs and individual doctors might consider providing low-cost veterinary services for adoption agencies.

7. Veterinary hospitals ought to consider using surplus greyhounds as blood donors. This would not preclude attempts to place these animals for adoption. One innovative program coordinates the adoption of greyhounds to families in an area, and uses these dogs as donors for small, regional blood banks.[108]

8. States that promote greyhound breeding through cash prizes or other incentives for owners should require those who receive such subsidies to pay part of their rewards into the greyhound adoption fund. Additionally, state encouragement of breeding ought to be modified or withdrawn if it is determined that the state's policy is contributing to the destruction of an inappropriate number of unadoptable animals. It makes no sense for a state to promote adoption and at the same time encourage overbreeding that contributes to an increased need for adoption programs.

9. Each racing state must place at least as much importance upon the adoption of retired and surplus greyhounds as on encouraging the breeding and racing of faster animals. In other words, if the quality of racing dogs must be compromised to control the number of animals euthanized, so be it. Owners and bettors should be able to live with somewhat slower dogs so that fewer animals have to be killed. A state policy refusing to tolerate increased euthanasias to improve dog "quality" might stimulate the search for breeding techniques that will not produce so many surplus dogs.

The Use of Surplus Greyhounds in Research

Some greyhounds find their way into scientific research facilities. Some animal welfare advocates find this fact even more disturbing than the euthanasia of surplus animals.

Chapter 24 argues that it is preferable to use existing unwanted dogs in biomedical research than to kill existing animals and require the breeding of new animals that will be treated exactly as would those that are killed. I would apply the same general argument to surplus racing dogs. Indeed, using such animals in research might answer one complaint about the use of animals from pounds and shelters: the objection that former members of human-animal bonds ought not to be subjected to laboratory and experimental conditions. Nevertheless, because racing dogs have already been used for human purposes (many quite vigorously), I would argue that it is wrong to automatically and routinely use them in research. Given what they have already provided, no greyhound ought to be released for research until serious attempts have been made to place it for adoption.

The Massachusetts Advisory Committee recommended permitting the use of retired dogs in research provided that they are (1) eventually scheduled for euthanasia; (2) used in approved kinds of nonsurvival projects; (3) donated and not sold for research; (4) "not used in safety evaluation or toxicity research projects, or in any medical research involving recovery from anesthesia or the consciousness of pain"; and (5) "disposed of humanely at the completion of any research exercise."[109] It is a legitimate ethical principle that retired greyhounds used in research be given special consideration for their previous service. However, several of the Massachusetts Committee's recommendations are not reasonable applications of this principle. Some research necessarily involves recovery from anesthesia, and some involves pain that is brief and trivial. Nor is it obvious why all greyhounds used in research are better off being killed than recovering from anesthesia or experiencing some pain or distress. Indeed, some relatively benign uses of research dogs (for example, as long-term experimental blood donors) seem far better than automatic euthanasia. Killing all dogs would also preclude their being adopted after a research project is completed, a goal that I argue in Chapter 24 ought to be given more serious consideration by researchers.

Euthanasia

Rumors and reports surface periodically about owners and trainers who kill or dispose of euthanized dogs in unacceptable ways. If racing dogs do have to be killed, they must be euthanized according to approved methods and by personnel (such as trained animal shelter technicians) who can assure a painless death. If there is inhumane killing of greyhounds, state authorities must make it a major priority to find, punish, and prevent it.

Other Ethical Issues

Greyhound racing presents other important ethical issues, some of which are similar to those arising out of the use of horses in racing and show competitions. For example, there are legal restrictions on drugs that can be used in dogs prior to competition. These rules are not always followed. As is the case in horse racing, an attending veterinarian can play an important role in advocating the interests of the animal athlete. State laws require the presence of an official track veterinarian to protect the interests of the wagering public as well as the animals. As is the case in horse racing, some states expect more of dog track veterinarians than others, and some track veterinarians are more conscientious than others in protecting the welfare of the animals.

According to one opponent of dog racing, "no issue damages greyhound racing more" than the use of live animal lures, mainly rabbits, in the training of racing dogs.[110] The National Greyhound Association opposes this practice, and it is prohibited by state animal cruelty laws. A cruelty investigator employed by the Humane Society of the United States contends that 90% of trainers use live rabbits and that 100,000 animals are killed each year by pursuing dogs. Many trainers dispute this figure.[111] Because mechanical lures are available, allowing dogs to chase and kill rabbits is unacceptable and should be subjected to severe criminal penalties.

Challenges for the Profession

Research concerning race horses and their welfare has long been accepted as a legitimate part of the mission of the veterinary schools. Several veterinary schools are now undertaking serious work on racing greyhound medicine and welfare. The number of practitioners who have special expertise in the medical problems of racing dogs is increasing steadily. Among the goals of the growing body of racing dog practitioners are the following:

- Improvement in basic knowledge of racing greyhound kinetics, physiology, and biochemistry

- Development of track materials and design to enhance performance and provide greater protection against injury
- Continuing development of training techniques to prevent and assist in the treatment of injuries
- Systematic study of racing dog nutrition to enhance performance and welfare
- Investigation of scientific breeding techniques to reduce scattershot searches for the "magic" dog and unnecessary surpluses of animals
- Improved and more conscientiously applied measures for testing for prohibited substances. Effective training and state racing commission supervision of track veterinarians

~ RODEO
The Importance of Rodeo

More than 2,500 rodeos are held in the United States and Canada each year. The Professional Rodeo Cowboys Association (PRCA), the leading official organization for professional rodeos, sanctions approximately 800 performances each season. The largest rodeos, such as Cheyenne (Wyoming) Frontier Days, the National Western Stock Show and Rodeo, the U.S. National Finals Rodeo, and the Calgary (Alberta) Stampede, attract hundreds of thousands of spectators and are themselves gigantic cultural and economic events. Many high schools, colleges, and communities organize their own rodeos. The PRCA estimates that some 30 million people view rodeos annually either in person or on television.

Rodeo is much more than a source of entertainment or profit. As veterinarian and anthropologist Elizabeth Lawrence observes, rodeo is:

> …a quintessential part of that complex (and perhaps indefinable) mystique which we call the American West. As the cowboy sport of rodeo developed out of frontier experience, so it also shaped and continues to shape our perceptions of all that the Western frontier has come to symbolize.[112]

Rodeo proclaims and promotes such values as individualism, independence, egalitarianism, courage, toleration of pain and injury, and the desire to tame the wild. It provides "an opportunity for members of the contemporary society which support it to bring out and set forth for display and exploration the various themes still central to their occupation and ethos."[113]

Ethical deliberation about rodeo cannot underestimate the great importance the sport has to participants and spectators. Nor should those for whom rodeo is unimportant overlook the cultural diversity to which the sport contributes. At the same time, however, the interests of rodeo animals do not disappear because these animals are utilized in a culturally significant activity.

Welfare Issues: The Current Climate

Rodeo is anathema to many animal welfare advocates. The sport is regularly accused of offenses ranging from deliberate and willful cruelty to the corruption of U.S. and Canadian youth. In a joint statement, the Humane Society of the United States and the American Humane Society demanded complete abolition of rodeo. They claimed that rodeos "result in torment, harassment, and stress being inflicted upon the participating animals and expose rodeo stock to the probability of pain, injury, or death…Rodeos are not an accurate or harmless portrayal of ranching skills; rather, they display and encourage a sensitivity to and acceptance of brutal treatment of animals in the name of sport."[114]

The following are among the features of rodeo some animal welfare advocates find objectionable:

- The use of the flank strap to stimulate bucking in horses and bulls. The tightening of the strap around the animal's abdomen is often characterized as causing excruciating pain to the genitalia.
- Use of an electric cattle prod ("hot shot")
- Spurring of bucking horses and bulls
- The fact that much of the animals' time is allegedly "spent in transit or in tiny enclosures behind the chutes [and that]…these animals are not being 'saved' from anything, since the slaughterhouse is almost always their final destination after they have outlived their rodeo usefulness."[115]
- The calf-roping event, in which a rope is thrown by a mounted cowboy around the neck of a calf, which is then taken down to the ground and tied. This event has been called "a brutal mockery of western heritage."[115]
- The single cowboy steer-roping event, in which a rider ropes a steer around the horns, hits the steer with his rope as he turns thereby taking it to the ground, and ties the animal's feet
- The steer-wrestling event, in which a mounted cowboy jumps from his horse, grabs one horn and the jaw of a running steer and throws the animal on its side or back. This event has been characterized as pitting "man against animal in hand-to-hand combat."[115]
- The fact that spectators cheer for the cowboys to subdue the animals, which (with the exception of the cowboy's horse) are typically viewed as "the enemy"
- Mexican-style *charreada* rodeos, which have recently appeared in the United States. Charreadas typically include bucking events in which the cowboy (*charro*) rides a bareback bronc or bull with both hands on the ropes; the *Paso de la muerte* (ride of death) in which a charro jumps from one running bareback horse onto another; and, where it is not prohibited by law, the roping of running horses by the front legs.

As shall be discussed, many of these criticisms are mistaken. But far worse is the uncompromising assault by certain groups upon the entire sport of rodeo. This stance often makes it impossible for rodeo enthusiasts who are concerned about animal welfare to participate with humane societies in meaningful dialogue. It is not surprising that the rodeo community's response to demands that the entire sport be terminated is vigorous defense of rodeo as a whole. Humane societies might ask how they would react if they were told that *their* "piece of Americana" should be relegated to the history books where it belongs."[115]

Responses to Criticisms

Many objections to rodeo are incorrect or grossly exaggerated. For example, it is often alleged that the flank strap is impermissible because it induces horses and bulls to behave in ways they would not otherwise. Accordingly, rodeo people have been drawn into a debate about whether the strap enhances what these animals would do anyway or provides an external, "unnatural" stimulation. But this is not the most important issue. Sporting animals are often called on to behave in ways that are not completely "natural" to their species. The issue is whether the strap is sufficiently invasive of the animals' interests to render it unacceptable. PRCA rules require that the flank strap be lined with sheepskin, have a quick-release mechanism, and not contain any sharp or cutting objects.[116] As equine practitioner Dr. Frank Santos observes, the strap is not placed on the genitals, and horses or bulls do not behave as if tortured by pain for the 8 seconds or so during which the strap is tightened. If the animals were in significant pain, they would either "go into a wild frenzy, tearing up the chute, stampeding and crashing into fences, and throwing themselves down. Or they would simply lie down and sulk... ."[117] The strap is undoubtedly irritating. However, it is hard to conclude that this short-lived stimulation is so horrendous as to make bucking events immoral. Indeed, such a conclusion can only appear reasonable to someone who has *already* decided that artificially inducing an animal to buck (if this is what the flank strap does) is enormously disrespectful and greatly invasive of its interests.

Likewise, several other objections to rodeo seem understandable only if one supposes that they reflect an already-reached condemnation of the sport. How, for example, can a humane society that would not denounce the use of animals for food object to the eventual slaughter of rodeo animals, unless it believed that rodeo is inherently disrespectful to animals? (In fact, many rodeo animals have it much easier than their agricultural counterparts.) Similarly, those who find the spurring of horses or bulls offensive may not think it important that sharp spurs are prohibited and that injuries to animals from spurs are rare. To these people it is still the *spurring* of a horse or bull. Likewise, those who object to the use of an electric prod may view the application of an electric shock to an animal as inherently evil. They may not care that the stimulation is not painful even to people whose skins are literally a great deal thinner than those of stock animals. They may not care that PRCA rules prohibit using the prod in the arena to stimulate performance, allow for its use only to move animals into the chutes, and even then require that the prod be used on the less sensitive areas of the hips and shoulders.[118] They may not care that the prod is commonly utilized in ranching to move cattle and is far more humane than other methods such as whipping, beating, or twisting the animals' tails. Characterizing steer wrestling as "hand-to-hand combat" is more reflective of a conclusion about the appropriateness of such an event than of the facts. As Dr. Santos notes,[117] such a description gives more equality to the participants than they really have. The human participant in a steer wrestling event is more likely to be the one injured. Indeed, most rodeo animals are far more dangerous to cowboys than the cowboys are to the animals.

Many rodeo enthusiasts are seriously concerned about animal welfare. Participants who use their own horses in various events take great care of these animals, which are often the key to success and can require years of training. Stock contractors who provide animals to rodeos have a strong economic incentive to maintain them in good condition. Insistence upon proper treatment of the animals is a routine feature of instruction at organized rodeo schools. Rules of rodeo competition also address welfare considerations. For example, the PRCA prohibits excessive use of the electric prod. Other practices that have been criticized by animal welfare activists but are in fact prohibited and penalized by rodeo association rules include abruptly "jerking" roped animals and holding a horse by the ears or nose during the wild horse race event. At the time of this writing, the PRCA rule book contained 59 rules relating to animal welfare. These rules cover matters such as the inspection of animals for illness or injury prior to competition, the conditions of chutes and the rodeo arena, prohibition of the use of stimulants or hypnotics on animals, minimum and maximum weight for calves used in calf-roping events, length of time and conditions of confinement and transportation of animals, and the availability of veterinary care. Violators of PRCA rules can be disqualified on the spot by an officiating judge and are subject to substantial fines.

Rodeo enthusiasts with whom I speak appear eager to reduce hardship imposed on the animals. The PRCA worked with the legislature of one state to require the use of a padded flank strap after a law was passed prohibiting the strap (Max Etienne, attorney: Personal communication). The Salinas, California rodeo found that it could reduce calf hind leg fractures significantly by making the footing in the arena firmer (Dr. Gary Deter, equine practitioner: Personal communication). At many rodeos veterinarians are present to provide medical care for animals and to assure that they are not being overworked or mistreated.

Nor does it follow from the fact that some rodeo events pit cowboys against animals that the sport encourages cruelty to or dislike for animals. Most team sports invite spectators to pose the "good" team against the "bad." This practice does not appear to promote general cruelty or disrespect toward people.

It is difficult not to be impressed by the spirit of professionalism many rodeo enthusiasts express. Stated time and again is the desire to maintain rodeo as a family sport that rejects inappropriate treatment of animals. Many in the rodeo world support efforts to train cowboys and cowgirls who are technically proficient and who take a serious view of their responsibilities to the animals.

The rodeo world is not monolithic. There exist significant differences regarding the appropriateness of certain activities and practices. Rodeo people readily admit that some in the sport do not demonstrate sufficient respect for the animals. (This fact does not distinguish rodeo from any other animal sport or general use of animals.) Many cowboys criticize the traditional steer-roping event as inhumane. It is not allowed on the programs of many rodeos, and some states prohibit it by law.[119] Some rodeo people want to shorten the distance calves in roping events are permitted to run before they can be chased to reduce the potential for injury (Deter G: Personal communication). Female participation in some of the traditionally male-dominated events appears to be on the increase, although in general, rodeo still limits the activities in which women are permitted to participate.[120] The growing popularity of the sport may provide impetus for diversity and change. Rodeo has attracted participants and spectators who have geographic, cultural, and economic roots quite different from those of the traditional rodeo cowboy. For some of these people, athletic aspects of the performance might be more important than its cultural and economic underpinnings. They might take a different view of what the sport may demand of the animals.

Animal Welfare and Veterinarian Participation

As emphasized in this book, ethical deliberation regarding animal welfare often depends on the availability of sound empirical data regarding what actually happens to animals. Otherwise, opinions turn into empty bluster that derives more from preexisting positions than sound scientific knowledge. The PRCA has undertaken several studies to determine the incidence of animal injuries at its events. One survey was conducted by on-site veterinarians at 28 PRCA-sanctioned rodeos in 1993 and 1994. Of the 33,991 animals that were entered in the arenas only 16, or 0.47 %, were injured.[121] Between August 15 and December 31, 1994 the PRCA asked on-site, independent veterinarians to report on the effects of calf-roping at 28 California rodeos. The veterinarians were asked to note the condition of calves from their arrival at the rodeo to their departure. The study found that in 915 calf-roping runs, only one problem occurred, a minor stifle injury that the attending veterinarian indicated would heal completely. No other rodeo-related injuries were reported for the remaining PRCA-sanctioned events at these rodeos (Terri Greer, PRCA humane issues officer: Personal communication).

Although the animal welfare problems of rodeo have undoubtedly been exaggerated by its opponents, it is also clear that more can be done to improve the welfare of rodeo animals. (This statement can be made about any animal sport, and rodeo enthusiasts should therefore not find it offensive.) One important issue relates to the presence of veterinarians at rodeo events. Rodeo differs from horse and dog racing in that an official veterinarian is not required by law in all states. PRCA rules require that "a veterinarian shall be present or on call for every performance and/or section of slack."[122] The PRCA makes clear that it would prefer to have a veterinarian at all times at each of its events. It estimates that 86% of its sanctioned rodeos have a veterinarian on site; rodeos that utilize veterinarians on an on-call basis tend to be smaller, rural events (Greer T: Personal communication). The PRCA's approach to this issue is reasonable. Its sanctioned rodeos that do not have an on-site veterinarian are still required to adhere to its animal welfare rules. It is far better that such rules be in force than to have smaller rodeos forsake the rules because these rodeos cannot or will not employ on-site veterinarians.

Clearly, veterinary presence can be assured at all rodeos (including amateur rodeos as well as professional events not sanctioned by PRCA or similar organizations) only if state laws require the presence of an official, independent on-site veterinarian. Rodeo animals deserve no less protection than racing horses or dogs. It is difficult to argue that a sport which attracts some 30 million observers annually is not of sufficient importance to merit some government supervision of its use of animals. If rodeos were required by law to have an on-site veterinarian, veterinarians capable of doing the job and funding sufficient to pay them would be found. Whether their presence is required by law, official rodeo veterinarians must have sufficient training and expertise in the medical problems of rodeo animals. Thus small animal practitioners are not appropriate rodeo veterinarians. On-site veterinarians should have substantial experience in the medical problems of stock animals that are part of rodeo events as well as of horses.

Having a veterinarian at each and every rodeo will have a wider effect than providing veterinary care for individual animals in need of it. The very presence of a veterinarian will impress upon the organizers of even the smallest rodeos that the eyes of the entire veterinary profession are upon them. Abuses will be noticed and will not be tolerated. The entire sport will benefit from public knowledge that veterinarians are on the scene at all rodeos protecting the animals and looking after their welfare.

State legislatures should also consider requiring that all rodeos be sanctioned by or adhere to the humane standards of the PRCA or other organizing bodies. The PRCA, whose animal welfare rules are the most stringent of any rodeo organization, sanctions 30% of the professional rodeos in the United States. Another 50% are sanctioned by smaller rodeo organizations which also have animal welfare standards.[123] Thus approximately 20% of all U.S. professional rodeos are not sanctioned by any organization with rules for humane care and treatment of animals. This is unacceptable. At the very least, people who attend rodeos should be vigorously informed about the humane standards imposed by organizing groups, and should demand that rodeos they attend adhere to humane standards such as those of the PRCA.[124]

Some rodeo events, such as steer roping, subject animals to significant physical force. Lawrence reported that during one 9-day rodeo, more than 27 animals were lost, including nine steers that had to be destroyed as a result of steer roping, one of which suffered a broken neck.[125] As the reduction in leg fractures achieved by the Salinas rodeo demonstrates, steps can sometimes be taken to decrease the risk of injury while not materially altering an event. Research can be conducted to find less dangerous ways of approaching some rodeo events and practices. However, if an event is inherently and irreparably dangerous to the animals, it ought to be eliminated. The fact that some states prohibit steer roping proves that changes can be made without ruining the sport.

Charreada rodeos will require special attention. At the time of this writing, they were not on the PRCA circuit and thus were not subject to its animal welfare rules. In 1994 California enacted a law prohibiting the intentional tripping of horses in entertainment, thus outlawing the charreada horse-roping event in that state. With its own distinctive flavor and history, charreada may be able to tap into much of traditional Western rodeo's appeal to pageantry and regional tradition. Especially in areas of the United States in which Western cowboy and Mexican cultures thrive together, charreadas are likely to become extremely popular. This fact was demonstrated by the enormously favorable audience reaction to the charreada events held at the National Western Stock Show and Rodeo in Denver for the first time in 1995.[126] In my view, it would be unwise for supporters of traditional rodeo, veterinarians, or animal welfare advocates to look down upon charreada as uncivilized or inferior. (This is a piece of behavior traditional rodeo enthusiasts rightly resent when directed at their sport by some supposedly more "civilized" Easterners.) At the same time, animals used in charreadas must be treated no worse than animals at traditional Western rodeos. This may mean that certain charreada events in addition to horse-roping (such as grabbing running steers by the tail and perhaps even untimed horse and bull bucking) may have to be eliminated or substantially modified. If charreadas are unwilling or unable to adequately protect their animals, they may provide the impetus for state governments to require minimum animal welfare rules and veterinarian presence for all rodeos.

More evidence of the effects of rodeo events and conditions on the animals should be gathered so that animal welfare problems can be detected and addressed. The organized veterinary profession and the veterinary schools have not done enough in this area. An AVMA policy statement on the welfare of animals in spectator sports "recommends that all rodeos abide by rules to ensure the humane treatment of rodeo livestock, such as those established by the Professional Rodeo Cowboy's Association and the International Rodeo Association." The policy also "supports continued research into sport animal medicine to reduce injury for both contestants and animals."[127] The PRCA has utilized members of the AAEP and individual veterinary school clinicians to assist in PRCA animal welfare studies and to provide medical care for rodeo animals. Nevertheless, while veterinary schools now devote considerable energy to the study and promotion of the welfare of race horses and racing dogs, relatively little sustained scientific attention has been paid to rodeo animals. If veterinary science is only now beginning to obtain reliable scientific knowledge regarding horse and dog athletes, can anyone doubt that much remains to be learned about rodeo animal welfare?

Veterinary schools in states with substantial public attendance at rodeos should make it part of their academic mission to engage in the serious study of rodeo animal welfare. Leading conventions and conferences should include seminars in which practitioners who serve at rodeos can share knowledge and suggestions with other veterinarians. The more veterinarians know about the sport, the greater will be the likelihood of promoting rodeo animal welfare. Rodeo will continue to attract many millions of spectators and to involve many thousands of animals. The veterinary profession must give this unique and enormously popular sport the attention it and its animals deserve.

REFERENCES

[1]Fetrow J, Madison JB, Galligan D: Economic decisions in veterinary practice: A method for field use, *J Am Vet Med Assoc* 186:792, 1985.

[2]*Id*, p 794.

[3]Van Saun R, Bartlett PC, Morrow D: Monitoring the effects of postpartum diseases on milk production in dairy cattle, *Compend Cont Ed Pract Vet* 9(6):F212-220, 1987.

[4]*Id*, p F212.

[5]For example, Friend TH and others: Adrenal gluticocorticoid response to exogenous adrenocorticotropin mediated by density and social disruption in lactating cows, *J Dairy Sci* 60:1958-1963, 1977.

[6]Straw B, Friendship R: Expanding the role of the veterinarian on swine farms, *Compend Cont Educ Pract Vet* 8:F69, 1986.

[7]Stein TE: Marketing health management to food animal enterprises, Part II, *Compend Cont Educ Pract Vet* 8(7):S331, 1986. Stein cites with approval another proposed redefinition of health as "the level of production that the animal's owners have set as their objective and which is consistent with humane practices." This definition, also, errs in making productivity part of the very essence or definition of health. Nor is it helpful to include reference to humane practices in a definition of health. To ask whether some husbandry practice is "humane" is to ask whether it is, all things considered, morally appropriate. Neither medical diagnosis nor ethical analysis will be served by putting off all decisions regarding whether an animal or a group of animals is "healthy" until after one has answered the ethical question whether they are being treated properly.

[8]Curtis SE: Animal well-being and animal care, *Vet Clin North Am Food Anim Pract* 3(2):373-374, 1987.

[9]*See*, for example, Husmann RJ: Dairy cow herd health management. In Howard JL, editor: *Current Veterinary Therapy: Food Animal Practice 2*, Philadelphia, 1986, WB Saunders, p 123; Erb HN: The teaching of animal health economics at the undergraduate level. In: *Third International Symposium on Veterinary Epidemiology and Economics*, Edwardsville, KS, 1983, Veterinary Medicine Publishing, p 343.

[10]Brambell FWR: *Report of the Technical Committee to Enquire Into the Welfare of Animals Kept Under Intensive Livestock Husbandry Systems*, London, 1965, Cmnd. 2836, Her Majesty's Stationery Office.

[11]Jacobs FS: A perspective on animal rights and domestic animals, *J Am Vet Med Assoc* 184:1344-1345, 1984.

[12]For an excellent discussion of behaviorism and its flaws, *see* Rollin BE: *The Unheeded Cry*, New York, 1990, Oxford University Press.

[13]For example, Hart BL: *Behavior of Domestic Animals*, New York, 1985, WH Freeman, p 353 (stating that because of correlations between processes in human and nonhuman subcortical areas of the brain, "in dealing with stimuli that we relate to the production of pain or fear we feel somewhat justified in assuming that animals are experiencing some of the same emotions as we would").

[14]*J Am Vet Med Assoc* 191:1184-1298, 1987.

[15]*J Am Vet Med Assoc* 191:1187, 1987.

[16]Nielsen M, Braestrup C, Squires RF: Evidence for a late evolutionary appearance of brain-specific benzodiazepine receptors: An investigation of 18 vertebrate and 5 invertebrate species, *Brain Res* 141:342-346, 1978.

[17]Gray JA: *The Neuropsychology of Anxiety: An Enquiry into Functions of the Septo-Hippocampal System*, Oxford, 1982, Oxford University Press.

[18]Curtis SE: Animal well-being and animal care, *Vet Clin North Am Food Anim Pract* 3(2):373-377, 1987.

[19]Fox MW: *Farm Animals: Husbandry, Behavior, and Veterinary Practice* (hereinafter referred to as Fox: *Farm Animals*), Baltimore, 1984, University Park Press, p 94.

[20]American Veterinary Medical Association: Positions on Animal Welfare, Animal Agriculture, "Castration and Dehorning of Cattle," *1994 AVMA Directory*, Schaumburg, IL, 1993, The Association, p 58.

[21]Fox, MW: *Farm Animals*, p 99.

[22]Id, pp 98-105.

[23]Id, pp 99-101.

[24]Scher G: Facts about Veal Production and the Economic Impact of H.R. 2859 on Veal Farmers, Dairy Farmers, Consumers, North Manchester, IN, undated, American Veal Association, unpaginated.

[25]American Veterinary Medical Association: Positions on Animal Welfare, Animal Agriculture, paragraph 12, *1994 AVMA Directory*, Schaumburg, IL, 1993, The Association, p 58.

[26]American Veterinary Medical Association: *Guide for Veal Calf Care and Production, 1994 AVMA Directory*, Schaumburg, IL, 1993, The Association, pp 58-59.

[27]*See*, for example, Veal crate ban—We are still waiting, *Agscene* June 1987:8 (reporting support by the Animal Welfare Committee of the British Veterinary Association for a government proposal to prohibit veal crates).

[28]Fox MW: *Farm Animals*, p 138; Johnson DE: Extra-label drug use—veterinary practitioner views: Food animals, *J Am Vet Med Assoc* 202:1645-1647, 1993.

[29]Wise JK: *The US Market for Food Animal Veterinary Medical Services*, Schaumburg, IL, 1987, American Veterinary Medical Association, p 53.

[30]*Id*, p 91-92.

[31]*Id*, p 74-76.

[32]*Id*, p 53.

[33]*Id*, p 92, emphasis added.

[34]For a history of the FDA policies and the AVMA legislative proposal, *see* Kram MA: The AVMA legislative initiative, *J Am Vet Med Assoc* 202:1668-1670, 1993. *See generally, Symposium: Use of FDA-Approved Drugs in Veterinary Medicine: Prohibitions, Prerogatives, and Responsibilities, J Am Vet Med Assoc* 202:1601-1745, 1993.

[35]21 U.S.C. § 360b(a)(1988).

[36]FDA Compliance Policy Guides, Guide 7125.06, Chapter 25, *Animal Drugs*, November 11, 1986, emphases added.

[37]Young FE, FDA Commissioner: Letter to Representative Ted Weiss, Subcommittee on Intergovernmental Relations and Human Resources, US House of Representatives, January 9, 1987.

[38]Weiss T: Chairman, Subcommittee on Intergovernmental Relations and Human Resources, US House of Representatives: Letter to Frank E. Young, FDA Commissioner, November 17, 1986.

[39]For a history and summary of the Animal Medicinal Drug Use Clarification Act, *see* Brody MD: Congress entrusts veterinarians with discretionary extra-label use, *J Am Vet Med Assoc* 205:1366-1370, 1994.

[40]Quoted in Brody MD: Congress entrusts veterinarians with discretionary extra-label use, *J Am Vet Med Assoc* 205:1369, 1994.

[41]All the ethical issues mentioned in the above paragraphs also apply to the subtherapeutic use of antibiotics or other drugs in food producing animals. There is disagreement in the scientific community about whether the use of subtherapeutic levels of penicillin, tetracyclines, and other drugs in animal feed is already posing a threat to human heath by promoting the spread of drug-resistant bacteria. For example, *Antibiotics in American Feed: A Threat to Human Health?* Summit, NJ: American Council on Science and Health, 1985, p 24 (stating that there is "no evidence of a current or imminent human health hazard from penicillin and the tetracyclines in animal feed"). But compare Spika JS and others: Chloramphenicol-resistant Salmonella newport traced through hamburger to dairy farms, *N Engl J Med* 316(10):565-570, 1987. For a reasoned discussion from the veterinary standpoint, *see* Herrick JB: Have we created antibiotic-resistant monsters? *J Am Vet Med Assoc* 205:1396-1397, 1994.

[42]For example, the FDA has prohibited compounding of animal drugs by veterinarians, in part on the grounds that this constitutes extra-label use and in part on the view that "practicing veterinarians do not possess the pharmacologic training, experience or equipment necessary to compound...drugs with any assurance of safety and effectiveness..." Letter to an unnamed veterinarian, quoted in Signer AW: Has the Food and Drug Administration abused its authority to regulate veterinary compounding? *J Am Vet Med Assoc* 205:243, 1994. For an invaluable collection of arguments for and against animal drug compounding by veterinarians, and of possible approaches by the profession and the FDA, *see* Symposium: Compounding in Veterinary Medicine, *J Am Vet Med Assoc* 205:189-303, 1994.

[43]21 U.S.C. § 353(f). In 1994 the AVMA adopted a revised policy explaining and providing suggestions to practitioners regarding the new legal category of "veterinary prescription drugs." AVMA Guidelines for Veterinary Prescription Drugs, *J Am Vet Med Assoc* 992:[inserted supplement]1, 1994.

[44]Wise JK: *The US Market for Food Animal Veterinary Medical Services*, Schaumburg, IL, 1987, American Veterinary Medical Association, p vi.

[45]*Id*, p 143-147.

[46]Johnson DE: Extra-label use—Veterinary practitioner views: Food Animals, *J Am Vet Med Assoc* 202:1645, 1993. Dr. Johnson also maintains that there is still a "remarkably low prevalence" of drug residues because producers have used what is available in the marketplace and allowed by the system.

[47]*Id*, p 1647.

[48]*See*, Tannenbaum J: *Veterinary Ethics*, ed 1, Baltimore, 1989, Williams & Wilkins, pp 266-267.

[49]Accreditation of veterinarians and suspension or revocation of such accreditation, 9 CFR § 160.1 *et seq.*

[50]For example, just the issue of whether genetically engineered animals, plants, or microorganisms should be the subjects of patents has generated prodigious debate on the scientific, ethical, religious, and economic implications of granting people property rights in life forms. In 1980 the U.S. Supreme Court held that microorganisms are patentable. *Diamand v. Chakrabarty*, 447 U.S. 303 (1980). In 1988 Harvard University was granted a patent for a genetically-engineered mouse prone to cancer (the famous so-called "Harvard mouse" or "oncomouse"). This patent rekindled the debate about the morality of patenting life and led to unsuccessful attempts in Congress by opponents of animal patents to impose a temporary moratorium on such patenting. Many of the arguments raised then, and now, against animal patenting are similar to those made against genetic engineering in general. However, patenting of life strikes a number of philosophers and theologians as especially objectionable because it reflects the view not just that people may manipulate forms of life, but also that they can own and profit from these forms of life. For useful discussions of the history of animal patenting, and of ethical and legal issues, and descriptions of positions taken by various sides in these debates, *see* Barton JH: Patenting life, *Sci Amer* 264(3) March 1991:40-46; Adler RG: Biotehnology as an intellectual property, *Science* 224:357-363, 1984; Adler RG: Controlling the applications of biotechnology, *Harvard J Law Tech* 1:1-61, 1988; Dresser R: Ethical and legal issues in patenting new animal life, *Jurimetrics J* 28:399-435, 1988.

[51]*See*, for example, Kang Y, Jimenez-Flores R, Richardson T: Casein genes and genetic engineering of the caseins. In Evans JW, Hollaender A, editors: *Genetic Engineering of Animals*, New York, 1986, Plenum Press, p 102, citing Palmiter RD, Brinster RL: Transgenic mice, *Cell* 41:343-345, 1985.

[52]Headon DR: Biotechnology: Endless possibilities for veterinary medicine, *J Am Vet Med Assoc* 204:1597, 1994.

[53]Hullar TL: Putting it in context. In Macdonald JF, editor: *Agricultural Biotechnology: A Public Conversation about Risk*, Ithaca, NY: National Agricultural Biotechnology Council, 1993, p 13.

[54]Anderson WF: Genetic engineering of animals. In Evans JW, Hollaender A, editors: *Genetic Engineering of Animals*, New York, 1986, Plenum Press, p 7.

[55]Rollin BE: The "Frankenstein thing": The moral impact of genetic engineering of agricultural animals on society and future science. In Gendel SM and others, editors: *Agricultural Bioethics*, Ames, 1990, Iowa State University Press, p 300.

[56]*Id*, p 308.

[57]Morton D, James R, Roberts J: Issues arising from recent advances in biotechnology, *Vet Rec* July 17, 1993:53-56. This article provides an excellent summary, from the veterinary perspective, of ethical issues in biotechnology and genetic engineering, as well as sound common-sense responses to commonly asked questions.

[58]Increases of 10% to 25% extra milk in a 305-day lactation were reported by the Animal Health Institute, and 10% to 15% by the Council for Agricultural Science and Technology. Kronfeld DS: Health management of dairy herds treated with bovine somatotropin, *J Am Vet Med Assoc* 204:117, 1994. Monsanto advertised that "Posilac® increases milk response 5 to 15 pounds per cow, per day." *Hoard's Dairyman* 139(4):140-141, 1994.

[59]Balk RA: Public values and risk assessment. In Macdonald JF, editor: *Agricultural Biotechnology: A Public Conversation about Risk*, Ithaca, NY, 1993, National Agricultural Biotechnology Council, pp 87-96.

[60]For an example of such an argument, which also defends a larger social context of which family farms are a part, *see* Comstock G: The case against bGH. In Gendel SM and others: *Agricutural Bioethics*, Ames, 1990, Iowa State University Press, pp 309-339.

[61]Kronfeld DS: Health management of dairy herds treated with bovine somatotropin, *J Am Vet Med Assoc* 204:116-130, 1994.

[62]*See*, Willeberg P: An international perspective on bovine somatotropin, *J Am Vet Med Assoc* 205:538-541, 1994; Post D and Colbert JL: Letter, Comments on bovine somatotropin, *J Am Vet Med Assoc* 204:508-509, 1994.

[63]For example, DeGroff LE: Letter, Positive experience with bovine somatotropin, *J Am Vet Med Assoc* 204:1000-1001, 1994.

[64]They've used BST, *Hoard's Dairyman* 139(4):134-135, 175-176, 1994.

[65]Seidel GE: Characteristics of future agricultural animals. In Evans JW, Hollaender A, editors: *Genetic Engineering of Animals*, New York, 1986, Plenum Press, p 302.

[66]In 1994 Monsanto advertised an incentive program for dairy farmers that offered a $150 voucher toward payment of a veterinarian's professional services with the first purchase of Posilac®. The program was advertised to veterinarians, *J Am Vet Med Assoc* 204:860-861, 1994, as well as directly to farmers, *Hoard's Dairyman* 139(4):140-141, 1994.

[67]*See*, for example, Rollin BE: The "Frankenstein thing": The moral impact of genetic engineering of agricultural animals on society and future science. In Gendel SM and others, editors: *Agricultural Bioethics*, Ames, 1990, Iowa State University Press, pp 306-307.

[68]Huxley A: *Brave New World*, New York, 1932, Random House.

[69]Donnelly S: The ethical challenges of animal biotechnology, *Livestock Prod Sci* 36:98, 1993.

[70]Rose RJ: Foreword, "Symposium on Equine Physiology", *Vet Clin North Am Equine Pract* 1(3):437, 1985.

[71]Dalin G, Jeffcott LB: Locomotion and gait analysis, *Vet Clin North Am Equine Pract* 1(3):568-569, 1985.

[72]American Horse Council: *1994 Horse Industry Directory*, Washington, DC, 1994, American Horse Council, p 5.

[73]For an excellent discussion supporting controlled precompetition medication approaches *see* Tobin T, Heard R: *Drugs and the Performance Horse*, Springfield, IL, 1981, Charles C Thomas; for a contrary approach *see* Baker RO: *The Misuse of Drugs in Horse Racing*, Barrington, IL, 1978, Illinois Hooved Animal Humane Society. For a comprehensive survey of drugs and methods used to detect doping of horses, *see* Sams RA, Hinchcliff KW: Drugs and performance. In Hodgson DR, Rose RJ, editors: *The Athletic Horse*, Philadelphia, 1994, WB Saunders, pp 439-467.

[74]Baker RO, *op. cit.*, p xxv (stating that "undoubtedly, track veterinarians often find it difficult to follow the dictates of their own conscience and the ethics of their profession").

[75]*See*, for example, O'Connor JT: The untoward effects of the corticosteroids in equine practice, *J Am Vet Med Assoc* 153:1614-1617, 1968; Galley RH: The use of hyaluronic acid in the racehorse. *Proceedings of the 32nd Annual Convention of the American Association of Equine Practitioners*: 657-661, 1986.

[76]For a critique of the usefulness of such terms as "restorative" versus "additive" in the use of drugs by human athletes, *see* Fost N: Banning drugs in sports: A skeptical view, *Hastings Center Rep* 16(4):5-10, 1986.

[77]There is substantial disagreement among equine practitioners and pathologists about whether, or to what extent, the administration of corticosteroids and other drugs actually contribute to break-downs, and more scientific data are needed. *See*, for example, Munson L: Deciperhing a death. *Sports Illus* 79(18):81, 1993; Verdon D: DVMs play pivotal role in horse racing ethics, *DVM* 22(3) March, 1991:1,59; O'Connor JT: The untoward effects of the corticosteroids in equine practice, *J Am Vet Med Assoc* 153:1614-1617, 1968; Galley RH: The use of hyaluronic acid in the racehorse, *Proceedings of the 32nd Annual Convention of the Annual Convention of the American Association of Equine Practitioners*, 1986, The Association, pp 657-661.

[78]Nack W, The breaking point, *Sports Illus* 79(18):80, 1993.

[79]*Id*, p 84.

[80]*Id*, p 85, emphasis in original.

[81]Vecsey G: Racing can't afford more tragedies, *New York Times* June 6, 1993, Section 8, p 1. This column, the stimulus for which was the breakdown and death of Prairie Bayou in the 1993 Belmont Stakes, does not mention overmedication as a possible cause of the breakdown problem.

[82]Kingsbury MD: Pleasure and show horse preventive medicine. In Mansmann RA, McAllister ES, Pratt PW, editors: *Equine Medicine and Surgery*, ed 3, Santa Barbara, 1982, American Veterinary Publications, pp 60-65.

[83]Nack W, Munson L: Blood money, *Sports Illus* 77(21):19-28, 1992.

[84]*See*, for example, Hrehocik M, Stultz TB: Two DVMs indicted in equine fraud scam, *DVM* 25(9):1, 1994; Sprague K, Shields C: Ward, Lindemann among 23 indicted for fraud in connection with horse killings, *Chron Horse* 57(31):58-59, 1994.

[85]Strassburger J: Horse showing is now paying for its past, *Chron Horse* 57(42):4-8, 1994.

[86]Bixler T: Intentionally killing horses is only one kind of equine insurance fraud, *DVM* 24(3):27, 1993.

[87]Bixler T: DVMs can help prevent equine insurance fraud, *DVM* 24(3):62, 1993.

[88]Bixler T: Murdering for money: Equine DVMs react to insurance fraud investigation, *DVM* 24(3):1, 1993.

[89]Mackay-Smith M, Cohen M: Exercise physiology and diseases of exertion. In Mansmann RA, McAllister ES, Pratt PW, editors: *Equine Medicine and Surgery*, ed 3, Santa Barbara, 1982, American Veterinary Publications, p 128.

[90]Nack W. The breaking point, *Sports Illus* 79(18):90, 1993.

[91]Bixler T: AAEP writes guidelines concerning pre-race inspections, *DVM* 24(2):1, 1993.

[92]American Veterinary Medical Association: Guidelines for Horse Show Veterinarians, *1994 AVMA Directory*, Schaumburg, IL, 1993, The Association, p 68.

[93]In Deutschmann K: *Fairgrounds Thoroughbred Horse Racing in Massachusetts*, Boston, 1986, Massachusetts Society for the Prevention of Cruelty to Animals, App B.

[94]Bixler T: Racing commissions: Suspensions draw criticism on medical decision-making authority, *DVM* 23(7):1,27, 1992.

[95]American Horse Shows Association: *1994 AHSA Drugs and Medications Rule and Its Practical Application*, Hilliard, OH, 1994, The Association.

[96]Lengel JG: Understanding the 1994 AHSA drugs and medications rule. In *1994 AHSA Drugs and Medications Rule and Its Practical Application*, Hilliard, OH, 1994, American Horse Shows Association, p 11.

[97]15 U.S.C. § 1821 *et seq.*

[98]9 CFR § 11.1 *et seq.*

[99]9 CFR § 11.7(a)(1).

[100]9 CFR § 11.21.

[101]Tye L: Greyhounds pay the price of racing's shadow world, *Boston Globe* November 8, 1992, p 65.

[102]*Report of the Advisory Committee on the Adoption and Humane Disposition of Greyhounds*, (hereinafter referred to as *Massachussetts Advisory Committee Report*), Boston, 1987, Commonwealth of Massachusetts Executive Office of Consumer Affairs and Business Regulation, p 1.

[103]*Id*, p 12.

[104]Romano R: Owners of racers take responsibility, risk, *Boston Globe* November 8, 1992, p 67.

[105]Tye L: Greyhounds pay the price of racing's shadow world, *Boston Globe* November 8, 1992, 1-2.

[106]*Massachussetts Advisory Committee Report*, pp 6-7.

[107]Nassar R, Fluke J: *American Humane Animal Shelter Reporting Study: 1988*, Denver, 1990, American Humane Association (estimating that of the 10.3 to 17.2 million dogs that enter pounds and shelters each year, 5.8 to 9.6 million are euthanized).

[108]Kahler S: Banking on greyhounds, *J Am Vet Med Assoc* 204:1295-1299, 1994.

[109]*Massachussetts Advisory Committee Report*, p 16.

[110]Maggitti P: See how they run: A look at the hidden side of greyhound racing, *Anim Agenda* March, 1992:13.

[111]Tye L: Live lures remain an issue, *Boston Globe* November 8, 1992, p 65.

[112]Lawrence E : *Rodeo*, Knoxville, 1982, University of Tennessee Press (hereinafter referred to as Lawrence: *Rodeo*), p 10.

[113]Lawrence: *Rodeo*, p 269.

[114]Joint Statement of the HSUS and AHA. Quoted in Drennon C: Rodeo: Cruelty, not sport, *Calif Vet* 37(1):65, 1983.

[115]Drennon C: Rodeo: Cruelty, not sport, *Calif Vet* 37(1):65, 1983.

[116]Professional Rodeo Cowboys Association: *Humane Facts: The Care and Treatment of Professional Rodeo Livestock*, Colorado Springs, CO, undated, The Association, (hereinafter referred to as PRCA: *Humane Facts*), pp 8-9.

[117]Santos FK: Is rodeo really cruel? *Calif Vet* 37(1):66, 1983.

[118]PRCA: *Humane Facts*, p 9.

[119]Lawrence: *Rodeo*, p 177.

[120]Lawrence: *Rodeo*, pp 119-121.

[121]PRCA: *Humane Facts*, p 4.

[122]PRCA Rule 9.1.1, quoted in PRCA: *Humane Facts*, p 13.

[123]PRCA: *Humane Facts*, p 3.

[124]The 1994 American Horse Council *Horse Industry Directory* lists the following rodeo organizations and the number of rodeos sanctioned by each in 1993: American Professional Rodeo Association (109 rodeos), Canadian Professional Rodeo Association (65 rodeos), International Pro Rodeo Association (520 rodeos), National High School Rodeo Association (920 rodeos), National Intercollegiate Rodeo Association (109 rodeos), National Little Britches Rodeo, Professional Rodeo Cowboys Association (791 rodeos), and Women's Professional Rodeo Association (700 rodeos). American Horse Council: *1994 Horse Industry Directory*, Washington, DC, 1994, The Council, p 102.

[125]Lawrence: *Rodeo*, p 125.

[126]Lipsher S: Mexican rodeo an extravaganza, *Denver Post* January 10, 1995, p 1AA; Lipsher S: Mexican rodeo rousing success, *Denver Post* January 11, 1995, p 1AA.

[127]American Veterinary Medical Association: AVMA Policy on Animal Welfare, Welfare of Animals in Spectator Events, paragraph I.8, *1994 AVMA Directory*, Schaumburg, IL, 1993, The Association, p 56.

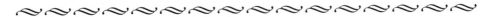

CHAPTER 24

Animal Research

Relatively few veterinarians engage in animal research. Biomedical and scientific research accounts for a very small fraction of all animals used by society. Nevertheless, a discussion of professional veterinary ethics must consider issues relating to the use of animals in research.

First, there exists a sizable body of work addressing the ethics of the use of animals in research. Many of the questions discussed in this literature bear upon animal welfare, which is a general concern of the veterinary profession.

Moreover, continued progress in preventing and alleviating animal and human disease depends upon the ability of veterinarians, physicians, and biomedical scientists to use animals in research. Promoting the interests of their patients, clients, and profession requires veterinarians to support animal research. This, in turn, means that veterinarians must know about current controversies and must be able to participate in them persuasively.

Finally, no one can speak more convincingly than veterinarians about the legitimate needs of all those affected by animal research, including research animals. The veterinary profession possesses great knowledge about animals, science, and human and animal disease. The deepest values of the profession include a recognition of the legitimacy of the human use of animals, as well as a desire to treat animals fairly.

This book focuses on ethical issues faced by veterinarians in private clinical practice. Therefore I cannot attempt to discuss in detail all the ethical questions posed by the use of animals in research. My aims here are to provide helpful information about some of the more important current issues and to apply principles developed in this book to some of these issues.

∼ WHAT IS ANIMAL RESEARCH?

Animal research can be defined as the search for or investigation of facts through scientific inquiry that utilizes animals. Research (regardless of whether it uses animals) can be "basic," in the sense of being motivated by a desire to obtain knowledge irrespective of any practical applications or benefits, or "applied," in the sense of being aimed at obtaining such results. One important justification for basic research is the desire to understand our world and its components. But because making the world better almost always requires knowledge of it, basic research frequently stimulates, or eventually becomes of direct use to, applied research.

There is great variety in activities that are properly called "animal research." This fact is not always appreciated or emphasized by opponents of the use of animals in research. Animal research does not necessarily involve manipulating animals or their environments; ethologists or psychologists can sometimes do research on animals by observing them in their natural habitats. Animal research need not involve causing animals pain or distress; indeed, many research animals fare much better in laboratories than they would in the wild. Animal research is not directed solely at benefiting human beings; much animal research helps animals. Animal research does not necessarily involve sacrificing the interests of a research animal for the good of people or other animals. A great deal of animal research is conducted by veterinary clinicians and is directly beneficial to animals undergoing experimental procedures.

It is also important to understand that activities which, strictly speaking, might not be termed "research" are often important components of the general research enterprise—either because they can be involved in particular parts of research projects or because they provide training for those who do, or will eventually do, animal research. A complete account of the ethics of the use of animals in research must therefore include consideration of the employment of animals in the production and standardization of drugs and biologicals, the diagnosis of human and animal diseases, toxicity testing, and education.

∾ HOW MANY ANIMALS ARE USED IN RESEARCH?

Much attention has been paid by both supporters and opponents of animal research to the question of how many animals are actually used in research in the United States. This is a legitimate question. Unfortunately, at least at present, it is extremely difficult to answer it.

A 1986 study by the U.S. Congress Office of Technology Assessment estimated that between 17 and 22 million animals are utilized in research and testing annually.[1] This estimate is still cited frequently. However, its reliability is undercut not just by the passage of time but also by the fact that it could not accurately calculate the number of mice and rats, even though such animals probably account for between 80% to 90% of research animals. Research facilities have not been required to report the number of mice, rats, birds, reptiles, and amphibians they use. It has therefore been impossible for any study to estimate with any degree of precision the total number of animals used in research. The difficulty in accurately estimating the number of research animals is compounded by the fact that laboratories operated by the federal government (including military medical and research facilities) are not required to report animal numbers. A 1994 analysis of various data sources concluded that between 14 and 21 million animals were used for research in 1992.[2] Although this study complained about the lack of reliability of reporting statistics, its estimate of the numbers is probably as accurate as is possible at the present time.

However difficult it may be to determine how many animals are used in research, several important facts are noteworthy.

1. **The total number of animals used in research annually appears to be declining.** The 1994 analysis cited above concluded that animal use has fallen "by at least 23% and maybe as much as 40% since 1967."[3] An earlier study conducted by the National Research Council Institute of Laboratory Animal Resources (ILAR) estimated that there was a 40% decrease in annual use between 1968 and 1978.[4] Statistics from countries whose laws require accurate estimates of research animal use also indicate declining numbers.[5]

2. Although the total number of research animals used anually appears to be falling, there has also been a shift from some species toward others. The USDA's 1992 figures show that since 1979 the number of dogs has declined 41%, the number of cats 44%, guinea pigs 18%, hamsters 12%, and rabbits 20%.[6] At the same time, National Institutes of Health (NIH) funding statistics indicate an increase in the number of funded projects utilizing mice, rats, and fish.[7] USDA figures show a dramatic increase in farm animals (such as pigs and goats) used in nonagricultural research from, 54,000 in 1990 to 365,000 in 1993.[8]

3. It is extremely difficult to predict long-term trends in research animal use. Features inherent in biomedical research may result in some increases. As Dr. Louis Sibal of the NIH observes, the apparent trend toward "lower" or less controversial species such as rats, mice, farm animals, and fish may eventually require some expansion in the use of other species. When researchers achieve promising results in mice or rats, for example, some will be required for scientific reasons to move up the phylogenetic ladder to verify these results in species closer to humans.[7] Additionally, attempts by granting agencies to encourage "alternatives" to research utilizing animals (see below) may increase animal use at least temporarily. Animals may be required to verify that certain nonanimal or reduced-animal methods are as reliable as more traditional animal techniques. It is also possible that the growing use of transgenic (that is, "genetically engineered") animals will substantially increase research animal numbers—by enabling the utilization of lower species such as mice and rats to study diseases that could formerly be studied only in more expensive or controversial species and by resulting in the development of animal "factories" for various drugs, biologicals, tissues, and body parts.

4. The attention given to controversies involving research animals—by animal activists, biomedical researchers, veterinarians, veterinary school ethics courses, legislators and regulators, and the public at large—is out of proportion to the numbers of these animals. It seems safe to say that most, perhaps the great majority, of debates and disputes about animals involve animal research. Yet, if one were to take the best contemporary upper estimate of approximately 21 million animals used each year in research, one would still be talking about a minuscule fraction of animals used annually. Over 6 billion broiler chickens were raised in 1991 in the United States.[9] If one adds to this figure just the 116 million laying hens and pullets of laying age,[10] the 75 million pullets not of laying age,[11] the 100 million cattle and calves on farms and ranches,[12] the 10 million milk cows,[13] the 57 million hogs and pigs in production facilities,[14] the 285 million turkeys,[15] and the 11 million sheep,[16] it would be difficult even to place research animal numbers on a pie chart of total annual animal use in this country.

Scientists, veterinarians, and government regulators have no choice but to respond to attacks on animal research. However, it is interesting to speculate about why so many people are concerned about animal research, when so many more animals are used for other purposes, and when most of these other animals are not nearly as well protected by laws or public concern. The following are some possible explanations:

• Many people may be more susceptible to opposition by activists to animal research than to, say, the use of animals for food, because doing without meat and other animal products would be inconvenient or bothersome, but animal research may seem to them to provide less clear and direct benefits.

- Many people may be ignorant about the benefits of animal research to people and animals, about how scientists actually treat animals, and about laws and institutional practices that protect research animals.
- Some people may be prepared to believe that animal researchers either deliberately torture animals or at the very least allow experimental animals to suffer horribly, because of a mistrust of scientists and of science.
- Animal activists have been able to utilize sensationalistic photographs and "horror stories" to convince some people that research typically causes substantial animal pain and suffering.
- Many people may think that research animals are particularly helpless and susceptible to painful procedures because these animals do tend to be confined and subjected to activities that are not natural for them. This view may be coupled with ignorance or unrealistic views about how farm and other kinds of animals are treated.

～ DEFENDING ANIMAL RESEARCH: THE ARTICULATION OF STANDARDS

The contributions of animal research to the health, safety, and well-being of people[17] and animals[18] have been enormous. There are countless people and animals alive and healthy today because of advances that would have been impossible if not for the use of animals. To stop or seriously curtail animal research would wreak unspeakable and intolerable evil.

The important activity of articulating good reasons for animal research has been hindered by the fact that many proponents of animal research are preoccupied with responding to attacks by abolitionists and other kinds of critics. Proponents of research often permit critics to choose the premises, indeed the very language, around which argument turns.

For example, I speak often with animal researchers about their work. I would be happy to have a dollar every time I hear that a particular project is "necessary" for the attainment of some crucial advance in medical knowledge. The literature defending animal research is filled with statements about the indispensability of animal research to every medical advance beneficial to humans and animals.[19] Such claims seem to be in response to critics who charge that animal research is *not* "necessary" because, in their view, almost every important biomedical advance would have been or would be possible without it.[20] There are, surely, some animal experiments that have been "necessary" in the sense that important advances in medical knowledge could not have occurred without them. Such necessity, when it exists, would constitute a strong argument in favor of a research project. But why should defenders of research accept the premise that any use of animals is unjustifiable unless it some day can be shown to have been "necessary?" We do not require farmers or meat-eaters to prove that hamburger or chicken is "necessary" for human well-being, health, or survival, or even for great esthetic pleasure.

The attainment of a modest piece of medically relevant knowledge or a moderately useful medical technique is surely far more important than the eating of even the most artfully prepared hamburger or chicken wing. Indeed, attempts to make advances in treating disease and illness, even when they *fail*, are far more valuable than the eating of any particular kind of food or the use of a myriad of animal products. Because science does not always succeed in producing significant or useful knowledge and because the implications of scientific research are often unpredictable, animal researchers should not always feel compelled to demonstrate that their experiments are "necessary."

If proponents of animal research sometimes make their task overly difficult, they sometimes make it too easy. The primary example of this is the widespread acceptance in the research community of the anticruelty position, and its implication that animal welfare consists entirely of freedom from unnecessary pain or other negative states (see Chapters 11 and 13). This view rejects the intuitively appealing notion that we sometimes are obligated to give animals we use for our own purposes some measure of happiness. The anticruelty position also implies that all animal experiments that do not cause *any* pain are justifiable.[21] This is too simplistic an approach. I know very few researchers who believe that it is appropriate to experiment upon or kill an unlimited number of chimpanzees or monkeys, for example, so long as this is done painlessly. With regard to some animals at least, there seems to be a higher burden of proof before even a completely painless experiment seems justified.

∾ ANIMAL RESEARCH ETHICS: BASIC PREMISES

Ethical issues relating to research animals are similar in important respects to issues involving agricultural animals. Many laboratory animal veterinarians take a herd health approach to research animals. Like farm and food animals, animals used in research are often kept in groups. Their usefulness typically derives from the role they play in relation to what can be gained from other animals. Because of similarities in laboratory and agricultural animal use, it is helpful for normative veterinary ethics to approach animal research with a set of basic premises similar to those it would apply to agricultural animals. I therefore want to set out the 10 basic premises developed in Chapter 23, modified for the area of animal research and with some additional discussion.

1. **It is not inherently wrong to use animals in research.** If some animals may be used in the production of food and clothing for humans, some animals surely may be used in the prevention and cure of human and animal disease. At the same time, defenders of animal research should not be too hasty (as some are) to assume that direct benefit to people or animals is the only justifiable purpose of animal research. Understanding basic features of our world and taking pleasure in such understanding is no less valuable than taking pleasure from an animal food or clothing product. It follows that the search for basic knowledge—even when it does not present an immediate or clear prospect of applied benefits—can also be a legitimate use of animals. To be sure, there are additional considerations. I would argue that in general, a stronger showing of the importance of a piece of basic research must be made when that work would cause pain or discomfort to animals than when the research shows great prospect of providing practical medical benefits. Considerations regarding other interests of the animals involved must also be taken into account. However, it is both inconsistent and antiintellectual to accept ordinary uses of animals for food and other consumer conveniences and to require animal researchers to always show that their work must have some (usually enormously important) practical benefit.

2. Researchers may factor research and management considerations into decisions regarding the use, care, and treatment of their animals. Because some animals may be used in research, it follows that optimal animal welfare sometimes may be compromised in animal experimentation. Otherwise, some legitimate research projects would be impossible. At the same time, one must ask whether any given level of welfare associated with an experiment is morally justified by the expected results (practical or theoretical) of the research.

3. The role of public needs and interests in the determination of how research animals are treated must not be underestimated. Animal researchers tend to be the targets of activist attacks, even though most research is done because of what is perceived to be in the public interest. Government and private agencies do not fund animal research on cancer, diabetes, heart disease, or AIDS to provide amusement for scientists. Ordinary citizens are not as actively involved in the choice of the employment of animals in research as they are in market forces that influence the use of agricultural and performance animals. Many people may not know why animal research is important for themselves and their loved ones. Scientists and the government are morally obligated to inform the public about what is being done with *its* tax dollars to support animal research. The case for such education becomes even stronger when activists seek to persuade people that animal research is inherently cruel and useless. Ultimately, the most effective protection for animal research and research animal welfare may come from an informed public that will demand both.

4. Research animals have interests that must be taken into account. Research animals, like those used for companionship and in agriculture and entertainment, have legitimate interests that must be taken into account in determining what may be done to them. Taking research animals' interests seriously does not mean always giving their interests priority over the interests of others. But it does mean rejecting the notion that such other interests automatically must prevail. There is a variety of both human and animal interests, some of which are weightier than others. The avoidance of pain, for example, is clearly a very important interest of research animals. Overriding this interest will, in general, require the presence of important countervailing interests.

The concept of ethical costs is important in the research animal area. As is generally the case, the need to consider ethical costs does not imply the legitimacy of a "cost-benefit" or utilitarian approach (see Chapter 5). Utilitarianism is no more theoretically or practically satisfactory in dealing with laboratory animals than it is in deciding how to treat agricultural animals. It is no more possible to quantify with rigorous precision the mental states of research animals than it is to do so for other animals. Utilitarianism also refuses to recognize that it is sometimes just *unfair* to treat research animals in certain ways (for example, by performing multiple major invasive procedures on animals to save costs by using fewer animals) even if such treatment could be shown to maximize the total pleasure or happiness of all affected.

5. Individual animals count.

6. Research animals have certain basic moral rights. The fact that individual research animals can experience such states as pain and stress means that their interests must be taken into account. Moreover, like domesticated agricultural and performance animals, research animals are not without moral rights because they may have been bred for suitability for certain uses. They are sentient beings with interests of their own, interests that sometimes cannot be overridden just because doing so would be expedient.

There remains significant opposition to the concept of animal rights within the biomedical and scientific research community. I suggest in Chapter 12 that much of this opposition stems from identification of the concept of animal *rights* with certain particular claims of the so-called animal rights *movement*. However, as I argue there, the concept of animal rights does not imply the anti-research platform of the animal rights movement. Like it or not, recognition of the existence of some animal rights will be a necessary part of any satisfactory approach to the ethics of the use of animals in research. As Chapter 12 suggests, veterinarians and scientists who insist on rejecting rights language altogether are probably fighting a losing battle, wasting time that could usefully be spent reconciling animal research with reasonable characterizations of animals' rights, and risking alienation from a public that appears comfortable both with animal research and the term "animal rights."

7. **Although assessment of mental states is an important component of determining research animal interests, we must avoid exaggerated claims about these mental states.** As is the case regarding other animals, identifying and assigning proper moral weight to the legitimate interests of research animals requires accuracy about what mental states they experience. As is the case generally, determining what mental states research animals have, either normally or in response to experimental environments, raises difficult conceptual and factual issues. Some of these issues are discussed below.

8. **All other things being equal, a research or husbandry method or course of veterinary care that causes a research animal less pain, suffering, distress, or discomfort is preferable to one that causes it more.**

9. **All other things being equal, a research or husbandry method or course of veterinary care that gives a research animal more positive mental states is preferable to one that gives it fewer.** These are intuitively appealing principles that sometimes cut against certain current assumptions and positions. But they are minimal principles. They do not address the issues of when animals *ought* to be subjected to less pain or be allowed to experience greater pleasure when these options would impose extra costs on experimenters in terms of expense, inconvenience, or the prospects of success of a research project. Moreover, as we shall see, sometimes all other things are *not* equal; there can be important scientific and therefore ethical reasons why a given individual animal may have to experience more distress or less pleasure than might otherwise be acceptable.

10. **It is almost always unhelpful to maintain that research animals should not be caused "unnecessary" pain, suffering, distress, or discomfort, or that they should be treated "humanely."** As I discuss in Chapters 11 and 23, typically, to say that a certain treatment of animals is "necessary" or "humane" is to claim that it is justified. However, determining what treatment is justified is precisely the task of ethical argument.

The limited usefulness of the notions of "necessary" pain and "humane" treatment is illustrated by the following statements of two thinkers at distant poles in the research animal issue. According to philosopher Carl Cohen, "(i)n our dealings with animals, few will deny that we are at least obligated to act humanely—that is to treat them with the decency and concern that we owe, as sensitive human beings, to other sentient creatures. To treat animals humanely, however, is not to treat them as...the holders of rights."[22] Dr. Michael Fox, who opposes much current animal research, disagrees. He insists that because animals, too, have "intrinsic value and thus rights within themselves," we must "if we are to be humane stewards judge [between competing human and animal rights] with caution and humility."[23] Clearly, the concept of "humaneness" is not doing argumentative work in these statements. Rather, the concept is being used to summarize positions about the proper treatment of animals that have already been reached for other reasons. Likewise, Cohen and Fox doubtlessly would disagree about whether certain animal research projects are "necessary," in part because they would disagree about whether any pain that might be associated with these projects is justified by their intended aims.

∼ THE ETHICS OF ANIMAL RESEARCH: POLITICAL CONSIDERATIONS

Serious investigation of animal welfare requires attention to difficult conceptual, factual, and ethical issues. In the area of research animal welfare, there is another important consideration—politics. Government (and those who attempt to influence government) are exerting ever greater influence on how research animals are treated. As a result, investigations of research animal welfare can be affected by political tests and demands. This happens in several ways.

1. Researchers are finding themselves compelled to explain their work and its effects on animals in terms understandable to laymen. My own experience serving as a nonscientist member and chairman of an animal care committee has been that researchers are perfectly capable of doing this. Indeed, they seem to be stimulated to think more clearly about scientific, practical, and welfare aspects of their experiments by having to explain their work to a layman.

2. The biomedical research community (as well as professional veterinary associations and veterinary schools) must devote already scarce resources to public relations and lobbying in support of animal research. Money and effort that might otherwise be spent on research, and indeed on research aimed at improving laboratory animal welfare, must be diverted into the political arena.

3. The necessity of addressing political issues can lead supporters of animal research to make decisions based not solely on logic, empirical evidence, or ethical argument, but on political expediency. For example, there have been prolonged efforts to convince state legislatures and Congress to prohibit the release by public pounds and animal shelters of abandoned dogs and cats for research. As I argue below, grave questions can be raised about the wisdom of such laws. Nevertheless, some scientists and veterinarians have concluded that they cannot prevail on this issue and that they only risk more general hostility to animal research if they raise the opposing arguments. This approach may or may not be justified on the grounds of expedience. But at the very least, some people who would like to be making certain arguments and developing certain positions are wary of doing so. Such a climate is not conducive to the search for truth.

4. The entry of politics into animal welfare investigations poses questions and imposes answers that are not always entirely justified ethically or scientifically. Some legislators and regulators may be accustomed to ordering what they want done, whether anyone knows how to do it or what it even means to do it. For example, the 1985 amendments to the federal Animal Welfare Act require that measures be taken to assure the "psychological well-being" of primates.[24] In fact, a great deal remains to be learned about what constitutes psychological well-being, for primates in general and various species of primates in particular. What mental states do these animals experience? How would one distinguish various levels of psychological well-being, and what moral weight might be assigned to these levels? Are certain practices (for example, restraint for long periods of time) really required for certain experiments, and if they are not, what approaches would have less negative impact on the animals' psychological well-being while permitting important research to continue?

Legislation and regulation is a double-edged sword. It can promote animal welfare by requiring that important questions be asked and overdue steps be taken. It can also discourage continuing progress, by imposing answers before they may be justified. Premature regulation can stifle serious animal welfare research by allowing those who do not care about animal welfare to rest on minimal government standards when much additional work is required. For example, if regulators declare that larger cages and "enrichment toys" in which primates fit nuts or pieces of fruit into holes in a board, are sufficient to promote primate psychological well-being, will that be the end of serious research into primate psychological well-being? Will the requirement that primates enjoy psychological well-being discourage funding of research directed at improving psychological well-being for nonprimates?

⁓ RESEARCH ANIMAL WELFARE: GENERAL CONSIDERATIONS
Housing, General Care, Environment

The conditions under which research animals are kept is obviously crucial to their welfare.[25] Among relevant issues are the size and construction materials of cages; temperature; ventilation; quantity and quality of food; lighting; the nature and quantity of bedding for nesting animals; density of animals within cages; ability of animals to come in contact with other animals; opportunities for adequate exercise; group housing of social species;[26] segregation of controls from sick and distressed animals; and opportunities for contact with technicians and handlers.[27]

Much more needs to be learned about all of these considerations. Researchers, ethicists, and regulators must be wary of approaches that seem intuitively appealing to someone who seeks to imagine what it would be like to be a laboratory animal, but may have little basis in fact. As is always the case in animal welfare science, assessing the effects of certain environmental conditions on welfare is rarely the end of the matter. The appropriateness of welfare-improving or welfare-lessening conditions cannot be evaluated without considering their impact on research protocols. However, such deliberations must leave open the possibility that the interests of research animals require certain basic conditions irrespective of their cost, inconvenience, or impact upon a research project.

Pain and Other Negative Mental States
Ethical issues

Although pain is a relevant moral variable, assessing its proper relevance is not always a simple matter. Some researchers appear to accept as obvious an obligation to minimize the total amount of pain experienced.[28] This is a utilitarian approach. It is overly simplistic and does not recognize certain morally important factors. The utilitarian must favor an experiment that causes a very small number of animals extremely severe pain over one that might cause a larger number of animals much less pain if the former experiment would cause on balance less total pain than the latter. However, this approach ignores the intuitively appealing principle that animals have a much greater interest in avoiding very severe or prolonged pain than in avoiding trivial or fleeting pain. Therefore it may sometimes be preferable to cause more *total* pain if doing so will cause less pain to each individual animal. Another morally relevant factor that cannot be recognized by a utilitarian is the issue of the fairness of subjecting an animal to more pain after a certain point. The utilitarian must recommend continuing to cause pain to animals that have already been experimented upon, rather than using new animals, if the former approach will cause less total pain or will be less expensive than the latter. However, at some point it just may be unfair to subject an individual animal that has already undergone severe deprivations of its interests to any more. The very plausible objection to repeated survival surgeries on individual animals is based upon this nonutilitarian principle.

Conceptual issues: Defining pain and negative mental states in research animals

Like their counterparts in farm animal welfare, some investigators in the research animal area appear to have an irresistible urge to quickly set forth definitions of animal mental states that may not always clarify or stimulate important empirical and ethical questions.

The proceedings of the landmark AVMA *Colloquium on Recognition and Alleviation of Animal Pain and Distress*[29] contain examples of problematic definitions of exceedingly complex concepts relating to negative mental states in research animals. Kitchell offers the following "working definition" of pain in animals: "an aversive sensory and emotional experience (a perception), which elicits protective motor actions, results in learned avoidance, and may modify species-specific traits of behavior, including social behavior."[30] This definition seems to exclude one phenomenon that clearly has important applications for animal welfare: "learned helplessness," in which an animal responds to repeated or severe pain or distress by "giving up" and doing nothing.[31] A second paper in the *Proceedings* asserts that pain "is a perception or unpleasant sensation arising from noxious stimuli that are actually or potentially damaging to tissues and is a subjective perception that is accompanied by feelings of fear, anxiety, and panic."[32] As I argue in Chapter 23, it is far from obvious that all animals that feel pain can also be said to experience mental states such as anxiety or fear. Including such states within the definition of pain will either make of pain more than it need be or render such concepts as "anxiety," "fear," and "panic" less descriptive and distinctive than they now are.

Another discussion in the *Proceedings* states that "suffering can be defined as a severe emotional state that is extremely unpleasant, that results from physical pain, emotional pain, and/or discomfort at a level not tolerated by the individual, and that results in some degree of physiologic distress."[33] Yet, people commonly speak of endurable suffering. Indeed, one of the most important ethical issues regarding suffering is how long an animal may be forced to tolerate it. Moreover, as we ordinarily speak of it, "suffering" does not require observable physiological distress. The proposed definition also ignores the fact that we do not always distinguish two mental states, pain and suffering, and say that the former causes the latter. Commonly, we regard an experience of pain as itself being sufficiently intense, lengthy, or bothersome to become an instance of suffering. This linguistic fact has great moral significance. As we use the term, "suffering" does seem to denote a mental state much more intense and longer-lasting and therefore worse to the individual than pain. Therefore in general, the imposition of suffering upon an animal would appear to require greater justification than the imposition of pain alone. The fact that pain can itself become suffering means that sometimes nothing extra need be done to animals in addition to causing them pain to bring into play the stronger ethical requirements required for justification of suffering.

Many opponents and supporters of animal research toss about the word "suffering" altogether too liberally. *Suffering* is a serious matter. We have an ethical obligation to prevent or alleviate suffering of research animals whenever possible. However, if every kind of negative or unpleasant experience, or every instance of pain, is termed "suffering," either the problems experienced by research animals will be greatly exaggerated, or the term "suffering" will lose its distinctive meaning and significance.

Scientific issues

There are many unresolved factual issues relating to pain and other negative mental states experienced by research animals,[34] among them the following:

- Learning more about the extent to which the degree of pain perception varies among species and individuals of the same species.[35] Research indicates that procedures that cause little or no pain in humans may cause significant pain in animals, and *vice versa*.[36]
- Obtaining greater knowledge and appreciation of the effects of previous experiences of research animals upon their perception of pain and other negative states[37]
- Finding anesthetics, analgesics, and tranquilizers and methods of administration of these substances that will lessen pain, discomfort, or distress in research animals without interfering with experimental protocols or producing undesirable side effects. It is already known that effectiveness and side-effects of anesthetics and analgesics vary widely among different species.[38]
- Developing new techniques to monitor pain and pain control in animals subjected to surgical and other procedures[39]
- Developing nondrug approaches (for example, exercise, socialization, contact with human handlers) to the control of stress and other negative mental states[40]
- Learning more about behavioral signs of pain and other unpleasant mental states
- Increasing our sophistication in distinguishing pain from other negative states. This is important, in part, because sedatives and tranquilizers, which lessen distress, might either have no effect on pain or might increase pain perception.

- Exploring environmental and behavioral measures (such as return to a familiar environment and control of unpleasant visual, auditory, olfactory, and tactile stimuli) to minimize pain associated with surgical or other procedures[41]
- Developing restraint systems for primates and other animals that minimize pain, distress, or discomfort and maximize comfort while being consistent with important experimental aims[42]
- Minimizing pain and distress associated with the enhancement of antibody production through the use of adjuvants[43]

Practical issues

PAIN CATEGORIZATION. Researchers, veterinarians, and animal care committees must be able to apply in the laboratory setting the best available knowledge regarding animal pain and other negative mental states. To facilitate practical application of such knowledge, several pain categorization schemes have been proposed. These systems attempt to set forth the degree or severity of pain associated with experiments and procedures commonly utilized in animal research. The best known system was developed in Sweden. It divides research techniques into six categories: (1) those causing no pain or negligible pain (for example, injections, blood sampling, some dietary experiments); (2) those involving anesthetized animals that are not permitted to revive or are killed painlessly; (3) those involving surgery under anesthesia from which the animal recovers and where the surgery or procedure causes minimal postoperative pain; (4) those involving surgery under anesthesia from which the animal recovers and where the surgery or procedure causes considerable postoperative pain (for example, major surgeries, certain skin grafts); (5) experiments on conscious animals involving pain, or in which the animals are expected to become seriously ill or suffer pain (for example, toxicity studies, tumor transplants); and (6) experiments on unanesthetized animals paralyzed by curariform agents.[44] A similar pain categorization system, proposed by the Scientists Center for Animal Welfare, has been adopted by many institutional animal care and use committees in the United States.[45] Another approach, mandated by law in the United Kingdom, calls for "severity banding" of various procedures, with the aim of comparing their "cost" against their "benefits." "Severity is seen as a spectrum of adverse effects, but being broadly divisible into mild, moderate, substantial, and severe bands. If an animal is considered in the fourth category…steps will have to be taken to alleviate the pain or distress or the animal will have to be euthanatized even though the experiment has not been completed."[46]

Such ways of categorizing procedures can stimulate researchers, veterinarians, and committee members to ask about what experiments are likely to do to the animals. However, classifications are only as good as the factual evidence supporting them. Premature "scoring" can discourage further scientific research and can result in sloppy thinking regarding the degree of pain associated with already-categorized procedures. Many animal care committees have suffered through endless discussions about whether a given experiment should be classified as a category "2," "3," or "4" (or whatever). Such discussions can distract members from careful consideration of the protocol before them in favor of abstract considerations of whether certain kinds of procedures are inherently painful or about how much pain they usually cause. Categories can also be used as rationalizations for avoiding serious thought about particular cases. A researcher who is not inclined to worry about the welfare aspects of an experiment may find it convenient, and legally sufficient, to point to a category rather than ask about what is actually happening to *these* animals.

ESTIMATING THE TOTALITY AND DISTRIBUTION OF ANIMAL PAIN. The USDA requires all institutions to report annually about painful procedures in animals subject to the jurisdiction of the Animal Welfare Act. Facilities must indicate how many animals are not exposed to or are involved in painful procedures; how many are exposed to painful or potentially painful procedures but receive anesthetics or pain-killing drugs; and how many animals are exposed to painful procedures but do not receive anesthetics or analgesics because of the nature of the research or testing. The USDA considers any procedure that requires anesthesia (thus any surgery) to be painful or potentially painful even if anesthesia in fact prevents the experience of significant pain.

USDA statistics for fiscal year 1992 showed that, according to these annual pain reports, 58% of all animals were not exposed to any pain, 36% were involved in painful or potentially painful procedures but did not experience pain or distress, and 5.63% experienced pain and distress not relieved by drugs.[47] Such figures are of limited usefulness. First, pain in mice and rats need not be reported. Second, the USDA does not provide clear guidance about how institutions should define "pain" and about what kinds of procedures should or should not be considered painful. An analysis of the 1992 USDA statistics showed that in some states fewer than 1% of animals were reported to have experienced unrelieved pain, while in others the figure exceeded 25%.[48] Third, it is extremely difficult to find guidelines that will produce consistent reports about pain, not just because experiments vary widely, but more importantly because even scientists who specialize in animal pain disagree about how to define and measure it.

Pain research

Pain that is an unfortunate and necessary consequence of an experimental procedure is bad enough. Some animal research involves the intentional infliction of pain. This typically occurs when the object of research is to understand or prevent pain itself.

From the point of view of an animal, it cannot matter whether pain is an unfortunate by-product or is induced intentionally. However, investigators who intentionally inflict pain know that this is what they are doing. Therefore they have a clear obligation to pay unswerving attention to signs of pain or distress and to try to assure that no more is being caused than is absolutely necessary for the conduct of a justifiable research protocol. Dresser suggests two general guidelines: (1) any painful stimulus should be kept well below the animals' pain tolerance threshold, and (2) animals should be given control over stimulus intensity and duration by enabling them to terminate or escape it.[49] The International Association for the study of pain recommends that, where possible, investigators first try out on themselves any painful stimulus to be given to an animal.[50]

Pleasure and Other Positive Mental States

Relatively little work has been done to explore pleasure and other positive mental states in research animals and methods of promoting such states. The difficulties of verifying the presence of positive states should not be underestimated. Nevertheless, it seems clear that the major reason for the paucity of serious thought about promoting pleasure and other positive mental states in research and other animals is the prevalence of the anticruelty position (see Chapters 11 and 13). As long as animal "well-being" is identified with the absence of pain, suffering, or distress, animal welfare science will not find it relevant to investigate animal pleasure or happiness. Investigators will also continue to view such things as weight maintenance, reproductive success, freedom from disease, and normal behavior not as signs of the presence of something good, but of the absence of something bad.

Cancer and Immunology Studies

Research aimed at the prevention and cure of cancer and immunological disorders is of great importance and may therefore justify treatment of animals that would not be appropriate in other kinds of research. Nevertheless, researchers are obligated to reduce, as much as possible, pain or suffering that can be associated with cancer and immunological research.[51] Tumors implanted in animals must be monitored carefully so as not to grow beyond a size that is necessary for the study. It is also important that such tumors be placed in areas where they are least likely to cause debilitation or discomfort and that they not be permitted to grow too large. The use of adjuvants to stimulate antibody production also raises serious issues. Injection of Complete Freund's Adjuvant in the footpads of mice and small rodents and the feet of rabbits has been found to be distressing, and single rather than multiple injection techniques may also prove adequate and less problematic for the animals. Great care must also be taken in monitoring animals used in hybridoma antibody production.[52]

Behavior and Psychology Research

Few areas of animal research have aroused more criticism than behavioral and psychological experiments. Part of this opposition stems from the fact that such work often employs stimuli that are painful or distressing, such as electric shock or deprivation of food or water. Some critics find the use of these techniques especially disturbing because they doubt the value of the research itself. Rollin, for example, states that "it is difficult to defend such research on the grounds that it will help people or even help to understand such people. Few people would give much credence, for example, to the claim that blinding hamsters to see if it will increase their territorial aggression has positive implications for human welfare."[53]

In fact, as Rowan notes, substantial benefits have come from behavioral experimentation on animals, including "major advances in the understanding and treatment of epilepsy, stroke, language disorders, and brain damage."[54] However, there has been behavioral research that does seem aimed at discovering what will happen if terrible things are done to animals.[55] It is dangerous to jump from superficial descriptions of behavioral experiments without an appreciation of their underlying aims or justifications to condemnation of these projects or behavioral research in general. However, I submit that it is impossible for even a sympathetic supporter of animal research not to be deeply distressed by some of the things that are done to animals in the name of behavioral science. Theoretical foolishness and inattentiveness to animal interests in any area of animal research strengthens the hand of research abolitionists. For it helps them to argue that all animal experimentation is pointless and immoral.

As is generally the case, the articulation of appropriate standards for the use of animals in behavioral and psychological research will reflect a balancing of the potential results of research against the effects on the animals. Part of this task will be to consider how to apply the minimum amount of aversive or painful stimulation (including deprivation of food or water) and to substitute positive reinforcement or nonexperimental observation wherever possible.[56] A strong argument can also be made that the most effective way of assuring morally appropriate animal research in the behavioral area will be to differentiate good from bad science.[57]

Euthanasia

One of the most important ethical decisions researchers face concerns the appropriate time for euthanasia. Making morally correct decisions requires knowledge not just of what the animals may be experiencing but also of when keeping them alive is no longer required by an experiment. An animal's interests may require euthanasia even if it would cause the researcher additional expense, inconvenience, or difficulty using other animals to achieve desired results.

As discussed in Chapter 21, the choice of how to perform euthanasia is in part an ethical decision because researchers are ethically obligated to use a method that will, if at all possible, induce a completely painless death. Federal Animal Welfare Act regulations and Public Health Service Policies require researchers to use methods of euthanasia approved by the AVMA *Panel Report on Euthanasia*, unless it can be demonstrated to the institutional animal care and use committee that a departure from these guidelines is scientifically justified.[58] Also critical is adequate training for and supervision of personnel who perform euthanasia. These people often are not veterinarians, but veterinary technicians, investigators, or employees or students of investigators. As the AVMA Panel Report on Euthanasia emphasizes, methods of euthanasia that are ordinarily appropriate can cause pain if not performed properly.

Lack of further usefulness of an animal is typically viewed as sufficient justification for euthanasia. However, some animals used in research are capable of being rehabilitated and placed privately or in settings (such as zoos, science museums, schools, and nursing homes) in which they can lead happy lives. The argument for at least trying, within reasonable economic limits, goes beyond the wastefulness of ending animal life with little attendant human benefit. An animal that has been used in a research project has (ideally) given something to the researcher. It is not too much, I submit, for the research community to think more creatively about how something might be given back, even if only a small proportion of research animals can be saved.

The Concept of "Alternatives"

In recent years, much attention has been given to so-called "alternatives" to the use of animals in research and testing. As explained by one of its leading advocates, Andrew Rowan, the concept refers to the "three Rs":

> ...those techniques or methods that: replace the use of laboratory animals altogether, reduce the number of animals required, or refine an existing procedure or technique so as to minimize the level of stress endured by the animal. These three Rs provide a broad-based approach to reducing both laboratory animal numbers and laboratory animal suffering.[59]

Among the alternatives that are often touted as replacements, reductions, or refinements are physiochemical testing techniques (for example, gas-liquid chromatography and mass spectroscopy rather than animals for assay of substances), computer and mathematical models of biological organs or systems, use of microbiological systems (for example, tests for detecting mutagens that utilize bacteria rather than animals), and tissue culture.

The concept of "alternatives" as defined above has a number of severe limitations.

1. The concept cannot be applied unless there are at least two options (one a so-called "alternative") that can be predicted to have identical or sufficiently similar theoretical results or practical benefits. This can be a major difficulty. The results of scientific research—whether or not animals are employed—are often unpredictable. An item of knowledge or a technique may find its way into unexpected areas of inquiry and application. Thus it often is impossible to assert at a given time that an approach which does not use animals (or uses fewer animals or subjects those used to less distress than another) really will in the long run prove to be an "alternative." This is not to say that "alternatives" in Rowan's sense are never available. But they are likely to be available when (1) researchers know precisely what they want or will obtain, or (2) they are close to an endpoint in some stage of a research project and can be sure that a nonanimal or reduced-animal approach would also be sufficient. For example, genetic engineering of bacteria or tissue culture may sometimes provide a cost-effective nonanimal "alternative" for the production of a specified substance. However, many research projects or general areas of inquiry in biomedical research are in their beginning stages. Precisely what will happen and what questions will have to be asked down the line are not yet known.

2. Because so much is yet to be done in biomedical research, it is scientifically and practically dangerous to now call for a drastic reduction in animal research. As Carl Cohen observes, biomedical research is constantly searching for better approaches to dreaded diseases. These approaches often must be tested before they can be utilized generally. But because it can be the case that "initial trials entail great risks, there may be no forward movement whatever without the use of live animal subjects."[60] It is often immoral to attempt a trial, experiment, or technique on humans before doing it on animals.

3. There are other ethical limitations on the use of reduced-animal alternatives, even when identical or sufficiently similar results can be expected. As we have seen, it may sometimes be morally obligatory to use more animals to spare fewer individual animals a higher degree of stress or deprivation. Additionally, the expense of an alternative is a legitimate consideration in determining its advisability. Techniques that use fewer animals are often less costly than those using more, but this is not always the case.

4. Paradoxically, the vigorous search for "alternatives" might sometimes increase the number of animals used in research. It will sometimes be impossible, without using animals, to verify whether a nonanimal or reduced-animal approach is as good as some animal technique. For example, it might be impossible to determine whether computer modeling of an animal system can generate the same kinds of results as investigation of living systems without comparing the computer data against a large amount of animal-based data.

5. Finally, the concept of alternatives as it is typically understood is employed in ways that do not square with other widely held attitudes regarding animals. The ultimate aim expressed by this concept is the replacement of animals, that is, eventual cessation of their use in research. Rowan asserts that researchers:

> ...readily admit that they would prefer not to use animals if it were not necessary. In other words, they would, in a perfect world, like to see the elimination of animal research. Therefore their ultimate goal is the same as that of the most ardent [research animal use] abolitionist.[61]

The eventual cessation of animal research—*all* animal research, whether or not it causes animals any pain, distress, or discomfort—is stated as an intrinsically desirable goal, one that does not require any further justification. But why should cessation of the use of animals in research be such a goal? Most of us do not regard termination of the use of animals for food, fiber, or entertainment as a fundamental, intrinsically desirable component of a perfect world. Why then should we regard cessation of the use of animals in research a necessary component of such a world?

Proponents of *this* concept of "alternatives" appear to have two options. They can view their aversion to the use of animals in research as part of a general dissatisfaction with the use of animals for any purposes. Or they can approve of at least some traditionally accepted uses of animals but call for the eventual elimination of the use of animals in research. If they choose the former option, they favor animal-use abolitionism at least as an ideal and must be prepared to defend that position. If they choose the latter option, they are being unreasonable. For it surely is unreasonable to consider the use of animals in the prevention and alleviation of disease less important than their use for such things as food, fiber, or entertainment.

The term "alternatives" does have intuitive appeal. The concept can be used to express the following eminently reasonable principle: if there is more than one way of using animals to attain a given legitimate goal and one of these ways will achieve the very same goal while treating the animals better than would the other ways, we ought to choose the way that treats them better. We can call this better way an "alternative." However, saying that we may sometimes be able to treat research animals better by not using them or using fewer of them or causing those we use less pain or distress is *not* the same thing as saying that we have a fundamental, independent obligation to try to eliminate or reduce their use in research. There are reasons researchers should sometimes seek replacement of animals, reduction in their numbers, or refinement in techniques so as to cause less distress. These reasons include the fact that some (but by no means all) research projects cause animals pain, suffering, distress, or discomfort. These reasons can also include (where appropriate) the cost-effectiveness or scientific advantages of not using animals or of using fewer animals.

The articulation and defense of good reasons for replacement, reduction, or refinement will be part of the general endeavor of exploring the ethics of the use of animals in research. This enterprise must consider a wide range of interests and morally relevant considerations. This enterprise can sometimes be expected to conclude that certain uses of animals in research just are not objectionable, and that other uses with negative impact on the animals should be continued. Talking about "alternatives" can play a role in stimulating such ethical and scientific investigations—but only if the concept is purged of the implication that the use of animals in research is intrinsically evil and something to be tolerated only if absolutely "necessary."

Weighing the potential results of research against effects on animal interests

The major ethical question that must be faced in the evaluation of any piece of animal research is whether the potential results of the work justify its likely effects on the animals. As we saw in Chapters 13 and 23, animal welfare science and ethics have a long way to go in understanding how animals are affected in ways that are relevant to their welfare and interests. Neither should one underestimate the many difficult issues involved in assessing the likely value or importance of animal research projects.

For example, at first glance, it might seem plausible to think that an experiment that would benefit many people would have greater value than one that would benefit just a handful, and might therefore justify a greater amount of animal distress. But it is not always so simple. If this handful is suffering greatly, if there is no effective treatment for their condition, and if there are already ways of helping the many people who are suffering from another condition, a strong case can be made for concluding that animal research on the rarer condition has greater value and urgency than work on the more common one. However, this also may not be the end of the matter. If a proposed project on the illness suffered by the many might illuminate and eventually lead to the treatment of other conditions, this may provide stronger justification for it. And there are still other factors that can be relevant in determining the value of these proposals, including their expense, whether they promise a significant improvement of the lives of sufferers, and the likely ability of the researchers proposing the projects to achieve valuable results.

Table 24-1 sets forth some of the factors that are relevant in assessing the value of an animal experiment for the purposes of determining whether that experiment justifies its likely effect on the animals. The table divides issues into questions relating to aims of research and the likelihood of success. Both kinds of considerations must be addressed in evaluating the relative weight or value of a research project. One must concede that the unpredictability of the results of scientific experiments is an important issue that raises problems in assessing the value of proposed animal research projects. Nevertheless, overblown exaggerations[62] about unexpected results of scientific investigation will not do. As the table suggests, relevant questions *can* be raised regarding the likelihood of potential theoretical or practical results. Because animal interests are often compromised in animal research, we need to try to think more critically about predictability of the results of various kinds of such research.

The table does not indicate who might bear the burden of proof regarding whether a proposal is morally justified, for example, whether it is the task of a researcher to show that a proposed use of animals is justified or that of someone with doubts (such as an animal care committee or granting agency) to prove that it is not. Nor am I suggesting here who should make such determinations and how or what general principles should be employed in making them.

I will not address these issues here because I do not think animal welfare science and ethics are yet capable of tackling them systematically. We need more conceptual and factual analysis of what promotes and hinders research animal welfare. We need more sustained ethical analysis of considerations such as those listed in the table. We will also need time to see how effectively institutional committees and facility veterinarians can monitor and assure animal welfare. We may not know for some time what kind of job they are doing. It will also take time for committees to share with each

TABLE 24-1

Some issues relevant to assessing the value of proposed animal research

Aims of the Research

How many people or animals does the project aim to benefit?

How serious is the problem that is experienced by potential beneficiaries of the research?

To what extent is their problem presently treatable?

To what extent is their problem transmissible to other persons or animals?

What are the side-effects and dangers of present treatments?

What are the present or projected costs and burdens of the condition upon the economy or the health care system?

To what extent is the project aimed at understanding or treating several diseases or conditions?

To what extent is the project aimed at understanding a problem, condition, or area about which there is little good or useful knowledge?

To what extent is the research aimed at providing knowledge that could be relevant to several areas or fields of theoretical or practical importance?

Is the research proposed as part of, or is it aimed at enabling, a progression toward experimentation, testing, or use upon the ultimate intended beneficiaries of a proposed treatment or technique?

Does the proposed project seem sound from a scientific point of view, or does it rest on questionable premises or assumptions? (For example, does it propose the use of too many or too few animals to achieve meaningful results? Is a proposed animal model scientifically sound?)

Is the proposed project aimed at confirming an important research result or resolving inconsistent or disputed results or conclusions of important experiments?

To what extent does the project have a clearly defined purpose and rationale, as distinguished from being a scattershot attempt to see "what will happen if" certain things are done to animals?

To what extent is the project aimed at providing a required educational exercise or funding for the person conducting the work?

Has the question posed by the researcher already been sufficiently settled or investigated so that there may be insufficient scientific justification for the project, much less for its potential effects on the animals?

Likelihood of Achieving Stated Aims

What are the general educational qualifications of the investigator proposing the project?

How knowledgeable in this area is the researcher?

Does the investigator's laboratory have a record of success of fruitful results?

To what extent does the researcher possess equipment and support personnel adequate for pursuing the project's stated aims?

Is funding likely to be sufficient to continue to support the work so that animal use will have a chance to achieve the desired aim or results?

To what extent have projects such as the one proposed provided good knowledge or useful techniques?

---

other and government regulators different approaches they may be taking to various kinds of issues.

We are now just beginning to scratch the surface of theory and practice in the promotion of research animal welfare.

SOME CURRENT CONTROVERSIES
The "Pound Seizure" Debate

There are many controversies relating to animal research about which veterinarians should be aware. One of the most important concerns so-called "pound seizure," the practice of allowing or requiring pounds and animal shelters to give or sell unadoptable animals to research facilities. (The general acceptance of the term "seizure" reflects the extent to which opponents of pound release have succeeded in framing the terms of the debate. "Seizure" conveys the false impression that all states in which pound animals can be released compel pounds to do so and that all pounds would prefer not to release them.) Opponents of "pound seizure" have had some success in convincing state and local legislatures to prohibit the release of pound animals to researchers. As of this writing, 13 states and several counties and localities have prohibited pound release.[63] Supporters of such laws often call them "pet protection" measures.

By all accounts, the use of pound animals in research (mostly dogs) has always accounted for a small fraction of the number euthanized. In 1974, prior to laws prohibiting pound release, the Humane Society of the United States estimated that between 13 and 14 million dogs and cats were euthanized in pounds and shelters annually. About 6.5 million of these were dogs. In the late 1960s approximately 105,000 dogs used in research came from pounds.[64] A 1994 study by the National Association for Biomedical Research[65] estimates that approximately 50% of the 124,000 dogs and 39,000 cats used in research in 1992 were random source animals, that USDA-licensed Class B dealers supplied about 40% of these animals to laboratories, and that research facilities received just over 10% of dogs and 16% of cats directly from pounds or shelters.

Opponents of pound release offer the following arguments:

1. *"Pound animals are inferior to purpose-bred animals for research purposes because they are genetically more variable and tend to have diseases and infirmities that compromise their usefulness."* This claim cannot be made about all pound animals used in research, especially those utilized in certain investigations of surgical techniques and cardiovascular disease. There may well be some use of pound animals that is scientifically questionable. But the most direct (and scientifically sound) way of preventing such situations would be for investigators not to use pound animals when such use is scientifically questionable—not an absolute ban on all use of pound animals.

2. *"Pound release discourages people from turning in strays they find."* As Rowan observes,[66] there is little evidence supporting this claim.

3. *"Pound release subjects animals to torture and abuse."* This assertion is false as a general characterization. Moreover, if a researcher does abuse or perform unjustified experiments on animals, that they might come from a pound is irrelevant. Abuse of research animals is wrong because it is wrong, not because some animals that might be abused come from pounds. The most direct way of preventing such abuse would be to prevent it, not to cut off the supply of pound animals.

4. *"Pound release is inconsistent with the primary task of humane societies as 'effective promoters of animal welfare.'"*[66] It is difficult to understand how the killing of thousands of unwanted animals each year that could otherwise be used in research, thus requiring the breeding of additional animals for research, constitutes effective promotion of animal welfare.

A rational approach to pound release

The strongest argument against pound release is that it may well be unfair to subject animals that have been part of a human-animal bond to kinds of treatment research animals receive. Such treatment sometimes involves distress and almost always greater confinement and a less pleasurable life than that to which a valued pet has been accustomed. This argument can be made with or without the premise that a former beloved pet appreciates the change in its condition; if true, the latter premise would add to the forcefulness of the argument. One problem with this argument is that many, perhaps most, pound animals did not "enjoy" a rich human-animal bond; many are strays or were abused, neglected, or abandoned by their owners. Nevertheless, I think there is some plausibility to the desire to protect animals that have participated in a meaningful human-animal bond or that did lead a relatively pleasant life from conditions that are likely to be far less enjoyable.

However, what follows from this argument is that reasonable attempts ought to be made to enable owners to locate lost animals or to place them with other owners. In contrast, total prohibition of pound release is illogical and wrong for many reasons.

First, many of the animals that would be released by pounds are not significantly different from purpose-bred animals. Many have led no better a life prior to use in research, and they are just as capable of feeling pain or distress and of enjoying human companionship. It makes no sense to "protect" such animals by killing them and replacing them with other animals that will be used exactly as the "protected" (dead) animals would have been.

Second, although permitting pound release is bound to result in the release of some members of human-animal bonds, and this is unfortunate, absolutely precluding such situations through total prohibition of pound release is not preferable to the wastefulness of total prohibition. It is costly to euthanize and dispose of pound animals, which are of use to no one as a result of the process. The effect of a total prohibition of pound release would be to make much animal research more expensive than it need be. Even though total abolition of pound release might benefit some former beloved pets, this benefit would not be so important as to outweigh the horrendous waste of total prohibition. For purpose-bred animals are not drastically different from even the most beloved of pets. There does not seem to be such a chasm of difference between these two kinds of animals to justify concluding that it is right to use one but not the other, if the consequence of this is that one group of animals will be substituted (at great cost) for another.

Third, protection of pets is not the aim of many who oppose pound release. Many of these people hope that the increased cost associated with purpose-breeding will reduce the number of animals used in research. Indeed, for many activists, "pet protection" laws are just the first step toward ending all animal research. As one animal rights organization declared, "when the supply of dogs and cats from pounds and dealers is finally cut off, the animal rights field will then be able to address cutting off the supply of all purpose-bred species of animals for scientific purposes."[67]

The only straightforward and effective way to address abuses in animal research is to openly identify and prevent them. It is folly to suppose that increasing the cost will stop research that uses dogs or cats. A few relatively poor institutions may be forced to reduce their use of such animals; but even so, there is no assurance that the least valuable or distressful experiments will be the ones sacrificed. In the most prestigious and best-endowed institutions, animal research will continue—as it should. Increased expenses for purpose-bred animals will be borne by taxpayers or others who ultimately pay for the costs of research (such as health insurance companies, medical patients, and veterinary clients). Imposing additional costs on biomedical research by forcing all unadoptable animals to be killed will not give pet owners sufficient time or means to locate their animals from shelters. It will not reduce society's enormous burden of dealing with our millions of unwanted animals. It will not eliminate unjustifiable animal research or protect research animals from neglect or abuse. These worthy goals can be achieved only if they are sought directly.

Toxicity Testing

An issue that has connections with research and that has aroused significant controversy concerns the use of live animals in toxicity testing of drugs, pesticides, chemicals, and various consumer products. The two main targets of criticism have been the LD_{50} test, which determines the dose of a substance that will kill 50% of test organisms, and the Draize test, in which a substance is placed in one eye of rabbits (the other eye serving as an untreated control) to determine its irritating effects. These tests can cause animals substantial pain and distress.

An important ethical question that must be asked about any test which can cause distress is whether, even if the test provides satisfactory evidence regarding the safety of a substance, the distress of the animals is justified by the importance of the substance being tested. This question is especially significant with regard to nonmedical household or personal items. The marketing of a new consumer product may be important to those who might profit from it. However, it is extremely difficult to maintain that yet another shade of makeup or a new toilet bowl cleaner is of sufficient general importance to require any significant amount of animal suffering or distress.

It seems clear, however, that compelling objections to the LD50 and Draize tests can sometimes be made without judging the worth of a particular substance or product to be tested. There is substantial scientific evidence that these tests do not establish the safety of certain substances, or make determinations with a degree of precision that is unnecessary for an assurance of safety. Rowan has estimated that if regulatory bodies required the submission of LD50 figures only when there is scientific justification for the test, the number of animals used in determining lethal doses would be reduced by between 80% and 90% worldwide. This would represent an annual saving of between 2 and 4 million animals.[68]

Because toxicity testing can involve animal pain and consumers do have a legitimate interest in safe products even when such products are not essential for life or happiness, the search for nonanimal alternatives seems especially important in this area. Such work is proceeding.

The Use of Animals in Education

There has been considerable discussion among veterinarians and members of the public about the appropriateness of the use of animals in education. Among the targets of critics has been the use of animals in elementary and high school courses, science fairs and competitions; college biology courses; the training of graduate biology and psychology students; medical school courses; and continuing education courses for physicians. Several lawsuits have been brought against elementary and secondary schools, colleges, and veterinary schools on behalf of students who have refused to participate in required educational exercises employing live or dead animals. There is also controversy about the use and euthanasia of animals in veterinary school surgery exercises. Some argue that this practice is inconsistent with the veterinarian's commitment to alleviate animal pain and suffering.[69]

At least two very different questions can be raised about a given educational animal use: (1) whether it is permissible, and (2) whether a student in a given educational setting may be compelled to participate in the animal exercise if he or she does not want to receive a reduced or failing grade. Addressing each of these issues requires consideration of the educational importance of a given animal experience. Nevertheless, the two issues should not be confused. There are undoubtedly certain educational uses of animals that are not sufficiently objectionable to render them impermissible but are at the same time not sufficiently important to justify compulsory student participation.

Disputes about the educational necessity or value of various animal educational experiences are long-standing[70] and cannot be resolved here. I offer the following observations to stimulate the reader's consideration of this issue.

1. Demands that students at lower educational levels simply *must* kill, dissect, or use animals in other ways are often almost always highly overblown and usually appear motivated more by a rejection of animal-use abolitionism than by demonstrable educational needs. It is extremely difficult to maintain, for example, that most elementary, high school, or even college students would suffer an irreparable or important blow to their understanding of biology (or whatever) without hands-on animal experience. For most students, photographs, videotapes, or models of animal parts or procedures are adequate for their educational needs. An English major who is taking a biology course to meet his college science requirement need not actually dissect a frog to learn what a properly educated English major or college student really must know about animal anatomy.

2. Although arguments for requiring animal use by all students are overblown, so are claims that all such use is profoundly immoral and must be stopped. It is unreasonable to contend that, for example, high school students ought not to be allowed to dissect a frog because this is a horrible waste of animal life—but allow these same students to retire after biology class to the school cafeteria for a lunch of frankfurters. Dissecting a frog might not be a momentously important experience. But neither is eating a frankfurter. Indeed, the benefits of dissection might well be greater, if even a small proportion of students who dissect animals become motivated to take a serious interest in biological science. At the same time, because serious scientific training typically is not provided in elementary or secondary schools, such institutions should not engage, or allow students to participate, in animal use (including various kinds of "experiments") that causes any animal pain, stress, or discomfort. As observed in Chapter 11, animal pain must be justified by strong reasons, and lower school educational exercises just do not provide such reasons.

3. Because certain hands-on animal experiences at least at the high school and college levels are neither momentously important nor immoral, many such students ought to be allowed to decline such experiences if this is their choice and to participate if that is their choice. Educators who oppose such options (for example, by insisting that students "knew before they signed up for the course that a dissection laboratory was required") usually accomplish little more than affording publicity to animal activists, and wasting resources on legal expenses.

4. Nevertheless, hands-on animal experience is sometimes reasonably required of students, especially at higher educational levels where the purpose of a course

or program is to train people to understand or use animals. Thus although a college English major may not need to participate in the dissection of a frog or fetal pig, it is probably reasonable to require biology majors to do so—and it is surely appropriate to require students preparing for or pursuing graduate work in biology to do so. The latter need to know a great deal about animal anatomy, not for their general intellectual edification, but as part of their chosen careers.

5. Progress is sometimes hindered by a highly charged atmosphere in which opposing parties approach the situation with an uncompromising general attitude that leaves no room for examination of relevant facts. This sometimes seems to be the case when veterinary educators and students argue about required surgery exercises on live animals. Some educators refuse to entertain any suggestions regarding different ways of doing things. On the other hand, some veterinary students base their opposition to surgery laboratory on the principle that it is always morally wrong for a veterinarian to kill or perform procedures upon healthy animals. Neither of these uncompromising positions permits careful examination of the factual issues regarding the usefulness of educational exercises for the variety of students a veterinary school must train.

6. The key factual question relating to veterinary school surgical exercises is whether they are useful in the training of veterinarians. The following principles are suggested for approaching this question, and to provoke readers to sharpen their own views.

A. Veterinary educators should not abdicate their responsibility to determine whether live-animal exercises, nonsurvival surgeries, or any other kind of animal experience should be required of students. If such experiences are important, it would be wrong from an educational and ethical standpoint to allow students to decide whether to engage in them. Educators are supposed to know more about their field (and how to teach it) than students; this is why they are the educators.

B. Members of the public and their animals rely on the veterinary schools to train competent practitioners. Any veterinary school which would even consider compromising the interests of animals and veterinary clients to satisfy the perceived needs of some students or animal activists should be shut down, forthwith. Eliminating or allowing students to opt out of surgery or any other kind of animal experience can be justified only if it can be demonstrated that such an approach will not compromise these students' training. The schools should err, if at all, on the side of protecting animals and clients. Therefore the burden of proof must be on those who would change approaches that have provided Americans and their animals the competent veterinary services to which they are accustomed.

C. At the same time, veterinary schools may legitimately explore approaches that would accomplish this goal while satisfying the desires of some students. Several schools now have regular or alternative programs which involve spays and neuters on animals that will not be killed after the procedure but will be adopted. If such approaches provide equivalent educational experiences afforded by nonsurvival surgeries, it is difficult to see what is wrong with them, provided a school can sustain the effort and expense.

D. In providing alternative educational experiences, veterinary schools should not endorse (explicitly or by implication) the view of some advocates of these alternatives that is wrong to kill animals or to use animals as means to benefit people or other animals. The schools can respect the right of students to have and express such views—consistent with their obligation to assure that all graduates can practice veterinary medicine competently. However, veterinary educators should not fall prey to those whose underlying aim is to make everyone feel guilty about using animals. If it is not immoral to kill some animals for leather and food, it cannot be wrong to kill some animals to train people to help countless other animals. If it is morally acceptable to kill animals to find cures for animal diseases, it is morally acceptable to kill animals to train future battlers of animal diseases. As long as there is a reasonable probability that live-animal exercises provide educational benefits that alternatives do not, such exercises are not only morally acceptable, they are morally obligatory. If some of these exercises must be done on animals that must be euthanized (either because no one can be found to adopt them or because the exercises require the death of these animals), euthanizing these animals is also morally acceptable.

Laws Affecting Animal Research
State and local laws

ANTICRUELTY STATUTES. At the state level, an interesting current controversy concerns whether anticruelty statutes should be capable of being applied to animal research. Such application would permit criminal prosecution of researchers who neglect or abuse their animals, or whose experiments cause unjustifiable pain or suffering. As of 1993, 26 states and the District of Columbia specifically exempted activities by researchers from the application of their anticruelty laws.[71] Elsewhere, neglect, abuse, or unjustified distress caused by a researcher is a prosecutable criminal offense.

Realistically, inclusion of animal research within the purview of a state's anticruelty statute is unlikely to have much general effect on the conduct of research. Even in states without research exemptions, prosecutions of researchers are rare. This is so not only because most prosecutors' offices do not attach a high priority to animal cases but also because it usually is extremely difficult to convict a researcher of cruelty. Although most states do not require willful animal abuse for a conviction of cruelty, the government must still prove, beyond a reasonable doubt, that the manner in which a researcher treated an animal was unjustified. In many cases, investigators may be able to be sufficiently persuasive about justification to cast some doubt in the minds of a jury or appellate court. Cruelty convictions of researchers are likely only in cases of extreme neglect or malicious abuse.

An argument can, nevertheless, be made for including animal research within the application of cruelty statutes. This would permit criminal prosecutions when appropriate and feasible. Including research within the scope of a state cruelty statute also makes a symbolic statement that it is part of the official public policy of the state that researchers, like other people, must not subject animals to unjustified pain, distress, abuse, or neglect.

STATE AND LOCAL LICENSING AND REGULATION PROGRAMS. As of 1993, 20 states and the District of Columbia had laws imposing some kind of licensing or regulation upon animal research facilities.[72] These laws, and the extent to which they are enforced, vary. (For example, some jurisdictions require licenses for the use of dogs or cats, and others require licenses only for facilities receiving impounded animals.) Time will tell whether states implement programs that promote animal welfare without infringing unduly upon research. It also remains to be seen whether the courts will invalidate state or local regulation programs that might attempt to restrict certain kinds of animal research permitted by federal law, on the grounds that such regulation is preempted by federal law.

Federal law

THE ANIMAL WELFARE ACT AND REGULATIONS. Robust debate is likely to continue for some time regarding the proper extent of federal regulation of animal research. The federal Animal Welfare Act applies to research facilities using laboratory animals in basic or biomedical research, education, and product safety testing. In 1985 the following important amendments were added to the Animal Welfare Act.[73] Researchers must consult with a veterinarian to assure that pain and distress will be minimized. Tranquilizers, anesthesia, analgesia, or euthanasia of animals in pain or distress may be withheld only when "scientifically necessary," and any unavoidable pain or distress may be permitted to continue "only for the necessary period of time." Multiple surgeries on animals are to be done only when "scientifically necessary." The "psychological well-being" of primates and appropriate exercise for dogs is to be assured. Each facility governed by the Animal Welfare Act must have an institutional animal care and use committee. At least one member of the committee must be a doctor of veterinary medicine. At least one member must not be affiliated with the institution and must represent "general community interests" in the proper care and treatment of animals. It is the responsibility of this committee to assure compliance with the provisions of the Animal Welfare Act, to "minimize pain and distress to animals," and to "represent society's concerns regarding the welfare of animal subjects used" at the facility. Facilities must train researchers and support personnel in "the humane practice of animal maintenance and experimentation" as well as in "research or testing methods that minimize or eliminate the use of animals or limit animal pain or distress."

As required by the Animal Welfare Act, the USDA has issued specific regulations explaining and amplifying upon these statutory provisions.[74] Two features of these regulations are particularly noteworthy.

1. As of 1995 the regulations did not include mice, rats, and birds within the statute. In issuing its standards pursuant to the 1985 amendments, the USDA reiterated its long-standing positions that the Animal Welfare Act's definition of the term "animal" gives the Department discretion whether to include these species and that the Department lacks sufficient funds and manpower to regulate the use of these animals. In 1992 in response to a lawsuit brought by animal activists, a federal judge ruled that the USDA had misinterpreted the Animal Welfare Act and ordered the Department to include mice, rats, and birds. A federal appellate court overturned this ruling on the grounds that the plaintiffs lacked legal standing to challenge the Department's decision not to regulate the use of these animals.[75]

2. In another lawsuit brought against the USDA by activists, the same federal district court judge overturned the Department's regulations concerning psy-

chological well-being of nonhuman primates and exercise for dogs. The Department had decided to forego so-called "engineering standards," specific and potentially lengthy regulations intended to dictate acceptable approaches by all research facilities. Instead, the USDA opted for so-called "performance standards," allowing veterinarians in each facility (subject to Department review) to determine how to afford adequate exercise for dogs and psychological well-being for primates. The judge found that performance standards violated the intent of Congress by allowing the regulated to regulate themselves. This ruling also was overturned on appeal and on the grounds that the plaintiffs in the lawsuit lacked standing to object to the regulations.[76]

OTHER FEDERAL LAWS. The other major federal apparatus for the regulation of research animal care aside from the Animal Welfare Act is the Public Health Service (PHS) Act[77] and the associated PHS *Policy on Humane Care and Use of Laboratory Animals.*[78] These cover all vertebrate animals and apply to all institutions that receive PHS funds. The Public Health Service Act requires an animal care and use committee similar to that required by the Animal Welfare Act, the filing of an Animal Welfare Assurance document with the National Institutes of Health, and adherence to animal care standards contained in the *Guide for the Care and Use of Laboratory Animals.*[79] Other federal laws affecting animal research include the Endangered Species Act[80] (which requires permits for the possession of species classified as endangered or threatened); the Marine Mammal Protection Act;[81] and the "Good Laboratory Practice" (GLP) standards promulgated by the Food and Drug Administration for conducting studies pursuant to the Federal Food, Drug, and Cosmetic Act,[82] and by the Environmental Protection Agency for conducting studies pursuant to the Toxic Substances Control Act[83] and the Federal Insecticide, Fungicide, and Rodenticide Act.[84] These GLPs cover a wide range of animal care and handling issues, are enforced by agency inspectors, and if violated, can result in refusal of an application for drug approval or disqualification of a testing facility.

QUESTIONS ABOUT CURRENT FEDERAL APPROACHES. The following are among the questions raised most frequently about current federal regulations.

1. Should mice and rats be included within the scope of the Animal Welfare Act? Does it make sense not to include these animals if they constitute at least 80% of all animals used in research? Can the federal government speak credibly about the humane treatment of research animals if the major legal vehicle for regulating animal research does not include the great majority of research animals?

2. How should institutions decide who should serve as a representative of "community interests?" Should these persons have some background in research animal welfare? Should they be "advocates" for the animals? Can institutions be trusted to appoint appropriate persons, with (as at present) no government oversight of their choices?

3. What qualifications should be required of veterinarians who serve in research facilities governed by the Act? Is licensure to practice veterinary medicine in any state sufficient, or must the veterinarian be licensed in the state in which he or she functions? Should laboratory animal veterinarians be required to demonstrate competence in the area of laboratory animal medicine, and if so, how might this be done? The AVMA has opposed accreditation of facility veterinarians by the USDA.[85]

4. *To what extent should animal care committees, research proposals, and decisions by committees be open to observation or discovery by members of the public?* Several states require that animal care committee meetings at state-owned research institutions (such as state universities and medical schools) be open to the public. Many researchers believe that permitting public attendance of committee meetings or access to research protocols stifles committee debate and discussion.

5. *Should certain members of the public have legal standing to sue institutions for alleged violations of the Animal Welfare Act, or should legal action be restricted, as it is presently, to the USDA?* Many researchers believe that standing for private citizens will result in harassment of institutions, committees, and researchers by animal activists. Other people believe that it is not fair (to the animals) to await changes in policy by the USDA or the Congress; they maintain that unless regulations are open to review in the courts, there will be little incentive for improvement of regulations and their enforcement.

6. *To what extent should animal care committees review the scientific soundness of research proposals?* Some contend that such review is improper on the grounds that the task of the committee is only to assure adequate animal welfare. But this position seems untenable. Committees must sometimes ask whether animals are being subjected to *justifiable* pain or distress. It is impossible to make such a determination without considering whether proposals are sufficiently strong scientifically to provide such justification.[86] It is not altogether clear, however, what kinds of soundness review by animal care committees are appropriate. For these committees are not intended, and are typically not qualified, to provide another forum for a complete review of the scientific soundness of experiments.

7. *To what extent may government regulation be permitted to increase the costs of running a research facility?* Where, if at all, should compromises be made in regulation or assurance of animal welfare on the grounds of cost? How much paperwork may reasonably be imposed upon researchers and animal care committees? Should costs attributable to federally required animal welfare measures be paid by individual grant recipients, their academic departments, the institution, the animal care committee budget, granting agencies, or the federal government?

Illegal Activities

Any discussion of contemporary issues must mention the extent to which some animal activists engage in unlawful behavior. In 1987 the NIH reported a total of 26 incidents in which animals had been stolen from research facilities.[87] A 1993 publication of the National Association for Biomedical Research states that "over the past ten years, there have been more than 90 reported arsons, break-ins, and bomb-threats 'in the name of animal rights.'"[88] The following are a few examples.

• In 1984, members of the Animal Liberation Front broke into the Experimental Head Injury Laboratory at the University of Pennsylvania. They stole videotaped records of experiments showing the induction of head trauma upon restrained baboons. The break-in eventually led to suspension of NIH funding for the laboratory and a $4,000 fine by USDA for violations of the Animal Welfare Act.[89]

- In 1986, activists broke into a facility at the University of Oregon, stole over 150 animals, and caused more than $50,000 in property damage. Animal activist groups held a news conference at which they distributed several hundred photographs allegedly taken during the break-in. These photographs were in fact from another university and did not clearly show any abuses.[90]
- In 1987, an animal rights group calling itself the Band of Mercy stole 37 cats from the USDA Animal Parasitology Institute in Beltsville, Maryland. Eleven of the cats were infected with *Toxoplasma gondii*. The "liberators" of these highly infectious animals stated that their purpose was to obtain veterinary care for the cats and to place them in "caring, permanent homes." The theft caused the loss of 3 years of research on the transmissibility of toxoplasmosis after cessation of immunity.[87]
- In 1987, activists broke into and set on fire the veterinary diagnostic laboratory under construction at the University of California at Davis. The fire caused over $3.5 million in damages. The facility was to have been part of a reorganization of the California diagnostic laboratory system for the control of animal disease.[91]
- In 1989, a fire set at the University of Arizona caused property damage estimated at $100,000.[88]
- In 1992 a firebombing of a laboratory and faculty member's office at Utah State University caused damage estimated at $100,000.[88]

Although advocates of law-breaking and violence may prefer to cite their success at the University of Pennsylvania, the other incidents related above are more indicative of what happens when true believers consider themselves above the law. Innocent people and animals can be harmed. Property is mindlessly destroyed. What may have been motivated at first by high ideals begins to resemble common thuggery. As of 1993, 30 state legislatures,[92] as well as the U.S. Congress[93] had passed laws making it a criminal offense to commit certain kinds of acts against research facilities, farms, ranches, and other institutions that utilize animals.

Not all members of the animal rights movement condone violent or unlawful behavior. However, law-abiding activists will find it increasingly difficult to convince the public that theft and violence is not an integral part of the program of the animal rights movement. Eventually, some people may come to associate such tactics with the concept of animal rights itself. This could well be the most destructive legacy of the lawbreakers.

∽ THE ROLE OF LABORATORY ANIMAL VETERINARIANS
Promoting the Importance of Institutional Veterinarians

Not all laboratory veterinarians have been successful in promoting animal welfare in their facilities. The USDA reported that during preliminary investigations prior to the promulgation of its Animal Welfare Act regulations, it found that:

> Some facilities have not provided required veterinary care and others have switched veterinarians every few months causing confusing situations that are difficult to trace...
>
> Many other veterinarians...indicated that they felt their efforts were a waste of time as their recommendations concerning the health care of the animals were ignored, and they had no authority to see that such recommendations were carried out.
>
> Veterinarians at many research facilities indicated that often they did not have the authority to enter the animal facilities of certain Departments or investigators and thus could not certify what conditions might be at those animal sites. Many of these veterinarians also indicated that due to

various local political or managerial systems, their jobs would be in serious jeopardy if they tried to force adequate veterinary care in certain instances or if they refused to certify that all was in compliance at the facility when they, in fact, had no such knowledge.[94]

My own conversations with laboratory animal veterinarians confirm the accuracy of these observations even today. I am told repeatedly that there are two main reasons laboratory animal veterinarians can find it difficult to function effectively. Some investigators do not want anyone to interfere with their work. Some investigators do not have great respect for veterinarians and use this attitude to ignore or belittle the laboratory animal doctor's efforts to improve the treatment of research animals.

Problems laboratory animal veterinarians have in assuring adequate animal welfare will not disappear overnight. The profession can help by promoting the expertise of laboratory animal doctors. This must be done not only through public relations, but by encouraging the training of specialists in this area, and supporting laboratory animal welfare research that will enable veterinarians to play a preeminent role in the protection of research animal welfare. Yet, history already shows that laboratory animal veterinarians will not achieve the respect and influence they deserve, and that the animals need, without the vigorous assistance of government.

Academic institutions can take an important step to assist their veterinarians. At too many universities and professional schools, laboratory animal doctors occupy non-faculty staff positions. Institutional veterinarians (at the very least, the institution's chief veterinarian) should have academic appointments, indeed, tenure track appointments. Veterinarians are more likely to be taken seriously where they are co-equal members of the faculty.

Potential Conflicts of Interest

Ironically, laboratory animal veterinarians who do occupy positions of influence often face ethical problems caused by these positions of influence. At many of the finest institutions, laboratory animal doctors head the animal care facility. In principle, this seems good both for animal welfare and the effectiveness of the veterinary staff. Unfortunately, veterinarians who run these facilities can have conflicting interests. As protectors of animal welfare they sometimes ought to ask investigators whether various experiments can be done using fewer animals or perhaps no animals at all. At the same time, the fiscal health of the animal facility often calls for maintaining or even increasing the number of animals and associated charges paid by investigators. In principle, such conflicts of interest could be alleviated by a strong institutional animal care and use committee (IACUC), which can focus on the interests of the animals. In fact, veterinarians who run the animal facility almost always are appointed to the institution's IACUC. Often these veterinarians, because of their expertise and prominence in the field, exercise enormous influence on the committee.

Another potential conflict of interest faced by veterinarian directors of animal facilities stems from their sometimes unpleasant task of having to set and collect *per diem* and other animal care and use charges. More than a few veterinarians have found themselves blamed by investigators for what are perceived to be high fees. Some veterinarians may feel the necessity of smoothing ruffled feathers by not objecting too strenuously to proposed or actual experimental procedures.

Because it is extremely important—for reasons of animal welfare—that veterinarians run animal facilities where possible, the conflicts of interest faced by veterinarian-directors are probably unavoidable. These conflicts of interest must be confronted by ethical institutional veterinarians and strong, independent IACUCs.

WHAT THE PROFESSION CAN DO

This is an exciting time in laboratory animal medicine. Many important scientific and practical breakthroughs are being made. Continuing progress will require the efforts of the entire profession, including veterinary clinicians who utilize the products of research for the benefit of their patients.

First and foremost, the profession must encourage, promote, and fund first-class research in the area of laboratory animal welfare. The biomedical research community cannot be counted on to do this work by itself. Animal welfare studies conducted by or with the active participation of veterinarians will also enable the development of techniques that can be applied by laboratory animal doctors in the research setting.

Conceptual and ethical investigations must be made an important component of research into laboratory animal welfare conducted by veterinarians. These investigations should include participation by ethicists committed to the study of animal- and veterinarian-related moral issues.

The veterinary schools must make it a major priority to encourage students to consider a career in laboratory animal medicine. Training in this area must include substantial exposure to animal welfare science and to veterinary and animal ethics.

Finally, veterinarians should participate actively in discussions regarding laboratory animal welfare. All practitioners should be able to discuss with clients, community leaders, and politicians the benefits and justifications of animal research.

REFERENCES

[1] U.S. Congress Office of Technology Assessment: *Alternatives to Animal Use in Research, Testing, and Education,* Washington, DC, 1986, US Government Printing Office, 1986.

[2] Rowan A, Loew FM, Weer JC: *The Research Animal Controversy,* North Grafton, MA, 1994, Tufts University School of Veterinary Medicine Center for Animals and Public Policy, p 14.

[3] *Id,* p 17.

[4] Department of Health and Human Services: Institute of Laboratory Animal Resources: *Fiscal Year 1978 National Survey of Laboratory Animal Facilities and Resources,* Washington, DC, The Department, NIH Pub No 80-2091, p 21.

[5] For example, animal use has fallen approximately 50% in the United Kingdom since the mid1970s; in the Netherlands animal use declined from 1.57 million in 1978 to approximately 850,000 in 1991; in Italy research animal numbers fell by 55% to 1.9 million from 1978 to 1989; and in France numbers declined by 25% to approximately 3.5 million from 1984 to 1990. Rowan A: Laboratory animal numbers: Trends and problems, *Tufts University School of Veterinary Medicine Center for Animals and Public Policy Animal Policy Report* 8(1):1-2, 1994.

[6] *Lab Animal Use Declines,* (brochure), Washington, DC, 1993, Foundation for Biomedical Research, p 1.

[7] Sibal L: NIH Plan for Use of Animals in Research: Fostering the 3Rs, (Presentation), NIH-OPRR Regional Workshop on the Use of Animals in Research, New Orleans, September 30, 1994.

[8] Rowan A, Loew FM, Weer JC: *The Research Animal Controversy,* North Grafton, MA, 1994, Tufts University School of Veterinary Medicine Center for Animals and Public Policy, p 13.

[9] US Department of Agriculture: *Agricultural Statistics 1992,* Table 506, "Chickens: Broiler production and gross income by States, 1990 and 1991," Washington, DC, 1992, US Government Printing Office, p 342 (1991 preliminary figure of 6,138,350,000 broilers).

[10] *Id,* Table 497, "Chickens: Hens and pullets of laying age by States, Dec 1, 1989-91," p 334 (1991 figure of 116,289,000).

[11] *Id,* Table 498, "Chickens: Pullets not of laying age, and other chickens, by States, Dec 1, 1989-91," p 335 (1991 figures of 33,450,000 pullets 3 months old and older not of laying age and 40,785,000 pullets under 3 months old).

[12]*Id*, Table 385, "All cattle and calves: Number, by classes, United States, Jan 1, 1977-92," p 246 (1992 preliminary figure of 100,110,000).

[13]*Id*, Table 468, "Milk and milkfat production: Number of milk cows, yield per cow, and total quantity produced, by States, 1991 (preliminary)," p 306 (preliminary 1991 figure of 9,990,000).

[14]*Id*, Table 401, "Hogs and Pigs: Number and value, by States, Dec 1, 1989-91," p 260 (1991 preliminary figure of 56,974,000).

[15]*Id*, Table 514, "Turkeys: Production and value, United States, 1976-90," p 346 (1991 preliminary figure of 285,000,000).

[16]*Id*, Table 420, "Sheep and lambs: Number of stock sheep and sheep on feed, by States, Jan 1, 1990-92," p 271 (preliminary 1992 figure of 9,042,900 for stock sheep and 1,807,000 for sheep and lambs being fattened for slaughter).

[17]*See*, for example, National Academy of Sciences and Institute of Medicine Committee on the Use of Animals in Research: *Science, Medicine, and Animals*, Washington, DC, 1991, National Academy Press, and references cited therein; Gay WI, editor: *Health Benefits of Animal Research*, Washington DC, undated, National Association for Biomedical Research.

[18]*See*, for example, AVMA Council on Research: Contributions and needs of animal health and disease research, *Am J Vet Res* 42:1093-1108, 1981; Ewald BE, Gregg DA: Animal research for animals. In Sechzer JA, editor: *The Role of Animals in Biomedical Research*, New York, 1983, New York Academy of Sciences, pp 48-58; Loew FM: Animals as beneficiaries of biomedical research originally intended for humans, *ILAR News*, Fall 1988:13-15.

[19]For example, Raub W: Foreword. In Gay WI, editor: *Health Benefits of Animal Research*, Washington, DC, undated, National Association for Biomedical Research, p i (stating that "(v)irtually every medical innovation of the last century—and especially of the last four decades—has been based to a significant extent upon the results of animal experimentation").

[20]For example, Kuker-Reines B: *Psychology Experiments on Animals*, Boston, 1982, New England Anti-Vivisection Society, p 67 (stating that "the animal modelling technique has proved virtually useless against the *bona fide* noninfectious diseases including cancer…"); Ryder R: Experiments on animals. In Godlovitch S, Godlovitch R, Harris J, editors: *Animals, Men, and Morals*, London, 1971, Victor Gollancz, p 78 ("The probability of unequivocal benefits arising out of any individual animal experiment is so small as to be negligible. …We can far better benefit our species, as well as the others, by effectively disseminating the enormous technology and materials we already possess rather than by striving cruelly to extend our knowledge a little further.").

[21]For example, Hewitt HB: The use of animals in experimental cancer research. In Sperlinger D, editor: *Animals in Research*, Chichester, England, 1981, John Wiley & Sons, p 170 ("The question the prospective animal experimenter has to ask himself is whether he considers that the painless taking of animal life is itself an immoral act. For me it is not…").

[22]Cohen C: The case for the use of animals in biomedical research, *N Engl J Med* 315(14):865, 1986.

[23]Fox MW: What future for man and earth? Toward a biospiritual ethic. In Morris RK, Fox MW, editors: *On the Fifth Day*, Washington, DC, 1978, Acropolis Books, p 226.

[24]7 U.S.C.A. § 2143(a)(2)(B).

[25]*See*, for example, *Guide for the Care and Use of Laboratory Animals*, NIH Pub No, 86-23, 1985; Animal Welfare Institute: *Comfortable Quarters for Laboratory Animals*, Washington, DC, 1979, The Institute.

[26]For example, Reinhardt V: Advantages of housing rhesus monkeys in compatible pairs, *Scient Center Anim Welf Newslet* 9(3):3-6, 1987.

[27]For example, Wolfle T: Laboratory animal technicians: Their role in stress reduction and human-companion animal bonding, *Vet Clin North Am Small Anim Pract* 15:449-454, 1985.

[28]For example, Morton DB: Epilogue: Summarization of colloquium highlights from an international perspective, *J Am Vet Med Assoc* 191:1292, 1987 (calling for "the minimum amount of pain consistent with a scientific objective").

[29]*J Am Vet Med Assoc* 191:1184-1298, 1987.

[30]Kitchell RL: Problems in defining pain and peripheral mechanisms of pain, *J Am Vet Med Assoc* 191:1195, 1987.

[31]Seligman MEP: *Helplessness: On Depression, Development and Death*, San Francisco, 1975, WH Freeman; Fox MW: *Farm Animals*, Baltimore, 1984, University Park Press, pp 237-249.

[32]Benson GJ, Thurmon JC: Species difference as a consideration in alleviation of animal pain and distress, *J Am Vet Med Assoc* 191:1227, 1987.

[33]Spinelli JS, Markowitz H: Clinical recognition and anticipation of situations likely to induce suffering in animals, *J Am Vet Med Assoc* 191:1216, 1987.

[34]*See* National Research Council Institute of Laboratory Animal Resources: *Recognition and Alleviation of Pain and Distress in Laboratory Animals*, Washington, DC, 1992, National Academy Press; Short CE, Van Poznak A, editors: *Animal Pain*, New York, 1992, Churchill Livingstone.

[35]Benson GJ, Thurmon JC: Species difference as a consideration in alleviation of animal pain and distress, *J Am Vet Med Assoc* 191:1227-1230, 1987.

[36]*The Biomedical Investigator's Handbook*, Washington, DC, 1987, Foundation for Biomedical Research, p 4 and references cited therein.

37Loew FM: The challenge of balancing experimental variables: Pain, distress, analgesia, and anesthesia, *J Am Vet Med Assoc* 191:1193, 1987.

38For example, Thurmon JC, Benson GJ: Pharmacologic consideration in selection of anesthetics for animals, *J Am Vet Med Assoc* 191:1245-1251, 1987; Stanley TH: New developments in opioid drug research for the alleviation of animal pain, *J Am Vet Med Assoc* 191:1252-1253, 1987; Crane SW: Perioperative analgesia: A surgeon's perspective, *J Am Vet Med Assoc* 191:1254-1257, 1987.

39Smith NT: New developments in monitoring animals for evidence of pain control, *J Am Vet Med Assoc* 191:1269-1272, 1987.

40Wolfle TL: Control of stress using non-drug approaches, *J Am Vet Med Assoc* 191:1219-1221, 1987.

41*The Biomedical Investigator's Handbook*, Washington, DC, 1987, Foundation for Biomedical Research, pp 5-6 and references cited therein.

42Morton WR and others: Alternatives to chronic restraint of non-human primates, *J Am Vet Med Assoc* 191:1282-1286, 1987.

43Amyx HL: Control of animal pain and distress in antibody production and infectious disease studies, *J Am Vet Med Assoc* 191:1287-1289, 1987, and references cited therein.

44Rowan A: *Of Mice, Models, and Men*, Albany, 1984, State University of New York Press, (hereinafter referred to as Rowan: *Of Mice, Models, and Men*), p 282.

45Orlans FB, Simmonds RC, Dodds WJ: Effective Animal Care and Use Committees, *Lab Anim Sci* 37:11-12, 1987.

46Morton DB: Epilogue: Summarization of Colloquium highlights from an international perspective, *J Am Vet Med Assoc* 191:1295, 1987. For a useful discussion of other systems for categorizing pain or invasiveness, *see* Orlans FB: *In the Name of Science*, New York, 1993, Oxford University Press, pp 86-90, 134-135.

47US Department of Agriculture: *Animal Welfare Enforcement, Fiscal Year 1992: Report of the Secretary of Agriculture to the President of the Senate and the Speaker of the House of Representatives.*

48Rowan A, Loew FM, Weer JC: *The Research Animal Controversy*, North Grafton, MA, 1994, Tufts University School of Veterinary Medicine Center for Animals and Public Policy, p 21.

49Dresser R: Assessing harm and justification in animal research: Federal policy opens the laboratory door, *Rutgers Law Rev* 40:795, 1988.

50Rowan A: *Of Mice, Models, and Men*, pp 281-282.

51*See* generally, Hewitt HB: The use of animals in experimental cancer research. In Sperlinger D, editor: *Animals in Research*, Chichester, England, 1981, John Wiley & Sons, pp 141-174.

52Dresser R: Assessing harm and justification in animal research: Federal policy opens the laboratory door, *Rutgers Law Rev* 40:792, 1988.

53Rollin BE: The moral status of research animals in psychology, *Am Psychol* Aug 1985:925.

54Rowan A: *Of Mice, Models, and Men*, p 134. *See also*, Gallup G, Suarez S: On the use of animals in psychological research, *Psychol Rec* 30:212, 1980.

55For a description of some of these "experiments" that is balanced by acknowledgment of important psychological animal research *see*, Drewett R, Kani W: Animal experimentation in the behavioural sciences. In Sperlinger D, editor: *Animals in Research*, Chichester, England, 1981, John Wiley & Sons, pp 175-201 (summarizing an experiment in which conscious rats were taped to a restraining board and driven to epileptic fits with a combination of a convulsive drug and a 90 dB sound).

56Rowan A: *Of Mice, Models, and Men*, pp 147-148.

57Drewett R, Kani W: Animal experimentation in the behavioural sciences. In Sperlinger D, editor: *Animals in Research*, Chichester, England, 1981, John Wiley & Sons, pp 175-201.

58*1993 Report of the AVMA Panel on Euthanasia, J Am Vet Med Assoc* 202: 230-249, 1993.

59Rowan A: *Of Mice, Models, and Men*, pp 261-262. The terms "replacement," "reduction," and "refinement" were first proposed in Russell WMS, Burch RL: *The Principles of Humane Experimental Technique*, London, 1959, Methuen, p 64.

60Cohen C: The case for the use of animals in biomedical research, *N Engl J Med* 315(14):865, 1986.

61Rowan A: *Of Mice, Models, and Men*, p 3.

62For example, Thomas L: Hubris in science, *Science* 200:1461, 1978 (stating that "committees cannot formulate the ideas or lay out the plans; this is work that can only be done in the mind of the investigator himself. ...Sometimes an idea emerges from what can only be called intuition, and when the mind producing the idea is very imaginative, and very lucky, the whole field moves forward in a quantum jump."). What was true regarding Lewis Thomas does not necessarily apply to a more typical scientist or graduate student.

63National Association for Biomedical Research: *Regulation of Biomedical Research Using Animals*, Washington DC, 1993, The Association, p 4. In 1988, 12 states prohibited the release of pound animals for research. What appeared in the 1980s to have been a trend toward such laws has apparently subsided. Indeed, in response to "pound seizure" laws, several states (five at the time of this writing) and the District of Columbia now require the release of pound animals for research and several others (nine at the time of this writing) have laws that specifically permit such release.

64Rowan A: *Of Mice, Models, and Men*, pp 155-156.

[65]National Association for Biomedical Research: *1994 Survey on Laboratory Dogs and Cats*, Washington, DC, in press, The Association. Cited in Foundation for Biomedical Research: *Lab Animal Use Declines*, Washington, DC, 1994, The Foundation.

[66]Rowan A: *Of Mice, Models, and Men*, p 161.

[67]Two-fold effect in stopping use of pound animals for labs, *Int Soc Anim Rights Rep* May 1986:6.

[68]Rowan AN: The LD50—The beginning of the end, *Int J Stud Anim Prob* 4(1):6, 1983.

[69]For example, Dodds WJ: Letter. Use of animals in the education of veterinary students, *J Am Vet Med Assoc* 190:1372, 1987.

[70]*See* Rowan A: *Of Mice, Models, and Men*, pp 93-108.

[71]National Association for Biomedical Research: *Regulation of Biomedical Research Using Animals*, Washington, DC, 1993, The Association, p 4.

[72]National Association for Biomedical Research: *Regulation of Biomedical Research Using Animals*, Washington, DC, 1993, The Association, p 4.

[73]7 U.S.C. § 2131 *et seq.*

[74]United States Department of Agriculture, Animal Welfare Regulations and Standards, 9 C.F.R. , Chapter 1, Parts 1, 2, and 3.

[75]*Animal Legal Defense Fund* v. *Madigan*, 781 F. Supp. 797 (D.D.C. 1992), *rev'd*, 29 F. 3d 496 (D.C. Cir. 1994).

[76]*Animal Legal Defense Fund* v. *Espy*, 813 F. Supp 882 (D.D.C. 1993), *rev'd*, 29 F. 3d 720 (D.C. Cir. 1994).

[77]Health Research Extension Act of 1985 (Pub. L. No, 99-158), 42 U.S.C. § 290aa-10.

[78]PHS *Policy on Humane Care and Use of Laboratory Animals*, Washington, DC, 1986, US Department of Health and Human Services, Public Health Service, National Institutes of Health, Office of Protection from Research Risks.

[79]*Guide for the Care and Use of Laboratory Animals*, NIH Publication No 86-23, 1985.

[80]16 U.S.C. § 1531 *et seq.*

[81]16 U.S.C. § 1361 *et seq.* 1994 amendments to the Marine Mammal Protection Act delegate to the USDA the responsibility to establish and regulate conditions of care and maintenance of these animals under the Animal Welfare Act.

[82]21 U.S.C. § 321 *et seq.*; 21 C.F.R. § 58.

[83]15 U.S.C. § 2603 *et seq.*; 40 C.F.R. § 792.

[84]7 U.S.C. § 136 *et seq.*; 40 C.F.R. § 160.

[85]AVMA comments on Animal Welfare Act amendments, *J Am Vet Med Assoc* 191:510, 1987.

[86]For a persuasive argument in favor of this position *see* Prentice ED, Crouse DA, Mann MD: Scientific merit review: The role of the IACUC, *ILAR News* Winter/Spring 1992:15-19. Most discussions of this issue speak of "merit" or "scientific merit" review. This is not a useful way of speaking, because the merit of an experiment or protocol often cannot be adequately judged until well after it is completed, when additional evidence or the work of other researchers shows its results to be correct or valuable. It is preferable to speak of the *soundness* of an animal use protocol. Soundness can be judged when an experiment is proposed. A determination of scientific soundness turns on whether, given the facts, data, and science available at the time a piece of research is begun, the research appears directed at valid scientific questions and is constructed in a manner that will properly address these questions. Committees that believe they are evaluating *merit* rather than soundness may also believe, erroneously, that they are qualified to predict the likely theoretical or practical results of experiments.

[87]Infected laboratory cats stolen by activists, *J Am Vet Med Assoc* 191:1536, 1987.

[88]National Association for Biomedical Research: *Animal Rights Extremists: Impact on Public Health*, Washington, DC, 1993, The Association, p 2.

[89]Sun M: USDA fines Pennsylvania animal laboratory, *Science* 230:423, 1985.

[90]National Association for Biomedical Research: *1987 Annual Report*, Washington, DC, 1988, The Association, p 11.

[91]Terrorist group suspected in fire that ravages UC-Davis laboratory, *J Am Vet Med Assoc* 191:174, 1987.

[92]National Association for Biomedical Research: *Animal Rights Extremists: Impact on Public Health*, Washington, DC, 1993, The Association, p 2.

[93]Animal Enterprise Protection Act of 1992, 18 U.S.C. § 43.

[94]*Federal Register* 52(61):10303, 1987.

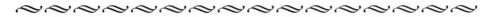

CHAPTER 25

Employer-employee Relations
Ethics in the Workplace

The field of veterinary ethics must include consideration of how practice owners and employees treat each other. If employees are mistreated or are unhappy, the interests of patients and clients can be compromised. Veterinary employees have legitimate interests of their own. So do employers. The body of professional ethical responsibilities includes the obligations of employers to employees, of employees to employers, and of all who work in or for a veterinary practice to each other.

This chapter considers some of the ethical issues that arise in relations between practice owners and their employees. The term "employee" will be used in its ordinary, nonlegal sense, in which an employee is any nonowner of a practice who works on a regular basis for and is paid by a practice owner or owners. In some contexts, the law defines an employee as any person who works for salary or wages. In this sense, owners of a veterinary professional corporation are also employees of the practice; and because all members of a professional partnership are legal agents of each other, there is a sense in which they also can be called "employees" of one another. There are many important ethical issues arising out of relations among practice owners, but they will not be discussed here.

This chapter also focuses on ethical issues that arise between *veterinarian* employers and their employees. As discussed in Chapters 16 and 17, some veterinary practices are now owned by nonveterinarians. This development will have significant (and if my arguments are correct, detrimental) effects on veterinarians—*most* of whom may become not only employees, but also employees of laymen. However, because the great majority of veterinary practices are still owned by veterinarians, this discussion will restrict itself to relations between veterinarian owners and their employees. It can be expected that the expansion of practice ownership by nonveterinarians will bring new and distinctive ethical issues in employer-employee relations. Some of these issues are mentioned in Chapter 16.

∼ LEGAL CONSIDERATIONS
Virtually every aspect of the employment relation is affected by law. Federal or state laws prohibit discrimination in hiring and firing on the basis of race, religion, color, national origin or age; sexual harassment; and employment of undocumented aliens. Other statutes cover minimum wages, payment for overtime work, health insurance benefits, pension and profit sharing plans, and maternity leave. Federal and state laws and regulations protect employees from environmental work hazards such as x-rays,

chemicals, and poisons. Words and deeds exchanged privately between employer and employee can create legal rights and duties. For example, if an employer agrees with a worker, either verbally or in writing, to pay a certain salary or to extend certain benefits, there might arise a contractual obligation on the doctor's part, a violation of which could support a lawsuit by the employee.

It is not possible to summarize here all laws relating to employer-employee relations, although salient aspects of some important legal principles will be mentioned. In general, whenever one deals with an ethical issue involving employee relations, it is always advisable to ask whether the law has something to say about the matter (see Chapter 4).

∼ VETERINARIAN EMPLOYEES
Are veterinarian associates unhappy about their employment status?

It is difficult for a veterinary educator to remain in contact with former students and not come to the conclusion that many new doctors are unhappy about their employment status. I hear regularly from recent graduates who complain about long hours, disrespectful employers, restrictive covenants (see Chapter 19), and low salaries. Dr. James Wilson writes about "the vast number of unhappy associate veterinarians."[1] A 1993 *Veterinary Economics* survey of associate (that is, nonowner) veterinarians found widespread dissatisfaction.[2] It is unclear whether the views gathered were representative of associates in general, because the survey was based on responses of 216 doctors to a questionnaire in the magazine.[3] Surveys that rely solely on volunteered responses are notoriously unreliable, because they cannot provide scientific assurance that the response pool reflects the larger population. Nevertheless, detailed comments by the respondents reflected complaints about which many veterinary educators and observers of the profession have long been aware, including low salaries, lack of fringe benefits such as malpractice and health insurance, imperious owners, sexual harassment, owners who do not listen to associates' opinions about medicine or management, and owners who regard new doctors as a disposable resource with no prospect of advancement in the practice. The survey found that 66.7% of the respondents were no longer with the first practice they joined, 72.4% left within 2 years, and 45.8% either found that their first job was "much worse" than expected or "not at all" what was expected.

In an analysis of the survey results, Dr. James Brockmeier interviewed several associates, veterinary educators, and management consultants.[4] He concluded that:

> ...*at least* 20 percent of practice owners do, in fact, abuse their associates in some way. They sign contracts they don't honor; they make verbal promises they break; they let such personal problems as drug abuse, burnout, and family trauma affect their practice personalities; they verbally abuse their staff members and associate doctors. Many would defend their behavior to the death—especially if they grew up in abusive households or were treated badly themselves as associates—but they obviously don't know how to appreciate and nurture their associates, or to act as their mentors.[5]

In the remaining 80% of cases of associate dissatisfaction, Dr. Brockmeier believes there are a wide range of problems, including insufficient research by associates about practices they join and lack of clear communication between employer and employee about the nature of the practice and the job. However, Brockmeier places a great deal of the blame for associate dissatisfaction upon the veterinary schools, which, he asserts, do not prepare students adequately for the kinds of problems and issues they will face in practice, do not always instill self-esteem or self-confidence in students, and too often discourage students from pursuing private practice.

One possible response to Dr. Brockmeier's diagnosis of the shortcomings of veterinary education is to devote more time to practice management in the curriculum. This approach is sensible, provided instruction about "the real world" does not become synonymous with promotion of the model of veterinary practice as a business. Such identification is objectionable, and not just because of the serious ethical shortcomings in this view of private practice (see Chapter 16). One recurring theme in the *Veterinary Economics* survey is the complaint of associates that they do not wish to be seen merely as revenue generators. Many want to be treated as fellow professionals and doctors whose primary concern is helping animals. If veterinary schools attempt to prevent associate dissatisfaction by trying to convince students to become businesspeople, they will unleash a tide of complaints that will make the results of the *Veterinary Economics* survey pale by comparison. Moreover, if many new doctors do not like being used as revenue generators by veterinarian-owners, what will happen if a large number of new—and experienced—doctors become employees of entrepreneurs who are not even veterinarians?

Compensation and Benefits
What is a fair salary?

Practice owners are morally required to compensate their employees fairly. Each of the following are among the relevant considerations in determining whether compensation is fair.

1. The extent of the doctor's training and experience. Clearly, veterinarians have some moral entitlement regarding compensation because of the considerable time and expense they have invested in their skills. All other things being equal, a doctor with more or better education and practice experience deserves a higher level of compensation than one with less.

2. The salary level of other professionals with comparable training, experience, and value to society. Some new veterinary school graduates believe they are being paid unfairly because members of other professions with training, skill, and responsibility no more important than their own are sometimes paid much more than they are paid. In the abstract, it does seem unfair that the typical new veterinarian is paid much less than a new lawyer because the lawyer has had only 3 years of professional schooling to the veterinarian's 4 years and is not likely to be as quickly entrusted with weighty matters of life and death. However, this argument does not show that all veterinarians must be paid as much as members of other valued professions. Veterinarians cannot earn more than their practices can pay them, and as we shall see, there are other fair limitations on associates' salaries. What the argument shows is that there is strong moral weight in favor of a salary commensurate with a veterinarian's training and skills.

3. The amount and difficulty of the doctor's work. All other things being equal, a doctor who works 5 or 6 days per week merits more than one who works 4 or 5 days. This is so not just because she probably is contributing more to practice revenues but also because she deserves more for her greater effort.

4. The quality of the doctor's work. It is also fair to reward doctors for the quality of their work. A doctor who performs flawless surgeries that subject patients and clients to a minimum of complications may be rewarded for a job well done. This is so not just because he is likely to increase practice revenues but also because quality performance is a good in itself that can merit monetary reward.

5. The ability of the practice to pay the doctor's salary, benefits, and support (including ancillary staff) required for his employment. A doctor's actual compensation must conform to the economic limitations of his practice. There undoubtedly are many fine veterinarians who in the abstract merit a higher salary than they are receiving but whose earnings are restricted by the financial capabilities of their clients. Other limitations on veterinarians' salaries that derive from the economic facts of life of their practices include the cost of labor for ancillary personnel such as receptionists and technicians, the indebtedness of the practice, and the costs of insurance and facility maintenance.

6. The right of the owner(s) to gain a fair profit from the practice. The moral right of practice owners to gain a fair return on their investment must also be factored into the determination of the fairness of an employee doctor's compensation. Owners are obligated to share some of the fruits of an associate's labor with the associate. However, because they have invested their time, efforts, and money in the practice and are its legal owners, they often are entitled to allocate the greater portion of revenues and profits to themselves.

7. The cost of living in the community. In determining an associate's compensation, owners must take into account the cost of living in the community, even if this sometimes means receiving a smaller return on their investment. It might sometimes be necessary to adjust an associate's compensation for the cost of living so that she can remain an employee. But it is sometimes also a matter of fairness to make such adjustments. One of the legitimate rewards of working as a professional is being able to live decently where or near where one works. This is something veterinarians deserve, even though they bear little responsibility for the level of the cost of living in the communities in which they practice.

8. The compensation levels of other doctors in the practice. A particular doctor's compensation can be unfair if it is disproportionate to that of other doctors in the practice. A practice's existing compensation levels can place severe constraints on the weight owners are able to give to other considerations relevant to fairness. For example, a practice with a large number of doctors might find it extremely difficult to adjust upward all the salaries of present doctors so that a newcomer can be given a salary that considered by itself might be more fair.

9. The doctor's present contribution to the gross revenues of the practice. The more an associate contributes to gross revenues, the more he is paying his own way and that of personnel and facilities required for his support. He also is contributing more to the profits of the owners and is therefore entitled to receive in return some of the fruits of his labor. Nevertheless, a doctor's "productivity" is only one factor in determining the fairness of his compensation. New doctors typically need to be trained not just in the ways of a practice but also how to practice veterinary medicine under real conditions. It can be unfair to new doctors to tie their compensation strictly to their contribution to gross revenues, because their need for an adequate income will exist before their capacity for significant productivity does. Tying compensation strictly to productivity can also be unfair to more experienced associates. Doctors can become ill, have personal problems or commitments (such as giving birth), or might, through no fault of their own, just not have a good run of profitable cases.

10. The doctor's potential contribution to practice revenues. It can be unfair to pay associates a low salary during the time they are training to be able to make more substantial contributions to practice revenues. Novice doctors have legitimate economic requirements of their own. Moreover, they are training not just for their own benefit but also for the benefit of the owner who hopes to profit from their employment in the future. Owners often must expect to invest considerable money and effort in new doctors, patiently awaiting the time when associates can pull their own weight. An owner's obligation to pay starting associates more than they might be worth at the time gives rise to a moral duty on the part of associates to try to return the owner's investment in them. To leave a practice soon after being trained at someone else's expense can be profoundly immoral. It can also strengthen any inclination owners might have to hold inexperienced associates to salaries tied strictly to their present "production."

11. The extent to which the doctor is building equity in or is likely to become an owner of the practice. It can be appropriate to pay associate doctors less than they might otherwise receive if they are working toward becoming an owner of the practice. If, for example, deferring an increase in an associate's salary is necessary to enable the practice to purchase equipment that will eventually inure to the associate's benefit when she becomes an owner, it might be reasonable for the owners to ask her to agree to such a sacrifice—provided that they, too, share in the burdens. An owner and associate may decide that part of the latter's payment for progressive increments in ownership will be somewhat lower compensation in the short term.

Fairness by formula?

It is impossible to reduce fairness in compensation to a single consideration or criterion, with or without accompanying mathematical formulae. Dr. Ross Clark has recommended that employee doctors be paid a gross pretax income including fringe benefits of approximately 20% of their contribution to gross practice revenues. "Twenty percent of individual production," Dr. Clark states, "is fair."[6] There are doubtlessly many practices in which paying associates 20% of "production" would be fair. But there is no reason in principle why one should expect any percentage of "production" to be the sole measure of fairness. There is no guarantee—indeed, it seems highly unlikely—that such a figure will necessarily reflect some of the other factors identified above. For some of these factors have no intrinsic relationship to generation of revenues. A new graduate who joins a sophisticated specialty practice in a city in which living expenses are extremely high might be treated unfairly if restricted at the start to 20% of actual "production". Moreover, even when considering an associate's contribution to gross practice income as a relevant factor, it is far from clear that one can settle on an appropriate percentage figure before looking at all the relevant factors bearing on fairness in the particular practice. For a practice earning minimal profits that is located in a community in which living expenses are low, 20% of an inexperienced associate's contribution to gross income could be excessive. On the other hand, it might be unfair for the same practice to pay 20% to an extraordinarily skilled surgeon who has the potential to generate substantial new revenues.

Bonuses and fringe benefits

In determining the fairness of benefits apart from salary, one must ask whether a particular form of compensation inures as much to the benefit of the owner as it does to the employee or is essential to the associate's continuing employment. In both kinds of cases, fairness can require the practice to extend such compensation. Among the things that benefit owners directly is malpractice insurance, which typically protects the owner or the practice as well as the associate. Among employee benefits essential to maintaining morale and productivity are adequate health insurance and vacation time.

Some forms of compensation are better categorized as rewards rather than necessities. Such compensation may often be given differently (or not at all) to certain associates and still be fair. For example, it can be fair to give 3 rather than 2 weeks paid vacation only to associates who have worked for the practice for a certain number of years. Likewise, more senior associates may be afforded payment of professional association dues or continuing education fees as a token of appreciation for their time in the practice.

Certain kinds of compensation that are optional in one practice might be required as a matter of fairness in another. It is difficult to maintain that fairness requires all practices to pay professional association dues or continuing education fees for all associates. However, in a practice that does routinely cover such items, it would be unfair not to do so for a particular doctor who works as hard and well as the others.

Also relevant to whether a certain kind of compensation that might generally be regarded as a "fringe benefit" must, in fairness, be given to a particular doctor is whether that kind of compensation is really part of straight salary. Some owners prefer to pay a somewhat lower than base salary during the year and to supplement this salary with a larger end-of-year bonus. In such a practice, a "bonus" may not be an optional payment but rather deferred salary. Likewise, if a practice decides to make up for a somewhat lower salary with generous contributions to a pension or profit sharing plan, such compensation also can become an entitlement of associate doctors who work under the assumption that they will receive it.

Are associates' salaries fair?

Starting salary for 1993 graduates of U.S. veterinary schools employed in private practices was $29,888, an increase of 3.3% from the previous year. The average starting salary in private practices for 1993 female graduates was more than $1,500, or 5%, less than the mean starting salary for male graduates.[7] In 1986 starting female graduates in private practice averaged 4.6% less than the male counterparts.[8] Thus as the proportion of female graduates increases, the relative earning power of new female doctors appears to be decreasing. The mean educational debt of the 81% of 1993 graduates who indicated having debt was $39,197, up 10.6% from 1992[9] and 67% from 1986.[10]

Many associates appear to believe that they are working very hard to generate revenues which go in disproportionate measure to their employers. Unfortunately, the facts support this belief, at least regarding private practices generally. It is extremely difficult to determine, in general, whether associate veterinarians are being paid fairly. However, a good test of fairness in compensation is whether increases in employer earnings translate into some increases for employees. One cannot say that practice owners are ethically obligated to match each percentage of increase in their earnings with the same percentage of increase for employees. It is often appropriate for owners to take for themselves a larger proportion of the increased gross revenues, as a reward for the work that went into establishing their practices, and as just compensation for their assumption of the risks as well as the rewards of ownership. Nevertheless, fairness would appear to require *some* correspondence between increased profits for owners and compensation for employees. Moreover, it would definitely be unfair if increases in employer earnings were accompanied over a sustained period of time by decreases in employee earnings.

This latter situation appears to be precisely what has been happening, at least until quite recently. Between 1983 and 1991, the real mean income (adjusted for inflation) of practice owners rose by 32%, while the real mean incomes of associates fell by almost 1%. Between 1991 and 1993, the real mean income of owners declined by 15%, while associates' real mean income increased by 6%.[11] Only time will tell whether the developments of these latter 2 years represent a new trend or will prove an aberration. Clearly many associates, and even some specialists in practice management, are asking whether employee veterinarians are receiving a fair "piece of the pie." According to management consultant Cynthia Wutchiett, one cause of low associate compensation may be management consultants themselves, many of whom have advised owners to hold an associate's salary at 22% of revenue generation. Wutchiett contends that the percentage paid to associates has actually increased from an average of 16% to 17% in the 1980s to 19% to 22% by 1994. However, the idea that associates should be paid 22% of their contribution to gross revenues:

> ...originated in the early 1980s at a time when the profit-to-revenue ratio (profit from operations before veterinary compensation divided by total revenue) for the small animal practice averaged 30 to 36 percent. But if the profit-to-revenue ratio in the well-managed practice is currently averaging 42 to 45 percent, does the 22 percent figure still apply?[12]

The fact that nonowner veterinarians earn less than physicians, dentists, and lawyers may be unavoidable in light of the revenue veterinary practices can generate. However, if the real incomes or profit-to-revenue ratios of practice owners is increasing, and the real or relative earnings of associate doctors is remaining stagnant or is decreasing, something is very wrong.

Commission or Proportional Compensation

Serious ethical questions are raised by the apparently growing practice of basing all or part of employee doctors' compensation on a percentage of their contribution to gross revenues. This can be done either by offering a straight percentage commission of contribution to revenues,[13] or by paying a base salary plus a certain percentage of a doctor's contribution to revenues above a specified level.[14] Such compensation plans are said to provide associates motivation to generate revenues. New doctors are supposed to learn much more quickly about the procedures of the practice and to waste less time in nonproductive activities. It is argued that paying both doctors and support staff on a commission basis will prevent doctors from undercharging clients or reducing fees they regard as excessive.[15]

Not in the interests of many doctors

However well-intentioned they might be, such methods of compensating doctors pose a grave moral threat to the profession. Associates paid in these ways might compete among themselves for higher-dollar clients and cases, thus leading to difficult relations among doctors. Some who refuse to sell unnecessary services could find themselves working so many extra hours or packing so many extra patients into the work day that they risk premature burn-out.

Not in the interests of clients and patients

Most important, tying compensation directly to "production" places enormous pressure on doctors to make recommendations and decisions based not on the needs of patients but on their own pecuniary interests. Some doctors might be able to resist such pressures. But others will not, and there will often be a strong potential conflict of interest between a doctor's desire to earn more and one's obligations to patients and clients. There will be pressure to recommend the most expensive procedures clients can afford, even if less expensive ones would do. There will be pressure to advise that a procedure be done immediately even if time might prove it unnecessary. There will be pressure to recommend unnecessary procedures. There will be pressure to counsel longer and more expensive hospital stays. There will be pressure to dispense the most expensive drugs the client can afford and to dispense as much of these drugs as possible. In practices with their own testing laboratory or that charge clients a mark-up on outside tests, there will be pressure to recommend as many tests as the traffic will bear. In practices that sell nonprofessional goods and services, and credit such sales to a doctor's "account," there will be pressure on the doctor to move these items also, regardless of whether they are in the best interests of patients and clients. And all of these pressures will be greatest on recent graduates, whose lower base salary and ability to generate revenues will act as still further inducement to sell, sell, and sell again.

Not in the long-term interests of the profession

In addition to threatening harm to the interests of patients and clients, proportional or commission salaries subject the entire profession to potentially irreparable damage. People are accustomed to the automobile or household appliance salesman who is paid on commission. We begin our dealings with such people with skepticism, and a firm grip on our wallets. Today most people approach their veterinarian with precisely the opposite attitude: they trust that a veterinarian will recommend something because it is right medically and not because it will earn him or her a larger salary.

I submit that if the public learns that a significant number of veterinarians are being paid on commission, the entire profession will find it more difficult to persuade clients of the need for legitimate medical procedures. Once lost, the image of the trusted medical professional might be impossible to regain.

A doctor's contribution to practice revenues is one legitimate factor in determining a fair level of compensation. But the unavoidable link between revenues and compensation already places a heavy moral burden on veterinarians to assure that they are working primarily for their patients and clients. Proportional or commission compensation makes every dollar brought into the practice a matter of direct benefit to a doctor. This, I submit, creates too great a risk that the veterinarian's interests will come before those of patients and clients.

"Production" as an incentive

Dr. Clark maintains that "a straight salary does little to provide associates with the incentive to produce."[16] One practice management consultant believes that, at least in certain circumstances, money is the only possible incentive.

> I believe the only fair way to pay associates is based on individual production. After all, if the associate surpasses his or her production responsibilities, he or she deserves to be compensated accordingly—and the practice stands to benefit as well.
>
> I realize that money alone may be viewed as a negative motivator, but I think this mindset often is unrealistic. What incentive, for example, does an associate who's paid a flat salary have to see emergencies?[17]

STRAIGHT OR FLAT SALARY VERSUS PERCENTAGE COMPENSATION? Percentage compensation is *not* the only alternative to "straight" or "flat" salary. Many practice owners begin with a base salary to which they add bonuses or rewards contingent on the ability of the practice to afford them. Such additions to base salary need not be tied, dollar by dollar, to a doctor's total "production." In determining bonuses, some practices will take into account cases especially well-handled or achievements of special distinction (such as publication of a paper in an important journal or assumption of an important post in a professional association). Some practices pay associates a percentage of the yearly gross; some practices pay all associate doctors the same percentage, while others pay doctors with different levels of experience different percentages. Other practices make a less precise division of a total bonus pool by determining what proportion of this pool individual doctors appear to deserve.

All these approaches differ markedly from paying associates a straight percentage of "production" or a base salary plus a percentage of "production." Even if a percentage of the gross is distributed as an incentive, the practice is still not motivating doctors to ratchet up each client's bill so that they can be credited the largest possible amount. Doctors in such practices can still concentrate on providing good and necessary services for each patient, knowing that if they all work hard to help patients and clients they can all share in the just rewards of the practice's general success.

MONEY THE ONLY INCENTIVE? It is not, I believe, hopelessly old-fashioned to suppose that many veterinarians are motivated not just by money but also by a desire to help animals and clients. However, even if doctors sometimes need financial incentives to approach difficult or routine situations with vigor, it does not follow that money is the *only* incentive—or, that money should be viewed only as an incentive. Compensation is better viewed as part incentive and part something doctors *deserve* in return for competent and ethical service. Percentage compensation schemes not only tend to view money as the only incentive, they tend to encourage doctors to regard money as the only incentive. These schemes link every decision and action to the prospect of benefiting oneself. For each additional $10 one can get clients to spend, there can be an extra $2 for me, and if one can build one's "production" in a given case up another $20, why, here's an additional $4! Slowly but surely, as doctors come to appreciate their own pecuniary interests in *everything* they do, their consideration of these interests will intrude more and more into *anything* they do. The *Principles of Veterinary Medical Ethics* take a decidedly different approach. They remind us that:

> Veterinarians should consider first the welfare of the patient for the purpose of relieving suffering and disability while causing a minimum of pain or fright. Benefit to the patient should transcend personal advantage or monetary gain in decisions concerning therapy.[18]
>
> Determination of therapy must not be relegated to secondary consideration with remuneration to the veterinarian being the primary interest.[19]

"PRODUCTION" VERSUS SERVICE. The *Principles* also ask veterinarians to "accept the Golden Rule as a guide for general conduct."[20] One implication of the Golden Rule is that veterinarians should not hide from clients key aspects of how they deal with clients and their animals. If something about the way they are being treated would upset clients, veterinarians are probably not treating clients as they would want to be treated if they were clients.

Veterinarians and management consultants who are used to the term "production" may not realize how offensive the term—and more importantly, that for which the term stands—is likely to be to clients. As it is commonly used in the management literature, "production" means revenue generation pure and simple. "Production" is not tied inherently to good and necessary services. To say that one will pay a certain percentage of "production" is to say that one will pay a percentage of total revenues attributable in some manner to a doctor, regardless of whether these revenues derive from services patients and clients need or should have.

Some defenders of percentage of production compensation may say that, *of course*, it goes without saying, associates should not be paid a percentage of revenues associated with unnecessary or inappropriate services. But if it is supposed to be so obvious that doctors are to be paid only for providing necessary services, why is it so difficult to find any such qualification in discussions recommending percentage compensation? Indeed, why does not *every* discussion of percentage payments remind practice owners that their *first* responsibility is to their patients and clients and that percentages should only be based on services that serve the true needs of patients and clients?

More importantly, speaking of "production" distorts the kind of relationship most clients assume they have with their veterinarian. Most clients believe that veterinarians respond to their needs and the needs of their animals. The concept of "production" is tied not to what patients and clients need but to the efforts of the producer. To impose upon associate doctors "production responsibilities" seems to be to require the generation of a certain amount of revenue. Clients who learn that their veterinarian is expected to tally up a certain amount each week or month may wonder what role *they* and their animals are supposed to have in this process. Are they just the stuff out of which a sufficient amount of "production" is to be extracted? Where do their needs fit into this process? What if they and their animal happen to see a veterinarian when she is lagging behind her "production responsibilities?" Is this a time to be less trusting of her recommendations? And if she is paid a percentage of "production," is it *ever* safe to be trusting of her recommendations?*

There is an important difference between the concepts of production and professional service. Pencils and tires are produced. Veterinary clients and patients should be served. Production is typically a linear, quantifiable process—the faster or longer one works, in general, the more one produces. One can often set a numerical minimum as a production responsibility because one can often reasonably require the pencil or tire worker to turn out so many units per hour or day. One can demand this because, all other things being equal, the amount of total production depends on the efforts of the worker.

In contrast, professional service does not depend solely on the efforts of the server. To *serve* means to help those one serves, to provide what *they* need, for *their* benefit. Service is *responsive* to the needs and desires of those being served. Sometimes, better service means taking more time, seeing fewer patients, and generating less revenue. If patient and client needs are down, revenues will be down—as they should be. Fortunately for veterinarians, there is a very large, often untapped, pool of true need for good veterinary professional service (see Chapters 17-19). However, if veterinarians view what they do as "production" rather than service, they will subvert the essence of the professional relationship. Such a change will not forever be lost on clients.

To advocates of percentage of "production" compensation I raise the following questions:

- Would you be willing to inform your clients that doctors in the practice are paid a percentage of the revenues they generate for the practice? If not, why not?
- Would you be willing to inform your clients that doctors in the practice are paid a percentage of their "production?" If not, why not?
- Even if you do not pay associates on a straight or modified percentage basis, would you feel comfortable using the word "production" in speaking with clients about your fees or that of the practice? If not, why not?
- Would you want your child's pediatrician or your own physician to earn a percentage of "production?" If not, why not?

Working Conditions and Environment

Just as owners have an obligation to provide fair salaries for their employees, so must they attempt to offer working conditions and a general practice environment that respects an associate doctor as a colleague and fellow professional. Among the complaints I hear most frequently from new doctors are that their employers do not give them enough time to have lunch, that they are always the ones who must endure weekend or night duty, and that their vacation plans can be canceled at a moment's notice. Many novice doctors have also told me that they are restricted to tasks they can already perform and are not being trained to assume the duties of more senior doctors. New doctors must understand that they cannot be permitted to do certain procedures until they are ready, and that it is often fair to assign less pleasant jobs to more junior associates. However, owners must understand that many recent graduates are working at relatively low salaries precisely because they can convince themselves that they are invest-

---

*In 1994 a large national home supply chain began advertising that its salespeople are not paid on commission. Therefore, the advertisement stated, all customers receive the same attention and service whether their needs are great or small, and salespeople never try to sell items customers do not need. Is there a message here for veterinarians?

ing in their own training. Some new doctors suspect that they are being relegated to routine tasks because their employer expects to turn them out when they can no longer stand the drudgery and to hire another new graduate who is willing to do such jobs until he tires of them, and so on.

Practice Philosophy

The philosophy of a practice can be defined as its most central values, regarding both the goals of the practice as well as the procedures by which its day-to-day management is accomplished. Even when not adopted deliberately, practice philosophies tend to emerge from the values and personalities of owners. Some practices place great emphasis upon generating revenues and expect doctors to work aggressively at promoting services. In other practices, doctors place a higher value on leisure time and might be satisfied with less revenue. In some practices, veterinarians and support staff treat each other with formality, while in others, a looser camaraderie is accepted or expected.

It is in both an owner's and a prospective associate's interests that the latter be informed prior to employment about the owner's practice philosophy. The following are among the questions relating to practice philosophy that veterinary students and recent graduates tell me are of greatest interest to them in approaching prospective employment:

- How many hours per week will I be expected to work? Will I often have to work nights or weekends? How flexible is the practice in excusing or rearranging work schedules for personal reasons?
- How vigorously must I sell services and products to clients? Will my economic "productivity" be monitored precisely? May I adjust fees to what seems fair or reasonable in particular circumstances?
- How often and under what circumstances will my performance be evaluated? Will I be given the opportunity to respond to criticisms or problems?
- What is the view of the practice concerning such procedures as ear-cropping, tail-docking, declawing, and euthanasia of healthy animals? If I object to any or all of these procedures, how shall I proceed if they are requested by clients?
- Will I be expected to sell nonprofessional goods and services?
- To what extent are important practice decisions made democratically, by all doctors in the practice? Am I expected to "grin and bear it," or will my opinions regarding problems be welcomed or accepted?
- Am I expected to become friendly with other doctors in the practice after work hours, or will my relationship with them be strictly professional?
- How long will I perform routine or menial tasks? To what extent does the practice believe in training new associates to handle difficult cases and to service more valued clients? If I believe I am not yet ready to handle certain kinds of cases, how will the practice respond?

∽ THE FEMALE VETERINARY ASSOCIATE

Few phenomena pose more important ethical issues for the profession than the fact that two-thirds of veterinary school students are now women.[21] Because the great majority of female veterinarians do not yet own their own practices, many of the ethical issues relating to women veterinarians involve their relations with employers.

The Uncertainties

Ethical issues relating to the status of female doctors are difficult, in part because it is not yet clear what the profession (including its growing female component) wants for its women doctors. Nor is it clear how the profession might be able to accommodate these desires. We just do not know how many female doctors (or male doctors in an era of shared parental responsibility) will want to work part-time during a substantial portion of their careers. There are very few role models of the long-term successful female veterinarian that can be relied upon by either new female associates or male practice owners. The profession does not know how easy it will be to arrange careers and practice economics around the various issues posed by pregnancy and childrearing. In short, although history appears to be in the making, it is still too early to predict how the story will turn out.

Speaking Openly about Important Issues

Because so much is yet to be learned—because we do not even know all the questions that will need to be asked—it is extremely important that all who raise ethical issues relating to women veterinarians feel free to express their views openly. Many male practice owners tell me that they would like to discuss moral issues regarding women doctors with their colleagues and with prospective female associates, but are afraid to do so lest they be accused of "sexism."

The danger of substituting accusation for argument is illustrated by an observation of that perspicacious observer of the profession, Dr. Robert M. Miller. He reported that many male college students with whom he spoke decided not to enter veterinary school because of the profession's low salaries. On the other hand, women veterinary students "often remark…that they are willing to endure this because they want to work with animals and realize that what they earn will probably be a second income if they marry."[22] Miller concluded that the influx of women who might be able to tolerate lower salaries could be discouraging some qualified males from becoming veterinarians.

Dr. Miller's remarks evoked the anger of some who saw in them a prejudice against women.[23] In fact, there was nothing antifemale in Miller's observations. They raised three important points the profession cannot afford to ignore. First, the proportion of male veterinary students is not just falling, it is falling dramatically. Second, if veterinary medicine is to remain a first-rate profession, it must attract the most qualified people of both sexes. Anything that prevents the entrance of qualified males into the profession will lower the quality of the general body of practitioners. Third, some qualified males who would seek to become the major breadwinner of their family might not enter the profession if it cannot provide them with a reasonable income.

Dr. Miller did not claim to know how the profession should deal with these matters. But dealing with them (and other issues relating to the changing face of veterinary medicine) must not be hindered by accusations of antifemale prejudice. It is no better to treat a legitimate, good-faith question about the impact of women on the profession as evidence of an antifemale attitude, than it is to think that women veterinarians are inferior.

The Law of Sex-based Discrimination

The task of normative veterinary ethics in considering sex-related issues is complicated enormously by federal, state, and local laws prohibiting discrimination on the basis of sex. Owners must know precisely what laws apply to their practices. This is not always an easy task because some of the federal laws do not apply to all practices, and state and local laws vary greatly. One must also be sensitive to the fact that some moral questions that seem perfectly reasonable might be prohibited by certain laws. The following discussion presents an overview of the most important laws that can affect consideration of moral issues regarding female veterinarian (or nonveterinarian) employees.

1. The federal Equal Pay Act[24] prohibits an employer from paying employees at a lesser rate than "he pays wages to employees of the opposite sex" for "equal work on jobs the performance of which requires equal skill, effort, and responsibility, and which are performed under similar working conditions." The law permits pay differentials based on "any other factor than sex," including seniority, merit, and quantity or quality of production. As noted above, in fact, not only do newly graduated female veterinarians earn less than their male counterparts, the difference in their earnings appears to be increasing.

2. Title VII of the Federal Civil Rights Act[25] provides that employers may not hire, discharge, or otherwise discriminate against any individual (male or female) "because of" or "on the basis of" sex. (Title VII also prohibits discrimination on the basis of race, religion, national origin, and age.) All aspects of the employment relationship are covered, including advertising for employees, interviewing applicants, hiring, salaries, benefits, working conditions, reassignment, and discharge. Unlike the Equal Pay Act, which applies irrespective of the number of employees, Title VII only covers practices with at least 15 employees who work for at least 20 weeks a year. The statute is enforced by the federal Equal Employment Opportunity Commission (EEOC). The following aspects of the law are noteworthy:

A. Pregnancy. One part of Title VII, called the Pregnancy Discrimination Act,[26] prohibits discrimination based upon or because of "pregnancy, childbirth, or related medical conditions." A woman may not be denied employment, discharged, or compelled to take maternity leave simply because she is or might become pregnant. All decisions regarding pregnant or potentially pregnant employees must be based on a good faith determination of whether prospective or present female employees can do the job.

The statute considers pregnancy to be a "disability," and all employers subject to the act must treat pregnancy as they would any other temporary disability. Thus if an employer would reassign any employee to another task because of some temporary infirmity or disability, he must do so for a pregnant employee. An employer may ask a pregnant employee to stop work or may deny a leave to one who claims she can no longer work, but only if he uses the same procedures (for example, acceptance of statements by an employee's personal physician) to settle such issues as he would use to determine whether an employee with another kind of disability must or may stop work. An employer must hold open a pregnant employee's job for her return "on the same basis as jobs are held open on sick or disability leave for other reasons."[27] If employers provide disability insurance or income maintenance for any worker with a temporary disability, they must do the same for a pregnant employee.

B. Sexual harassment. Title VII also prohibits sexual harassment, which is defined by the EEOC as:

...(u)nwelcome sexual advances, requests for sexual favors, and other verbal or physical conduct of a sexual nature...when (1) submission to such conduct is made either explicitly or implicitly a term or condition of an individual's employment, (2) submission to or rejection of such conduct by an individual is used as the basis for employment decisions affecting such individual, or (3) such conduct has the purpose or effect of unreasonably interfering with an individual's work performance or creating an intimidating, hostile, or offensive working environment.[28]

C. Reproductive and fetal hazards. The U.S. Supreme Court has ruled that the Pregnancy Discrimination Act prohibits employers from excluding pregnant or potentially pregnant employees from jobs or tasks to protect their fetuses. The Court held that exclusion is permitted only where it can be shown that pregnancy or the capacity to become pregnant prevents an employee from satisfactorily performing her duties. Even when working at a given task might impose risks on her unborn child, the Court said, the decision to work is "for each individual woman to make for herself."[29] One cannot conclude that the Supreme Court's interpretation of federal law would be endorsed by courts in states that have their own pregnancy discrimination law and where a state's law would apply to a veterinary practice.

D. Preemployment inquiries. Title VII permits employers to inquire about the sex of job applicants, unless such questions are asked for a discriminatory purpose. The EEOC has ruled that an employer may not ask a female job applicant about possible problems she might have with child care, at least if the same inquiries are not made of male applicants.[30]

3. State and local laws. Most states, as well as some municipalities and local governments, have their own fair employment practice laws that prohibit sex-based discrimination. These laws apply in addition to federal statutes. When, as is sometimes the case, a state's law is stricter or more comprehensive than federal requirements, employees or potential employees covered by state as well as the federal laws are entitled to the greater protection of the state standards. The number of employees required before state laws apply varies greatly. States also differ regarding whether countable employees must have been employed for a minimum time for the statute to take effect. In addition to fair employment acts prohibiting sex discrimination, many states have equal pay acts analogous to the federal statute. Some states also have constitutional provisions (such as equal rights amendments) that prohibit sex-based discrimination.[31]

Additional Employee Protection Laws

Laws other than those prohibiting sexual discrimination can protect employees of veterinary hospitals and thus can affect choices employers can make regarding the management of their practices. Detailed consideration of these laws is beyond the scope of this discussion. They are mentioned briefly here to assure that practice owners are aware of the need to attend to them and the ethical principles they embody.

The federal Family and Medical Leave Act[32] requires 12 weeks unpaid leave because of (1) "the birth of a son or daughter of the employee and to care for such son or daughter;" (2) "because of the placement of a son or daughter with the employee for adoption or foster care;" (3) "to care for a spouse, or a son, daughter or parent, of the employee" if such person "has a serious health condition;" (4) and "because of a serious health condition that makes the employee unable to perform the functions of the position of such employee." Although this law applies only to employers with 50 or more employees, several states have similar laws whose application requires fewer workers.

The federal Occupational Health and Safety Act[33] provides that each employer "shall furnish to each of his employees employment and a place of employment which are free from recognized hazards that are causing or are likely to cause death or serious physical harm to his employees." The statute permits the states to develop their own job safety and health programs, and various states have adopted somewhat different standards. Practice owners must be aware of applicable federal and state standards because these laws cover risks to employees from zoonoses, animal-inflicted injuries,[34] and chemicals. The AVMA has adopted guidelines to assist employers to design and implement the required written plan to assure compliance with the Federal Hazard Communication standard.[35] The AVMA guidelines specifically address issues relating to occupational risks for pregnant employees.

The federal Americans with Disabilities Act (ADA) applies to employers who have 15 or more employees for each working day in each of 20 or more calendar weeks. The ADA prohibits such employers from discriminating against qualified persons on the basis of a physical or mental impairment. The ADA covers many aspects of the employment relationship, including hiring and firing, compensation, job tasks, and promotion. Employers covered under the ADA are permitted to make employment decisions based on the physical or mental ability to do relevant tasks, provided the same standards are applied to all actual or prospective employees. The ADA also prohibits discrimination against disabled clients and members of the public. The law requires that all premises subject to the statute make "readily achievable" accommodations to physically impaired clients and other members of the public in new construction and major renovations.[36]

～ NONVETERINARIAN EMPLOYEES

Many of the same considerations relating to the ethical treatment of associate doctors apply to nonveterinarian employees. However, because of the differences in training and duties between veterinarians and nonveterinarians, these considerations sometimes have different implications.

Salary and Benefits

Because they are less skilled than veterinarians and are not responsible for the great bulk of practice revenues, generally, nonveterinarian employees cannot expect to earn as much as doctors, even after years of service. Nevertheless, just as is the case with veterinarian employees, in establishing salaries and benefits for nonveterinarian workers, practice owners are obligated to consider such factors as the length and quality of their educational experience, the amount and difficulty of their work, the quality of their work, and the extent to which they participate in activities that contribute to practice revenues.

Veterinarians are obligated to hire nonveterinarian employees who are qualified and caring. However, because many practice owners face economic challenges (not the least of which can be the need to pay veterinarian employees fairly), there can be pressure to keep nonveterinarian compensation levels as low as possible. A number of states still do not register technicians. Even in states that do, people without a technician's education or skills are sometimes permitted to engage in many of the same activities as trained technicians. The most talented veterinary technicians will have little bargaining power if they can be replaced with people with much less skill willing to work for less. The fact that the overwhelming majority of technicians and other nonveterinarian employees are women makes it still easier for those who think that women ought to earn less than men to rationalize depressed salaries for nonveterinarian workers.

Proportional or Commission Compensation

If nonveterinarian employees work hard, and the practice prospers, it is fair that the owners share some of the bounty with them and use such compensation as an incentive for further good work. However, paying nonveterinarian employees a direct percentage commission of the sales of goods or services for which they are responsible raises the same problems for clients and the long-term image of the profession as does paying doctors a percentage of their contribution to revenues. If veterinarians are to retain their image as trusted medical professionals, the public must remain confident that the primary goal of everyone who works in veterinary practices is first and foremost service to patients and clients.

Understandings and Restrictions

Like associate doctors, nonveterinarian employees have an interest in understanding the conditions of their employment, including vacations, health insurance, maternity leave, required notice for termination of employment, and severance pay. As is the case with doctors, probationary periods of employment may be used to permit employer and employee to judge their suitability for each other. The understandings of the parties may be set forth in a written contract or in an employment manual. Owners must be careful in composing such manuals, for they can sometimes constitute the terms of a contractual agreement between the practice and the employee, even if no formal document labeled "contract" is ever signed. Violations of the terms of the manual, or indeed of any employment policies in whatever form they are stated, might subject the owners to a lawsuit for breach of contract.

One issue about which practices must be especially sensitive is termination of employment. It is unfair to a prospective employee to state or imply a longer term of employment than the owners really intend. If the practice does intend what the law calls "employment at will"—employment that can be terminated by the employer at any time and for any reason—this should be made clear to the prospective employee. Owners can find themselves subjected to legal action if they have indicated to an employee that her employment was not at will (whatever the employment manual might state) or if they fire her for a reason (such as age or sex) that the law does not recognize as a valid reason for termination even for employees at will.

Sex-related Issues

Sexual discrimination or harassment is no less illegal or immoral when directed at nonveterinarians than at licensed doctors. Male veterinarians may not treat nonveterinarian women employees in demeaning or degrading ways because they are not veterinarians. (I know one veterinarian who speaks of his female technicians, but not his female veterinarian associates, as "girls.")

The Face of a Practice

Nonveterinarian employees have important obligations relating to clients and other visitors to the practice. A frequent observer of veterinary facilities, I am appalled by the number in which clients who sit in the waiting room are confronted by a loud radio, boisterous behavior behind the reception desk, loud conversations of a personal nature among employees, and employees who are chewing gum or are dressed in dirty or disheveled attire. Working in a veterinary facility need not and should not be a solemn and somber undertaking. Nevertheless, veterinary employees must understand that they play a vital role in presenting their practice's face to the world. Undignified and disrespectful behavior directed at or done in the presence of clients is offensive to clients, can harm the image and earning power of a practice, and ultimately makes it more difficult for the profession to maintain an elevated image.

Technicians
Is veterinary technology a profession?

The most significant recent development in the area of nonveterinarian employment has been the emergence of veterinary technicians as a distinct category of non-doctor employee. In veterinary practices both large and small, technicians have established themselves as an essential part of the animal health care team. Indeed, it is difficult to look at veterinary technicians who have completed AVMA-approved degree programs and who assist surgeons in administering and monitoring anesthesia, nurse critically ill patients back to health, give medications, perform essential theriogenology services, assist in the care of laboratory animals, instruct clients about nutrition and pet care, and not conclude that many are as important to veterinary medicine as nurses are to human medicine.

Many veterinary technicians consider themselves members of the *profession* of veterinary technology. Accordingly, technicians have a national association analogous to the AVMA, the North American Veterinary Technician Association (NAVTA). NAVTA has adopted a Code of Ethics and a Veterinary Technician's Oath. The latter calls upon each technician to "accept my obligations to practice my profession conscientiously and with sensitivity, adhering to the profession's Code of Ethics." A prominent educator of veterinary technicians includes technicians within the profession of veterinary medicine.[37] The AVMA defines veterinary technology as "the science and art of providing professional support service to veterinarians in the practice of their profession."[38] Although this definition states that technicians provide professional service, it appears to fall short of calling veterinary technology a profession.

Inclusion of veterinary technicians within the profession of veterinary medicine is in my view neither feasible nor wise. There is too great a disparity in the educational backgrounds and skills of technicians and doctors of veterinary medicine, which is why only veterinarians are allowed to practice veterinary medicine and are subject to the ethical and legal obligations veterinary practice entails. This is not, however, to say that veterinary technology ought not to be regarded as a separate profession, as human medicine and nursing are regarded as separate professions.

Speaking of themselves as members of a profession gives technicians a measure of self-respect which they rightly deserve. Nor will veterinarians, the public at large, or the legal system ever view veterinary technology as a profession unless technicians do so themselves. However, at present, it is difficult to regard veterinary technology as a profession in the same sense in which law, medicine, veterinary medicine, or nursing are professions. Veterinary technology does not have as long a history as callings that are classified as professions; its members are not as well known to the public; they do not have the same kinds of advanced education; and they are not as well compensated. But things can change. For many years physicians refused to call nurses professionals and spoke of them as the "handmaidens" of medicine. Today nursing is universally regarded as a profession. It is therefore quite possible that veterinary technology will some day be regarded as a profession.

There is no discernible or magical event that takes place when an occupation becomes recognized by the legal system and members of the public at large as a profession. It took nursing many decades to reach professional status. Whether or how long it takes veterinary technology to reach this goal will depend on a number of factors, including the following:

- *Whether technicians continue to advance in the level of their importance.* At many small animal practices, veterinary technicians perform critical tasks in providing patient care and advice to clients. Veterinary technicians are becoming increasingly important in research facilities, some of which are managed by technicians. Many veterinary practices are seeking to reduce costs by utilizing technicians as extensively as possible. This economic impetus may speed the development of technology as a profession but may also cause strains with the veterinary profession, if doctors are displaced by technicians.
- *Whether members of the public become sufficiently aware of the role played by technicians in caring for animals.*
- *Whether technician organizations continue to increase in influence and importance.* Like the AVMA, NAVTA and state technicians' associations are active in the continuing education of technicians and the promotion of their competence and ethical responsibilities.
- *Whether technician training programs continue to advance in their breadth and depth and are able to attract bright, dedicated students.* The AVMA assures that accredited institutions maintain quality standards. A few institutions now offer or are planning to institute 3- and 4-year programs in addition to the standard 2-year program. It may be difficult to convince the public and the legal system that veterinary technology should be regarded as a profession as long as students can complete technician education in 2 years after high school.
- *Whether technicians develop specialized areas of expertise that enable them to perform certain important tasks better or more efficiently than many veterinarians.* For example, many technicians who function as intensive care nurses and assistants to laboratory animal doctors possess considerable skills without which their facilities could not function.
- *Whether the compensation of technicians improves.* Some technicians are compensated at a level that members of the public would associate with a profession, but many more are not.[39] Veterinarians must be encouraged to employ technicians in important tasks and to pay them fairly.

• *Whether technicians are registered and regulated by state veterinary licensing boards.* Such registration indicates that technician status should be granted only to those who meet certain qualifications. Registration also indicates that technicians are sufficiently important to require government assurance of their competence.

Should technicians be registered, certified, or licensed?

Many states certify, register, or license veterinary technicians. (The terms "certification," "registration" and "licensing" are used in various states, and none of these terms has special significance.) There are different possible kinds of registration, among them the following:

Option 1 A nonveterinarian employee is prohibited from calling herself a "veterinary technician" or "animal health technician," unless registered as such with the state board of veterinary medicine. Such registration requires graduation from an educational program approved by the board and demonstration (for example, by examination) of a level of knowledge or competence required by the board. Several states apply different titles depending on one's level of education. For example, a state might reserve the term "veterinary technician" or "veterinary technologist" to a graduate of an AVMA accredited program who has passed an examination approved by the board, but might allow people who have passed this examination and have not graduated from a technician program to call themselves "veterinary assistants."

Option 2 Option 1 plus continuing supervision of registered technicians (for example, by requiring continuing education, or through on-the-job inspections of the technicians' work conducted by the state board).

Option 3 Option 2 plus prohibition of certain activities (for example, assisting in surgeries or administration of anesthesia) by nonveterinarian employees who are not registered technicians.

All three of these options could benefit patients, clients, and doctors because they can all assist veterinarians to assure that qualified persons are hired as technicians. However, all the options have potential drawbacks. Among such drawbacks is not that registration entails the authorization of technicians to provide services directly to the public. There is nothing inherent in "certification," "registration," or "licensing" that requires giving technicians permission to act other than in the employment and under the supervision of veterinarians.

Options 1 and 2 can afford the public and its animals the benefits of more highly qualified registered technicians only if doctors choose to hire people who can call themselves registered technicians. Option 3 avoids this difficulty and might give technicians greater bargaining power to obtain decent salaries. On the other hand, Option 3 could harm those practices unable to afford higher technician salaries that might result from an Option 3 registration program. Ironically, Option 3 might also lead some practices to hire a new veterinarian rather than a registered technician, on the theory that if more must be paid to an employee, he might as well be a doctor.

Although Option 2 might appear to be a reasonable compromise, like Option 3, it would require resources in funds and personnel that some state veterinary boards do not yet have. Unless a state allocates sufficient funds to an Option 2 program, intolerable additional demands could be placed on the board. It might have difficulty adequately regulating veterinarians. More likely, the board would be unable to enforce the technician registration program or might not take it seriously.

The issue of whether technicians should be considered members of a profession is distinct from the question of whether they ought to be registered by state authorities. Members of some professions (for example, clergy and in some states psychotherapists) are not licensed and regulated by state authorities, and some persons who must have licenses (for example, cosmetologists and electricians) are not considered members of one of the professions.

Some Basic Ethical Principles Regarding Veterinary Technicians

In Table 25-1, I propose several general ethical principles relating to veterinary technicians. These suggestions are based upon considerable discussion with veterinarians and technicians and reflect many basic concerns of both. Some of the principles are quite general, and are intended to permit further refinement or elaboration of appropriate subprinciples. For example, much more can be said about the ways in which technicians ought to be honest with their employers and about how veterinarians can exhibit respect toward technicians. Some of the principles follow from others of the standards, elaborating upon an ethical requirement to address more explicitly a concern of doctors or technicians. The principles are also general in the sense that some might admit of exceptions in extreme or special circumstances. For example, the principle that technicians ought not to criticize a doctor to clients might conceivably be overridden in a case in which the only way a technician can prevent heinous suffering of a patient would be to tell the client that something is amiss. But because such a case would be highly unusual, it is still possible to suggest a general rule prohibiting technicians from complaining about doctors to or in the presence of clients.

The suggested principles make two fundamental assumptions. First, the actions of technicians must be based on the best interests of patients and clients. This, in turn, implies that technicians must always be under the supervision and control of veterinarians and must never be permitted to engage in activities that for medical reasons ought to be reserved for a veterinary medical doctor.

Second, because technicians are legal agents of their veterinarian employers, these employers can often be held liable for, or as a result of, their actions. This not only requires technicians to act diligently and competently. It also explains the appropriateness of a general prohibition against their complaining about doctors or other employees to or in the presence of clients. An inadvertent, misinformed, or malicious comment by an employee can subject a practice and its doctors to undeserved legal problems.

〜 INTERPERSONAL RELATIONS

Many difficult ethical issues can arise out of relations among owners and employees. Owners can face difficult choices when one or more of them cannot get along with or have a legitimate complaint about the performance of an associate doctor. Problems can also arise when any of the doctors in the practice have poor relations with a non-veterinarian employee, or when employees, veterinarian or nonveterinarian, have difficulties in their relations with each other. Any of these kinds of problems can be exacerbated when a client complains about an employee. The owners can be faced with a dilemma between satisfying a client for whom the practice works, and protect-

TABLE 24-1

Ethical principles regarding veterinary technicians

1. Technicians shall serve their employers loyally and faithfully.
A technician shall follow all orders and instructions given by doctors.
A technician shall take no actions regarding any patient or client unless properly authorized to do so. When in doubt about the propriety of any action, the technician shall, whenever possible, ask for direction from a doctor or appropriate supervisory personnel.
A technician shall not criticize any doctor or any employee of the practice to or in the presence of any client, but shall bring complaints or concerns to the attention of a doctor or other appropriate personnel.
A technician shall not make any decisions or take any actions bearing upon the economic affairs of the practice unless authorized to do so. For example, the technician shall not change without permission the normal fee for a particular client or dispense gratuitous medications, goods, or services.
A technician shall not take or use for any unauthorized purpose or in any unauthorized manner any patient or client records or any information contained in such records.
A technician shall work diligently, carefully, and competently, with the understanding that her employer can be held liable at law for the actions of employees.
A technician shall always act on the highest plane of honesty and integrity.
A technician shall treat all doctors and employees of the practice with courtesy and respect.
2. Technicians shall serve clients loyally and respectfully.
A technician shall treat all clients courteously and respectfully.
A technician shall comport herself in a dignified manner as befits an employee of a medical office.
A technician shall respect the professional and personal confidences of clients. Nor shall she reveal to any one, unless authorized by an appropriate member of the practice or required by law to do so, any information revealed to or in the possession of any doctor or employee of the practice regarding any patient or client.
3. Technicians shall serve all patients with dignity and respect.
A technician shall treat all patients humanely and respectfully. The technician shall never inflict unnecessary pain or discomfort on any animal for the purpose of rendering that animal tractable or for any other purpose.
A technician shall attend promptly to the needs of all patients and shall fulfill all orders and instructions regarding patients with the highest degree of diligence.
4. Technicians shall strive to improve the knowledge, technical skills, and moral character of themselves and their fellow technicians.
A technician shall keep informed of developments in knowledge and techniques relating to her duties and shall fulfill all educational requirements of her technician association and state board of veterinary medicine.
A technician shall strive to promote the entrance into employment as veterinary technicians persons of high competence and good moral character.
A technician shall obey the veterinary practice act of her jurisdiction and all other laws governing or pertaining to her medical duties.
5. Veterinarians shall treat technicians fairly and respectfully.
Veterinarians shall compensate all technicians in their employ fairly.
Veterinarians shall strive to utilize technicians in their employ at tasks appropriate to their level of competence.
Veterinarians shall encourage all technicians in their employ to maintain and improve their technical knowledge and skills.
Veterinarians shall treat all technicians respectfully, as valuable members of the veterinary medical team.

ing the employee in whom the owners might have invested a good deal of time and effort and whose continuing service is probably more important to the practice than any single client.

As is often the case in ethics, there is no simple rule that does justice to the variety and complexity of situations in which problems involving employees can arise. For example, regarding complaints against employees by clients, one cannot say that "the client is always right." Clients are sometimes wrong. And even if a client is correct that an associate or nonveterinarian employee acted incompetently or unethically, it does not follow that the owners must take some drastic action demanded by the client and thereby lose or seriously impair the effectiveness of a valuable employee. Likewise, when there are interpersonal difficulties within the practice, one cannot say that the owners should always favor the person with the greatest economic value to the practice, or should favor an associate doctor with greater seniority over one with less, or an associate over a technician, or a technician with greater seniority over one with less, and so on. Blaming or disciplining someone who is not at fault based on some preordained hierarchical scheme is unfair. It can also have disastrous effects, if employees come to think that they are likely to receive certain kinds of treatment not because they deserve it, but on the basis of their status or importance.

Whoever in the practice is authorized to deal with a problem involving employees must consider the first order of business to ascertain the facts. If one allows devotion to or economic interest in a particular employee to cloud one's judgment about who is responsible for a problem, one risks all sorts of bad results. One might unfairly blame the wrong person. One might fail to discourage a tendency in an employee that will recur in the future, to the detriment of others in the practice as well as to clients and patients.

At the same time, owners have a legitimate interest in keeping their practices comfortable and profitable places in which to work. They are entitled to protect even those employees who deserve criticism from unreasonable demands of clients or other employees. If an employee treats a client or another employee improperly, and the situation must be addressed, the owners should strive to cause as little bad feeling or disruption as possible. There is no legal or moral principle requiring, for example, that an unhappy client participate in or observe the disciplining of an errant employee.

Finally, moral deliberation must pay due regard to legitimate hierarchies. The most important moral distinction in a veterinary practice is that between owners and nonowners. Owners should never permit their preeminent legal status to lead to self-deception about their own professionalism or ability to deal fairly with others; this can lead to as much harm to others in the practice, clients, and patients as blaming the wrong person for some problem. However, when an owner just cannot get along with an associate or nonveterinarian employee, and someone must either change or leave, it is the owner who has the right to prevail. He has this moral right in virtue of his legal position as owner as well as his investment in time and money that this legal status reflects.

A distinction that in my view is too often overdone in veterinary practices in approaching issues of an interpersonal nature is that between veterinarians and technicians. Many technicians tell me that when a problem arises between them and a doctor, they have little chance getting their side of the story heard impartially and sympathetically. Indeed, a common complaint of technicians is that they are rarely treated with respect, and that feelings of inferiority and subservience are almost a part of their job description. For practical as well as moral reasons, technicians and other nonveterinarian workers must be respected by all doctors as important members of the veterinary medical team. This means respecting them both as valuable workers and as valued people.

REFERENCES

[1]Wilson J: Is your non-compete clause too restrictive? *Vet Econ* March 1994:64.

[2]Lofflin J: Unhappy associates, *Vet Econ* June 1993:26-38.

[3]Calling all associates, *Vet Econ* April 1992:85-86.

[4]Brockmeier J: To *all* concerned: It's time to ask some tough questions, *Vet Econ* June 1993:42-47.

[5]*Id*, p 44, emphases in original.

[6]Clark R: What's a DVM worth? *Vet Econ* March 1987:28.

[7]Wise JK, Yang J-J: Employment of 1993 male and female graduates of US veterinary medical colleges, *J Am Vet Med Assoc* 204:217-218, 1994. In 1993 female veterinarians in private practice earned a median income of $37,764 compared to $54,583 for male veterinarians. Wise, JK: *Economic Report on Veterinarians and Veterinary Practices*, Schaumburg, IL, 1994, American Veterinary Medical Association, p 13. This document suggests that there may be explanations (such as differences in the number of hours worked by male and female veterinarians and the preponderance of male practice owners) that account for the striking difference in median incomes. Such an interpretation seems to be undercut at the very least by the fact that in their first jobs, which tend to be full-time, female veterinarians earn significantly less than their male counterparts.

[8]Wise, JK: Employment of 1986 male and female graduates of US veterinary medical colleges, *J Am Vet Med Assoc* 190:449-450, 1987.

[9]Wise JK, Yang J-J: Employment, staring salaries, and educational indebtedness of 1993 graduates of US veterinary medical colleges, *J Am Vet Med Assoc* 203:1687-1688, 1993.

[10]Wise JK: Employment, starting salaries, and educational indebtedness of 1986 graduates of US veterinary medical colleges, *J Am Vet Med Assoc* 190:209-210, 1987.

[11]Wise JK: *Economic Report on Veterinarians and Veterinary Practices*, Schaumburg, IL, 1994, American Veterinary Medical Association, p 12.

[12]Wutchiett CR: Who is responsible for low associate pay? *Vet Econ* March 1994:24.

[13]Davis J: Discover the 15 percent solution, *Vet Econ* July 1987:77.

[14]Clark R: How much should I pay? *Vet Econ* July 1990:30-33.

[15]Incentives speak louder than words, *Vet Econ* June 1987:46. For various reactions to percentage payment, *see* Compensation tactics: Finding a plan that works for you, *Vet Econ* July 1990:34-44.

[16]Clark R: How much should I pay? *Vet Econ* July 1990:31.

[17]Opperman M: Stopping trouble before it starts: How to keep your associates happy, *Vet Econ* June 1993:48.

[18]American Veterinary Medical Association: *Principles of Veterinary Medical Ethics*, 1993 Revision, "Guidelines for Professional Behavior," paragraph 2, *1994 AVMA Directory*, Schaumburg, IL, The Association, p 42.

[19]American Veterinary Medical Association: *Principles of Veterinary Medical Ethics*, 1993 Revision, "Therapy, Determination of," *1994 AVMA Directory*, Schaumburg, IL, The Association, p 44.

[20]American Veterinary Medical Association: *Principles of Veterinary Medical Ethics*, 1993 Revision, "Attitude and Intent," *1994 AVMA Directory*, Schaumburg, IL, The Association, p 42.

[21]Veterinary medical degree enrollment, 1992-1993, *J Am Vet Med Assoc* 202:1954, 1993. *See also*, Enrollment declines in DVM-Degree programs, *J Am Vet Med Assoc* 192:1028,1988 (reporting that women comprised 50.8% of the total student body of U.S. veterinary colleges in 1985-1986; 53% in 1986-1987; and 55.03% in 1987-1988). In 1980, 10% of veterinarians were female; by 1991 their proportion had risen to 27%. American Veterinary Medical Association: *Veterinary Demographic Data Resource*, vol 1, Schaumburg, IL, 1992, The Association, pp 2-5.

[22]Miller RM: Response, *Vet Econ* June 1986:7.

[23]Violante J: Letter. Free shovels to dig your own hole, *Vet Econ* August 1986:4.

[24]29 U.S.C. § 206(d)(1).

[25]42 U.S.C. § 2000e.

[26]42 U.S.C. § 2000e(k).

[27]29 C.F.R. Pt. 1604, App., Ans. 9. (1993).

[28]29 C.F.R. § 1604.11(a) (1993).

[29]*International Union, UAW* v. *Johnson Controls, Inc.*, 111 S.Ct. 1196, 1207 (1991).

[30]EEOC Dec. No. 72-0386 (Aug. 24, 1971), *CCH EEOC Decisions* ¶ 6295 (1973).

[31]For a discussion of state sex discrimination laws, see Larson A: *Employment Discrimination*, New York, 1994, Matthew Bender.

[32]29 U.S.C. § 2611 *et seq.*

[33]19 U.S.C. § 654.

[34]*See* Tannenbaum J: Medical-legal aspects of veterinary public health in private practice, *Sem Med Surg (Sm Anim)* 6:175-185, 1991.

[35]American Veterinary Medical Association: Guidelines for Hazards in the Workplace, *1994 AVMA Directory*, Schaumburg, IL, 1993, The Association, pp 82-83, and references cited therein.

[36]For an excellent overview of the Americans with Disabilities Act in the context of veterinary facilities, *see* Emswiller BB: Impact of the Americans with Disabilities Act on veterinary medicine, *J Am Vet Med Assoc* 205:1129-1132, 1994.

[37]Lukens R: Veterinary technician demographics, *Vet Tech* 12:118, 1991 (speaking of the need to "recruit for our small profession [37,000 active veterinary practitioners and 10,000 active veterinary technicians])."

[38]AVMA recognizes NAVTA, *Vet Tech* 14:9, 1993 (official AVMA policy on veterinary technology).

[39]The 1991 AVMA survey of veterinary technology educational programs found that average starting salaries ranged from $12,475 to $18,380 per year. Average salaries for experienced graduates of accredited programs ranged from $13,160 to $28,604 per year. American Veterinary Medical Association: Veterinary Technology as a Career, *1994 AVMA Directory*, Schaumburg, IL, 1993, The Association, p 234. The 1983 AVMA survey of accredited animal technology programs found that average starting salaries for their graduates ranged from $8,583 to $12,500. Salaries of experienced graduates of these programs averaged from $9,133 to $17,735 per year. American Veterinary Medical Association: Animal Technology, *1988 AVMA Directory*, Schaumburg, IL, 1993, The Association, p 628.

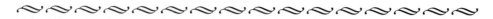

CHAPTER 26

Veterinary Ethics, Wildlife, and the Environment

*T*here appears to be virtually universal enthusiasm among veterinarians about the profession's growing involvement in the treatment and protection of wildlife. This attitude is understandable.

Veterinarians like and benefit from favorable publicity and a good image. The public loves to see veterinarians helping wildlife. Television and the print media present unforgettable portraits of selfless dedication: veterinarians tirelessly attempting to rescue marine birds and mammals from an oil spill, struggling to help back to sea whales that have mysteriously beached, performing sophisticated dental work on a zoo tiger to enable it to eat, repairing the broken wing of an eagle so it can return to its mountain habitat. Such images make people feel good about veterinarians, and make veterinarians feel good about their profession.

The public's concern about protecting the environment will surely enhance not just the public image but also the real influence of the veterinary profession. Wild animals are a major part of the environment. If people and government are to protect the environment, they will need the assistance of veterinarians. The importance of pets and the human-companion animal bond has enabled the profession to portray its members as ministers to human as well as animal health. The growing appreciation of the environment may enable veterinarians to become agents of ecological diversity and stability.

Unfortunately, the increasing involvement of the profession with wildlife and the environment also presents many difficult ethical issues. There is significant discussion and disagreement among ecologists, biologists, ethicists, and policy makers about what goals should be sought and how agreed-upon aims should be effected. Veterinarians will find themselves enmeshed in many of these debates. Veterinarians who cannot articulate defensible positions on these issues will not be effective or may do serious harm to the environment.

This chapter provides some basic tools for approaching ethical issues relating to veterinary practice on wild animals. The chapter is necessarily limited in scope for several reasons. First, it will take time, as veterinarians interact more regularly with wildlife, to obtain a comprehensive picture of the kinds of ethical problems that occur with sufficient regularity to make them of general interest. Second, considerations of space prevent full discussion of broader ethical issues into which veterinarians who deal with wild animals must inevitably be drawn. For example, a significant and growing body of veterinarians treats animals in zoos and aquariums. Although there are a number of specific questions relating to the treatment of such animals, there is an underlying ethical issue that all zoo and aquarium veterinarians must consider: Is it morally acceptable to keep animals, or certain kinds of animals, in zoos or aquariums in the first place? I offer an answer to this question, but the issue of the appropriateness of such facilities and certain of their activities is a large one, if only because so many people appear to be concerned about the issue. Finally, because veterinarians have a professional interest in animal welfare, they are interested in many ethical questions relating to wildlife that do not directly involve veterinary practice. Thus in 1993 the AVMA adopted an official policy condemning as inhumane the use of steel-jaw leghold traps.[1] It is tempting to move from any discussion of this policy to a more general consideration of trapping of animals, and then to the question of whether sport hunting is morally appropriate. Indeed, it can be argued that any ethical issue in environmental ethics relating to the welfare of animals should interest veterinarians, from which it would follow that much of environmental ethics should interest veterinarians. This book cannot offer a general survey of environmental ethics, nor can it consider wildlife issues far removed from actual veterinary practice such as the morality of sport hunting and fishing, or of trapping or raising animals for their fur.

∾ WHAT IS A "WILD" ANIMAL?

There are different possible definitions of the terms "wild animal" and "wildlife." For example, some veterinarians maintain that ferrets kept as pets in areas of the United States in which these animals cannot survive in the wild should not be classified as wild, precisely because these animals cannot live in the wild. To facilitate discussion this text uses the sense of "wild" generally employed by American law. The law defines a "wild" species as one that is not domesticated, that has not been tamed for economic uses, or typically does not live in association with people. The legal definitions of "wild" and "domestic" are not entirely biologically based. Although an elephant in the United States will be classified as a wild animal, American law considers the same elephant when located in India a domestic animal, because in that country, elephants are commonly used as beasts of burden. Whether an animal is classified as "wild" does not turn on whether it is "tame" in the sense of being safe to people or other animals or under complete human control. An iguana that barely moves in its terrarium and a tiger that always obeys human commands are both wild animals because they are members of species classified as wild. An "exotic" species can be defined as a wild species not native to a particular area. (Thus a rattlesnake is an exotic wild animal if kept in Maine but a wild animal when in southern Arizona; a cockatoo in either state would be an exotic wild animal.) American law regards as wild animals ferrets, parrots, parakeets, cockatoos, robins, iguanas, snakes, and gerbils. Using the legal definitions of "wild" and "exotic" is helpful because these definitions reflect what many people mean by these terms and because everyone who interacts with wild animals must know how the law conceives of such animals and what the law says about appropriate dealings with them.

∾ LEGAL CONSIDERATIONS

As discussed in Chapter 4, veterinarians must always consider whether their activities are affected by legal requirements or prohibitions. This is especially important when veterinarians treat wildlife.

The basic principle of American law relating to wildlife is that the state and federal governments own all wild animals on their respective lands in trust for the people. These governments may, and frequently do, give private citizens permission to possess or own members of wild species. Such permission can take the form of a general law, regulation, or policy decision allowing people to own certain species and exempting them from the general requirement of seeking permission to own a wild animal. (States typically provide blanket permission to own exotic birds commonly kept as pets or typical home aquarium fish.) Permission can also be granted by the issuance of written licenses or permits, which allow people to possess or deal with identified animals or species in designated ways. The authority of the federal or state governments to control the possession of wildlife extends to exotic as well as indigenous wild species. For example, a Northeastern state can dictate whether, or under what conditions, anyone within its territory may possess a boa constrictor just as it can dictate whether, or under what conditions, skunks or squirrels native to the state may be possessed.

The power of government to restrict or impose conditions on the ownership or possession of wildlife is extremely broad, and courts will not overturn such government decisions unless fundamental constitutional or legal principles are violated. (For example, a state could not prohibit only members of a racial or ethnic group from owning certain kinds of wildlife, because this would constitute unconstitutional discrimination.) This explains why one state can prohibit the possession of ferrets by private citizens, another state can condition such possession on the issuance of a license, and a third may allow anyone to possess a ferret. If a state decides that it shall allow ownership or veterinary treatment of certain wild species, or certain species under certain conditions, its decision will stand as long as it can articulate a defensible reason related to its interest in controlling wildlife for the public benefit. The power of the states to dictate under what conditions wild animals may be possessed is illustrated by a decision of the Massachusetts government. The state fish and wildlife agency enacted a regulation allowing veterinarians to temporarily treat sick and injured wild animals.[2] This decision resulted from complaints by Massachusetts veterinarians that the state's general prohibition against veterinary treatment of nonpermitted wild species prevented practitioners from providing emergency care to animals in the wild.

Veterinarians in private practice who treat wild or exotic animals kept by clients as pets often need not be concerned about these legal principles, for many such patients are lawfully possessed. However, some veterinarians do treat members of species that are not lawfully kept by clients and are not lawfully treated. These veterinarians may be subject to criminal prosecution as well as action from state veterinary licensing boards, which typically include within grounds for discipline violation of any law relating to veterinary practice (see Chapters 4 and 7).

Supplementing the fundamental authority of state and federal governments to control possession of wild animals within their borders are a host of other laws, mainly federal. The U.S. government has entered into treaties with other nations relating to wildlife, and pursuant to various constitutional powers has enacted many statutes that enable the federal government to exert control over the possession of wild animals even when these animals are not on federal land. The authority of the states to allow possession or veterinary care of certain wild species is therefore often contingent on decisions by federal wildlife authorities to allow anyone to own, possess, or interact in various ways with these animals. Moreover, some wild species come under the auspices of both federal and state governments. In such cases, veterinarians who treat such animals often must receive permission from both their state and the federal government. For example, the federal Endangered Species Act and associated regulations do not allow veterinarians to treat designated species without permission from federal authorities. Many states also have their own endangered species laws, and when certain species are designated by both federal and state laws as endangered, veterinarians who want to treat such animals typically must receive permission from both state and federal officials.

Veterinarians should not treat any wild animal without knowing whether they are permitted to do so, and they should obtain permits when these are required. Veterinarians who treat or want to treat wildlife should have in their practices up-to-date copies of all applicable federal and state regulations, including their state's lists of permitted and nonpermitted species. The many federal laws that can affect the possession and veterinary treatment of wildlife include the Endangered Species Act,[3] Migratory Bird Treaty Act,[4] Marine Mammals Protection Act,[5] Bald Eagle Protection Act,[6] and the Convention on International Trade in Endangered Species of Wild Fauna and Flora (CITES). Some of these laws or treaties, and others, apply to zoos, aquariums, and wildlife rehabilitation facilities. There is often shared responsibility and coordination among federal agencies. For example, the U.S. Department of Interior administers the Endangered Species Act and the Marine Mammals Protection Act. However, the latter law also requires the Department of Agriculture to determine and assure proper conditions of captive marine mammals pursuant to the Animal Welfare Act.[7]

∿ THE POSSESSION AND VETERINARY CARE OF WILD OR EXOTIC ANIMALS KEPT AS PETS

One ethical issue relating to veterinary practice on wild animals can be considered without addressing complex philosophical questions: Should people keep as pets members of wild or exotic species when allowed by law to do so, and should veterinarians enable and in effect encourage the keeping of such animals by providing routine medical care for them?

For many years, the AVMA has opposed the keeping of wild or exotic animals as pets. In 1973 it adopted an official policy recommending that "all commercial traffic of these animals for such purposes should be prohibited." This policy was defended on the grounds that (1) people "acquire skunks, raccoons, monkeys, alligators, and other exotic species because they like to possess unusual pets or regard them as status symbols;" (2) exotic species create "disease, diet, and exercise problems" different from those in dogs and cats; and (3) disposing of such animals "can be a traumatic experience, with difficulty in relocating such animals."[8] Interestingly, the policy did not appear to include exotic caged birds, perhaps because many veterinarians were already treating such animals.

The AVMA's policy was well-intentioned, but prevented the organized profession from fulfilling its rightful role in promoting good medical care for wild and exotic pets. Opposing private ownership of all wild species is like banning the consumption of alcoholic beverages. It simply will not work. Because many such animals are in homes around the country (and are there lawfully), the interests of these animals and their owners will only be served by the availability of first-rate veterinary care. A policy discouraging practitioners from treating these animals may drive owners to seek medical advice from less qualified pet store operators and self-styled lay "experts."

Moreover, the 1973 policy prevented the articulation and promotion of discriminating policies regarding these animals. The public and government undoubtedly need guidance about what species can make good pets, and about what owners must do to care for them properly. However, the organized profession will play no role in the determination of rational distinctions and standards if it opposes the keeping of all such animals. Nor will the profession be able to exert substantial influence to assure technical competence and ethical behavior on the part of those veterinarians who are in fact treating wild or exotic pets if its approach to the keeping of these animals is opposition.

In 1990 the AVMA modified its position, as follows:

> RESOLVED, that the American Veterinary Medical Association recognizes that: (a) Wild animals are often maintained in captivity as companion animals, for breeding purposes, for research activities, and for exhibition, and (b) Certain species of wild animals, when maintained under responsible ownership, may constitute no significant hazard to human health, other animal species, the environment, or to the animals themselves.
>
> It is FURTHER RESOLVED that certain species, or individual animals of most species, when maintained under irresponsible ownership may, in fact, be a hazard to human health, other animals, and/or the environment.
>
> It is FURTHER RESOLVED that the American Veterinary Medical Association strongly opposes the keeping of wild carnivore species of animals as pets and believes that all commercial traffic of these animals for such purposes should be prohibited.
>
> It is FURTHER RESOLVED that the American Veterinary Medical Association strongly opposes keeping as pets those reptiles and amphibians that are considered inherently dangerous to humans and believes that all commercial traffic of these animals for such purposes should be prohibited.[9]

At first glance, this policy seems to mark a significant departure from the old condemnation of private ownership and veterinary treatment of all wild species. Unfortunately, the new policy is less tolerant of ownership of wild animals than it might at first appear, nor does it attempt to place the organized profession in a leadership role in advocating good veterinary care for wild animal pets. The policy ends with an explanatory "Statement about the Resolution," which, in effect reinstates the old blanket opposition. This statement speaks disapprovingly not just about the possession of certain kinds of wild and exotic species, but also wild and exotic species in general. It is asserted that "people acquire wild animals as pets because they like to possess unusual pets or regard them as status symbols. …Veterinarians should exert their influence to discourage the keeping of wild animals as pets."

There are too many different kinds of wild and exotic species to make it possible to brand all equally as inappropriate pets. Surely, there are some exotic animals that can be kept healthy and safe by some knowledgeable and careful owners. If this were not the case, all states would prohibit the possession of all wild species. Moreover, although there undoubtedly are some people who acquire certain wild animals as status symbols or for certain strange psychological reasons, the same is true of some people who own dogs or cats.

At veterinary schools and private practices around the country more is continually being learned about how to treat these animals. Such progress will benefit the animals. Advances in treating wild and exotic pets will also benefit practitioners by providing another source of revenue. Disseminating knowledge about treating these animals might not be easy. Some doctors will need further training before they can competently treat some of these species. Already overburdened veterinary students will be required to learn about even more kinds of animals. Undoubtedly, certain species must remain off-limits to owners and veterinarians alike. But for reasons I have already discussed in this book, it is far better for veterinarians to address the need to generate practice revenue by increasing the range of patients for which they can provide competent medical care than by turning to activities such as merchandising nonprofessional goods and services.

∽ A PRELIMINARY VENTURE INTO DARK WATERS

Although medical treatment of wild animals kept as pets raises distinctive ethical issues, these questions pale in comparison to those presented by veterinary practice on wildlife that is not owned by private citizens. A brief glimpse of the potential problems is illustrated by the following case:

> *Case 26-1 Save the robin?* You are a private practitioner with a mixed animal practice. Many of your patients are exotic birds. You also have appropriate licenses to treat and rehabilitate nonendangered wildlife and are permitted, at your option, to rehabilitate and reintroduce into the wild or to euthanize certain species of migratory birds including robins.
>
> One late summer morning you are brought a female robin by a client whose cockateels you have been seeing for years. Less than an hour ago, as she was sitting in her living room, the client saw the robin crash headlong into her plate glass window. She placed it in a small cardboard box, resting on a cloth towel. The bird is breathing but otherwise is virtually motionless. Preliminary examination of the head, eyes, nares, and ears does not indicate fractures, hemorrhage, or bruising.
>
> The client is extremely upset and feels guilty because it was her window into which the robin crashed and because she treats her own birds so well. She wants you to save the animal if you can. She hopes it can be released back into her neighborhood, and offers to pay up to $200 for treatment of the bird if you think you could help it.
>
> It is possible that the bird will regain consciousness and can be brought back to health. The treatment, IV or IM corticosteroids and placing the bird in a dark chamber at a cool temperature for a day or two, would be covered by what the client is willing to pay. You have a general interest in such cases because some of your pet avian patients suffer such head trauma. Moreover, you can euthanize the robin at any time if its recovery appears unlikely or you believe you are spending too much time and effort in its care.
>
> Should you attempt to save the bird, euthanize it immediately, or give it back to the client (perhaps with instructions about what she might do to assist it to regain consciousness)?

This apparently simple case raises difficult issues. Put aside for a moment the potential benefit to the client of feeling good about attempting to alleviate a problem for which she feels responsible. One possible response to the case is to say that there is absolutely no reason to try to save the bird. It is not a member of an endangered or threatened species, nor will its death be a significant loss to the local or global environment. Indeed, one could argue that it is positively wrong to treat the bird, because the client surely must have better potential uses for her money and you might have better things to do with your time, including attending to other patients and clients.

Such responses to the case rest on a principle that some veterinarians find self-evident: there is no reason to treat unowned wild animals that are not members of endangered or threatened species, that are not important to the environment, or that do not serve another useful, more general purpose (such a being an inhabitant of a zoo). According to this position, in general, species and not individual wild animals are important. It may sometimes be appropriate to treat an unowned wild animal, but this is usually so only when treatment is important to maintaining the species or some larger entity such as the animal's immediate environment.

Other people would not agree with this approach. To them, the robin is still an individual animal that has been injured and that might be helped. That the bird is unowned is a significant fact, but not a fact affecting *its* interests. Surely, these people would say, this bird has an interest in living and returning to the wild. Are not veterinarians committed to serving the interests of individual animals? Is this bird different in significant anatomical respects from other birds treated by this practitioner? How, then, could it be inappropriate for a veterinarian to try to save this bird? The position that it is acceptable, admirable, or even obligatory to try to help the robin can be asserted without claiming that the client was somehow at fault for the bird's injury (say, because she has a plate glass window) and is therefore obligated to help the animal.

This little case raises issues that go beyond whether veterinarians should want to protect individual unowned wild animals or their species. Even if we suppose that it would be appropriate to try to save the robin, there are vastly different reasons one could come to this conclusion. One could assert that wild animals have value only insofar as they benefit human beings. Thus one could conclude that it might be worthwhile to try to treat the robin if by doing so one might obtain knowledge which could contribute to one's ability to treat birds owned by clients, or to treat injured birds the return of which to the environment is important to people. On the other hand, one could insist that if this robin should be treated, it should be treated, at least in part, simply to help it, for its own sake, irrespective of whether it will be of use or benefit to any human beings.

∼ APPROACHES TO UNOWNED WILD ANIMALS IN CONTEMPORARY ENVIRONMENTAL ETHICS

It is impossible to adequately consider the alternative approaches to Case 26-1, or many other kinds of ethical choices raised by the medical treatment of wildlife, without having some knowledge of current discussions in the field of environmental ethics. Positions that have been developed in this field illuminate ethical issues faced by veterinarians who want to provide medical care to wild animals. Moreover, decisions veterinarians make, either individually or as a profession, relating to the treatment of wildlife, will be scrutinized by thinkers in the field of environmental ethics. Because environmental ethics is itself a complex and rapidly growing discipline, the following discussion is intended as an introductory and broad summary. Not all positions advanced in environmental ethics relevant to the questions discussed are mentioned. The approaches described here have been supported by various kinds of arguments, which cannot be done justice in this brief survey.

Human-oriented Environmental Ethics
Traditional anthropocentrism

For many years, among philosophers, theologians, and policy makers, one view of the environment—and of wild animals that constitute an important part of the environment—has predominated. This view can be called "traditional anthropocentrism."* According to this approach, the environment and its components have no intrinsic value but are valuable only insofar as they can benefit human beings. Most proponents of this position do not advocate disregard for the environment. Quite the contrary. They argue that if people disregard or wantonly destroy the environment people and human society will ultimately be harmed. Advocates of traditional anthropocentrism can, and often do, oppose deforestation and replacement of complex animal and plant ecosystems with human agriculture or industry, on the grounds that in the short or long term, such behavior will harm people. Advocates of traditional anthropocentrism can support environmental policies that would compromise certain interests of people presently alive, to protect or benefit future generations of people. Traditional anthropocentrism can offer different kinds of arguments for preserving endangered or threatened species, including the contentions that (1) the more species that exist, the more interesting and beautiful the environment will be for people; (2) extinction of animal and plant species could cause the loss of material useful in treating human diseases; and (3) the loss of species is an important barometer of the general stability of the environment, and the less stable the environment, the more people are likely to be harmed.

The philosopher John Passmore is a leading proponent of traditional anthropocentrism. He writes that:

> The traditional moral teaching of the West…has always taught men…that they ought not so to act as to injure their neighbors. And we have now discovered that the disposal of wastes into sea or air, the destruction of ecosystems, the procreation of large families, the depletion of resources, constitute injury to our fellow-men, present and future. To that extent, conventional morality, without any supplementation whatsoever, suffices to justify our ecological concern, our demand for action against the polluter, the depleter of natural resources, the destroyer of species and wildernesses.
>
> …[A]n 'ethic dealing with man's relation to land and to the plants and animals growing on it' would not only be about the behavior of human beings, as is sufficiently obvious, but would have to be justified by reference to human interests. The land which a bad farmer allows to slip into a river did not have a 'right' to stay where it was. The supposition that anything but a human being has 'rights' is, or so I have suggested, quite untenable.[10]

Proponents of traditional anthropocentrism can conclude that it is important to protect wild animals and to provide them with medical treatment. However, doing so would be justified not because it might help the animals, but if it benefits people. Among the reasons advocates of traditional anthropocentrism can give for protecting and treating certain kinds of wildlife are the following:

- Protecting and sometimes providing medical care for animals in the wild can make these areas more interesting and enjoyable to people who visit them.

---

*Anthropocentrism in its various forms should not be confused with anthropomorphism, which can be defined roughly as attributing human characteristics or mental capacities to animals. The views associated with the term "anthropocentrism" are so named because they assert that human beings are in some sense at the *center* of things, at least regarding ethical obligations toward elements of the environment.

- Preserving and treating wildlife can bring economic benefits from tourism.
- Preserving and treating animals in zoos enhances the enjoyment people have visiting zoos, which, in turn, enhances their concern for wild animals and the environment, which, in turn, helps all people by helping to protect the environment.
- Protecting and sometimes providing medical care for wild animals can help to preserve wild areas that serve as a barrier or check to unbridled human overpopulation or overindustrialization, which is important to protect the health and well-being of people.
- Protecting and sometimes treating animals in the wild can enhance veterinarians' understanding of how to treat wild animals kept as pets or wild animals which should be treated because of their value to people.

Traditional anthropocentrism is consistent with the view that some wild animals such as the robin in Case 26-1, might have interests of their own. However, traditional anthropocentrism does not believe that animal interests should be furthered because it is independently valuable to do so—but only if some human interest would be furthered. Thus an advocate of traditional anthropocentrism could accept as a justification for treating the robin in Case 26-1 that doing so might improve the veterinarian's ability to treat owned birds, but would reject the position that this bird ought to be treated just because it is an individual animal the interests of which could be furthered by treating it.

Extended or modified anthropocentrism

Traditional anthropocentrism has certain counterintuitive implications, which have led a number of philosophers and environmentalists to modify it. Traditional anthropocentrists assert that people do not have any direct ethical duties to animals, but only have ethical duties regarding animals. However, most people do believe they have ethical duties *to* animals. Most people believe, for example, that they should not cause animals unnecessary or unjustifiable pain not just because treating animals inhumanely might lead to inhumane treatment of other people, but because doing this is wrong and unfair to the animals themselves (see Chapters 11-13). Just as most people would say that they have an obligation to give their pets nutritional food and appropriate veterinary care, so would most people say that, for example, wild animals kept in zoos ought to be given adequate food, water, and care. This is owed *to them* because they are being used by people for our own purposes.

Traditional anthropocentrism has other odd consequences. Imagine that there is a species of wildlife (say, a species of whales known only to yourself with very few members and that lives in a far-off isolated habitat) the extermination of which would not have any negative consequences on any people or any part of the environment that could eventually affect people. You can exterminate this entire species. Would it be wrong to do so? According to traditional anthropocentrism, there would be no ethical problem in doing this, provided there is built into the hypothetical situation an iron-clad assurance that the disappearance of the species could never have any negative effects on people. (In fact, it is often difficult to maintain that the disappearance of a species will not have wider effects, something that anthropocentrists of various persuasions can use to argue in favor of species preservation.) However, exterminating this species seems wrong. Surely, most people would say, these animals should just be left alone. They are certainly not harming any people. They surely have some interests of their own. It seems not just uncharitable but barbaric not to let them survive.

Environmental ethicists Richard and Val Routley suggest another hypothetical case which shows that animals (and, the Routleys argue, other parts of the environment as well) can have some value irrespective of their benefits to people.[11] Imagine that you are the last human being on earth. You have the power to exterminate all living things just before you die. Would it be wrong to do so? Surely this seems wrong, at the very least because the remaining animals would have lives of their own, including, for some of them, pleasures and sophisticated experiences. But if it would be wrong to deprive them of these experiences, it follows that these animals' lives do have some value independent of people. And if this is so of these animals, it must also be so of at least some animals that now inhabit the planet with people.

Many people believe that we human beings are stewards of the Earth and that we are ethically obligated to take care of it and to pass it on so that it can be inhabited and enjoyed by others. (One can adopt this position with or without a religious belief that God ordered humankind to be stewards of His creation.) However, if this is so, and traditional anthropocentrism were correct, the only justification for accepting the role of such stewardship would be to benefit present and future generations of people. This may be one good reason to take care of the planet, but it cannot be the only reason. Surely, there is intuitive force to the notion that we should take care of the planet because *it* (and certainly, at the very least, some of its animal inhabitants) is worth taking care of in its own right.

A number of philosophers and environmentalists have been led by such objections to traditional anthropocentrism to adopt a position I shall call "extended" or "modified" anthropocentrism.[12] Extended anthropocentrism still views human interests as greatly more important than animal interests. Extended anthropocentrism also accepts traditional justifications for various approaches to wild animals in terms of their overall impact on people and human societies. However, extended anthropocentrism concedes that animals (including wild animals) can have interests of their own, that people sometimes do have ethical obligations *to* animals (including some wild animals), and that these obligations sometimes demand a balancing of human and animal interests that can require some compromise of human interests. Extended anthropocentrism also asserts that certain approaches to wild animals are appropriate because they are good for, or are owed to, the animals themselves.

For example, an advocate of extended anthropocentrism can support keeping animals in zoos, on the grounds that zoos encourage an appreciation of wildlife by people and can help sustain endangered or threatened species—both of which inure to the benefit of people. However, a proponent of extended anthropocentrism can also assert that zoo animals deserve certain kinds of environmental conditions, in their own right, and that if such conditions cannot be provided, it may be wrong to keep them in zoos.

The following examples illustrate the difference between traditional and extended anthropocentrism. I recently visited a zoo which had in its collection a group of White rhinoceroses, a species endangered by hunters who seek their horns. Among these animals was a calf recently born in this zoo. The rhinos lived in a large area that permitted them to move about for some distance. A veterinarian companion pronounced the animals apparently healthy and noted that the calf resting placidly on a bed of straw next to its mother provided strong evidence that these animals were experiencing a satisfactory level of welfare. Contrast these rhinos with another exhibit at a zoo I visited, this one of animals for which large people like myself appear to have some affinity but which have not received as much publicity as the vanishing rhinoceros. Here were two Nile hippopotamuses in a pool that was sufficiently deep to allow them to submerge but was barely wide enough to afford either animal more than a few seconds' travel time from one end to the other. It seemed to me that the treatment of the rhinoceroses described above was acceptable, in light of the precarious future of the species, the fact that the conditions were conducive to breeding, and the ability of these animals to move about relatively freely. Now I happen to be a proponent of extended anthropomorphism. I support zoos because I believe they can play an important role in protecting and promoting public appreciation of wild species. However, I was troubled by the hippos. This species is not on the verge of extinction. Even if it were, I would wonder whether the conditions in which these hippos were kept was sufficiently attentive to their needs. The pool was large enough to fit them, and given the general hardiness of hippos and the clear dedication of this zoo to caring for its animals, I had no doubt that they were physically healthy. But hippos in the wild spend much of their time in the water, and the pool simply bore very little resemblance to a natural hippo habitat. I am no expert in hippopotamus mentality and behavior, and I would welcome an argument that the well-being of these animals was appropriately protected. Nevertheless, the example is useful to illustrate features of extended as distinguished from traditional anthropocentrism. A traditional anthropocentrist would probably find nothing wrong with this hippo pool, especially if visitors to the zoo enjoy looking at the animals and the hippos' health allows them to continue to serve this function. A traditional anthropocentrist would not care (except insofar as the viability of the exhibit might be affected) whether hippopotamuses can be "bored" or whether these hippos were bored. In contrast, I was inclined to think that even if this exhibit gave a very large number of people considerable pleasure, it might not have been fair to the animals, and that if the zoo wanted to display the hippos, it had an obligation to enlarge the pool. In sum, extended anthropocentrism bases the treatment of wildlife on human interests, but believes that animal interests can also count, though usually to a lesser extent than human interests.

Extended anthropocentrism shares one view with traditional anthropocentrism. It believes that people do not have ethical obligations to plants, inanimate parts of the environment, ecosystems, or the planet. Extended anthropocentrism advances ethical concern beyond people and human society only to certain other animals on the grounds that (1) only beings with interests have moral claims against people; and (2) plants and inanimate objects are not sentient beings, they do not feel or experience anything, and therefore cannot be said to have interests and goods of their own.

Human-Animal Egalitarianism
Utilitarianism

Two ethical theories relating to animals must be considered in this brief survey, even though these theories were not developed in the context of environmental ethics. As discussed in Chapters 5 and 12, utilitarianism asserts that people ought always to choose that alternative action (or rule) which, on balance, will produce no less utility (happiness, pleasure, satisfaction of preferences, depending on the variant of utilitarianism) than any other alternative.

The leading exponent of utilitarianism in animal ethics is philosopher Peter Singer.[13] Singer's view is that pain is pain, whether it is experienced by people or animals. Therefore in a utilitarian calculation, animal pain is to be counted no more nor no less than human pain. Thus according to Singer, people and animals are entitled to equal consideration. This does not mean that animals must be treated as well as people. Singer recognizes that humans are often able to experience more intense satisfactions than animals and that therefore a calculation of total human and animal satisfactions sometimes argues in favor of benefiting people rather than animals. Nevertheless, because Singer's utilitarianism does require equality of consideration, it is appropriately regarded as egalitarian.

Several features of utilitarianism as it applies to both wild and domestic animals are noteworthy. Because only individual animals feel pain or pleasure, groups or species of animals are not accorded independent value. Utilitarians can say that it is morally obligatory to preserve certain species, but only if doing so would, on balance, maximize utility for all individual sentient beings, that is, for individual people and animals. Thus one might be obligated to promote the health of a group of animals to benefit individuals in that group. According to utilitarianism, people cannot have obligations to groups or species of animals. Collections of animals (or humans) are relevant only insofar as their individual members contribute to the total aggregate of pain and pleasure. Utilitarianism is also consistent, at least in principle, with a variety of traditional approaches to wild animals, including veterinary care. A utilitarian could respond to Case 26-1 by urging the veterinarian to treat the robin, if treating it would make the client feel better and provide the veterinarian with useful knowledge regarding how to treat clients' birds.

Animal rights abolitionism

Like utilitarianism, animal rights abolitionism asserts that animals have interests irrespective of peoples' interest in them. However this view, as expressed by its leading proponent, philosopher Tom Regan, does not permit use of animals to benefit people even if such use would, on balance, maximize total happiness or utility. Regan believes that many animals have the same value as human beings, at least with respect to whether they may be used as means to benefit others. Just as people have a right not to be eaten, experimented on, killed, or otherwise used to benefit someone else without their consent, so it is a violation of an individual animal's rights to eat it, experiment on it, kill it, or otherwise use it for the benefit of people or other animals.*

According to Regan, only individual animals (or people) can have rights, because only individuals have interests and can be benefited or harmed. Therefore groups of

---

*This position is appropriately called animal rights abolitionism because it seeks to abolish the use of animals as means for the benefit of people or other animals. Because they oppose the idea that animals should be viewed as property, adherents of animal rights abolitionism see connections between their position and the historical abolitionist movement which succeeded in eliminating human slavery in the United States. I argue throughout this book that animal rights abolitionism should not be confused or identified with the view that animals can have moral or legal rights. One can assert that animals have rights without concluding that among these is the right not to be used for the benefit of people or other animals.

animals, or animal species, have no independent ethical significance. They have no rights. We have no obligations to them. We have obligations only to individual animals, domestic or wild. Wildlife management policies that manipulate animals or their habitats to protect groups or species use individual animals as means to benefit others and therefore violate these animals' rights. Regan believes that, in general, people will best respect the rights of wild animals by leaving them alone. Thus the:

> ...goal of wildlife management should be to defend animals in the possession of their rights, providing them with the opportunity to live their own life, by their own lights, as best they can...Being neither the accountants nor managers of felicity in nature, wildlife managers should be principally concerned with *letting animals be,* keeping human predators out of their affairs, allowing these 'other nations' to carve out their own destiny.[14]

While a utilitarian could approve of zoos if having zoos (or, perhaps, particular zoos or certain kinds of zoos) were, on balance, better for people and animals than not having zoos, Regan regards keeping animals in captivity to benefit people or other animals as a violation of the former animals' rights. However, it does not appear to follow from Regan's position that wild animals could never have the right to receive medical treatment. For example, one could argue that just as people whose rights are violated sometimes thereby gain the right to have the violation undone, so might wild animals sometimes gain this right. Thus an advocate of animal rights abolitionism might argue that otters mired in an oil spill resulting from negligent operation of a tanker have the right to veterinary care to undo the wrong done them.

Problems in utilitarianism and animal rights abolitionism

Both utilitarianism and animal rights abolitionism have difficulty accounting for strong moral intuitions many people have regarding the proper approach to wild animals. As ethicist Mark Sagoff has observed, if one really believes that animal pain is as important as human pain, or that humans and animals have equal value, the course of action seems clear: we should rescue as many animals from the wild as possible:

> Animal liberationists insist, as Singer does, that moral obligations to animals are justified by their distress and by our ability to relieve that distress. Accordingly, the liberationist must ask: how can I most efficiently relieve animal suffering? The answer must be: by getting animals out of the natural environment. Starving deer in the woods might be adopted as pets; they might be fed in kennels. Birds that now kill earthworms may repair instead to birdhouses stocked with food— including textured soybean protein that looks and smells like worms. And to protect the brutes from cold, we might heat their dens or provide shelter for the all too many who freeze.[15]

If, as egalitarianism asserts, animals and people must be given equal consideration, it seems at best callous and at worse wrong not to intervene as much as we can to help them. But most people do believe that wild animals should generally be left where they are. Moreover, the common view is that when intervention in their lives is justified, it may often take the form of attempting to save species or populations, even if doing this necessitates ignoring or even harming particular individuals. For example, most people would probably agree that if a population of deer has become so large that the individual animals are starving because there is not enough food for all, it is appropriate to cull some of the animals, to allow continuation of the population. Environmental management must often focus on sustaining groups or populations in ways that would be prevented by giving all wild animals the same consideration we give to humans, by giving all members of all species equal consideration, or by giving all members of a given group or species of animals equal consideration.

Biocentric Environmental Ethical Views

Some philosophers and ecologists reject anthropocentrism or egalitarianism in their various forms, on the grounds that all these positions fail to accord independent value to entities other than human beings or individual animals. Advocates of what are sometimes called "biocentric" or "deep ecology" ethical theories insist that there is value in, and human moral obligation to, nature, other than human beings and individual animals. According to biocentrism, people have obligations to nature, or at least to parts of it.[16]

There is a wide variety of biocentric approaches, and not all of them can be mentioned here. Some of these theories extend the range of direct ethical concern to groups or entire species of animals. Other biocentric views go even further, asserting that people have ethical obligations to plants, all living organisms, inanimate parts of the environment (such as rocks, rivers, and sky), ecosystems, and the entire planet. The following descriptions are intended only to indicate the range of possibilities—and to alert veterinarians who treat wildlife about the murky waters of environmental ethics into which they are unavoidably thrust. The different views presented here are not all incompatible, and some are endorsed (though with varying emphasis) by some of the biocentrists whose views are discussed.

Value in species

Some philosophers argue that people have ethical obligations to species as well as to individual animals. According to Holmes Rolston, for example:

> ...duties to a species are not to a class or category, not to an aggregate of sentient interests, but to a life line. An ethic about species needs to see how the species *is* a bigger event than the individual interests or sentience. Making this clearer can support a conviction that a species *ought* to continue.
>
> Events can be good for the well-being of the species, considered collectively, even though they are harmful if considered as distributed to individuals. This is one way to interpret what is often called genetic load, genes that somewhat reduce health, efficiency, or fertility in most individuals but introduce enough variation to permit improvement of the specific form.[17]

It need not follow from such a position that every species ought to be saved, or that assuring its survival is the only ethical obligation one might have to a species, or that all species are equally valuable. The view that there is value in species does imply that there is some good in a species independent of the value or moral claims of its individual members and that such species-good must be given some weight in determining a proper environmental approach.

Value in organisms

Philosopher Paul Taylor argues that each living organism has a good of its own entitled to respect by people. Moreover, because this good is the same for all organisms, including plants and bacteria, no living organism can be more valuable than another. According to Taylor, the good of any individual living organism consists of:

… the full development of its biological processes. Its good is realized to the extent that it is strong and healthy. It possesses whatever capacities it needs for successfully coping with its environment and so preserving its existence throughout the various stages of the normal life cycle of its species. The good of a population or community of such individuals consists in the population or community maintaining itself from generation to generation as a coherent system of genetically and ecologically related organisms whose average good is at an optimum level for the given environment.[18]

…Each individual organism is…a teleological center of life, pursuing its own good in its own way. …[T]he claim that humans by their very nature are superior to other species is a groundless claim…[that] must be rejected as nothing more than an irrational bias in our own favor.[19]

Taylor does not condemn people who defend themselves against other organisms such as animal predators or bacteria, because he believes that each organism may protect itself against threats to its basic needs. He does, however, reject human uses of animals that satisfy what he considers to be nonbasic human needs at the expense of what he considers to be basic needs of animals. On these grounds, he concludes that people should not "own caged wild birds, wear apparel made from furs and reptile skins, collect rare wildflowers, engage in hunting and fishing as recreational pastimes, buy ivory carvings, or use horn dagger handles…[because] every one of these practices treats wild animals and plants as if their very existence is something having no value at all, other than as means to the satisfaction of human preferences."[20]

Value in diversity, complexity, and stability of ecological systems

Some environmental ethicists, including several of the thinkers included in this discussion of biocentrism, argue there is value not just in individual people, animals, or even groups or species of animals, but also in ecological systems. This approach is sometimes based on the view that, in fact, systems comprised of interrelated plants, animals, and inanimate parts of nature are the "units" of biological functioning. Individual living beings cannot, it is argued, survive much less prosper outside of such systems. Among the "virtues" of ecological systems some ethicists have postulated are "diversity of systems and creatures, naturalness, integrity of systems, stability of systems, harmony of systems."[21] Philosopher Stephen Clark basis an argument for such values, in part on their role in perpetuating ecosystems. "The more sorts of creatures there are in an ecosystem, the more complex the interrelations and the more 'stable' the system…The climax community is, in Aristotelian (which is not to say 'animistic') terms, the final cause of the earlier stages: it is here that the diverse kinds all find their niche, and because there are such climax communities there are kinds available to repopulate the area if the community should be overthrown by outside influence."[22]

The "land ethic"

Perhaps the best known formulation of the idea that biological systems have value is what naturalist Aldo Leopold called the "land ethic." According to Leopold, this ethic "simply enlarges the boundaries of the community to include soils, waters, plants, and animals, or collectively, the land."[23] Leopold's often-quoted central ethical principle is that "A thing is right when it tends to preserve the integrity, stability, and beauty of the biotic community. It is wrong when it tends otherwise."[24] Unlike some advocates of respect for systems, Leopold does not urge leaving nature alone, nor does he believe that people cannot appropriate much in nature for their own benefit. Leopold speaks about the "biotic community," and pictures a "biotic pyramid," each successive layer of which:

> ...depends on those below it for food and often for services, and each in turn furnishes food and services to those above. Proceeding upward, each successive layer decreases in numerical abundance. Thus for every carnivore there are hundreds of his prey, thousands of their prey, millions of insects, uncountable plants. The pyramidal form of the system reflects this numerical progression from apex to base. Man shares an intermediate layer with the bears, raccoons and squirrels which eat both meat and vegetables.[25]

Although Leopold believes that human beings occupy but one level of this pyramid, he also insists that we may legitimately use many parts of the biotic community for our purposes, if the "land" is respected. Thus Leopold was an avid hunter. Philosopher J. Baird Callicott explains how Leopold's position sometimes justifies substantial human manipulation of wildlife and habitats. Callicott writes that:

> ...to hunt and kill a white-tailed deer in certain districts may not only be ethically permissible, it might actually be a moral requirement, necessary to protect the local environment, taken as a whole, from the disintegrating effects of a cervid population explosion. ...From the perspective of the land ethic, predators generally should be nurtured and preserved as critically important members of the biotic communities to which they are native. Certain plants, similarly, may be overwhelmingly important to the stability, integrity, and beauty of biotic communities. ...An example [of justifiable wildlife management] is trapping or otherwise removing beaver (to all appearances very sensitive and intelligent animals) and their dams to eliminate siltation in an otherwise free-flowing and clear running stream (for the sake of the complex community of insects, native fish, heron, osprey, and other avian predators of aquatic life which on the anthropocentric scale of consciousness are 'lower' life forms than the beaver).[26]

The Gaia Hypothesis

The culmination, perhaps, of environmental approaches that find physical coherence and ethical value in systems rather than individual animals or organisms is the Gaia Hypothesis. According to this view, the entire Earth is one living organism, named "Gaia" after the ancient Greek Earth goddess. Just as parts of a human's body function to support the whole, so do parts of the Earth, including inanimate things and physical processes, support the whole. Just as homeostasis is a goal, and therefore a good or value, for individual organisms, so is planetary homeostasis and stability a goal and a good for Earth, or Gaia. James Lovelock, an atmospheric chemist and creator of the Gaia Hypothesis, describes it as follows:

> But like one of those Russian dolls which enclose a series of smaller and still smaller dolls, life exists within a series of boundaries. The outer boundary is the Earth's atmospheric edge to space. Within the planetary boundary, entities diminish but grow ever more intense as the inward progression goes from Gaia to ecosystems, to plants and animals, to cells and to DNA. The boundary of the planet then circumscribes a living organism, Gaia, a system made up of all the living things and their environment. There is no clear distinction anywhere on the Earth's surface between living and nonliving matter. There is merely a hierarchy of intensity going from the 'material' environment of the rocks and the atmosphere to the living cells.[27]

Questions about biocentrism

It would be a mistake to assume that biocentrism in one of its forms will inevitably hold sway in the field of environmental ethics because biocentrism focuses directly on the clearly legitimate aim of preserving ecosystems and the planet as a whole. A substantial number of environmentalists and ethicists (including this author) find not just incorrect, but incoherent, the notion that people can have direct ethical obligations to all individual living organisms, groups or species of animals, plants, habitats, ecosystems, collections of ecosystems, or the planet.[28] As I have explained, traditional anthropocentrism, extended anthropocentrism, and utilitarianism are consistent with many policies directed at preserving species and the environment.[29] It is far from clear that it is coherent, much less factually correct, to speak of the entire earth as one living organism. Nevertheless, the popularity of biocentrism may well be on the rise. Moreover, any satisfactory account of our ethical obligations regarding the environment will undoubtedly have to be able to encompass approaches that sometimes sacrifice the interests of individual wild animals to preserve larger groups of animals, habitats, or ecosystems.

Issues and Positions in Environmental Ethics and Their Relevance to Veterinary Ethics

This brief tour of environmental ethics is not intended as general cultural enrichment. It is intended as a warning and a call to action. Like many members of the general public, many veterinarians immediately, enthusiastically, and almost instinctively approve of medical care for sick and injured wildlife. Whatever one thinks about particular positions advanced by environmental ethicists, these positions exist, and some have gained significant acceptance among environmentalists and philosophers. A heart-warming image of the compassionate veterinarian helping individual suffering wild animals will by itself be no match for theses in environmental ethics that do not accept this approach to wild animals or that accept it only in the context of broader ecological goals which transcend not just individual animals or groups of animals but also animals altogether. Veterinarians who treat wildlife must be prepared to deal with such positions and to justify their actions. Veterinarians must ask whether, for example, it really makes sense to expend valuable time and resources saving an injured rare bird that will never be able to be released back to the wild and must be kept in captivity until it dies, if for less money and time, a wild habitat in which more birds of its species live might be preserved. Veterinarians must also ask whether, given what really counts in the wild, uncompensated services sometimes devoted to treating wildlife would better be allocated to pet owners who cannot afford care for their animals.

⟳ THE CASE AGAINST MEDICAL TREATMENT OF WILD ANIMALS

The first question veterinary ethics must ask about animals in the wild is whether, and under what conditions, such animals should be given medical treatment. An incisive and unsettling argument if treating such animals is offered by philosopher Robert Loftin. He explains why anyone who regards ecosystems as more important than individual wild animals will view most veterinary treatment of wildlife with skepticism. Loftin tells of a sea turtle that lost its fins as a result of an attack by a shark. Veterinarians attempted to fasten artificial rubber fins on what was left, but the operation failed because there was insufficient bone for attachment.

...It is better, as I see it, to spend what time and energy I have to save more habitat for the benefit of healthy animals. To treat individual animals is merely a one-shot, short-term action. Even if I can save the life of an individual, that animal, like all of us, is doomed to die. Unless I can somehow return it to the breeding population, I have done nothing that will survive the death of that particular individual.

The chance of getting a sick or injured animal back into the breeding population is a slim one. Even if I keep it alive, I may never be able to release it. If I release it, it may not be able to care for itself in the wild. Only the fittest survive. Even if it can survive in fierce competition with healthier, more experienced animals, can it hold its own with them in the even fiercer competition to propagate genes? If it does, is it perpetuating less fit genes, say by replacing the genes of a sea turtle that somehow knows how to *avoid* shark attacks? Other turtles know how to do that. Sharks and sea turtles have lived side by side in the oceans for eons. Most birds' nests fail. Most of the fledglings do not make it through the first year. The same is true of most other groups of animals, including human beings under natural conditions. This is how the system works; that's what *makes* it work.[30]

Loftin is a biocentrist. He believes that the treatment of individual wild animals is sometimes justified, when such animals are members of endangered species, and when treatment is arguably necessary to save the species. However, such action, he insists, should not be aimed at serving the interests of the individual or even just of the species, but rather of larger ecological systems the existence of which depends in part on functioning species. Loftin asserts that people do have an ethical obligation to prevent injured or sick wild animals from suffering, by euthanizing them. He also concedes that publicizing certain stories of animal injuries and attempts at saving these animals may elevate people's regard for wildlife and the environment. Nevertheless, he believes that, in general, the great majority of medical treatment of animals in the wild is not an efficient way of protecting ecosystems and is a waste of time, money, and effort—however good it may make veterinarians or the public feel.

There are problems in Loftin's position. Like some other environmentalists, he appears to rely too easily what can be called the "evolutionary gambit," the assertion that a sick or injured animal might have gotten sick or been injured because of a genetic disposition or factor, and that allowing this animal to breed might perpetuate animals with less fit genes. This is sometimes a persuasive assertion. It may also make ecological sense to argue that when it is not clear whether fixing or treating an animal will perpetuate less fit genes, it is better to err on the side of not risking weakening the species and therefore not treating such animals and releasing them back into the wild.*

---

*For example, wildlife rehabilitation facilities commonly nurse young birds such as robins, which are brought in by people who find them on the ground or in apparently untended nests. Such "orphans" (as they are called by rehabilitators) have to be fed several times every hour, by hand, from morning until night. I would argue that unless it is known that such a bird has been "orphaned" because of some injury done to its parent by a person, it should not be saved. How can one know that its parent was not lost because of some genetic predisposition that rendered it less capable of finding food for its young, and that this predisposition will not be transmitted by the "orphan" to future generations? How can one know that the "orphan" did not fall out of its nest or did not get to wherever it was found because of a genetic predisposition and that this predisposition would not be passed on by it if it is rehabilitated? Does it make good ecological sense, indeed, is it fair to the animals to send back into the wild birds that may well generate more birds to rehabilitate, which may then generate still more birds to rehabilitate, and so on and so on? Young birds fall out of nests or lose their parents all the time in the wild. In light of the frequency of such events, there appears to be at least a reasonable probability that such occurrences are a routine part of natural selection. If only a fraction of the young "orphan" birds that rehabilitators are saving and releasing back into the wild do carry less fit genes, the compassionate activity of saving these animals could, on balance, be doing substantial damage to species and perhaps ultimately to ecosystems.

Loftin's hypothesis that the turtle with the failed prosthetic flippers might have passed on a genetic predisposition to fall prey to sharks is sheer speculation. This turtle just might have been at the wrong place at the wrong time—as might many animals that are injured or become ill. Moreover, when injuries or diseases of wild animals are caused by people, it is usually extremely unlikely that treatment and reintroduction into the wild will perpetuate "less fit" genes. Loftin also fails to appreciate positive reasons that can be given, even by biocentrists, in favor of treatment of wild animals. Nevertheless, Loftin's ecological doubts surely place the burden of proof on veterinarians to show why the treatment of animals in the wild, at least those that are not members of endangered or threatened species, is appropriate.

∼ THE CASE FOR MEDICAL TREATMENT OF WILD ANIMALS

As Loftin concedes, whether one finds any argument in favor or against the treatment of animals in the wild to be persuasive will depend in large measure on one's underlying ethical views regarding wildlife. For example, the position that people have an obligation to help animals they or other people injured or placed in danger presupposes the view that people have ethical obligations to individual wild animals other than a duty to alleviate their suffering, a view that Loftin apparently rejects. Therefore it may be impossible to suggest arguments for treating wild animals under certain circumstances that will satisfy proponents of all the various environmental ethical approaches described above. The following arguments in favor of medical treatment of animals in the wild are offered to assist veterinarians and others engaged in wildlife rehabilitation to answer Loftin's challenge.

1. Treatment of wild animals can enhance the ability of veterinarians to diagnose and treat illnesses and injuries in wild animals, which in turn can enable veterinarians to treat wild animals when it is appropriate to do so (for example, when they are appropriately kept as pets, used in captive breeding programs, members of endangered or threatened species, or kept in zoos). Although some biocentrists disagree, it is surely sometimes ethically acceptable for people to keep and care for wild animals. Many people enjoy the companionship of exotic birds, for example, and such relationships can benefit both the person and the animal. Zoos and captive breeding of wild animals can be (as will be argued below) ethically acceptable. However, if wild animals may sometimes be kept by people, veterinarians must learn much more about them and their medical problems than is currently known. Although knowledge in diagnosing and treating wild animals is advancing, veterinarians understand far less about many of these species than is known about domestic animals. A great deal can be learned from zoo and aquarium animals, but the number of animals that can (or should) be kept in such facilities is limited. Treating animals brought from the wild will therefore result in important knowledge that can be applied to wild and perhaps even domestic animals kept by people.

2. Treatment of wild animals, especially in veterinary school wildlife clinics or wildlife rehabilitation centers run by specialists in wildlife medicine, is necessary for the training of veterinarians in wildlife and exotic animal medicine. The profession cannot deal appropriately with illness and injury in wild animals unless it can train veterinary students and practitioners in wildlife medicine. Practitioners who wish to become board-certified in zoo and exotic medicine can receive much of their training at zoos. However, the majority of practitioners will have to receive their training at veterinary schools or other facilities that treat injured wildlife. Such facilities are also needed to train veterinarians who will engage in wildlife rehabilitation medicine that is appropriately done and does not involve zoo or aquarium animals.

3. Treatment of wild animals can enhance the public's appreciation of the environment and of wild animals. Although Loftin concedes that treatment of wildlife can enhance the public's appreciation of these animals and the dangers they face, he maintains that it would be less expensive and more effective to forego the treatments and deal directly with protecting habitats. However, these are not conflicting goals. Indeed, natural habitats will not be preserved unless people contribute to such efforts either voluntarily or through taxes. People will not contribute to these efforts unless they think preserving wildlife and the environment is important. It is impossible to overestimate the effects a professional and compassionate wildlife medicine program can have on people. My own veterinary school's wildlife center generates more publicity for the school than any of its other activities, and the publicity is not flash-in-the pan media stuff. It is positively electric and long-lasting. I have met animal owners and high school students who have seen one rehabilitated eagle or heron and are hooked—for life—on the idea of protecting wildlife.

4. Treatment of wildlife can often be done efficiently, at no sacrifice to other environmental programs, and can result in release of animals back into the wild with no likely effect on their ability to survive. Loftin underscores his argument against the treatment of wildlife with examples that are as unusual as they are dramatic. In addition to the story of the failed prosthetic turtle flippers, he cites veterinarians who transplanted the cornea of one eagle to the eye of another, and others who equipped a Laysan albatross found in San Francisco with new feathers and flew it to Midway Island 5,000 miles away for release. Such endeavors may well constitute an inefficient use of resources. However, the treatment of many wild animals is far less costly and far more likely to result in a normally functioning animal. It is often possible to attribute an animal's condition to an accident, or some human's behavior rather than inferior genes. Many rehabilitation centers will not undertake treatment of an animal unless they believe that it can be reintroduced into the wild. Moreover, as is discussed below, wildlife medicine sometimes involves treating individual or wild animals without taking them from their habitats or disrupting their natural behavior.

5. Even when treated animals cannot be released back into the wild and must be kept in captivity, treating and keeping them can provide continuing opportunities for veterinarians and others to learn about and appreciate these animals. Loftin observes correctly that some treated animals cannot be released because they are incapable of fending for themselves in the wild. Some of these animals can become pathetic hybrids, stuck somewhere between wildness and domesticity, a pale reflection of their original biological selves. However, sometimes it is possible to keep an animal that is not completely capable of normal behavior (for example, an owl that is unable to fly well but can still get around a spacious enclosure) but appears otherwise healthy and satisfied. It is sometimes possible to learn a great deal from such animals about animals of their species or about the behavior and needs of treated wildlife.

6. Treatment of wild animals is sometimes justified when these animals are intentionally or negligently harmed by human activities. If people should be concerned only about groups or species of animals, ecosystems, or the most efficient use of resources, it would always be inappropriate for veterinarians and wildlife rehabilitators to rush to the scene of an oil spill to save a relatively few gulls and sea otters from a painful death. It certainly might be easier and less expensive to kill them forthwith, and their ecosystem would probably survive quite nicely without them. However, the natural and almost unavoidable inclination to try to save these creatures surely reflects a moral truth—that people do sometimes have ethical duties to individual wild animals. It seems wrong not to sometimes try to help animals people have harmed, even if one could help more animals with the same amount of resources.

⤳ THE CHALLENGES FOR VETERINARIANS

Biocentrism is not alone in sometimes questioning the medical treatment of wildlife. Traditional and extended anthropocentrism also may often conclude that the interests of individual animals must be sacrificed or compromised so that appropriate attention can be directed to groups of animals, species, ecosystems, or the planetary environment as a whole. Environmental ethics therefore presents veterinarians several serious challenges:

1. Veterinarians must first ask themselves *why* they think it is appropriate to treat any individual wild animal. Veterinarians cannot simply treat such animals with the assumption that doing this is appropriate, or with the hope that someone else will demonstrate why it is.

2. Veterinarians must attempt to place any proposed course of action relating to the treatment of wild animals within the context of a well-reasoned and defensible ethical view relating to the environment in general and wildlife in particular.

3. Finally, and most importantly, veterinarians must articulate a role for themselves, as veterinarians, within prevailing approaches to wildlife and the environment that concentrate on populations, species, and ecosystems. For example, should wildlife veterinarians also focus on groups of animals and view themselves as practitioners of "population medicine?" Or should they retain the traditional concern of their profession on individual patients, seeking to assist individual animals when and in whatever manner is appropriate within the context of environmental policies that concentrate on groups or species of animals, or ecosystems?

⤳ BASING MEDICAL APPROACHES ON ETHICAL PRINCIPLES AND SCIENTIFIC KNOWLEDGE

Although there will sometimes be persuasive responses to questions about the wisdom of providing medical care for wildlife, there can be no doubt that too much treatment is occurring—and, more importantly, that too many veterinarians and laymen are treating animals without adequate attention to the wider environmental consequences of their activities. In a 1992 discussion of basic veterinary techniques in wildlife reha-

bilitation, wildlife veterinarian Dr. Stuart Porter estimated that American wildlife rehabilitation centers may be examining as many as 1.5 million wild animals yearly and that
some facilities receive from 2,000 to 6,000 animals per year. Yet, there were fewer than
six veterinarians in the country working full-time in the field. The vast majority of
rehabilitation clinics use the services of local veterinarians who, according to Porter,
"only see what they are brought and have little input as to the level of care the animals
receive."[31]

From Dr. Porter's account of wildlife rehabilitation there emerges a picture of
many well-meaning people doing what they can to help millions of animals in the wild,
often without coordination from sources that would assure their work makes coherent
ecological sense. Clearly, if even only a small proportion of animals treated and released
into the wild are being helped to propagate less fit genes, wildlife rehabilitation could
be responsible for releasing back into the wild tens of thousands, perhaps hundreds of
thousands, of animals that natural selection would handle otherwise. Clearly, if even
only a small proportion of the time, effort, and money devoted to wildlife rehabilitation would more efficiently be spent on habitat protection, tens of thousands, perhaps
hundreds of thousands, of dollars are being misallocated yearly.

Perhaps the worst feature of all this medical treatment of wildlife is that much of it
may be done without any clear, much less justifiable, underlying idea of its purpose.
The major impetus seems to be compassion, which, philosopher Holmes Rolston has
observed, may be a fine virtue when humans deal with each other but can wreak havoc
on the wild.[32] Dr. Porter recommends that veterinary practices that would like to
engage in wildlife rehabilitation establish a wildlife treatment plan, which includes how
the doctors will be remunerated, whether animals will be treated in the practice or elsewhere and who will be responsible for transportation and supervision of patients. The
problem with this recommendation and the general approach of so many veterinarians
and laymen who rehabilitate wildlife is that the approach is almost entirely instrumen-
talist. It is assumed that it is appropriate to treat and rehabilitate any sick or injured
animal that can be enabled to go back into the wild—if one *wants* to do it. The major
issue becomes how to do it effectively.

Dr. Porter does provide ethical justifications for this approach. It is important to
discuss his arguments because they reflect, I believe, the views of many wildlife rehabilitators. According to Dr. Porter:

> ...there are points in support of rehabilitation efforts worldwide. Wildlife rehabilitation is a
> humane activity. These animals have a biological right to survive. Because most of the reasons
> wild animals are injured are related to human interference, it cannot be said that we are interfer-
> ing with the natural order of things by rehabilitating the animals. They deserve to be humanely
> and correctly treated just as do our pets and to be given a second chance back in the wild. Some
> have even received third chances.[33]

Dr. Porter appears to believe that all injured wild animals (at least those capable of
being rehabilitated) have a "biological right" to survive and presumably a *right* to help
from wildlife rehabilitators. He does not explain what he means by a "biological right"
to survive. If he means that animals in the wild are somehow entitled, by natural biological processes, to survival, his claim is obviously incorrect, assuming it makes sense.
If anything, most animals in the wild would have a "right" to be preyed upon by other

animals because this is precisely the role nature appears to have assigned them. Nor can it be said that *species* have a "biological right" to survive, because the core principle of natural selection is that some species survive while others do not. If Dr. Porter means that all sick or injured wild animals have a moral right (derived somehow from biology) to assistance from people who know of or find them, he is surely incorrect. Although it can be argued that people sometimes are obligated to help wild animals injured because of human abuse or neglect, it is surely not the case that people have an ethical obligation to help *all* sick or injured wildlife. To do so would be to engage in a "human interference" more dangerous to wild animals and the environment than those human interferences to which Dr. Porter attributes most wildlife injuries: sending back into the wild genes and genetic predispositions that natural selection would eliminate.

Dr. Porter's suggestion that people are responsible—in the sense of being *morally* responsible—for most wildlife injuries is unacceptable. He maintains that wild animals "do get into trouble by getting hit by cars, gunshot, poisoned, caught in fences, flying into windows, being knocked out of fences, flying into windows, being knocked out of nests, and getting attacked by dogs and cats."[34] There is a potpourri of so-called human "interferences" here, but a brief discussion of the matter Porter mentions twice should suffice to illustrate the problem with the argument. In a sense, windows in human dwellings are an "interference" with birds that fly into them. But the apparent implication that windows are somehow a *wrong* for which we humans must atone by rehabilitating birds that fly into them is entirely unconvincing. Presumably, we humans also have a right to live on this planet and to construct for ourselves useful and pleasant habitations. It would be one thing to construct a giant window in the path of a bird migration, to build a house in a wildlife area critical for the preservation of an avian species, or to barbarically shoot at a flock of songbirds. However, it is quite another matter to build in a residential (or nonresidential) area a house into which some birds may occasionally crash. This is *our* habitat. If we are to feel guilty about our habitat or must set about repairing every animal that is harmed by it, we might as well close down human civilization forthwith so that we no longer "interfere" with any wild animals. Of course, even when people are appropriately blamed for wildlife animal injury or sickness—as we sometimes are—it still need not follow that we must try to save all animals we have harmed. As Loftin explains, sometimes it is so inefficient and expensive to try to help animals people have injured that, however sorry we may feel about it, we would still better devote available resources to assuring that such problems do not happen to other animals.

Nor is there merit to the argument (which I have heard from a number of wildlife rehabilitators) that many injured and wild animals are "just like" pets and like our valued dogs, cats, and caged birds, no less deserving of excellent veterinary care. Some pets may not be anatomically different from some wild animals, but there is a world of *ethical* difference between pets and wildlife. People take pets into their homes and their lives. We make them dependent on us. We often become dependent on them. They become part of lengthy and sometimes intense human-animal relationships (see Chapter 15), giving and receiving attention and love. As a result we owe them things we do not owe animals in the wild.

Wildlife rehabilitation is undoubtedly sometimes justified, as my response to Loftin argues. However, it will not do for veterinarian or lay rehabilitators to base their endeavors on feelings of compassion, scientifically insupportable views of animal or species "rights," exaggerated statements about human wrongdoing, or comparisons of sick or injured wildlife with family pets.

In his stimulating contribution to the 1991 AVMA Animal Welfare Forum on the welfare of wild animals,[35] Holmes Rolston sketched out the kind of ecological-ethical deliberation that is required in this area. One need not endorse all of Rolston's general positions on environmental and wildlife ethics, or even his conclusions regarding the cases he presents, to appreciate the value of his approach. Rolston seeks to apply reasoned and consistent general ethical principles to environmental science's best determinations of the factual implications of alternative approaches. He insists that we address particular problems involving identified groups of animals and habitats and remain open to the conclusion that, in light of all relevant considerations, animals should sometimes be helped but sometimes should be left alone. Rolston argues, for example, that it was appropriate for wildlife veterinarians to treat Colorado bighorn sheep that contracted lungworm from imported domestic sheep, by feeding the sheep apples laced with fenbendizole. Treatment was justified, he contends, because it was intended not to subvert but to promote processes of natural selection. Letting the lungworm take its course could have rendered a species extinct not because its natural habitat would have rendered it unfit but because something attributable to people placed it in danger. However, Rolston supports the decision not to treat bighorn sheep in Yellowstone National Park that contracted pinkeye (infectious keratoconjunctivitis) in the winter of 1981-82. He reports that while wildlife veterinarians wanted to treat the disease, which eventually caused the death of over 300 animals, "the Yellowstone ethicists knew that although intrinsic pain is a bad thing whether in human beings or in sheep, pain in ecosystems is instrumental pain, through which the sheep are naturally selected for a more satisfactory adaptive fit."[36] Rolston argues that a lame deer which had been attacked by a wolverine but escaped, injured and lame, onto the ice of a frozen lake was appropriately left by park officials to suffer for a day and to die, because the attack was an ordinary part of the competitive struggle for which humans were not in any way responsible. However, Rolston approves of the decision of the same park officials to quickly kill a bear that had been hit by a truck, on the grounds that:

> ...when human beings cause pain, they are under an obligation to minimize it. If we had thought that the wolverine failed to kill the deer because human beings interrupted the attack, that might have been cause to dispatch it, although even here consideration for the wolverine, as an endangered species, would probably have meant that the deer should be left in case the wolverine returned.[37]

⌒ THE VETERINARY PERSPECTIVE: INDIVIDUAL ANIMALS

Even when veterinarians *are* justified in treating wildlife, I would urge them to retain the traditional focus of their profession on individual animals. Even when sound environmental approaches determine that people should be more concerned about a group or species of animals or about larger ecosystems, the needs and interests of individual animals do not disappear. If, for example, some members of a population of wild animals should be killed to protect the herd and other animals and plants in its habitat, a veterinarian can be there to assure that this is done with minimal distress to the animals that will be killed and those that will remain. If members of a population should be moved to another area so that they and other members of their species can survive, a veterinarian can be there to assure that each animal is restrained and moved with minimal stress and discomfort. If animals should be tagged so that their movements can be followed or their history ascertained, a veterinarian can be there with the profession's best knowledge about how to tag animals with the least negative impact on their welfare. When a project is undertaken to conserve a species by general nonintensive maintenance of populations, such as in the gorilla conservation project in Rwanda, a veterinarian can be there to provide medical care for the animals consistent with the overall goals of the project.[38] Whenever an animal in the wild should be captured, restrained, or anesthetized, a veterinarian should be there to see that it is done with minimum stress and distress.[39] If a certain species should be propagated through a captive breeding program, a veterinarian should be there to assure proper care of all the animals in all phases of the process, including reintroduction into the wild.[40]

The concepts of "population health" and "population medicine"

Environmental programs and wildlife management are becoming high-visibility, high-prestige activities. These programs also, clearly, often focus on more than individual animals. Some veterinarians may therefore be tempted to try to include within their role (and their purported area of expertise) larger management decisions that depart from the profession's traditional role as protector of individual animals. Some wildlife veterinarians, like some farm and food animal veterinarians, are attempting to shift the emphasis of wildlife animal medicine—and indeed wild animal welfare—from individuals to groups. Wildlife medicine thus becomes population medicine, and wildlife animal health becomes population or species health. According to wildlife practitioner Dr. Victor Nettles, veterinarians must broaden the "stereotypic viewpoint" of a wildlife doctor as "a person who takes care of a sick or injured wild animal or an animal in a zoo."

> …The sheer number of animals makes us focus our attention on the health of a herd, flock, or group of wild animals to make certain that most of the animals in a wildlife population are healthy and that the species in question is able to reproduce in adequate numbers. …
>
> The wildlife veterinarian serves as a specialist/advisor to the wildlife management team in regard to health matters; however, the veterinarian's efforts are finally achieved through acceptance and actions of wildlife administrators, biologists, and law enforcement officers. Animal welfare, when defined in terms of healthy, sustained wildlife populations, is the common goal among wildlife managers and wildlife veterinarians.[41]

As I argue in Chapters 16 and 23, veterinarians can *talk* about group "health," "medicine," and "welfare," but they should understand that they may then be using the terms "health" and "welfare" differently from how these terms have been traditionally used. Group or species "health" is consistent with the sickness of many individuals. Group "welfare" is consistent with the misery of many individuals. I am not suggesting that it is always wrong to tolerate sickness or misery in individual wild animals (perhaps sometimes in many individual wild animals) to protect species or ecosystems. I do maintain that veterinarians should still retain their traditional focus on individual animals, and not attempt to become something that neither their training nor the language indicates they are, namely, "herd doctors," "flock doctors," "species doctors," and least of all, "ecosystem doctors."

Although there is a fair amount of talk about "population medicine" and "population health" in the veterinary wildlife literature, it is difficult to find clear and persuasive definitions of these terms. Repetition of these words may make them familiar, but it does not of itself clarify what they mean. Consider the term "population health." Imagine there are two herds of the same species with populations of approximately the same number. One herd has virtually no diseased animals, but in the other, 5% of the animals would be classified as suffering from an infection that some others in the herd will contract. Both herds are having no difficulty producing offspring. Indeed, let us suppose for the purposes of this hypothetical "thought experiment" that both herds are producing the same number of offspring, and that both will produce sufficient offspring to be able to continue indefinitely. Is the former herd "healthier" than the latter? If the ability to reproduce and continue its existence is the sole criterion of a population's health, then both herds are healthy, and perhaps equally healthy. But if this is what "population health" means, then it may sometimes be the case that widespread disease and illness is consistent with robust "population health" or "species health." This sounds odd and reasonably evokes the question as to why it is appropriate to use the term "health"—as distinguished, say, from population or species *stability*—in such cases. On the other hand, if the first herd described previously is deemed "healthier" than the second, the only reason this would be so is that the first has a larger number of healthier *individuals*. This kind of claim is perfectly understandable and does not appear to use the term "health" or "healthier" in an odd, counterintuitive way. But then "population health" seems to amount to no more than an accretion of the health of a number of individuals.

Definitions of "health" in terms of the survival of individuals or groups of animals or their ability to reproduce remind me of the story of the 90-year-old woman who visits her physician. After examining her, he states that he can give her "a complete bill of health." "A complete bill of health?" she asks. "I can barely walk because of my arthritis, I'm half-blind, my stomach hurts all the time, I itch all over, I have a pacemaker, and the only thing I hear clearly is the ringing in my ears. How can you talk about health?" The physician responds "For *you*, my dear, *this* is health!"

Calling a group or species of wild animals "healthy" or in a condition of good "welfare" simply in virtue of its having a relatively stable population, or being able to survive and reproduce is no less odd. Perhaps this is why some advocates of the new concept of "population health" themselves sometimes revert to more traditional ways of speaking. Note that, in the first passage quoted above, Dr. Nettles states that the aim of population medicine (and therefore the goal of population health) is "to make certain that most of the animals in a wildlife population are healthy and that the species in question is able to reproduce in adequate numbers." The first part of this quotation is understandable because it talks about the health of individuals. The whole statement appears to claim that the health of a sufficient number of individuals is conducive to the continuing reproduction of a species. This is a factual claim, the correctness of which must be established for different situations by empirical evidence, but at least it is an understandable claim. However, the problems and obscurity begin if the health of a sufficient number of individuals and the accompanying reproductive stability of a population or species are supposed to be transformed into a new kind of "health" or "welfare," namely population health or population welfare.

Wildlife veterinarians who insist on speaking about "population health" might want to exercise caution before attempting to emulate farm and food animal practitioners who are attempting to redefine health and welfare in terms of groups of animals. As I argue in Chapters 16 and 23, this latter approach may result in misuse of the terms "health" and "welfare," as well as treatment of individual animals that is sometimes improper. However, even if a definition of farm or food animal "health" or "welfare" in terms of the productivity and profitability of herds is defensible, defining the "health" and "welfare" of wild animals in terms of population or species stability is quite another matter. Herd management of farm animals aims at generating profits. Thus a "healthy" herd is viewed by those who want to redefine the term as a productive or profitable herd. It is not a major scientific undertaking to determine whether a herd is profitable or how profitable it is. Ascertaining the short or long term status of a population of wild animals, an ecosystem, or an entire species will rarely be so easy. Part of this determination may involve the difficult task of deciding what would constitute the "stability" of a given environmental entity. Then there will be the job of understanding, and perhaps manipulating, animal populations, plants, and inanimate components of ecosystems. Such tasks may involve difficult issues in zoology, botany, geology, and engineering. These are not fields in which veterinarians have special expertise. Such matters should be left to others, just as treating the animals medically should ideally be left to veterinarians.

Veterinary approaches to population management and stability

Nothing I have said is intended to question the importance of managing populations or the ability of veterinarians to apply their medical expertise to enable animal groups or species to reproduce and survive. Nothing I have said prevents wildlife veterinarians from exploring and understanding the behavior and habitats of groups and species of animals. The position expressed here is consistent with treatment of herds or groups of animals, in the sense of treating large numbers of animals in ways that do not involve providing medical care individually. In his discussion of wildlife diseases and population medicine, Dr. Nettles describes several different kinds of approaches aimed at maintaining populations of animals by application of pharmaceutical or medical techniques, including advocating steel rather than lead shot for hunters to prevent ingestion of the lead material and consequent poisoning of waterfowl, educating the public and the manufacturers of bird feeders and feeding products about the dangers of dirty feeders for bird populations, assuring that animals relocated to new habitats do not harbor diseases that can be transmitted to animals already inhabiting these areas, and administering rabies vaccine to entire populations of raccoons and foxes. Some or all of these approaches may well be appropriate from an environmental standpoint. They all involve special expertise possessed by veterinarians, as veterinarians. They also proceed by measures that transcend veterinary examination and treatment of individual animals one by one. They may also be aimed at something over and above the health of these individuals. But they still involve the health of individual animals— which is precisely why it makes sense to speak of them as *health* measures.

If I am correct, veterinarians should retain the view that the *veterinary* perspective is the health and welfare of individual animals that, in the wild, can constitute a population or species. Thus a wildlife population manager who is a veterinarian may well decide that, for ecological and therefore ethical reasons, it is best not to treat several sick members of a herd. However, when it is appropriately determined that individual sick or injured members of a group of wild animals should not be given medical treatment, as in the case of the Yellowstone sheep that were not treated for pinkeye, the situation would not be described as one in which the veterinary approach is to allow individual suffering for the sake of group health. Rather, this would be characterized as a case in which a *veterinary* approach is deemed *inadvisable*, to promote the ultimate survival of a population or species.

The claim that *veterinary* approaches contemplate individual animals, even if they do not involve the direct treatment of individuals and even if they sometimes are designed to promote the goals of population stability, is not a matter of semantics— that is, just an issue about definitions that can make no real practical difference. As I argue in Chapters 16 and 23, conceiving of "health" in terms of groups of farm or food animals can lead to minimizing the importance of the condition of individual animals. This is sometimes ethically wrong, in part, because it sometimes minimizes or overlooks ethical obligations to prevent individual suffering. From a purely technical standpoint, individual animals are what veterinarians know best, and what veterinarians know best about individual animals is how to make or keep them healthy. There is nothing wrong with this. Nor should the veterinary profession's traditional concern with individual animals be viewed as a "stereotype," or generate feelings of inadequacy or incompleteness in veterinarians. From an ethical standpoint, someone should always be present to speak for the interests of individual animals, *especially* in programs of wildlife management that concentrate on maintaining groups of animals or ecosystems and if it is decided to sacrifice the interests of individual animals. Like the environment itself, the field of environmental policy is large and complex. Expertise in many different areas is required. The whole will function more efficiently and humanely only if the various parts do their jobs well. The fact that the veterinary approach to wildlife management may often only be a part of the total picture does not render this part any less important.

⟋ ZOOS AND AQUARIUMS

Zoos are a favorite target of many animal activists. Moreover, some very sophisticated thinkers have said some exceedingly uninformed things about zoos. One philosopher, in the introduction to a major collection on animal ethics remarks that "zoos have helped to preserve species that would otherwise have become extinct, and have provided the resources necessary to teach us much we would not otherwise have known. But does this give us a blanket justification for sentencing wild creatures to a life in captivity?"[42] In other words, zoos, perhaps by their very nature, are prisons, places of severe confinement, and apparently for this philosopher, punishment. Philosopher James Rachels is more specific about the travails of these supposed prisoners. He asserts that many animals have a right to liberty, which he characterizes as the "right to be free of external constraints on one's actions." He decries the fact that zoo animals are among those:

> ...harmed by a loss of freedom. It is a familiar fact that many wild animals do not fare at all well in captivity: taken from their natural habitats and put in zoos, they are at first frantic and frustrated because they cannot carry on their normal activities; they then become listless and inac-

tive, shadows of their former selves. Some become vicious and destructive. They often will not reproduce in captivity, and when they do, their young often cannot survive; and finally, members of many species will die sooner in captivity than they would in their natural homes.[43]

In support of these observations, Rachels cites a 1968 report of animal disease in the Philadelphia Zoo and the failed attempt in 1932 by the London Zoo to keep captive baboons together in a large colony.

The contention that a wild animal kept in a zoo is thereby subjected to an unacceptable violation of its "right to liberty" can be made irrespective of the facts regarding how zoo animals are treated. One could conclude that zoo conditions apparently conducive to animal happiness violate this right to liberty (because these animals are in a *zoo*) and are therefore unethical. However, as contentions of *fact* Rachels' observations are inaccurate. Surely some zoo animals are not afforded sufficient freedom of movement. Some zoo animals are not provided the kinds of environments they ought to be provided. However, Rachels' generalizations bear little resemblance to conditions at many contemporary zoos. As philosopher Stephen Bostock observes in response to Rachels, today most zoo animals are born in zoos, and many are provided enriched environments that a person might find confining but in which the animals appear to do quite well.[44] Zoos are learning more about breeding, and the number of animals of various species born in zoos is increasing steadily. Zoo animals can become ill, sometimes with maladies some would not contract in the wild, but unlike their counterparts in the wild, they have veterinarians to treat these illnesses. Some zoo animals do die earlier than some animals in the wild, but many do not, either because they are spared from predation or because zoos have learned how to extend their longevity. Rachels' talk of the "natural homes" of wild animals evokes images of cozy places of prosperity and repose. For most species that spend a good deal of their time dealing with predators or engaging in a relentless pursuit of food—that is, virtually all species—life in a zoo can last longer and be far less stressful or painful than life in the wild. I recently visited the San Antonio, Texas Zoo, which is very proud of Lucy, the world's oldest known giraffe. About to mark her 40th birthday, Lucy was placidly eating her provisions, not at all listless or inactive, and hardly frantic or frustrated. I wonder whether Lucy, if she could express a choice, would ever have preferred a "natural home" afforded by her "right to liberty." I wonder whether, at her advanced age, she would want to spend her days in the wild finding enough nutritious food, or would rather have it readily available, at precisely the correct elevation, when she needs it.

Ethical Justifications for Zoos and Aquariums

For animal-use abolitionists, who believe that it is immoral for people to use animals as means for their own purposes or even to benefit other animals, zoos are inherently unethical, and this is the end of the matter. It is also possible to endorse more specific ethical principles, such as some "right to liberty," which can be employed to deny the appropriateness of keeping animals in zoos.

However, most people believe that is not necessarily wrong to use animals to benefit people or other animals and that it is not inherently wrong to confine animals or to subject them to conditions other than those they would experience in the wild. For most people, the ethical questions raised by zoos are the same ethical questions raised by many other uses of animals: Is what is done to the animals justified by what is gained from this use? Are the animals treated in ways that fulfill at least our minimum ethical obligations to them, that is, are they given what at the very least they ought to be provided? Is it possible to treat them still better than is minimally required?

These questions can often be answered but seldom with great precision. For example, as discussed below, it seems reasonable to justify the keeping of zoo animals because of their educational value to people who visit zoos. It also seems reasonable to require that, in return for this and other uses, zoo animals be afforded a life without undue distress or discomfort and with conditions conducive to an adequate level of welfare. But what is undue distress and adequate welfare? Assuming one knows what is conducive to a zoo animal's welfare, how high a level of welfare is ethically adequate? How large, for instance, must a hippo pool be, and how much space is minimally acceptable for rhinos, spider monkeys, or polar bears? There may be no clear answer to such a question. And there may be no clear answer to the question of how much stress or discomfort zoos may allow their animals to experience, in light of the fact that life in the wild is not always pleasant. Perhaps the best we can do is to adopt as an open-ended goal the continuing improvement of the conditions of zoo animals, and keep working further toward an ever-rising target as additional knowledge and funds become available. Many of today's zoos and aquariums are a far cry from the cramped and dingy facilities of the past. Tomorrow's facilities can be expected to be still better.

Knowledge and education

Much of what is known about diagnosing and treating medical conditions of wildlife has been learned at zoos and aquariums. Veterinarians can interact with animals over a lifetime, sometimes over generations, observing subtle behavioral and physiological signs of illness, injury, health, and welfare. Zoos are also places of education for members of the public. Good zoos do much more than exhibit animals. They offer people useful instruction, and they provide experiences and impressions available only when one sees animals in the flesh. As zoos and aquariums place their animals in more natural surroundings, these lessons become even more informative and valuable.

Perpetuation of vanishing species

One important justification for zoos is their role in breeding members of endangered and threatened species. So-called "captive breeding" is coordinated by international and national efforts, including the Species Survival Plans (SSPs) of the American Zoo and Aquarium Association (AZA).[45] At the time of this writing, these SSPs included 62 species. Populations of captive and wild animals are surveyed, and where it is deemed appropriate to attempt breeding in captivity, arrangements are made to promote genetic diversity so that animals, if introduced into the wild, will contribute to the species genetic pool as would animals that would have remained in the wild. The American Association of Zoo Veterinarians believes there are many essential functions veterinarians can fulfill in SSPs, ranging from providing medical care or consultations, to contributing to the SSP husbandry manual, to development of methods of contraception and enhanced breeding, to consulting about breeding soundness and potential health problems of introduction of new pathogens during transfer from zoo to zoo or into the wild.[46]

Captive breeding may result in adding animals to populations in the wild or in the re-introduction of a population or species into a habitat from which it has disappeared. Although the goal of captive breeding is eventually to place animals in natural habitats, even where this cannot occur (for example, because of irreversible human destruction of such habitats) captive breeding can be justifiable. Captive breeding programs allow veterinarians to perform genetic and nutritional analyses and behavioral and disease studies that would not otherwise be possible.[47] It is also appropriate to preserve species so that people can see and understand them, provided the animals are kept in conditions conducive to their welfare and also serve as a lesson why such species should not be permitted to become extinct. Species that can be perpetuated but cannot be returned to historical habitats need not be unhappy and need not live under conditions markedly different from such habitats. How wonderful it would be, if someone had been able to perpetuate species of dinosaurs, even in constructed (but sufficiently expansive) environments so that people could still see and study them!

Interests and Rights

The task of ethical analysis of zoos has been furthered substantially by the publication of Stephen Bostock's book *Zoos and Animal Rights*.[48] Bostock is a philosopher and Education Officer at the Glasgow Zoo. He offers perceptive discussions of many issues relating to zoos, including the ethics of taking animals from the wild, zoo animal welfare, and ethical questions raised by captive breeding. Bostock's treatment of these issues is required reading for anyone with a serious interest in this area; his historical and philosophical discussions cannot be done justice here.

Bostock argues that, although it is often ethically acceptable to keep animals in zoos, zoo animals have moral rights. This position accords with the conception of animal rights I have defended in this book, which maintains that while people may legitimately use animals for certain purposes, animals sometimes have moral claims that are so strong they can be overridden, if at all, only for the most important reasons. Bostock applies this intuitively powerful idea to zoos, arguing that there are moral constraints on what can be done to zoo animals. He also argues, as I have in this book regarding companion and farm animals, that zoo animals have moral rights to certain conditions of welfare in light of these animals' biological, physiological, and psychological needs. Bostock concedes that there might be a sense in which zoo animals might have a right to liberty, but argues with force and subtlety that such a right need not entail freedom from *all* constraints on freedom of movement or entitle all animals to a life in the wild. He argues that a zoo animal's fundamental interests can still be respected if it is afforded sufficient opportunities to behave in accordance with its nature, which in some animals requires a substantial amount of space in which to move.

Bostock's application of the concept of moral rights to zoo animals illustrates in yet another context how the concept of rights does not preclude many traditional human uses of animals. However, the concept of moral rights does put people on notice that even zoo animals have interests that must be respected. These animals must be provided adequate environmental enrichment and good veterinary care not because it makes people feel good to provide such things, or because providing such things makes for popular and profitable zoos, or even because providing these things might help the environment. Zoo animals have a moral claim on people to respect their basic needs because they have these needs *and* because people have chosen to keep them in zoos. There is thus an important ethical difference between wild animals in the wild and wild animals in zoos and aquariums. While one does not owe a lion or giraffe in the wild good food and good veterinary care, one does owe these things, and more, to lions and giraffes in zoos. They have an overriding moral claim—a right—to these things because people have voluntarily undertaken to make these animals their responsibility. Because zoo animals have a *right* to certain conditions, if people are not able or willing to provide these conditions, they are ethically prohibited from keeping these animals in zoos.

Zoo and Aquarium Animal Welfare

As discussed in Chapters 12 and 13, not all interests of animals rise to the level of rights. Moreover, as is the case with other animals, for zoo animals as well the realm of welfare intersects, but is also far larger in scope than, the realm of rights. (Thus one might say that while rhinos kept in zoos have a right to an enclosure large enough to enable them to move about sufficiently [and an enclosure of several thousand acres might be more conducive to their welfare than one of four or five acres] it would not follow that they have a right to an enclosure of several hundred acres, or even four or five.) The less a species resembles humans or animals with which people have had substantial contact, the more difficult it may be to ascertain whether such an animal is doing well or just is subsisting. In general, veterinarians and zoologists look to whether an animal is free from disease and engaging in behavior that is characteristic of members of its species in the wild. Other factors that may, but need not always be, associated with welfare are longevity, ability to reproduce, and absence of stereotypical behavior. As is the case with farm animal welfare, in the case of zoo and aquarium animal welfare, there is no substitute for sound scientific knowledge. The following are among the considerations that zoo veterinarians and managers give special attention in assessing and promoting the welfare of the animals in their charge:

- Range and kinds of movement and behavior allowed by the total area of confinement
- Size, design, and construction materials of housing areas
- Regulation of environmental conditions (such as temperature, ventilation, and ambient odors) of housing areas
- Provision of appropriate food
- Waste management
- Fences and barriers that do not endanger animals of particular species
- Ability of animals to choose what they shall do at any given time and opportunities for psychological enrichment
- Maintenance of general environmental conditions natural for a species or in which the animals can function normally
- Protection of animals from indigenous wildlife (such as birds, rats, and mice) and from intentional or negligent harm from zoo visitors
- Opportunities for companionship or interaction with conspecifics or other species when this is beneficial, and protection from other animals when appropriate
- Conditions of breeding, including protection of young from parents or other animals in certain species
- Protection of animals from annoying behavior by spectators

- Restraint during veterinary examination and treatment
- Preventive medicine, including general hygiene, adequate veterinary examination, and protection from trauma, poisoning, infectious diseases, and parasites
- Veterinary treatment of illnesses and injuries
- Careful transportation of animals from area to area in a zoo or to other zoos when necessary (for example, as part of a captive breeding program)
- Choosing and providing adequate compensation for skilled and compassionate support staff

Euthanasia and Proper Treatment of Surplus Animals

Dr. Murray Fowler has observed that culling of zoo animals can be so difficult for zoo personnel that "in zoological circles the word is shunned, as if it were unethical, immoral, or illegal to kill or alter any nondomestic animal. If zoos are to be successful propagators of some of the world's rare fauna, however, culling must be practiced."[49] Some people may think that when a zoo or aquarium obtains an animal it undertakes a corresponding ethical obligation to keep that animal alive as long as possible or at least until it can no longer live without pain or suffering. However, such a view does not always accord with the fundamental underlying ethical justifications of keeping such animals in zoos. As Dr. Fowler notes, one of these justifications is propagation of species. If zoos do not carefully select individuals for physical soundness and genetic make-up, the goal of species propagation can be seriously impaired. Animals that should not be selected for breeding but are sound and healthy can sometimes be sterilized. However, keeping an animal originally intended as part of a breeding program but no longer suitable for breeding can be extremely expensive and can impair a facility's ability to maintain a properly functioning program. It may sometimes be possible to transfer the animal to another zoo, but doing this will be unfair to the animal unless that facility can care for it properly.

Zoo animals that are not members of endangered or threatened species also reproduce, and their ability to do so is often a sign that they are being kept in conditions conducive to their welfare. This can also raise problems. If a given exhibit has reached the capacity or financial ability of a zoo to include additional animals, keeping offspring can harm other animals in the exhibit or zoo. Again, it may sometimes be possible to transfer offspring to another zoo. However, this presupposes the ability of another facility to care for them or to introduce them into its own populations, something that is not always possible or cost-effective.

Solutions to the problem of surplus animals short of euthanasia are sometimes possible. Animals that are not part of a breeding program can also sometimes be sterilized or temporarily rendered incapable of breeding. Unfortunately, sometimes it is cost-effective and humane to euthanize surplus animals.

The problem of surplus animals should never be addressed by transferring such animals to people who do not treat them properly. Some of these animals wind up in the hands of private collectors who are unequipped to provide appropriate conditions, or in small zoos or amusement parks not accredited and supervised by the American Zoo and Aquarium Association (AZA). Worst of all is the direct or indirect sale (through dealers or auctions) to hunting ranches, where hunters pay for the privilege of stalking exotic game in so-called "canned hunts." In the late 1980s and early 1990s stories about the sale of surplus animals for such hunts appeared in the written and broadcast media, implicating several leading zoos and dealers. As a result, the AZA incorporated into its code of ethics a prohibition against the sale or transfer of animals for the purpose of sport, trophy, or other kinds of hunting.[50] Whether or not sport hunting is morally acceptable, supporting the practice is certainly not among the fundamental aims of zoos and aquariums. When zoo and aquarium animals no longer serve their purpose and when reasonable efforts to place them elsewhere have been made, it is best that they be euthanized.

Ill, injured, especially dangerous, and elderly animals must also sometimes be euthanized. The purpose of most zoo or aquarium exhibits is to keep and display animals so that they look and behave like real wild animals. If an animal is elderly or infirm, or is changed markedly by medical treatment designed to save its life or cure it of some condition, it can cease to play this role. It can become a danger to itself and other animals with which it is kept. The cost of treatment can diminish the facility's ability to care for other animals. On the other hand, where animals are in short supply, or legitimate veterinary or scientific information can be gained, it may be appropriate to treat rather than euthanize. It is a fact of life, however, that zoos and aquariums often cannot keep animals alive as long as pet owners do.

Animal "Exhibits" and Performances

Among philosopher James Rachels' objections to zoos is that they *exhibit* animals. Rachels writes that "there is something very sad about a grand animal such as a lion or an elephant being put on exhibit at a zoo, and being reduced to nothing more than a spectacle for people's enjoyment." He compares these animals to human lunatics who used to be placed in cages for the amusement of passersby. Rachels condemns the "sadness and indignity of the spectacle" of exhibiting lunatics or lions.[51]

Some zoo animals undoubtedly are made unhappy by inadequate or inappropriate conditions, and when this occurs, it is wrong and ought to be changed. However, many animals (including many lions and elephants) seem to do quite well in zoos. Rachels, who insists that their right to liberty is still being violated, would probably still find them sad, but he would then be reporting his own reaction, which as Bostock notes,[52] is not everyone's! Emotion-laden terms such as "indignity" and "spectacle" may be intended to imply that the animals themselves are unhappy, even ashamed, about being viewed by people. However, there does not appear to be evidence for the notion that zoo animals *must* be made unhappy by being viewed, especially in modern exhibits designed to minimize the effects of visitors on the animals. (Some zoos have exhibits that confine visitors within a habitat in which the animals move freely.) Rachels' suggestion that all animals are kept in zoos merely for people's enjoyment is patently incorrect.

Of course, there is a sense in which it is possible to treat zoo or aquarium animals with *disrespect*, even if most or all of them are not sad or ashamed, or lack the mental capacity to understand that some people do not care about them or are treating them improperly. To treat an animal with disrespect is different from just treating it as one ought not to treat it. Lack of respect is an *attitude* that can include, among other things, not having sufficient appreciation for the worth or value of what one disrespects, and not caring to understand the nature of what one disrespects.

Performances involving captive animals are not inherently disrespectful. They can be designed to illustrate anatomy and behavior in ways that have the animals behave naturally, more or less. There are, for example, cetacean exhibits which reveal how these animals jump out of the water in the wild, their sounds, and how they use sounds to obtain food. Such performances can be educational, and enjoyable to watch. It can be argued that having cetaceans do remarkable "tricks" is unobjectionable, provided it does not harm or bother the animals. There are, however, at least two problems with this view. First, a dolphin or whale performance may leave the impression (especially with small children) that these animals always exist to make people happy. Second, there appears to be an almost inevitable tendency to have the animals do things that make them look or behave like human beings. People play with balls; dolphins in the seas do not. I once viewed a performance that included cetaceans rising out of the water at the close of the show and moving their flippers back and forth as the announcer intoned, "Good-bye kids, moms, and dads!" Such anthropomorphism is dangerous as well as foolish. Television, cartoons, and animated movies already foster the impression in young children that many kinds of animals are different-looking people, that they have human thoughts and emotions and do human things in the wild. It may be one thing to present such images in a form of entertainment that children may (perhaps) understand is fictional, but it is quite another to show a live animal behaving like a person. People need to know that wild animals do not live human lives. Moreover, if one of the major functions of aquariums and wildlife parks is to inculcate an appreciation of wild animals and their behavior, this function can be frustrated rather than furthered by portraying these animals in contrived anthropomorphic activities.

It is impossible to consider cetacean performances or exhibits without asking whether some or all of these species ought not to be kept in captivity at all. In my view, it is dogmatic and doctrinaire not to recognize that there are arguments on both sides of the question. Dolphins, orcas, belugas, and pilot whales can obviously delight their audiences. These spectators bring substantial revenues to aquariums and marine parks, many of which are then able to educate the public about these animals. Much is being learned by veterinarians and animal scientists from captive cetaceans. On the other hand, in the wild many of these animals travel distances that no captive environment can even begin to approximate. Many die in captivity well before they would otherwise. Cetaceans are obviously intelligent, but in (to us) a mystifying way that makes it likely that they are deprived of much of whatever mental life they have in the wild. It is not the purpose of this discussion or this book to proclaim easy answers to hard questions. However, it does seem to me that opponents of keeping wild animals in captivity have just as much cause to be skeptical about supporters of zoos and aquariums who never object to the keeping of animals as supporters have the right to be skeptical about people who always object. My own view (for what it is worth) is that the competing considerations tip the scales against keeping cetaceans in captivity. There may be certain exceptions, for example, when an injured or stray animal clearly will never be able to live in the wild. Perhaps a case can be made for keeping a very small number of dolphins or whales in a few locations for veterinary and scientific study—provided they are afforded expansive environments and are allowed to behave as naturally as possible. Some people will argue that such an approach would deprive many people of immense pleasure. But if it is wrong to confine these animals, this would just be an unfortunate consequence of doing what is right.

The Role of Zoo Animal Veterinarians

In 1963 the eminent zoo director and zoologist Heini Hediger published his classic description of the nature and function of zoos, *Man and Animal in the Zoo*. Hediger, a leader of the modern movement toward zoos and aquariums more accommodating to the needs of animals, expressed skepticism about whether veterinarians make good zoo directors. He noted that zoos are zoological parks and not hospitals for sick animals. Hediger believed that most veterinarians are unprepared even for treating zoo animals because zoos are populated almost entirely by wild animals and the "study and the curriculum of the veterinary surgeon…generally passes over zoology and zoologically oriented biology, because the veterinary surgeon is usually concerned with a few types of domestic animals and their diseases and not with wild animals." He complained that there "is no university yet which trains veterinary surgeons for zoo animals."[53] He related several stories in which veterinarians, ignorant about wild animals and their behavior, thought that perfectly healthy zoo animals were seriously ill.

Hediger was correct in warning that zoos have concerns about animals that go beyond matters of health and illness. However, his picture of zoo veterinarians is as far removed from today's zoo doctors as today's zoos are from those he rightly regarded as antiquated. Several veterinary schools now teach serious courses in zoo and aquarium medicine. The American College of Zoological Medicine was recognized by the AVMA in 1983 as a specialty board, and a number of veterinary schools and zoos around the country are training future members of this specialty. Veterinary organizations such as the American Association of Zoo Veterinarians promote and disseminate research in the field. At my own veterinary school, courses in zoological and wildlife medicine attract large numbers of enthusiastic students. Veterinarians occupy positions of leadership and influence at some of the world's greatest zoos and aquariums.

It is exciting to contemplate what zoos and aquariums and the field of zoological and wildlife medicine might be like 20 or 30 years hence. The future seems bright and exciting for veterinarians who are extending their profession's concerns to the wild animals with which people share the planet. The aim of this chapter has been to warn that with the all excitement will come some hard ethical issues. As I have argued, veterinarians who practice on wild animals in zoos, aquariums, wildlife rehabilitation facilities, or in the wild must function within the larger context of sound environmental policy. The fact that veterinarians can do this is already shown by their involvement in SSPs, which take into account global populations and habitats. I want to close with warnings about two general ethical problems that will inevitably accompany the growing importance of zoological medicine.

1. Veterinarians who occupy positions of leadership and influence in zoos, aquariums, and wildlife programs that depend upon public attendance or funding will face difficult conflicts of interest. As veterinarians, they have an interest in protecting and helping animals. As directors or policy makers, they may sometimes be asked to take actions to help or please people at the expense of certain animals. These potential conflicts of interest can become especially significant for veterinarians who direct or make general policy decisions for zoos. Hediger wrote that:

…The central problem in zoo biology is the reconciliation of the demands of the public and the requirements of the animals. For example: in some cases the animal wants cover whereas the public wishes to see it in the open; when an animal is ready for a period of rest the public wants to see it being active. In these circumstances a solution is arrived at by a prolonged and often extremely difficult search for a compromise in the fields of biology, management and organization.[54]

Reconciling the legitimate interests of the public and the animals is the central *ethical* problem in zoo management. Zoo directors may sometimes be called upon to spend funds to make the facilities more comfortable or appealing to the public, or to develop or stress animal exhibits that attract visitors but that, from a zoological or veterinary perspective would not constitute the best allocation of resources. (For example, Hediger complained that the governing boards of the zoos he directed regarded the public restaurant as the most important building in the zoo.) As this book discusses, veterinarians are often subjected to conflicts of interest because of the traditional concern of their profession for both people and animals. Veterinary training and experience may therefore provide an excellent background for dealing with competing legitimate interests of animals and people in zoos.

2. At the present time, there is clearly a need for more veterinarians with training in zoo and wildlife medicine. It is also important that the profession disseminate information about the treatment of wildlife to private clinicians who participate in ecologically appropriate wildlife management or rehabilitation activities. However, there is a potential danger in the creation of too large a population of veterinarians who treat wild animals as a major portion of their professional activity. As I have argued, sometimes (perhaps quite often) animals in the wild ought best not be treated. Veterinarians whose major activity is treating wildlife, or who just enjoy treating wildlife, will want to treat wildlife. The profession must therefore think about how situations can be avoided in which wild animals are treated not because they should be treated, but because there are veterinarians who need or want to or can treat them. The best way of preventing this problem is, I believe, to instill in zoo and wildlife animal doctors a sense of their ethical responsibilities within larger environmental concerns.

REFERENCES

[1]House tightens grip on leghold trap, *J Am Vet Med Assoc* 203:594, 1993.

[2]321 *Code of Massachusetts Regulations* § 2.12(11).

[3]16 U.S.C. § 1531 *et seq.*

[4]16 U.S.C. § 668 *et seq.*

[5]16 U.S.C. § 1361 *et seq.*

[6]16U.S.C. § 703 *et seq.*

[7]For a summary of federal laws, policies, and agencies relating to wildlife *see* Wells-Mikota SK: Wildlife laws, regulations, and policies. In Fowler M, editor: *Zoo and Wild Animal Medicine*, ed 3, Philadelphia, 1993, WB Saunders, pp 3-10.

[8]American Veterinary Medical Association: Wild or Exotic Animals as Pets, *1988 AVMA Directory*, Schaumburg, IL, 1987, The Association, p 489.

[9]American Veterinary Medical Association: Wild Animals as Pets, *1994 AVMA Directory*, Schaumburg, IL, 1993, The Association, p 93.

[10]Passmore J: *Man's Responsibility for Nature*, New York, 1974, Scribner's, pp 186-187.

[11]Routley R, Routley V: Human chauvinism and environmental ethics. In Mannison D, McRobbie M, Routley R, editors: *Environmental Philosophy*, Canberra, 1980, Research School of Social Sciences, Australian National University, pp 121-125. The Routleys do not accept extended or traditional anthropocentrism.

[12]*See*, for example, Feinberg J: Human duties and animal rights. In Morris RK, Fox MW: *On the Fifth Day: Animal Rights and Human Ethics*, Washington, DC, 1978, Acropolis Books, pp 45-69. Feinberg's version of this approach, like my own, includes the position that some animals (individuals, not groups or species of animals) have not only interests but also some moral rights.

[13]Singer P: *Animal Liberation*, New York, 1975, The New York Review of Books.

[14]Regan T: *The Case for Animal Rights*, Berkeley, 1983, University of California Press, p. 357, emphases in original.

[15]Sagoff M: Animal liberation and environmental ethics: Bad marriage, quick divorce, *Univ Maryland Center Phil Pub Pol Rep* 4(2):8, Spring 1984. *See also*, Sagoff M: Animal liberation and environmental ethics: Bad marriage, quick divorce, *Osgood Hall Law J* 22:303-304, 1984.

[16]For a comprehensive historical account of the development of views in environmental ethics *see* Nash RM: *The Rights of Nature*, Madison, 1989, University of Wisconsin Press.

[17]Rolston H: *Environmental Ethics: Duties and Values in the Natural World*, Philadelphia, 1988, Temple University Press, p 147, emphases in original.

[18]Tayor PW: The ethics of respect for nature, *Environ Ethics* 3:199, 1981.

[19]*Id*, p 207. Although Taylor believes that no individual organism is of greater inherent value than another, he takes a dim view of humans, or at least of the effects we have had on the "community" of living individuals. Taylor states that if humankind ceased to exist "and if we should not carry all the other [species] with us into oblivion, not only would the Earth's community of life continue to exist, but also in all probability, its well-being would be enhanced. Our presence, in short, is not needed. If we were to take the standpoint of the community and give voice to its true interest, the ending of our…epoch would most likely be greeted by a hearty 'Good Riddance!'" *Id*, p 209.

[20]Taylor PW: *Respect for Nature*, Princeton, 1986, Princeton University Press, pp 275-276.

[21]Routley R, Routley V: Human chauvinism and environmental ethics. In Mannison D, McRobbie M, Routley R, editors: *Environmental Philosophy*, Canberra, 1980, Research School of Social Sciences, Australian National University, p 170.

[22]Clark SRL: Gaia and the forms of life. In Elliot R, Gare A, editors: *Environmental Philosophy*, University Park, PA, 1983, Pennsylvania State University Press, p 187.

[23]Leopold A: *A Sand County Almanac*, New York, 1966, Oxford University Press, p 219.

[24]*Id*, p 240.

[25]*Id*, pp 230-231.

[26]Callicott JB: Animal liberation: A triangular affair, *Environ Ethics* 2:320-321, 1980.

[27]Lovelock J: *The Ages of Gaia: A Biography of Our Living Earth*, New York, 1988, Norton, p 40.

[28]*See*, for example, Feinberg J: The rights of animals and unborn generations. In Blackstone WT, editor: *Philosophy and Environmental Crisis*, Athens, GA, 1974, University of Georgia Press, pp 43-68.

[29]For an argument supporting species preservation on the grounds of the esthetic value of individual members of species to people, *see* Russow L: Why do species matter? *Environ Ethics* 3:101-112, 1981, reprinted in edited form in Regan T, Singer P, editors: *Animal Rights and Human Obligations*, Englewood Cliffs, NJ, 1989, Prentice Hall, pp 266-272.

[30]Loftin RW: The medical treatment of wild animals, *Environ Ethics*, 7:233, 1985, emphasis in original.

[31]Porter SL: Role of the veterinarian in wildlife rehabilitation, *J Am Vet Med Assoc* 200:634, 1992.

[32]Rolston H: Ethical responsibilities toward wildlife, *J Am Vet Med Assoc* 200:619, 1992.

[33]Porter SL: Role of the veterinarian in wildlife rehabilitation, *J Am Vet Med Assoc* 200:638, 1992.

[34]*Id*, p 634. Interestingly, among the kinds of care Dr. Porter discusses in his review of rehabilitation techniques is the nursing of "orphan" birds. It is unclear how most of such situations would be attributable to "human interference."

[35]Rolston HR: Ethical responsibilities toward wildlife, *J Am Vet Med Assoc* 200:618-622, 1992.

[36]*Id*, p 619.

[37]*Id*, p 620.

[38]Foster JW: Mountain gorilla conservation: A study in human values, *J Am Vet Med Assoc* 200:629-633, 1992.

[39]Jessup DA: Veterinary contributions toward improving capture, medical management, and anesthesia of free-ranging wildlife, *J Am Vet Med Assoc* 200:653-658, 1992.

[40]Bush M, Beck BB, Montali RJ: Medical considerations of reintroduction. In Fowler M, editor: *Zoo and Wild Animal Medicine*, ed 3, Philadelphia, 1993, WB Saunders, pp 24-26.

[41]Nettles VF: Wildlife diseases and population medicine, *J Am Vet Med Assoc* 200:648, 1992.

[42]Miller HB: Introduction. In Miller HB, Williams WH: *Ethics and Animals*, Clifton, NJ, 1983, Humana Press, p 10.

[43]Rachels J: Why animals have a right to liberty. In Regan T, Singer P, editors: *Animal Rights and Human Obligations*, ed 2, Englewood Cliffs, NJ, 1989, Prentice Hall, p 126.

[44]Bostock SS: *Zoos and Animal Rights*, London, 1993, Routledge, p 49.

[45]The AZA was formerly known as the American Association of Zoological Parks and Aquariums (AAZPA). In addition to supervising its SSPs, the AZA accredits and inspects member facilities in the United States and Canada, among which are all major zoos and aquariums.

[46]For a list of these suggestions and an overview of veterinary functions in species survival programs *see* Boever WJ: Medical input into species survival plans. In Fowler M, editor: *Zoo and Wild Animal Medicine*, ed 3, Philadelphia, 1993, WB Saunders, pp 11-14.

[47]Miller RE: Zoo veterinarians—doctors on the ark? *J Am Vet Med Assoc* 200:644, 1992.

[48]Bostock SS: *Zoos and Animal Rights*, London, 1993, Routledge.

[49]Fowler M: Preventive medicine. In Fowler M, editor: *Zoo and Wild Animal Medicine*, ed 2, Philadelphia, 1986, WB Saunders, p 15.

[50]For an interesting history of these events, *see* Easy targets: Did HSUS expose zoo links to canned hunts or just play to the grandstand? *Anim People* 3(8) October 1994:1.

[51]Rachels J: Why animals have a right to liberty. In Regan T, Singer P, editors: *Animal Rights and Human Obligations*, ed 2, Englewood Cliffs, NJ, 1989, Prentice Hall, p 129, emphasis in original.

[52]Bostock S: *Zoos and Animal Rights*, London, 1993, Routledge, p 48.

[53]Hediger H: *Man and Animal in the Zoo*, New York, 1969, Delacorte Press, p 10. Originally published as *Mensch und Tier im Zoo*, Zurich, 1963, Albert Muller Verlag.

[54]*Id*, p 4.

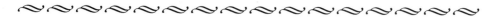

Cases in Veterinary Ethics

∾ ABOUT ETHICS CASES

The most distinctive recent development in the teaching of professional ethics has been the use of cases to stimulate in-class discussions. Many ethics instructors have found that cases can quickly provoke and excite. Cases are extremely useful in impressing upon students the fact that ethical issues do not arise in the abstract but grow out of real-life situations. Cases also help teach that the facts of a particular situation are crucial in determining an appropriate ethical approach; just a slight change in the facts can justify a different, sometimes an entirely different, response.

Unfortunately, there are also potential dangers in using cases. These dangers must be resisted vigorously, lest cases become a substitute for, rather than a stimulus to, ethical deliberation.

The Need for Preparation and Study

First, it is sometimes quite easy to fill a class hour (or an entire semester of class hours) by using cases without requiring any serious work by students. If a case is really interesting, and touches enough ethical nerves, all one need do is ask students what they think, and one will get 45 or 50 minutes of reactions. If the case is well-designed, some of these reactions will be interesting. Most students will leave the class believing that they had a wonderful time *and* that they learned a great deal. If the case is really well-designed, an instructor can produce these feelings without asking the students to do any reading.

Well-designed cases can sometimes elicit intelligent responses even from unprepared students. However, it is no more sensible to ask students to react to ethics cases without previous preparation than it is to have them begin doing surgery on live animals without first studying anatomy and surgical techniques. Ethical issues do not arise from nowhere. They grow out of behavior and predicaments of veterinarians, clients, and animals. Such behavior is often capable of different factual and ethical interpretations. Students *must* know about the ethical issues that underlie a case and about different positions that can be taken regarding these issues. Otherwise, they may react to the case in a way they might not react had they understood the background and contemplated the arguments. Their response may be less persuasive (sometimes much less persuasive) than it would otherwise be.

One example will suffice to illustrate. Case A-3 concerns a phenomenon that is of increasing concern to many veterinarians: Yellow Pages and newspaper advertising. One can ask students to discuss this case and its advertisement without previous reading, and one might obtain some interesting responses. But these responses will mean little unless the students are already prepared with background information about many issues, including the following: what state veterinary licensing boards say about acceptable advertising; how the AVMA *Principles of Veterinary Medical Ethics* deal with advertising; current legal constraints on how licensing boards and professional associations may and may not regulate advertising; how practitioners can get into various kinds of trouble if they attempt to stop or criticize certain kinds of advertising; what constitutes professional as distinguished from merely lawful advertising; and how the subject of advertising relates to the issue of competition. Understanding such matters, in turn, requires an appreciation of the differences between official, administrative, and normative ethics, as well as familiarity with the *Principles of Veterinary Medical Ethics* and applicable state licensing board ethical rules. To have students respond to a case without any preparation is simply to encourage the venting of preexisting and not necessarily reflective "gut feelings." I tell my students that if they want to express their "gut feelings" they belong in an gastroenterologist's office, not an ethics course. The purpose of an ethics course is not to express what one's feelings (gut or otherwise) already *are*, but to demonstrate that one's feelings, and more importantly, one's reasoned positions, are as they *ought to be*.

Making Cases Immediate and Relevant

Because classroom cases are hypothetical and are created by someone else, they do not grow out of—and need not be associated with—actual situations students have seen or experienced. Hypothetical cases are, by definition, someone else's cases. Students must be encouraged to understand that ethical questions are not something that happen to someone else, but will be an unavoidable feature of *their* professional life. This is why at Tufts University I use cases such as those in this book in required classroom courses on ethics. However, when I see students in their fourth year, when they are handling or observing real patients and clients, our roles are reversed. Now the students present *their* ethics cases, based on something they have seen or done, much as they present medicine or surgery grand rounds. This places ethics cases where they really belong, among the real situations veterinarians face daily.

A predisposition to center all discussion around hypothetical cases can also lead to inefficiency and artificiality. There are thousands of questions one can discuss with veterinary students. For example, I like to ask about the ethical appropriateness of nontherapeutic ear-trimming. The best way of addressing questions relating to ear-trimming and many other issues in veterinary ethics is simply to *ask* them: "Is nontherapeutic ear-trimming ethically acceptable? If so why? If not, why not? If you believe that nontherapeutic ear-trimming is not appropriate, what should you tell clients who request or demand it? How should you respond to a prospective employer who asks you during a job interview what you think about nontherapeutic ear-trimming?" I have seen instructors who feel compelled to invent something like the following "case": "You are employed by a practice that is trying to determine whether to provide nontherapeutic ear-trimming. What should the practice decide?" Putting all questions in the form of a cases is a waste of time. It does not add anything either to the discussion of all issues or to an appreciation of the importance of ethical implications of real cases.

~ SUGGESTIONS FOR USING THESE AND OTHER CASES

This appendix contains 30 cases for use in ethics classes or by readers who want to test their responses to the text against designed hypothetical situations. The cases in the appendix represent a range of typical ethical issues faced by veterinarians. These issues are all discussed in this book. There are an additional 23 cases in the body of the text. The text also relates a number of stories that can serve as a focus for classroom discussion. Because consideration of hypothetical cases can be an effective educational tool (or a waste of time) I want to suggest several guidelines for using cases. The suggestions apply to cases that instructors themselves supply for their classes as well as to the cases contained in this book:

1. Before reading or assigning a case, determine what would be appropriate background reading in this book, and do (or assign) this reading.

2. If the case suggests additional relevant reading, do (or assign) this reading as well.

3. In considering any case, use, at least initially, the proposed procedure for approaching issues in veterinary ethics set forth in Chapter 10.

4. Never restrict oneself to the questions asked in the formal presentation of a case. The best cases elicit original, unexpected responses. Encourage students to think about alternative approaches or issues not queried specifically.

5. As suggested by the decision procedure in Chapter 10, each student should have close at hand a copy of the *Principles of Veterinary Medical Ethics* and if possible, relevant standards of administrative veterinary ethics such as those contained in the state's veterinary practice act and state licensing board regulations.

~ ABOUT THE CASES IN THIS BOOK

The following table sets forth the cases presented in the body of the text classified by some of the topics raised in these cases.

With the exception of Case A-11, which relates events that are in the public record, all the cases in the book are fictional. They are constructed and presented as hypotheti-

TABLE A-1

~

Cases in the body of the text

TOPIC	CASES
Euthanasia	1-1, 4-2, 4-5, 4-6, 22-1, 22-2, 22-4, 22-6
Humaneness to the patient	4-2, 4-5, 22-1, 22-2, 22-4, 22-6, 22-7, 22-8
Humaneness to the client	4-5, 22-1, 22-2, 22-4
Client demands	1-1, 4-1, 4-2, 4-6
Affordability of veterinary services	4-5, 22-1, 22-3
High-tech, innovative, or experimental treatments	22-1 to 22-8
Scarce resources and "donor" animals	22-4, 22-5
Criticism of colleagues	19-1 to 19-7
Competition	19-1, 19-2
Honesty, trustworthiness, and loyalty	4-2 to 4-4, 4-6, 22-7, 22-8
Treatment of wildlife	4-1, 26-1
Law and ethics	4-1 to 4-6
Specialization and specialized services	19-3, 22-6

cal situations. Any resemblance between anything in these cases and any past, present, or future events is not intended and is entirely coincidental.

Some events in some of the cases in the body of the text and this appendix were suggested by ethics presentations of my fourth-year veterinary students at Tufts University. Several of the cases resulted from suggestions or stories of practitioners. However, to preserve the fictional character of the cases and to preserve confidentiality, features of actual events have been modified. Species, clients, medical conditions, doctors' reactions, and situations have been changed, rearranged and placed in different contexts, always with my own fictional embellishments. Because I cannot identify or thank by name the hundreds of students and practitioners whose thoughts and arguments over the years have probably had some influence on these cases, I want to thank them all here.

∾ CASE A-1 DOES KILLING AN ANIMAL HARM ITS WELFARE?

An anatomist studies the structure of the brains of monkeys. He utilizes monkeys of several different species and, within each species, animals of various ages. He is attempting to determine whether the brains of different species vary significantly and how age relates to brain structure. All the monkeys are euthanized with scrupulous attention to preventing any pain, distress, or discomfort other than the minimal sensation of receiving the injection of euthanasia solution. The researcher believes that this work will provide basic information about the neurological structure of the brains of monkeys. He cannot predict that the research will lead to practical benefits for monkeys or human beings, but he points out that anatomical studies of this sort have sometimes yielded or suggested knowledge that has proved useful in developing treatments for human neurological diseases.

- Does killing these monkeys have a negative impact on their welfare? If so, why? If not, why not?
- Would your answer to this question be any different if the animals used in the experiment were laboratory mice? If so, why? If not, why not?
- Would your answer to the question of whether the painless killing of these experimental subjects has a negative impact on their welfare be different if these subjects were cats or dogs? If so, why? If not, why not?
- What features of this research, other than the killing of the monkeys, might have an effect on the monkeys' welfare?
- Is the fact that this is basic research, that is, research aimed at obtaining knowledge irrespective of any potential benefits, relevant to the issue of whether killing the monkeys has a negative impact on their welfare? If so, why? If not, why not?
- Is the number of animals used relevant to the issue of whether animal welfare is affected or to the ethical apropriateness of the researcher's work? Is there any ethical difference between the painless killing of a few and of many monkeys? If so, why? If not, why not?
- Do you approve of the research described in the case? Do you need further information about the work before answering this question?
- Would you respond any more or less positively about the research if it had the following features:
  -The monkeys are killed painlessly, and the researcher can demonstrate the likelihood that the experiment will lead to treatments for epilepsy in human beings?

-The monkeys must be allowed to experience painful convulsions before they are killed, and the researcher cannot predict that the experiment will lead to practical benefits for monkeys or human beings?

-The monkeys must be allowed to experience painful convulsions before they are killed, and the researcher can demonstrate the likelihood that the experiment will lead to treatments for epilepsy in human beings?

∼ CASE A-2 SHOULD ANYTHING BE DONE ABOUT PETZILLA'S?

Please read the fictional story of Petzilla's, the Monster Pet Supply Store, and its in-store veterinary clinic, Vetzilla's the Monster Animal and Pet Repair Station, told in Chapter 16.

The Nowhere State Veterinary Medical Society (NSVMS) has called a meeting to discuss the problem of Petzilla's in particular and superstore veterinary facilities in general. You have been asked to make a presentation to the group to express your views about the situation.

The NSVMS does not wish to restrict the topics you discuss, but the members would like guidance on at least the following questions:

- What do you think about the various marketing practices of Petzilla's? Are they legal? Are they ethical?
- What do you think about the various medical practices of Petzilla's? Are they legal? Are they ethical?
- To what extent, if any, do the activities of Petzilla's illuminate issues relating to nonveterinarian ownership of veterinary facilities? Is Petzilla's an aberration, not representative of such ownership and therefore not to be worried about?
- How can the NSVMS, or those veterinarians who oppose Petzilla's or nonveterinarian ownership, stop it once and for all? Should Petzilla's or nonveterinarian ownership be stopped if that were possible?
- Are there lessons in this story for veterinarians about how they should conduct themselves in the contemporary marketplace? Are there lessons in this story regarding the future of the veterinary profession?

∼ CASE A-3 THE STATE-OF-THE-ART VETERINARY HOSPITAL

You are part owner of a small animal practice in the fictional state of Americania. Your practice has been flourishing in the large city of Americanopolis for 10 years. You and your co-owner doctors have prospered by offering excellent services in a dignified atmosphere. Your fees tend to be slightly higher than those of some other practices in the city. However, you pay all your doctors and support staff well and believe that your fees are fair in light of the high level of competence and dedication exhibited by everyone who works in the practice.

The practice decided years ago not to place advertisements in local newspapers but to rely on word-of-mouth referrals from your many satisfied clients. You have a small listing in the Americanopolis Yellow Pages that indicates only the name, address, and telephone number of the practice. Each doctor in the practice is also listed separately, and then only with his or her name, and the name, address, and telephone number of the practice.

Six months ago, Dr. Richard Smith and Dr. Judith Jones, who have been out of veterinary school for less than a year, opened a small animal hospital less than a mile from yours. To attract clients, they began to advertise aggressively in the local newspaper. They also placed a half-page advertisement in the Americanopolis Yellow Pages. Their facility is approximately one quarter the size of yours. Drs. Smith and Jones, like you and your co-owners, are general practitioners who refer cases when necessary to specialists at the state veterinary school.

Last week, the following advertisement appeared in the *Americanopolis Times* newspaper. It is similar to the advertisement that Drs. Smith and Jones have just placed in the Yellow Pages.

AMERICANOPOLIS ANIMAL MEDICAL CENTER
Doesn't YOUR pet deserve the best?

Richard Smith, DVM and Judith Jones, DVM
Graduates of Americania State University School of Veterinary Medicine

1000 Normal Street – Americanopolis
Telephone: 555-555-6666

SPECIALIZING IN SMALL ANIMAL MEDICINE, DENTISTRY, AND SURGERY!
COMPLETE, MODERN FACILITIES!
STATE-OF-THE-ART SERVICES FOR ALL YOUR PET'S NEEDS!
FREE ESTIMATES!
HIGH-QUALITY, AFFORDABLE CARE!
EFFECTIVE, AFFORDABLE VACCINATIONS!
SAFE, AFFORDABLE SURGERY!

A DIFFERENT KIND OF ANIMAL HOSPITAL, WHERE YOU AND YOUR PETS
ARE TREATED LIKE FAMILY, BECAUSE YOU ARE PART OF OUR FAMILY

"Check us out LAST for prices. We will NOT be undersold!"

You and your co-owners are now engaged in heated discussion regarding what to do about Smith's and Jones's advertising techniques. The Americania State Board of Veterinary Examiners has regulations prohibiting "false, deceptive, or misleading advertising" and engaging in "any conduct which reflects unfavorably on the profession of veterinary medicine." One doctor in your practice wants to file a complaint with the state board against Drs. Smith and Jones. Two other doctors want to meet the challenge head-on by having your practice begin an aggressive advertising campaign of its own. Another doctor wants to take the matter to the Americania Veterinary Medical Association "so that they can stop these [expletive deleted] hucksters!"

- What do you think about the advertisement and about the promotional approach of Drs. Smith and Jones? Are they legal? Are they ethical?
- What, if anything, should you or your practice do?

∾ CASE A-4 SECOND OPINION OR LONG RELATIONSHIP?*

A new client comes to you with her Golden Retriever, Rusty. The client tells you that she has consulted another veterinarian, Dr. X. Dr. X diagnosed an abdominal mass and wants to take radiographs, do tests, and possibly operate on Rusty to remove the mass. You are asked to render a second opinion.

You examine Rusty and determine that Dr. X was correct. As an ethical veterinarian, and a good colleague, you praise Dr. X for his acumen and suggest that the client return to him for further evaluation of Rusty's problem. The client responds by asking you to take over the case. Dr. X was very nice, she tells you, but she's here now and it would be easier just to leave Rusty here. Furthermore, she tells you that she likes your gentle manner with Rusty and would like to become your client.
  • What do you do?
  • Do you have an ethical responsibility to Dr. X? If so, does that take precedence over the wishes and convenience of the client?
  • How would you approach this case if you were Dr. X?

∾ CASE A-5 "YOU PEOPLE ARE THIEVES!"

You are presented with a new client, Mrs. Smith, and her 2-year-old female Yorkshire Terrier, Cindy. Mrs. Smith has just moved from another state to your town, and she is looking for a new veterinarian for her dog. Her next-door neighbors, who have been bringing their animals to your practice for years, suggested that she come to you.

Mrs. Smith is a conscientious client and has brought with her Cindy's medical records from the previous veterinarian. She now wants you to give Cindy "a complete physical exam" and make sure she is up-to-date on her vaccinations.

You find a healthy, alert, and adorable dog. You spend approximately 20 minutes with Cindy and Mrs. Smith, reviewing the records of her previous doctor, talking with Mrs. Smith about Cindy's history and her general behavior and personality, and giving her a thorough physical examination. You tell Mrs. Smith that you like to run a complete blood count test as part of a general physical examination, and she says that sounds good to her. You need to test Cindy for heartworms because the heartworm season is about to begin. Mrs. Smith can come by and pick up the heartworm medicine if the test is negative. A fecal examination would also be a good idea, and Mrs. Smith is already prepared with an appropriate sample. The records show that Cindy is due for her rabies vaccination and for her annual revaccination for distemper, hepatitis, parvovirus, parainfluenza, and leptospirosis. You administer the vaccines, and tell Mrs. Smith that you will have the rabies tag and proof of vaccination for her in a few moments so she can obtain a license for Cindy. You ask her to see your receptionist who will give her the tag, photocopy Cindy's records so that they can be placed in her file at the practice, and process the bill. You look forward to a long relationship.

A few moments later you hear Mrs. Smith yelling at your receptionist in your busy waiting room. You rush out to see what is wrong. She has just seen the bill. The total came to $125: $35 for the office visit, $10 for the fecal examination, $20 for the CBC, $20 for the heartworm test, $35 for the vaccinations, and your $5 initial registration fee

*This case was authored by Robert Weiner, VMD and appeared in the Winter 1990 issue of the *WRVMA News,* the newsletter of the Westchester-Rockland (New York) Veterinary Medical Association. ©1990 Westchester-Rockland Veterinary Medical Association. Reprinted with permission.

574   Appendix

for first-time patients to cover setting up the file. "All this money for what?!" she is shouting. "I wouldn't have been charged half this much at my old vet's. You've got to be kidding. You people are thieves!"

- What happens next?
- Does this story present any lessons?

⮟ CASE A-6 GIVING SOME CLIENTS A BREAK

You are the only associate veterinarian employed by a mixed animal practice. The practice is owned by two veterinarians. You are paid 22% of the gross revenues for which you are responsible. Last year you also received a $1,000 year-end bonus. The owners were convinced by a practice management consultant that paying you 22% of production would provide adequate incentive to you and a fair return for themselves.

Recently, the owners have become concerned that this method of paying you has not worked as planned. The owners believe that there has been a substantial amount of fee "slippage," that is, revenues the practice should earn but does not. The owners believe that you can probably recommend more services than you are now performing. They also believe that you have too often reduced the practice's customary fees for clients you think cannot afford to pay them. The owners believe that the present percentage compensation system still gives you too much leeway. They find it admirable that you are willing to forego some of your own compensation when you reduce fees for certain clients, but they are not pleased that this is being done at their expense.

To address the problem of reduced fees, the owners have instituted a new program. They have set aside for you a year-end bonus "fund" of $1,000. This will be your bonus for this year. However, whether you get all of this money is up to you. At the end of the year you will get to keep whatever is left in the fund. From now on, all reductions in the fees you would otherwise generate will be deducted from this fund. The owners have told you that if this system does not produce the expected upturn in revenues, they will consider imposing a "production goal" for you, that is, a level of gross revenues that you must generate if you are to remain with the practice.

You are now contemplating what to do about two clients. Both want to have their cats spayed. Both cats are the same age and size and would require the same amount of time and material. The first client, Mr. Blue, lives in a low-income housing project. He has told you that he likes your practice and believes that your services are better than those of a local humane society animal hospital, which would charge him $45 for spaying his cat. He would like you to do it, but says he cannot afford your $70 fee. Then there is Mrs. Gold, a wealthy client who has been bringing her animals to the practice for years and, you are convinced, would never go elsewhere. Money is never a problem for her. She never asks what the fee for a service is before it is done, and when it is explained to her what the charge will be for a service after it is done, she always believes that she has been charged reasonably and fairly by the wonderful doctors in the practice.

- Would it be proper to charge Mrs. Gold $95 and Mr. Blue $45 for the procedures on their cats? Mrs. Gold will not mind, Mr. Blue will be happy, both animals will be well served, and you will not lose any money from your bonus fund.
- Is it relevant to your consideration of this question that the service both clients want is one that is important to have done on their animals? Would you be less

willing to reduce a fee for Mr. Blue and make it up with an increase from Mrs. Gold if Mr. Blue wanted his cat spayed and Mrs. Gold wanted a root canal done on a tooth that could easily be extracted without significant effects on the cat? Would you be less willing to reduce a fee for Mr. Blue and make it up with a fee from Mrs. Gold if Mr. Blue wanted the root canal and Mrs. Gold the spay?

- If it is appropriate to reduce a fee for a client who has difficulty affording it, why would it not be appropriate to raise a fee for a client who can afford it, irrespective of whether a practice has such a "bonus" fund or pays its associates on a percentage basis?
- Are veterinary practices ever ethically obligated to reduce fees for needy clients? If they are so obligated, is it appropriate for practice owners to have associates (or all doctors in the practice) take such reductions out of their own compensation rather than out of the profits of the practice?
- Is it appropriate to pay associates on a percentage basis? What arguments might be advanced in support of or in opposition to doing so?
- Is it appropriate to set "production goals" for associate doctors? What arguments might be advanced in support of or in opposition to doing so?
- Suppose that you are the sole owner of a practice and that all reductions in your customary fees will come out of your pocket and only your pocket. Under such circumstances is it ethically appropriate to charge different clients different fees for the same procedures based on their ability to pay? To decrease one client's fee and make it up with an increase from another client? To generally charge clients more if they can afford to pay more?

～ CASE A-7 DR. SUE?

You have just returned to work invigorated from a weekend seminar on practice management. The speaker urged the attendees not to become too friendly with clients. Becoming too friendly, the speaker said, can make it difficult to charge clients what you deserve, to insist on acceptable payment terms, and to take necessary steps to effect collection. Becoming too friendly can make you feel guilty about your fees even when you have absolutely nothing to feel guilty about. The relationship with a client should be courteous, caring, and sincere, but it must remain a professional and not a personal relationship. Don't get too close. "Remember," you were advised, "you are *doctors!* You can be Dr. Jones, or Dr. Susan Jones—but you are *not* Dr. Sue."

Your first name happens to be "Susan," and as you begin your practice day you realize that some of your clients do in fact call you "Dr. Sue." Moreover, at times you encourage clients to view you as a friend. When clients request euthanasia of a pet and are distraught and in need of some emotional support, you tend to give them a genuine and friendly hug, and literally a shoulder to cry on. You display on a bulletin board letters from grateful clients praising you for being such a good friend to them and their pets in their times of need.

- Is it appropriate for veterinarians to view themselves as their clients' friend?
- To what extent might becoming friendly, or too friendly, with clients make it difficult to carry on a professional relationship?
- If veterinarians can (or should) view themselves as their clients' friend, should there be limits to this relationship? If so, where should these limits be drawn?

- To what extent is a veterinarian's status as a doctor undermined by friendship with clients or by appellations such as "Dr. Sue" or "Dr. Joe?"
- Is it appropriate to allow clients to refer to you just by your first name? Is it appropriate for you to refer to clients by their first names?

∾ CASE A-8 THE DIFFICULT BREEDER

You are a board-certified specialist in theriogenology (reproductive medicine) at a veterinary school hospital. Among your duties is conducting research into, and developing techniques to cure, sterility and infertility in large and small animals.

You are contemplating what to do about Roxanne Rumney, a breeder of German Shepherds referred to you by a local general practitioner.

Rumney has brought you three dogs. First there is Otto, a 2-year-old male with a history of unilateral cryptorchidism (one undescended testicle) up to the age of 5 months. At that time, the testicle descended into the scrotum and appeared normal.

Breed club standards prevent male German Shepherds from being shown unless both testicles are descended. Otto has been shown several times with great success, and Mrs. Rumney has accepted a number of offers to breed him. However, all attempts to breed Otto have been unsuccessful. The referring veterinarian wanted you to take a look at Otto to see if there is a medical explanation for his failure to breed successfully.

You have already collected and examined semen from Otto and made a tentative diagnosis of azospermia (no sperm). A biopsy of both testicles revealed normal spermatogenesis in all stages, leading to a tentative diagnosis of blockage in the sperm transport pathway. Surgical intervention to establish the diagnosis and reverse the condition is possible, but the prognosis for restoring fertility is poor. (Sometimes, a surgical approach will involve more than one attempt.) The cryptorchid trait is suspected to be genetically inheritable (something Mrs. Rumney knows), and it is therefore possible that some of Otto's offspring will also have the trait. Cryptorchid dogs are predisposed to developing testicular cancer in the undescended testicle. The standard approach to cryptorchidism is castration.

Then there are Fritzl and Schnitzl, the last two dogs in a litter of eight, the offspring of Mrs. Rumney's prize champions Eva and Hermann. Fritzl and Schnitzl, males, are 8 weeks of age. Until very recently, they have behaved normally but are very small compared to their littermates. Recently, they have been exhibiting some behavior not seen in the other puppies. They appear to have difficulty learning their names, and have a high-pitched bark that does not warm Mrs. Rumney's heart. The referring veterinarian did some blood work on the little puppies and found slightly lower than normal thyroid levels. Fritzl and Schnitzl were referred to you, for further testing and interpretation of thyroid function, to rule out a pituitary problem or some other medical cause of their small size, and to see if their growth can be improved.

Mrs. Rumney wants you to do everything possible to get Otto to breed. "Money is no object," she tells you, "They're breaking down my door for Otto's puppies, and I'd certainly like to mate him with Eva. I was really worried about Otto. Wow, was I lucky! His father, Bismarck, had one that never came down, but with a face like that, we just had to breed Bismarck, and I'm glad we did. Look at Otto! What a face! I've been thinking about the two runts. Sure, we could have them tested some more, but what's the point? Just more money down the drain. They'll never amount to much. I can't show them, and I can't sell them. I guess I could give them away, but if someone finds out that my Eva and Hermann had puppies with problems, I'll be ruined. No, *everyone* must know that *all* Eva's and Hermann's puppies and *all* my dogs are *always* perfect, that's what I always tell them! So, Doc, fix up Otto, whatever it takes, and put the runts to sleep, and if I like the way you treat me, you'll have a lifelong client in me and my breeder friends, you can bet on that. And by the way—not a *word* about any of this to *anyone*. In fact, let's not even write any of this in the records. I can't let anyone know about any of it, or I'll be ruined, I tell you. Ten years of work will go down the drain!"

• What should you say or do and why?

∼ CASE A-9 NOW THAT YOUR PATIENT IS DEAD, WHAT DO YOU TELL THE CLIENT?*

You are performing a mastectomy on a 9 year old dog. Physical examination of the patient was unremarkable except for the presence of a single mammary tumor and a 2/6 systolic cardiac murmur. The patient showed no evidence of cardiac decompensation. Preoperative blood counts, blood chemistries, urinalysis, chest radiographs, and electrocardiogram were all within normal limits. Anesthesia was induced by your standard anesthetic protocol. The patient is being maintained on inhalation anesthesia and intravenous fluids. You do not own an electronic cardiac monitor, but your most experienced licensed veterinary technician is monitoring anesthesia by observing respiration, color, pulse, etc., and by listening through an esophageal stethoscope.

You are closing the incision when your associate asks to borrow your technician to assist him with an emergency. Your patient is stable and doing well and you agree. The technician leaves and you concentrate on closing the wound with precision and dispatch. Ten minutes later you complete your closure, remove the surgical drape, and find that the patient is dead.

Naturally, you are shocked and angry with yourself for not having paid more attention to the patient's respiration.

• What do you tell the clients?
• Do you bill them for the surgery? If you offer a *post mortem* do you charge for that?
• Do you share your feelings of guilt with the owners or keep them to yourself?
• Would your answers to any of these questions be different if you determined that your technician had inadvertently turned off the oxygen instead of the nitrous oxide in her haste to assist your associate with his emergency case?
• Would your approach be different with an old established client as distinguished from someone to whom you consider yourself less close and who may be more likely to seek a legal remedy?

∼ CASE A-10 THE LUCKY PUPPY

You own a small animal practice. You employ as a full-time associate Dr. Cynthia Smith, who graduated from veterinary school 6 months ago. Also working at your hospital are two technicians, Betty Carter and Carolyn Ford.

---

*This case was authored by Robert Weiner, VMD and appeared in the Summer 1991 issue of the *WRVMA News*, the newsletter of the Westchester-Rockland (New York) Veterinary Medical Association. ©1991 Westchester-Rockland Veterinary Medical Association. Reprinted with permission.

Late one Friday afternoon there appeared in your waiting room a married couple and their two young sons, aged 7 and 9. You had never seen these clients before. The husband was holding what appeared to be a dead male puppy. You rushed the animal into your examining room. The animal was alive, but was barely breathing and was comatose. Blood was seeping from its mouth, and there was an enormous swelling on the right side of its head.

The owners explained that their sons were fighting again and that one of them apparently had thrown the puppy at the other. They weren't sure whether the puppy hit the wall or the floor, or had been kicked in the head. They explained that the boys fought frequently and that the puppy usually either wandered into these altercations or was thrown about by one or more of the boys during them.

You informed the owners that the puppy was in critical condition and required intensive care at least for several days. You told them that it might have serious internal injuries from which it would never recover. Intensive care would cost at least several hundred dollars. The owners stated that they did not have enough money to help the dog. They thought it would be best if the animal was put to sleep. When told what the fee for euthanasia was, they stated that they were not sure they could afford that either. In a moment of weakness, to put the dog out of its misery and to get these people out of your office, you agreed to do the euthanasia free of charge if they paid your $30 office visit fee. They agreed. Dr. Smith and Betty Carter were with you and the clients in the examining room during these events. Eager to get home for the weekend, after the clients left you told Dr. Smith to "take care of it."

Unbeknownst to you Dr. Smith examined the puppy further after your departure. She palpated the animal and found no signs of fractures. Although the pulse was weak, the seepage of blood appeared to have stopped, and examination indicated that there probably was no internal bleeding. At that point, Smith and Ms. Carter decided to try to save the puppy. They administered fluids, placed him on a heating pad, and fed him critical care solution every few hours. Ms. Carter telephoned Carolyn Ford who was then at home, and Dr. Smith and the two technicians agreed that one of them would stay with the animal at all times throughout the weekend.

It is now Monday morning. You arrive at the practice and notice the puppy during your visit to the inpatient ward. The puppy is not only alive, it appears to be making a miraculous recovery. At that moment, Dr. Smith enters the ward. She tells you what she and the technicians did and informs you, with mixed feelings of excitement and dread, that in her opinion the animal will probably survive. It may need nursing care while it heals, but most of this can be done after it is adopted by someone. She tells you that either she or one of the technicians would be glad to adopt the puppy and take care of it.

- How do you now respond to the actions of Dr. Smith and the technicians? Do you praise or reprimand them? Do you insist that they pay for the materials they used in caring for the puppy? What considerations are relevant in your determination of how to respond to what your employees did?
- Should you tell the clients anything? If so what?
- If you do not inform the clients about what has happened, should you allow Dr. Smith or one of the technicians to keep the puppy? Should you euthanize it as you told the clients you would?

- If you allow one of your employees to keep the puppy, should you ask them who will pay for further drugs and supplies that might be needed in its care or for additional time the animal would have to spend in the practice?
- Imagine now that you are Dr. Smith and not the doctor who owns the practice. How would you want the owner of the practice to respond to what you did? If called upon by the owner to defend your actions what would you say?
- What lessons might this case present regarding how a practice should be run, and about how issues of an ethical nature should be handled by those who work in or for it?

⮑ CASE A-11 IS A PET A PIECE OF PERSONAL PROPERTY, A PERSON, OR SOMETHING IN BETWEEN?

The following presents the opinions of the judges in two court legal cases, some background discussion, and questions.

The First Court Decision

William Smith v. *Palace Transportation Co. Inc.*
Municipal Court of the City of New York, Borough of Manhattan
Decided October 19, 1931
142 Misc. 93

Decision and opinion of Judge David C. Lewis:

Man's attachment for the dog is of old standing.

The auto has driven the horse from the highway, but even in this mechanical age the dog is no stranger on our streets.

Plaintiff was the owner of a five months old fox terrier. One day his wife brought the pup to the streets. The dog ran or romped to the children, and then, while in the One Hundred and Seventy-ninth Street roadway, close to the north curb, a taxi south bound on Pinehurst Avenue, after making a left turn, laid the little dog lifeless on the highway.

At this locality...the cross street was not then a much-traveled thoroughfare. The construction of the George Washington Bridge has cut off south bound traffic on Pinehurst Avenue, below One Hundred and Seventy-ninth Street, and obstructions in the highway had narrowed the lane of traffic going east. These facts and features in themselves called for cautious driving.

To take a pup from the household to the highway is a legitimate errand. To release it of its leash or muzzle is not in itself negligence. The ordinances requiring these precautions manifestly were adopted to protect the public from attack by the dog, not to protect the dog from assault by the public. ...

Naturally, one cannot exact or expect of a dumb animal that standard of prudence that marks the conduct of the average careful creature.

Aside from the question of negligence and contributory negligence, there is presented the question of damages.

A live dog is personal property. Its value is governed by the type and traits and pedigree of the dog. What one pays for property is of import in appraising its value, though not necessarily controlling. While one's feelings for a dog constitute a sentiment which we are inclined to value, it is not recognized as an element of damage.

Judgment for the plaintiff for seventy-five dollars.

The Second Court Decision

Kay Corso v. Crawford Dog and Cat Hospital, Inc.
Civil Court of the City of New York, Queens County
Decided March 22, 1979
97 Misc.2d 530

Decision and opinion of Judge Seymour Friedman:

The facts in this case are not in dispute.

On or about January 28, 1978, the plaintiff brought her 15 year old poodle into the defendant's premises for treatment. After examining the dog, the defendant recommended euthanasia and shortly thereafter the dog was put to death. The plaintiff and the defendant agreed that the dog's body would be turned over to Bide-A-Wee, an organization that would arrange a funeral for the dog. The plaintiff alleged that the defendant wrongfully disposed of her dog, and failed to turn over the remains of the dog to the plaintiff for the funeral. The plaintiff had arranged for an elaborate funeral for the dog including a head stone, an epitaph, and attendance by plaintiff's two sisters and a friend. A casket was delivered to the funeral which, upon opening the casket, instead of a dog's body, the plaintiff found the body of a dead cat. The plaintiff described during the non-jury trial, her mental distress and anguish, in detail, and indicated that she still feels distress and anguish. ...

The question before the court now is twofold. 1) Is it an actionable tort that was committed? 2) If there is an actionable tort is the plaintiff entitled to damages beyond the market value of the dog?

Before answering these questions the court must first decide whether a pet such as a dog is only an item of personal property as prior cases have held [citing *Smith* v. *Palace Transportation Co., Inc.* and other court decisions]...This court now overrules prior precedent and holds that a pet is not just a thing but occupies a special place in between a person and a piece of personal property.

As in the case where a human body is withheld [citations omitted], the wrongful withholding, or, as here, the destruction of the dog's body gives rise to an actionable tort.

In ruling that a pet such as a dog is not just a thing I believe the plaintiff is entitled to damages beyond the market value of the dog. A pet is not an inanimate thing that just receives affection; it also returns it. I find that plaintiff Ms. Corso did suffer shock, mental anguish, and despondency due to the wrongful destruction and loss of the dog's body.

She had an elaborate funeral scheduled and planned to visit the grave in years to come. She was deprived of this right.

This decision is not to be construed to include an award for the loss of a family heirloom which would also cause great mental anguish. An heirloom while it might be the source of good feelings is merely an inanimate object and is not capable of returning love and affection. It does not respond to human stimulation; it has no brain capable of displaying emotion which in turn causes a human response. Losing the right to memorialize a pet rock, or a pet tree, or losing a family picture album is not actionable. But a dog—that is something else. To say that it is a piece of personal property and no more is a repudiation of our humaneness. This I cannot accept.

Accordingly, the court finds the sum of $700 to be reasonable compensation for the loss suffered by the plaintiff.

Background

In asking whether the situation before him presented an "actionable tort," Judge Friedman was asking whether there was a recognized cause of action, or legal theory, that would entitle the plaintiff to relief. In the absence of an established cause of action, Ms. Corso's lawsuit would have had to be dismissed. Judge Friedman analogized her complaint to that of a person who is wrongfully denied possession of the body of a deceased relative, a situation regarding which the law allows legal remedy. It was not necessary for the Judge to appeal to this kind of legal theory to allow Ms. Corso to sue her veterinarian. It has long been held that even a dead animal is the property of its owner. Therefore Ms. Corso could have sued merely on the grounds that her property was not delivered to her as was agreed. Judge Friedman appears to have appealed to the legal theory of the wrongful withholding of a body to strengthen his argument that Ms. Corso was entitled to monetary compensation for her mental anguish. Such compensation is typically allowed in cases of the wrongful withholding of a person's body, but not where mere property is withheld. It is also important to understand that Ms. Corso did not sue her veterinarian for negligence. Rather, she alleged, and the Judge found, that the veterinarian had committed an intentional wrong. This distinction is important because when clients sue a veterinarian they usually allege negligence, that is, the failure to act as an ordinarily competent veterinarian would have acted under the circumstances.

Although Judge Friedman declared that he was "overruling precedent," this has not been the effect of his decision. First, he was a judge at the trial court level, and neither the intermediate nor highest appellate courts in New York have accepted or adopted his opinion. Second, in virtually all states, the law remains as it was stated by Judge Lewis in 1931. Clients who can prove they were damaged by a veterinarian's negligence, and have not suffered physical injury as a direct result of that negligence, are entitled only to compensation for economic damage. Such damage could include the fair market value of the animal at the time of its death (that is, what someone would be willing to pay in an arms-length transaction while it was alive), money paid to a second veterinarian to undue the negligence of a previous doctor, and loss of demonstrable earnings from the animal. However, mental suffering or anguish is not included within compensable damages, any more than someone whose sofa had been negligently destroyed by an upholsterer would be permitted to recover any damages for resulting mental anguish.

In recent years, a few courts have broken from this principle and have allowed animal owners or veterinary clients monetary awards for mental anguish caused by negligent destruction of an animal. The Supreme Court of Florida has held that an animal owner can recover for "mental suffering" when the defendant acted maliciously or demonstrated "an extreme indifference to the rights" of the owner. *La Porte* v. *Associated Independents, Inc.*, 163 So.2d 267 (1964). This decision was applied in another Florida case in which the court decided that leaving a dog unattended on a heating pad for over a day represented great indifference to the owners' property rights therefore entitling them to compensation for their mental suffering. *Knowles Animal Hospital, Inc.* v. *Wills*, 360 So.2d 37 (Fla. Dist. Ct. App. 1978). Several trial and appellate courts have indicated a willingness to include within the "actual value" of an animal some measure of sentimental value to its owner. *Jankoski* v. *Preiser Animal Hospital, Ltd.*, 510 N.E.2d 1084 (Ill. App. 1987); *Brousseau* v. *Rosenthal*, 119 Misc.2d 1054 (N.Y. Civ. Ct. 1980). However, in general, in states and courts in the United States the traditional rule not allowing recovery for mental suffering or anguish appears to remain firmly in place.

- Is *Corso v. Crawford Dog and Cat Hospital* an animal rights case?
- Do you agree with Judge Friedman's position that it is "a repudiation of our humaneness" to regard a pet such as Ms. Corso's dog as "a piece of personal property?"
- If you agree with the Judge, do you agree with his statement that, therefore, the law should regard pets such as Ms. Corso's dog as occupying "a special place in between a person and a piece of personal property?" Would you prefer animals such as Ms. Corso's dog to be regarded by the law as persons, the equivalent of persons, or something else?
- Is it relevant to your answers to the above questions that if the law no longer considered animals, or certain animals, to be personal property they could no longer be bought or sold?
- Judge Friedman characterizes the animals the legal status of which he wants to change in several different ways. He speaks about "a pet such as a dog," "a pet," and "a dog?" Do you think the Judge would have ruled the same way had Ms. Corso's pet been a cat? A pet ferret? A pet horse? A pet cow? A pet parakeet? A pet iguana? How would you have ruled regarding such animals had you been the judge? Why?
- If you agree with Judge Friedman's ruling about Ms. Corso's dog, would you extend it beyond pets and allow owners recovery for mental suffering relating to animals not kept as pets, such as racing horses and dogs, dairy cows, beef cattle, and farm pigs? If so why? If not, why not?
- Subsequent to Judge Friedman's decision, a lawsuit was filed in New York City after a dog died following electrolysis to remove a wart in its rectal area. The plaintiffs demanded $1 million for compensation to them, $4 million in punitive damages as punishment for the veterinarian, $98,000 as compensation for the dog's pain and suffering, and $2,000 in property damage. Does this lawsuit affect your opinion of Judge Friedman's decision? If so, why? If not, why not?
- Judge Friedman's decision caused great concern among veterinarians. The American Veterinary Medical Association Professional Liability Insurance Trust, which provides malpractice insurance for most veterinarians in the U.S., has vigorously opposed the awarding of compensation for mental suffering allegedly resulting from veterinary negligence. Why do you think many veterinarians oppose allowing such compensation? Do you believe this position is justified?
- Is it consistent for veterinarians to proclaim to clients the value of the human-companion animal bond and to insist that, when a pet is killed or seriously injured as the result of veterinary negligence, it should be treated simply as a piece of personal property? If you believe that there is a dilemma here, how do you think the law should deal with it?

~ CASE A-12 FOUND ON THE ROAD

It is late one afternoon and you are about to see another patient. Into your building rushes a distraught man with a badly injured female mixed breed puppy. "I just found it down by the side of road. It needs help, Doctor, real bad."

You take the puppy into your examining room, followed by the rescuer. The puppy is alert and responsive, but in pain. Her left rear leg has been injured. The femur may be fractured. There are abrasions on the right leg and rump. The signs are consistent with a possible automobile injury.

Your state and local laws allow you to stabilize injured cats and dogs that are found injured on the roads by passersby, but the owners of which are not known or cannot immediately be ascertained. There is no government fund that compensates you for such services, but you are entitled to compensation from the owner if he or she can be located. You are not, however, legally entitled to all fees from a located owner for all services required to keep the animal alive indefinitely or to cure it. Applicable laws give you the option to euthanize seriously injured unidentifiable animals found on town public roads without first notifying the town animal control officer or animal shelter.

You tell the rescuer that this animal can be put to sleep right away, or diagnostic work can be done to determine whether there are internal injures, whether the leg is broken, and whether and how the injuries can be repaired. There may be life-threatening internal injuries, but you just do not know yet. He tells you that this is not his puppy, he cannot pay for its care, and it is no longer his responsibility.
- What do you now tell the rescuer?
- What do you do after he leaves?
- What do the laws in your state and locality say about what veterinarians must or may do when an unidentifiable animal is brought to their facilities for emergency treatment?

～ CASE A-13 THE UNWANTED BEAGLE*

Mr. Smith presents his beagle dog, Sam. He tells you that he and his wife are no longer able to keep Sam. He is reluctant to elaborate on the details. He does not want Sam to go to a shelter, where his future would be uncertain, and has been unable to place 9 year old Sam in a home. You examine Sam and determine that he is healthy. Furthermore, he seems like a nice enough dog. You offer to try to place Sam in a home, but Mr. Smith politely declines your offer. Sam, he says, is his responsibility and he wants to be sure that Sam won't be abused by strangers or bounced from home to home. He insists on euthanasia, but does not want to be present.
- Does it bother you to euthanize this pet? If so, do you still do it?
- What are your alternatives?
- Is Sam "property?" Even if your state's law considers him to be property, should you? As a veterinarian, are there other considerations for you that supersede the law?
- If you refuse to euthanize Sam, a colleague might not. Have you helped Sam if you refuse to euthanize him and send him out the door with Mr. Smith, or have you just passed the problem on to another veterinarian?

～ CASE A-14 NOT IN *MY* LIFESTYLE!

You have been presented with Perry, a 6-year-old male domestic shorthaired cat and his owner, Penelope Weldworthy, Esq. Perry is a beautiful, well-behaved cat with two med-

*This case was authored by Robert Weiner, VMD and appeared in the Spring 1992 issue of the *WRVMA News*, the newsletter of the Westchester-Rockland (New York) Veterinary Medical Association. ©1992 Westchester-Rockland Veterinary Medical Association. Reprinted with permission.

ical problems: obesity and Type II (mature onset) diabetes. Your client does not yet know about the second of these problems.

You tell Ms. Weldworthy that you have some bad news and some good news. The bad news is that Perry has diabetes and that unless this problem is addressed, he will become extremely ill and will die. The extremely good news is that it may be possible to manage the diabetes by putting Perry on a diet to reduce his weight and balance his energy intake. This would mean careful periodic and controlled feeding, which Perry really needs anyway because of his weight. If this does not work, Perry would have to be given insulin injections together with a controlled diet. It is not as bad as it sounds, you tell Ms. Weldworthy. A number of your clients have diabetic cats. They get used to giving the shots in no time at all. It's just like having a diabetic human member of the family.

For Ms. Weldworthy, this sounds very bad. She is, she reminds you, an associate at a prestigious law firm. She works a 10- to 12-hour day, and during what little free time she has after work and on weekends she socializes with friends and colleagues. She tells you that she likes Perry very much, but she "got a cat in the first place because they are no bother at all. You put down enough food and water, change the litter box, and they take care of themselves. The perfect pet for the '90s, isn't that what they are supposed to be? All my colleagues have switched from dogs to cats." Ms. Weldworthy tells you that she does not have time to supervise Perry's eating, and certainly would not be able to give him periodic insulin injections. The very thought of giving injections makes her cringe. She tells you that it would be best if Perry were put to sleep now so that she can get another cat.

• What do you say or do?

∽ CASE A-15 PLAYING GOD?

You are a fourth-year veterinary student doing your clinical rotation in small animal medicine. This week you are assigned to the intensive care unit. Tonight you are on duty from 11 p.m. until 7 a.m., when the resident doctor assigned to the ICU reports to work. Another resident is available to you by telephone should you need him. Otherwise, you are alone in the unit.

There are currently three animals in intensive care. In one cage is a 14-year-old female Irish Setter diagnosed as having DIC, an often fatal condition marked by uncontrolled clotting and bleeding. This dog has had several plasma transfusions, none of which have improved her condition. Yesterday, she had a severe bleeding incident. In the past 3 days, she experienced cardiac arrest twice and was resuscitated by CPR.

In the second cage is a 5-year-old female cat with widely disseminated lymphoma and metastases to the lungs. Chemotherapy had been administered when the cat was 4 years of age. It produced a satisfactory remission of her lymphoma for about 9 months, but the cancer has returned and the prognosis is now extremely grave. The cat has difficulty breathing and is exhibiting renal failure. She is weak and anorectic.

In an isolation unit off the ICU is an 11-week-old mixed breed puppy with severe enteritis caused by a parvovirus infection. It is experiencing hemorrhagic diarrhea, and its dehydration is being treated with continuous fluid therapy. When it was admitted to ICU, the puppy's prognosis was poor, but earlier in the day it appeared to be improving. The puppy has become a favorite of the clinicians and technicians who work in the ICU, and who have placed a sign on its cage bearing the words "The Comeback Kid."

The ICU has a policy of asking clients whether they want the unit to attempt resuscitation if it appears necessary to save their pet's life and whether, in the case of heart failure, they want closed or open chest resuscitation should this appear medically feasible to the clinical staff. The owners of all three animals in the ICU this evening have requested that "everything possible" be done to save their animals, and the hospital has agreed.

It does not look like a good night. You are with the puppy monitoring the fluid therapy as the cat begins gasping for breath, and the Setter looks as if she may going into cardiac arrest.

- What should you do at this point?
- Is it appropriate to "prioritize" these animals, that is, to decide that it is better to save one rather than another, or that if two or all the animals need your attention simultaneously, one shall receive it? If you think such a decision is appropriate, which animal would you choose to favor in this case and why?
- If you believe that it is appropriate to give preference to certain patients in intensive care when you do not have the ability to provide the care each ideally would require, which, if any of the following criteria would be relevant to your choice?
  -Whether an animal has a pleasant personality or is vicious, disagreeable, or indifferent?
  -The extent to which you or your co-workers have become attached to the animal?
  -The extent to which the owner is attached and devoted to the animal?
  -The ability of the owner to pay for all the most sophisticated or extensive treatments your facility can provide?
- If you decide to prioritize patients in this case, how would such a decision accord with their owners' expectation that everything possible will be done to keep their animals alive?
- Is it right for veterinarians, veterinary students, or technicians working in an intensive care unit to decide which animals shall live and which shall die?
- Are there other lessons that this case presents?

∼ CASE A-16 "JUST LIKE PEOPLE"

You practice in a large specialty hospital with a well-equipped and staffed intensive care unit. You have just finished a telephone conversation with Dr. Nelson. He has referred a patient to you and wants to prepare you before you examine the animal and meet the client, Mrs. Rivers. Dr. Nelson tells you about Tabatha, a 20-year-old spayed female cat. She has a several-week history of dyspnea and anorexia and progressing respiratory distress, which is now severe. Blood work has indicated nonregenerative anemia and kidney failure. "This poor cat is dying; she's miserable. Mrs. Rivers absolutely refuses to consider euthanasia. I tried to convince her, but she won't hear of it. I told her I was referring Tabatha to you for additional diagnostic work, but I made it clear she probably won't last long. I'm hoping that *you* can convince her to do what's right."

As soon as you see Tabatha and Mrs. Rivers, you know that you are in for a difficult time. Tabatha is in dreadful condition. She is emaciated and extremely weak. She appears to have difficulty raising her head and is gasping for breath. You tell the client that you want to place Tabatha immediately under oxygen to see if her breathing can be made easier. As soon as she is in the ICU you will return and talk with her.

When you return, you find Mrs. Rivers in tears. "Poor Tabatha. She's been with me for 20 years. I love her so much. I know it's almost her time. I will miss her so very, very much. What can we do?"

You respond that Tabatha is a very sick cat. You do not know yet what the problem is. You can do further diagnostic work, but given her age and general condition, you do not think there is much hope.

"I know what you are going to say," Mrs. Rivers responds, "and I respect your position as you must respect mine. I'm a very religious person. I believe deeply that God made both people and animals. Animals are just like people. When their time comes is up to God and not man. No euthanasia! When Tabatha is called, she will die. Until then, please find out what is wrong with her, and keep her alive as long as you can. I'd want to be treated the same way. We all have souls, people and animals too. We're all God's creatures great and small."

Despite your misgivings, you proceed with further tests. Tabatha has carcinoma of the lungs with metastases to the diaphragm. She cannot survive the cancer and will never be able to be removed from oxygen. She might last in intensive care for a few days, or 1 or 2 weeks.

- What do you do now?
- How, in general, do you handle clients who will not authorize euthanasia when their animals are terminally ill and in great suffering?
- How do you respond to clients who have strong ethical or religious beliefs about euthanasia?
- As a veterinarian, how do you respond to clients who believe that it is no more acceptable to euthanize a pet than it is to euthanize a person?
- What do you say to clients who believe that animals are "just like people?"

～ CASE A-17 THE CLIENT WILL NEVER KNOW

Your client, Mr. Miller, has asked you to euthanize his 16-year-old male Boston Terrier, Buster. Six months ago, Buster began having seizures. Mr. Miller opted not to have a C-T scan done to try to determine the cause of the seizures because of Buster's advanced age and the cost of the scan. Treatment with phenobarbital prevented the occurrence of seizures for several months, but recently Buster has begun to have seizures again. The seizures are becoming more frequent, longer-lasting, and more violent. Mr. Miller tells you he does not want Buster to go through this any longer. You discuss with him the possibilities for handling Buster's remains. Mr. Miller requests that you have Buster cremated and Buster's ashes returned to him.

Buster was a long time patient. About a year ago, you palpated a mass in the area of his pancreas. Ultrasound revealed a cyst the likes of which you have never seen before. At the time of Buster's death, the cyst was almost the size of a golf ball. Before sending Buster's body for cremation, you would like to do a necropsy to examine the cyst. The client will never know.

- Is it ethically acceptable to do this? If so, why? If not, why not?
- Would the degree of devotion and attachment that Mr. Miller exhibited toward his pet be relevant to your answer? Would you be more inclined to do the necrop-

sy if Mr. Miller never appeared to care much about Buster than if he was extremely devoted to the animal?
- Would Mr. Miller's decision regarding what to do with Buster's remains be relevant to your answer? Would you be more inclined to do a necropsy if he told you just to dispose of the body? If he told you that he wanted to bury Buster?
- Would you feel more justified in doing the necropsy if the cyst might have been related to Buster's seizures than if it were just merely something of interest to you? If so, why? If not, why not?
- Would you feel more justified in doing the necropsy if you were a specialist in internal medicine or planned to have a specialist look at the tissue to determine whether it might provide useful information? If so, why? If not, why not?
- What lessons, if any, does this case provide?

⟶ CASE A-18 "DOCTOR, WHAT WOULD YOU DO IF THIS WAS YOUR ANIMAL?"

You are presented with Mr. and Mrs. Field and their 3-year-old male Labrador Retriever, Howard. Howard is a beautiful animal with a delightful personality. The Fields are very fond of him as, they have told you, is their 10-year-old daughter. You are now discussing treatment options for Howard. The small tumor on his right front leg has been confirmed as a spindle cell carcinoma. The good news is that the tumor is localized and has not metastasized. However, Howard's leg will have to be amputated. The prognosis is excellent that he can then live a normal life. You have a number of canine patients that have undergone amputations of one leg. You are about to begin a well-prepared presentation about how dogs can get along quite well without one leg.

Before you can start, Mr. Field expresses horror and disgust. He does not even want to think about amputation. "Howard loves to run and play. He just won't be the same. He might be a dog, but he won't be Howard. No, for his own sake, and ours, let's put him to sleep." Mrs. Field is angered by her husband's words. She insists that they will have no problem, Howard won't mind a bit, and their daughter would certainly prefer to have a three-legged Howard than no Howard at all. The Fields begin a discussion which then becomes an argument. Voices are raised.

At this point, Mr. Field appears to have found a solution to the problem. He turns to you and asks "Doctor, what would you do if this was your animal?" "Yes," Mrs. Field repeats looking at you for support, "what would you do if Howard was your dog?"
- How do you answer? What do you do?
- Suppose that you believe strongly that dogs that can be saved through amputation of one leg ought not to be euthanized. In fact, when you were a child you had a three-legged dog. On the other hand, a colleague in your practice does not oppose amputation but does not recommend it when at least one member of the family seems to have a problem with it. Suppose that you would answer the Fields' question by saying, "If Howard were my dog, I'd do the surgery and love him as never before." Suppose that if the Fields had been scheduled this morning with your colleague they would have heard the response, "Well, maybe in light of what Mr. Field is saying, it might not be such a great idea." Does the possibility that the clients might make a different decision based on which doctor is asked the question trouble you about the question?

• What do you think about the question, "Doctor, what would you do if this was your animal?" What good things can be said about the question? If there are bad things, what are they? Do you have, or should you have, a general response to this question?

∿ CASE A-19 "BOBBY, THE DOCTOR IS GOING TO TELL YOU WHY THIS IS BEST FOR KING."

King is an 7-year-old intact male Golden Retriever with secondary osteoarthritis associated with hip dysplasia. Both rear joints are severely affected. The clients, Mr. and Mrs. Black, have managed the situation as best they can during the progression of the disease. King has had a tolerable quality of life for the past several months, but he is now having difficulty functioning and is in severe pain.

During your last visit, you and the Blacks discussed seriously an option that you have mentioned from time to time, hip replacement surgery. A specialty practice in your area has had excellent results with this operation. King would need both hips done, at a total cost of well over $2,000. The Blacks have made another appointment to see you. With them is King and their 14-year-old son Robert.

The Blacks clearly have had a rough time. Robert has been crying. "Doctor," Mrs. Black says to you, "you know Bobby. Last night we all stayed up late talking about King. We love King very much, but it just isn't fair to him to put him through so much suffering. We explained to Bobby how King will be happier without all this pain. It's time for King to be put to sleep." Mr. Black puts his arm around his son and says "Bobby, the doctor is going to tell you why this is best for King. Doctor?"

• What do you say or do?
• Should your response depend on whether you believe that putting the dog to sleep is best for him?
• Should your response depend on whether you believe that, all things considered, euthanizing King is the right thing to do?
• Is there information you want about the Blacks before you decide whether you think euthanasia is appropriate or before you decide what to say to them?
• Suppose that King did not have hip dysplasia but suffered from a medical condition which could be cured with treatments costing $200. Would your response to the Blacks be any different if they now asked you to tell Bobby why putting King to sleep was the best thing for the dog? If your response would be different, why would it be different? If not, why not?
• To what extent should veterinarians attempt to support clients' decisions about treatment?
• What general lessons does this case present?

∿ CASE A-20 "I BELIEVE THAT IT IS UNETHICAL TO PUT THIS ANIMAL TO SLEEP."

You are presented with Tiger, a 4-year-old male domestic shorthaired cat, and his owner, Mr. White. Mr. White is in with Tiger for a consult after blood work taken as part of Tiger's annual checkup was positive for the feline leukemia virus. The news comes as a complete surprise to Mr. White because Tiger is his only cat, and generally never leaves the house, although he has gotten out on occasion to spend some time with a neighbor's cats. Other than testing positive for FeLV, Tiger is in excellent condition.

You explain to Mr. White that although there is no cure for feline leukemia, Tiger has no signs of the active disease and could live several years completely free of symptoms. Then, when Tiger does become sick, it might be possible to treat him with chemotherapy.

Mr. White responds very slowly and deliberately that he would like Tiger put to sleep now, before he becomes ill. "I don't want to see him get sick, and I don't want him to die a painful death, and that is all I have to say about the matter." You ask whether he would consider giving Tiger up for adoption. You tell Mr. White that your practice knows several people who adopt FeLV-positive cats. Mr. White refuses. "Do you have any objections?" he asks. "Well," you say, "since you have asked, I believe it is unethical to put this animal to sleep. I know what you must be going through, but I would no sooner put Tiger to sleep because he will eventually become sick than I would euthanize a relative of mine with Alzheimer's disease."

Mr. White politely picks up Tiger and leaves your examining room. "Well, I guess I need a different kind of veterinarian."

Unbeknownst to you, Mr. White's brother died 6 months ago from leukemia after considerable suffering. They were extremely close, and his illness and death have affected Mr. White enormously.

- Does the information about the client's brother make you feel any differently about Mr. White's decision? About what you said to him?
- How should veterinarians approach clients with animals that have tested positive for FeLV or FIV (feline immunodeficiency virus) and do not show any signs of active disease?
- Should veterinarians ever tell clients that what they are doing or want to do with their animal is unethical? If it is sometimes appropriate to say this, when would it be appropriate and why?
- Does this case suggest any lessons about how a veterinarian should deliberate about ethical issues? About how ethical issues should be discussed with clients? About how practitioners should speak with clients generally?

〜 CASE A-21 "DIDN'T SOMEONE HAVE A BABY TO GET BONE MARROW FOR A TRANSPLANT?"

Milton is a 3-year-old intact male domestic shorthaired cat that was diagnosed positive for FeLV last year. Milton's littermate Arnold died from leukemia-related complications 6 months ago. Milton now has the disease. His PCV is 10%. You inform the clients that Milton is succumbing to his leukemia. You could give him a blood transfusion, which would help his situation temporarily. However, he would then need additional transfusions. Assuming his leukemia did not have other manifestations, eventually transfusions would be ineffective. You explain to the clients that you can offer a transfusion now, but that your hospital sometimes has difficulty obtaining sufficient blood for all its feline patients, in which case it might not be possible to provide blood for Milton in the future.

The clients are extremely upset. Their previous veterinarian convinced them not to give Arnold transfusions, and they are now sorry they did not. They want to do everything possible to help Milton and to keep him alive as long as possible. One of them tells you that a friend of hers had a cat with leukemia that needed transfusions; she used her other cat as a blood donor. "We don't have another cat, but why can't we adopt one from the shelter as a pet and use it as a donor for Milton? They have lots of cats that are just going to be put to sleep. We'd love it every bit as much as Milton, and when poor Milton goes, we won't be alone. Didn't someone have a baby to get bone marrow for a transplant to save her other child? If that's OK, what's wrong with getting a donor for Milton?"

- What do you say?
- How do you answer the client's last question?
- Would the client's suggested course of action be fair to Milton?
- Would the client's suggested course of action be fair to the donor cat?
- Suppose the clients have a neighbor with a cat that is negative for FeLV and is a suitable donor for Milton. Would it be appropriate to use this animal as a donor for Milton?
- Suppose the clients tell you that they might be able to adopt as a donor and companion for Milton a cat that is negative for FeLV but has been vaccinated against feline leukemia. How should you respond to this suggestion?

⮑ CASE A-22 THE BEHAVIOR PROBLEM

Mr. and Mrs. Tucker have brought in their 1-year-old male intact Boxer, Major. Major has always had behavior problems. He growls and bares his teeth whenever someone tries to pet him. He goes berserk whenever the doorbell is rung, biting whatever he can get his teeth on. He howls at night, keeping the whole family awake. He has lunged several times at Mrs. Tucker, and the Tuckers are so afraid of him that they cannot leave Major and their 2-year-old child alone in the same room together. Last week, Major went after a package delivery man, who barely escaped with his life—or so he was reported to have said when the company called to inform the Tuckers that they can no longer deliver to their house as long as they own the dog.

"We've had it," Mr. Tucker tells you. "He's ruining our life. What should we do?" Although the Tuckers have complained about Major's behavior for the 3 months that he has been your patient, the issue of euthanasia has never been raised either by them or by you.

- What do you say? In formulating a response please make certain to consider both the legal as well as ethical implications of your approach to this situation.

⮑ CASE A-23 ARE SOME ANIMALS MORE EQUAL THAN OTHER ANIMALS?

The Americanopolis Veterinary Hospital ("Americanopolis") has agreed to participate in a program run by a local group to sterilize and vaccinate feral cats living in the community. The aim is to try to prevent these animals from reproducing and to provide them with a degree of protection from preventable diseases.

Because Americanopolis is not compensated for its services, it believes that it is justified in departing from certain aspects of its standard operating procedures in spaying these cats. To save money, surgical instruments are not autoclaved but are "cold-sterilized" with a disinfectant fluid. Less expensive suture materials are used.

Nothing has ever gone wrong as a result of these cost-cutting measures, and Americanopolis has spayed dozens of animals to the satisfaction of the volunteer group.

- Is it ethically appropriate for Americanopolis to depart from its standard procedures?

- Is the fact that nothing has ever gone wrong (and, let us suppose, that nothing will ever go wrong) as a result of the cost-cutting measures relevant to an answer to this question? If so, why? If not, why not?
- Is the fact that these are not owned animals relevant to the level of care that they should receive?
- Would it be appropriate to use the procedures used here, on cats that have been surrendered to a shelter for adoption, some of which will be adopted, but most of which will be euthanized anyway?
- Suppose you have several clients who cannot or do not want to pay your standard fee for spays. Would it be appropriate to tell them that you could do the procedure at a lower fee if you departed from your standard procedures? If you make such an offer, how much are you obligated to tell them about how far from your standard procedures you would depart and what you would do?
- There is a highly competitive market for spays and neuters. Some private practitioners find it difficult to meet the fees of humane society hospitals or of other practitioners who run spay and neuter clinics in which large numbers of animals are processed. Is it ever appropriate to "cut corners" in doing spays or neuters so that one can compete with other practices for the spay and neuter business? What arguments can be made against doing this? Are there any arguments that can be made for it? What kinds of "corners" might be "cut?" How much should clients be told about such measures?
- It may sometimes be lawful to offer clients a lower quality of service than the profession regards as good medicine, provided clients knowingly choose this level of care. For example, although it is good medical practice to do blood work on older animals prior to anesthesia to determine whether they are at risk, a veterinarian might not be held liable for malpractice if he or she clearly informs the client that blood testing would be advisable but the client exercises an "informed refusal." Even when it might be lawful for a veterinarian to offer a lower level of care, is it ethical to do so? What arguments can be raised for and against allowing clients to choose less expensive but also potentially less beneficial services for their animals?
- To what extent are the regulations or policies of your state veterinary licensing board relevant to your answers to any of the questions presented in this case?

⤳ CASE A-24 A NEIGHBORHOOD DOG

You are presented with Rover, a 7-year-old mixed breed intact male dog, and his owners, Mr. and Mrs. Johnson. Rover is limping badly from an apparent problem in his left rear leg. You immediately suspect a cruciate ligament injury.

On taking a history, you learn that the Johnsons received Rover as a present from Mrs. Johnson's sister when he was a year old. The Johnsons have never had him to a veterinarian. He has never been vaccinated, nor has he received heartworm preventative while owned by these clients. Mrs. Johnson tells you that "Rover is a neighborhood dog. He always knows he can come by for a good meal, but he likes to roam around the neighborhood. He comes home every couple of days. He's been no trouble at all, but he does get into a fight or two, I can tell you, and he holds his own, the rascal."

Examination reveals an alert and cheerful animal with a delightful personality. However, in addition to his apparent injury, his coat is in terrible condition, and he is emaciated.

Mr. Johnson tells you that they do not have a lot of money, but could scrape together $75. "He's a good dog. It's worth it to us to make him better."

You know that what the Johnsons say they can afford might not cover proper diagnosis of Rover's apparent leg injury and certainly would not cover surgery if this is required. You also believe that, in light of Rover's general condition and the fact that he has not been to a veterinarian for so long, competent medical practice dictates a thorough general examination, including blood work to see if Rover has heartworms, which are seen frequently among free-ranging dogs in your area. Then there is the matter of vaccinating the dog, including the legally required rabies vaccine. You are also concerned that Rover has not been neutered.

- What do you tell the Johnsons?
- Do you even consider helping them with the fee?
- What, if anything, can be done to make these clients responsible owners?
- What should be done about Rover?
- What, if anything, should be done about the Johnsons?
- Do you see any similarities between the Johnsons and Ms. Weldworthy in Case A-14? Are there important differences?

～ CASE A-25 SHOULD YOU CONTACT THE SPCA?

You are presented with a new client and his two male Pit Bull Terriers. One of the dogs appears to have multiple bite wounds on the face. The other has been bitten on his front left leg, around which has been tied a bloody piece of bed sheet. The client tells you that the dogs usually get along fine, but yesterday got into a bit of a spat. You examine both animals. Both will require minor surgery for their wounds. On examination you notice scars on both dogs that are consistent with previous bite wounds. One of the dogs has at least a dozen such scars on its face, belly, and legs.

Your state has a law making it a felony to "own, possess, keep, or train a bird, dog or other animal with the intent that it shall be engaged in an exhibition of fighting, or to establish or promote an exhibition of the fighting of birds, dogs, or other animals." Veterinarians who suspect that a patient is used for fighting may call the police in their town or their local Society for the Protection against Cruelty to Animals (SPCA). These persons are authorized to investigate and to seize animals they reasonably suspect are used for fighting. The animals are kept as evidence in potential criminal prosecutions and are almost always euthanized after a conviction or guilty plea. The great majority of animals seized in such cases are euthanized.

You suspect that these animals have been used for fighting.

- What do you do now?
- Do you try to discuss the matter with the client? If so, what do you say?
- Should you contact your local police or SPCA? What are the arguments for and against such an approach? In formulating your answer, consider the interests of at least the following three parties: (1) the dogs; (2) the client; (3) you and your practice.

- Suppose, either as a result of further examination of these animals or of what the client says, you become certain that these dogs are being used for fighting. Is an appropriate response to this conclusion refusing to treat them?
- Should your practice have a general policy relating to what should be done when animals are apparently used in illegal fights, or are neglected or abused in other ways that violate your state cruelty-to-animals laws? If you should have such a policy, what should it say?

~ CASE A-26 DO I DEFEND MYSELF?

Three weeks ago you saw Mr. Potts and Holly, his 2-year-old Labrador Retriever. Holly, the client reported, had been bothered for several days by a sore on her back. On examination, you discovered a circular lesion which you suspected to be a fungal infection. You informed the client of your suspicion and told him that you wanted to do a skin scraping and a fungal culture. Mr. Potts balked at the fee for the procedure and asked whether there was some less expensive way you could determine whether Holly had a fungal infection. You told Mr. Potts that you could look at the lesion under a Wood's light. A positive result would be a strong indicator of a fungus, but false positives are possible and a skin scraping and culture is the best method for diagnosis. Moreover, it would be good to be sure precisely what this was, which a scraping and culture can determine. You advised him again to authorize a skin scraping and fungal culture, and again he refused. Mr. Potts insisted on the Wood's light, which yielded a positive result. You dispensed an antifungal medication with appropriate instructions for its use and asked the client to check back with you in a few days.

You are now told that Mr. Potts is in your waiting room and that he insists on talking to you. You invite him into an examining room. Mr. Potts is quite irate. He informs you that a week after you saw Holly he took the dog to Dr. X, whose practice is on the other side of town. "I just didn't like that light business," he states, "and I wanted a second opinion." Mr. Potts explains that when Dr. X saw the sore, "he told me straight out that he had to culture the thing, that's all there was to it—that a good vet didn't stop with a light in a situation like this. And when I told him you thought Holly had a fungus he laughed and said that in all the years he's been around these parts, he never saw a fungus that looked like this." Growing more upset, Mr. Potts hands you a piece of paper, which was a copy of Dr. X's medical record for Holly. The record indicated that Dr. X had scraped the area on which Mr. Potts had used the antifungal medicine for a week and that the results of the fungal culture of the scraping were negative. "Now I want my money back. Dr. X told me to throw that cream away because it's useless, and that's exactly what I did."

You know that you acted properly in advising Mr. Potts to authorize a skin culture, and that the test probably came back negative because Dr. X took the scraping where the medication had been applied. You are troubled by his inaccurate recollection of your previous discussion with him and by the fact that Holly might still require further medication for the infection. You know that Mr. Potts believes that you are incompetent. He also wants his money back.

- What do you say or do?
- Do you give the client a refund?

- Do you defend yourself? If so, do you tell the client that you believe Dr. X did not act competently? Do you tell the client that you believe Dr. X's comments about you were unfair?
- Are you ethically obligated to speak to Dr. X before you tell the client what you think? If so, why? If not, why not?
- If you think you ought to talk to Dr. X, either before or after you tell the client what you think, what should you say to Dr. X?
- Does this case provide any lessons about how to handle situations in which clients refuse to authorize tests or procedures that would be dictated by good medical practice?

∾ CASE A-27 IS IT RIGHT NOT TO SHIP THE COW FOR SLAUGHTER?*

You examine a cow in late pregnancy that has keratoconjunctivitis, blepharospasm, and photophobia due to an ocular squamous cell carcinoma. You recommend enucleation or immediate slaughter. The owner wants the cow to calve, wean the calf, and then ship the cow. He does not want to invest in a surgery ($120) for a cow he is planning to ship, nor does he want to ship a cow that will soon calve. Is it ethically correct for the cow to be left untreated for several months?

∾ CASE A-28 "IF YOU DON'T DO IT, WE'LL FIND SOMEONE WHO WILL."

Lameness associated with tendinitis is a common, and can be a serious, problem in race horses. The acute phase is marked by swelling and pain. In the chronic phase, there can be localized or extensive swelling. The availability of ultrasound enables the equine practitioner to grade the lesion with regard to whether a fresh hematoma is present or the extent to which mature fibrous tissue has developed. A recent discussion presents a list of techniques for managing the problem, beginning with immediate cessation of exercise, followed by cryotherapy in the first 48 hours after injury, and then use of support bandages and nonsteroidal anti-inflammatory drugs (NSAIDs) such as phenylbutazone. The discussion states that "judicious use" of corticosteroids during the acute phase can limit inflammation. However, prolonged corticosteroid therapy "is contraindicated because of the inhibitory effect on many aspects of wound healing. The effectiveness of the reduction in inflammation and pain often results in overuse of the leg either because the horse feels better or because the trainer is misled by the apparently successful treatment. Intratendinous injection is contraindicated because of the tendency to produce necrosis and collagenolysis, as well as intratendinous calcification."† Surgical management of chronic tendinitis has been attempted. Percutaneous tendon stabbing or splitting has received some use, and superior check ligament (SCL) desmotomy is being investigated as a possible approach at various equine medical centers. According to the discussion quoted above, depending on the extent of fiber damage, a tendon may require 12 to 18 months to repair, and approximately 20% of animals are able to return to hoped-for athletic activity following conservative medical or surgical therapy.

---

*This case appeared in the *Canadian Veterinary Journal*, Volume 31, October 1990. Copyright ©1990 by The Canadian Veterinary Medical Association. Reprinted with permission.

†Speirs VC: Lameness: Approaches to therapy and rehabilitation. In Hodgson DR, Rose RJ, editors: The Athletic Horse, Philadelphia, 1994, WB Saunders, p 349.

You are 2 years out of veterinary school and have opened your own equine practice. You are holding your own. Slowly, you are building a clientele of pleasure horse owners, for whom you provide attentive and professional service. These people are willing to pay for your time and the best care you can provide because they value their horses as riding animals and companions. You have an excellent relationship with the equine medicine and surgery departments of the veterinary school from which you graduated. Your clients appreciate that their animals are referred to the school when necessary. However, you still need one or two big clients to enable you to pay some bills (including student loans) and to get the practice firmly established.

Your opportunity may have arrived. You have been called to Nicknacker Stables, which is owned by a local building contractor, Nick Ewing. Ewing meets you at the gate and introduces you to his trainer, Sammy. Ewing takes you on a tour of his facilities. He has about 2 dozen horses at a time, he tells you, mostly standardbreds, which he races at a track 20 miles away, but also some thoroughbreds. The thoroughbreds, he quips, "are on the downhill side of life you might say. They do all right for us, but most haven't got much left in them." Ewing explains that he is not a "high-class snob. If a horse can't make me money, I can't keep it. This operation isn't making me rich or famous, but it's enough for me."

Ewing explains that he is looking for a veterinarian who will help him out. His old veterinarian, who used to service the operation, just retired and moved down south. "A doc from the old school," Ewing said approvingly, "not one of these fancy-pants who doesn't know what it's like to run a business!" He explains that lameness is a special problem with his standardbreds, which are raced quite hard. Ewing relates that he recently had two doctors down to the stables, one from the state veterinary school and another from your town. Both told him that he had to rest his standardbreds with acute tendinitis, some for 6 months, some maybe for a year. The doctor from the school talked about some kind of experimental surgery they are studying. When Ewing asked for "the shots"—steroid injections—they both refused and looked at him with disapproval. "Are they crazy? I can't rest my horses for a year! OK, some of the standardbreds can be rested, but the thoroughbreds, no way! The thoroughbreds with bad joints, darnit, they do just fine on shots, they're up and about and earning their keep in no time at all. Sure, I could sell them to someone else, but they'll be treated worse than I treat them, I can tell you that. Is it better for them to be turned into steaks or whatever they do with horsemeat in France? Let them live a while, that's what I say, right Sammy? What's the big deal if I can get some more races out of them? How am I helping them by putting them down?"

You are then taken aside by Sammy, who explains that you have to understand that Nick isn't really a horse person, like you two. "Here's the bottom line. We have a decent operation here. We've got plenty of work for you here and at the tracks. I really love these horses, believe me. But we have to stay alive. I'll rest some, but for others I need steroids. If you don't do it believe me we'll find someone who will. Don't worry about Nick. He'll listen to me. Work with me, I'll work with you. Let's do what is best for all of us, including the horses. Think it over."

• What do you do?
• What arguments can be made for taking on Ewing as a client? What arguments can be made against it?

- How relevant would the following factors be in your decision whether to inject corticosteroids into one or more of Ewing's horses?
  -Whether a particular horse, if raced, is likely to earn a great deal of money for the client?
  -The general class of competition in which a particular horse races?
  -Whether a particular horse, unless raced, is likely to be shipped for slaughter?
  -Whether the client knowingly understands and accepts the risk that injection could cause an acute and irreparable breakdown?
- How should veterinarians approach situations in which animals cannot be kept or used in certain ways unless they earn money for their owners, when using the animals in these ways deprives them of appropriate medical care?
- Can you suggest any general approaches veterinarians might take, either as a profession or in their communities, to the issues presented by this case?
- What is your response to clients who say, in different contexts, "If you don't do it, I'll find someone who will?" How might your response be different depending on the kind of case or situation?

～ CASE A-29 WHEN DOES IT BECOME CRUELTY?

One Monday morning you received a telephone call from Mr. Jones, owner of a small dairy farm whose cows and one horse you have been seeing over the years. The horse, Sadie, is a 20-year-old Morgan mare kept as a pet. The Joneses are not well off, and generally, when they call, you know that something is wrong. "You'd better come, Doc, the mare's got colic."

On examination, Sadie was painful with a slightly elevated respiratory and heart rate, and negative gastric reflux. You advised Mr. Jones that it would be best if she were brought in to your hospital. Jones told you that he was "a bit short of funds" and wanted you to try to help Sadie at the farm. You palpated what seemed to be a mild cecal impaction, but you were puzzled by what you felt and were not certain. You made it clear to Jones that you were not sure what the problem was and a proper diagnosis could only be done at the hospital. You administered mineral oil through a nasogastric tube and told Mr. Jones to call you in the morning.

Two days later Mr. Jones called with the news that Sadie was much worse. She was kicking and appeared to be in great pain. When you arrived at the farm and saw Sadie, you advised Mr. Jones that unless she was brought to the hospital immediately she might die quickly. You told Jones that Sadie probably needed surgery, and at the very least fluids. "Doc, you know we can't afford surgery. We'll bring her in. Do what you can."

Sadie arrived at the hospital late Wednesday afternoon. Mr. Jones went home after she was admitted. Sadie was examined by your equine surgeon, who advised immediate surgery. He did not know precisely what the problem was, but was certain that unless they could look inside, Sadie would soon die, but not until after considerable suffering. Her pain appeared to be intensifying by the minute. There was no use trying to overhydrate her and somehow dislodge the impaction, or whatever was wrong with her.

At this point, you and the surgeon telephoned Mr. Jones and told him that the situation was grave. Sadie needed surgery right away. Otherwise, the only humane thing would be to put her down and spare her the suffering. "Doc," Mr. Jones said, "you know we can't afford the surgery. Do what you can." You then administered banamine to reduce her pain. Sadie calmed down for a few hours but then began kicking and pacing even more violently.

Early Wednesday evening you called Mr. Jones again and told him that Sadie was in agony and that unless she could be operated on, she had to be put down. You suggested that he and Mrs. Jones come to the hospital to see how much the horse needed to be put out of her misery. Mr. Jones informed you that he and his wife were discussing euthanasia. She was for it, he was against it. They just could not come to an agreement. Seeing Sadie was unthinkable. It would break their hearts to see her suffer.

It is now early Thursday morning. Sadie was pacing most of the night. She is now not responding to any of the various analgesics she has been given overnight, including xylazine and butorphanol. You call Mr. Jones and are told that he and his wife are still talking about whether to put Sadie down. She is now kicking and thrashing. Her agony can be heard all over the hospital. You and your colleagues are arguing with each other, not knowing what to do. You all want to euthanize Sadie immediately, before she literally drops dead. One doctor insists that it is illegal to euthanize an animal without the client's permission. A second asks "What about the cruelty law? When does something like this become cruelty?"

- What should you do?
- Are you legally obligated to wait until Sadie dies? What does the cruelty to animals law of your state say? Can it be interpreted to say that it is unlawful cruelty to allow an animal in terminal, agonal pain to continue to suffer? Is there anyone who might help you to answer this question?
- If euthanizing Sadie is illegal is it unethical? If the law tells you one thing in this case but your conscience tells you another, what should you do?
- Was it ethically wrong for the Joneses to refuse to authorize surgery? Is it ethically wrong for the Joneses to refuse to authorize euthanasia?
- If it is ethically wrong for the Joneses to refuse to authorize euthanasia, does it follow that it would be ethically correct for you to perform it without their authorization?
- Should you euthanize Sadie without the clients' authorization? May you euthanize her and tell them that she died? May you euthanize her and tell them that she died on her own?
- How should veterinarians try to deal with clients who will not authorize medical or surgical treatment but will also not authorize euthanasia, where failure to do either condemns the patient to unrelievable suffering?
- Can you make a list of kinds of situations in which failure to treat, or failure to perform a certain procedure or treatment, might constitute legal cruelty?
- Do you think a statute or veterinary licensing board regulation could assist veterinarians in such situations? If so, what kind of law or regulation would you suggest?

∾ CASE A-30 SAVE THE WHALES?

You practice in an eastern state with many miles of Atlantic Ocean coastline. In recent years there have been numerous beachings of pilot whales. Anywhere from a few to more than a dozen animals have swum onto beaches and appear either to be unable or unwilling to get back out to sea. The beachings often attract hundreds of spectators and always draw television and newspaper reporters. Most of the whales die after apparent considerable suffering. On occasion, a few can be coaxed or literally dragged back into the Ocean far enough and appear not to return to the beach.

You are now attending a meeting of your state Veterinary Medical Association, which has been convened at the request of the state and federal wildlife authorities. They, and the veterinarian and staff of the region's aquarium, can no longer handle all of the beachings. They need help, and they would prefer to get it from the state's veterinarians instead of volunteers from the public. They would like the VMA to solicit, on behalf of the state's veterinarians, practitioners who would be trained in basic aspects of whale anatomy and medicine and who can be called upon, if needed, to help in responding to the beachings. Veterinarians would be used to assist the animals that are beached to survive, to euthanize them when this appears necessary, and to participate in attempts to direct the animals back to sea.

Some of the members of the VMA are enthusiastic about this program. They assure other members that it will gain the VMA and the state's veterinarians good publicity. "What could be better," one doctor asks, "than the television news showing all our dedicated veterinarians dealing with these terrible situations? We have a chance to help the animals and the environment. This one is a no-brainer."

- Is this a "no-brainer?"
- Are there arguments that can be raised against the participation of veterinarians in these attempts to save the whales? Are there arguments that can be made in favor of the program other than those mentioned thus far?
- Are there arguments that can be raised against anyone, laymen as well as veterinarians, attempting to save such whales? What are the best arguments that can be made in favor of such attempts?
- Can you see any reason why these animals should not, at the least, be euthanized if they cannot be returned to sea? Before you answer this question consider the statement of philosopher Holmes Rolston (discussed in Chapter 26) that "pain in ecosystems is instrumental pain," through which animals "are naturally selected for a more satisfactory adaptive fit."*
- What facts about these whales or about treating them medically might be relevant in answering any or all of these questions?

---

*Rolston HR: Ethical responsibilities toward wildlife, *J Am Vet Med Assoc* 200:619, 1992.

INDEX

〜〜〜〜〜〜〜〜〜〜〜〜〜〜〜〜〜〜〜〜

A

AAHA; *see* American Veterinary Medical Association
Abolitionism
  animal-rights, 538-539
  animal-use, 10, 409
    greyhound racing and, 452
Abuse of animal
  case study of, 578-579
  in research, 488-489
Abusive client, 359-360
Academic veterinary medicine, 48-49, 401-407
  coerciveness of, 405-406
  communication in, 406
  criticism of colleagues and, 406-407
  justification for, 401-405
  quality of care and, 405
Accessories, selling of, 234
Accreditation program, federal, 432
Action, importance of, 38
Action-oriented ethics, 38
Action-oriented theory, 38-40
Active versus passive euthanasia, 359-360
Activism, animal, 10
Addiction, 66-67
Adenoma, perianal gland, 397
Adjudication, 82-83
Adjuvant cancer therapy, 481
Administrative agency
  nature and function of, 60-61
  nonveterinarian, 63
  standards of, 61-72
    advantages of, 71
    problems in, 72
    range of, 62
Administrative veterinary ethics, 16, 17, 60-73; *see also* Official veterinary ethics
Adoption, of greyhounds, 453-455
Advertising, 259-267
  broadcast and print, 262
  case study about, 571-572
  false, 67
  legal issues in, 259-260
  Supreme Court ruling on, 77
  Yellow Pages, 262-266
Advisory opinion, 82-83
Advocate
  for race and show horses, 445-446
  veterinarian as, 351
Affordability of high-tech procedures, 385-387
Aggressive competition, 283-284

Agricultural animal; *see* Farm animal
Alcoholism, 66-67
Alternatives to animal research, 482-484
American Animal Hospital Association, 81-82
American Association of Equine Practitioners, 451
  animal welfare committee of, 82
  rodeo and, 462-463
American Association of Zoo Veterinarians, 562
American Association of Zoos and Aquariums, 556
American Bar Association, 264, 266
American College of Veterinary Ophthalmology, 307
American Horse Shows Association, 450-451
American Veterinary Medical Association
  advertising and, 260-262, 281
    Yellow Pages, 263-264
  American College of Veterinary Ophthalmology and, 307
  animal rights movement and, 140, 144-145
  animal welfare and rights policy of, 150-151, 153-154
  antitrust law and, 278
  bond with companion animals and, 185
  competition and, 284-285
  corporate sponsorship and, 270-272
  de-clawing of cat and, 368-369
  ear-cropping and, 366
  euthanasia and, 340, 482
  extra-label drug use and, 429
  farm animals and
    husbandry methods and, 418
    underutilization of veterinary services and, 428-429
    veal production and, 426-427
  food animal services and, 239
  humane society and, 284-285
  lay administration of drugs and, 431
  oath of, 88-92
  official ethics and, 78-79
  policies and positions of, 83-86
  practice names and, 256
  Principles of Veterinary Medical Ethics of; *see* *Principles of Veterinary Medical Ethics*
  reports and statements of, 83
  research animals and, 477-478
    federal laws about, 494-495
  revision of *Principles* and, 94-102
  signs and logos and, 256-257
  specialization and, 307
  technicians and, 519-521
  third-party redemption program and, 268-269
  wild animals and, 530-531, 550
  zoo animals and, 562

Right and wrong of moral standards, 40-41
Right-hand merchandising, 202
Rights, animal, 133-149; *see also* Animal rights
Rodeo, 457-463
Role of veterinarian
  as businessperson, 199-204
  as friend and counselor, 196-197
  as healer, 195-196
  as herd health consultant, 197-199
Roping, steer or calf, 458, 462

S

Salaries, fees and, 318
Salary, fair, 504-507
Sale of animal, for nonpayment, 323-324
School, animals in education and, 489-492
Science
  animal welfare, 9-10
  professionalism and, 89
  pure science model of animal welfare and, 153-158
    mischief of, 162-164
Science fair, using animals in, 489
Scientific research; *see* Research animal
Second opinion
  case study about, 573
  client's request for, 305-306
Secular view of animals, 22-24
Self-awareness of animals, 125
Self-improvement, 89
Self-interest of veterinarian, 193-194
Self-regarding values, 46-47
Selling, 199-202
  of nonprofessional goods and services, 228-247; *see also* Nonprofessional goods and services, selling of
  of unadoptable animals for research, 486-489
  of zoo animals, 559-560
Sending of sympathy card, 254
Senility, 129-131
Services
  aggressive competition and, 283-284
  client as purchaser of, 176-178
  negligent, 300
  nonprofessional, 228-247; *see also* Nonprofessional goods and services, selling of
  productivity versus, 511-512
Sex differences, in salary, 508
Sex-based discrimination, 514-516
Sexual harassment, 515-516
Sheep
  animal welfare issues for, 423
  lungworm in, 550

Shelter animal
  as organ donor, 392
  as research animal, 486-489
Sherman Antitrust Act, 276-277
  specialization and, 307
Show dog, hormone therapy and, 394-396
Show horse, 442-451; *see also* Horse, race and show
Signs and logos, 256
Skepticism, 40
  rejection of, 41
Skunk, illegal possession of, 28-29
Society, professionalism and, 89
Solicitation, 264, 266-267
Spay and neuter clinic, 287
Specialist, misuse of term, 67-68
Specialization, as competitive weapon, 307
Species
  perpetuation of, in zoos, 556
  value in, 540
Species Survival Plans, 556
Splitting of fees, 324-325
Sponsorship, corporate, 270-272
Sport animal
  animal welfare issues relating to, 169-170
  greyhound racing and, 451-457
  horse racing and, 442-451; *see also* Horse, race and show rodeo and, 457-463
  veterinarian as advocate of, 9
Standard
  for animal research, 471-472
  breed, 362-368
    concealment of defects in, 368
  ethical versus legal, 26-27, 32-33
  official, 75-86; *see also* Official veterinary ethics
  professional, 7
  code and, 92-93
State law
  antitrust, 277, 280
  employment practice, 516
  wild animal ownership and, 529-530
State licensing agency
  animal research and, 492-493
  standards of, 61-72
State racing commission, 449-450
State veterinary medical association, 80-81
Statements of official bodies, 82-83
Steeljaw trap, 85-86
Steer roping, 458, 462
Steer wrestling, 459
Sterilization of defective animal, 366
Store, retail
  sale of professional products and services by, 241-243
  veterinarian-owned facility in, 220-223